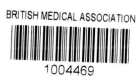

Histopathology of the Nail
Onychopathology

Eckart Haneke, MD, PhD
Department of Dermatology, Inselspital, University of Bern, Switzerland
Dermatology Practice Dermaticum, Freiburg, Germany
Centro de Dermatología Epidermis, Instituto CUF, Porto, Portugal
Kliniek voor Huidziekten, Universitair Ziekenhuis, Ghent, Belgium

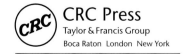

CRC Press
Taylor & Francis Group
Boca Raton London New York

CRC Press is an imprint of the
Taylor & Francis Group, an **informa** business

A FOCAL PRESS BOOK

CRC Press
Taylor & Francis Group
6000 Broken Sound Parkway NW, Suite 300
Boca Raton, FL 33487-2742

© 2017 by Taylor & Francis Group, LLC
CRC Press is an imprint of Taylor & Francis Group, an Informa business

No claim to original U.S. Government works

Printed and bound in India by Replika Press Pvt. Ltd.

Printed on acid-free paper

International Standard Book Number-13: 978-1-4822-1232-7 (Hardback)

Library of Congress Cataloging-in-Publication Data

Names: Haneke, Eckart, author.
Title: Histopathology of the nail : onychopathology / Eckart Haneke.
Description: Boca Raton, FL : CRC Press, Taylor & Francis Group, [2017] |
Includes bibliographical references and index.
Identifiers: LCCN 2016052973| ISBN 9781482212327 (hardback : alk. paper) |
ISBN 9781315184005 (ebook)
Subjects: | MESH: Nail Diseases--physiopathology | Nails--anatomy & histology
Classification: LCC RL165 | NLM WR 475 | DDC 616.5/47--dc23
LC record available at https://lccn.loc.gov/2016052973

Visit the Taylor & Francis Web site at
http://www.taylorandfrancis.com

and the CRC Press Web site at
http://www.crcpress.com

Contents

Foreword

A wonderful clinician, an excellent surgeon, an exceptional pathologist, Eckart Haneke deserves to enter the Pantheon of Dermatologists—unfortunately restricted to the dead…

I knew him to be one of the best dermatologists immediately after his talk, when I met him for the first time at the ISDS meeting in Morocco in 1978. We subsequently worked together for many years. He was a contributor, then a coauthor, and finally a coeditor of the several books we published together.

I owe him a lot and it is a tremendous honor for me to have been asked to write a Foreword to *the* greatest contribution to the nail pathology literature, appearing 40 years after Alkiewicz and Pfister's Atlas.

Robert Baran

Acknowledgments

My late father, who was my first teacher in dermatology, and my wife, who was often my discussion partner, greatly contributed to this book by their decade-long support in all respects. I am also indebted to Dr. Robert Baran, who motivated me to direct my clinical, surgical, and histopathological interests toward nails—something I enjoyed during the last 40 years. Further, I wish to thank my nail friends from all over the world for their invitations, discussions, and support. Last but not least, I want to thank the technicians of the histopathology laboratories who took great effort to provide me with good slides.

Introduction

The nail has gained much attention in clinical medicine in the last three decades. However, apart from the book of Alkiewicz and Pfister, which gave an overview of some clinicopathological facts known in 1975 and which appeared in German,[1] no comprehensive review of the histopathology of the human nail has been published. Short descriptions of the microscopic features of nail diseases can be found in modern nail diseases textbooks[2–7] and selective aspects of nail diseases in chapters in dermatopathology textbooks.[8,9] Curiously, even books on tumors of cutaneous appendages do not deal with nail tumors.

This book is written for all those dermatologists, dermatopathologists, and nail-interested pathologists who have to read histological sections of nail tissue. All of them are familiar with the difficulties of obtaining good biopsy and excision specimens, as well as of processing, cutting, and staining them. Furthermore, the clinicopathological correlation is often challenging and, for the inexperienced in nail pathology, confusing. Nail science also has its own specialized terminology and the onychopathologist has to be familiar with it. As is the rule in dermatopathology, knowledge of the normal appearance and microanatomy, the biology and growth characteristics, clinical diagnoses, and differential diagnoses is inevitable in order to reach a reliable histopathological diagnosis. Therefore, some clinical data are given with the histopathological description.

Even though the first monography on nail diseases appeared 115 years ago,[10] the science of nails is a relatively young part of dermatology. Unna coined the term of onychopathology 125 years ago.[11,12] Systematic histopathologic examinations have only been rarely performed in the past[13–18] though there is a huge body of literature on single cases and small case series. It is not possible to show photomicrographs of all the nail diseases and conditions ever described as most authors have relied on dermatopathology slides in the case of skin and nail lesions. Most physicians are still hesitant to take a nail biopsy, and many are even not aware of the diagnostic power of a nail clipping.

I am very grateful to all friends and colleagues who provided their slides and pictures for this book. We hope that this text will aid all readers to be better able to understand and read histopathological sections of nail specimens.

REFERENCES

1. Alkiewicz J, Pfister R. *Atlas der Nagelkrankheiten. Pathohistologie, Klinik und Differentialdiagnose.* Stuttgart, New York: Schattauer, 1976.
2. Baran R, Dawber RPR, eds. *Diseases of the Nails and Their Management.* Oxford: Blackwell, 1984.
3. Baran R, Dawber RPR, eds. *Diseases of the Nails and Their Management*, 2nd edn. Oxford: Blackwell, 1994.
4. Baran R, Dawber RPR, de Berker DAR, Haneke E, Tosti A, eds. *Baran and Dawber's Diseases of the Nails and Their Management*, 3rd edn. Oxford: Blackwell, 2001.
5. Baran R, de Berker DAR, Holzberg M, Thomas L, eds. *Baran and Dawber's Diseases of the Nails and Their Management*, 4th edn. Oxford: Wiley Blackwell, 2012.
6. Baran R, Camacho FM, Mascaró JM. *Oncología. Biología y alteraciones de la unidad ungueal.* Madrid: Grupo Aula Medica, 2006.
7. Scher RK, Daniel CR III. *Nails: Therapy, Diagnosis, Surgery.* Philadelphia: WB Saunders, 1990.
8. Elder DE, Elenitsas R, Johnson BL Jr, Murphy GF, Xu X, eds. *Lever's Histopathology of the Skin*, 10th edn. Philadelphia: Lippincott Williams & Wilkins, 2009.
9. André J, Sass U, Theunis A. Diseases of the nails. In: Calonje E, Brenn T, Lazar A, McKee PH, eds. *McKee's Pathology of the Skin.* Philadelphia: Elsevier, 2012;1051–1075.
10. Heller J. *Die Krankheiten der Nägel.* Berlin: Hirschwald, 1900.
11. Unna PG. Anatomisch-physiologische Vorstudien zu einer künftigen Onychopathologie. *Vjschr Dermatol Syph* 1881;8:3–24.
12. Unna PG. Beiträge zur Onychopathologie. *Vjschr Dermatol Syph* 1882;9:2–20.
13. Pinkus F. Anatomie des Nagels. In: Jadassohn J, ed. *Handbuch der Haut- und Geschlechtskrankheiten*, vol I/1. Berlin: Springer, 1927.
14. Alkiewicz J. Recherches histologiques sur les sillons transversaux des ongles (Beau). *Ann Derm Syph (Paris)* 1935;6:35–45.
15. Achten G. Normale Histologie und Histochemie des Nagels. In: Jadassohn J, ed. *Handbuch der Haut- und Geschlechtskrankheiten, Ergänzungswerk*, vol I/1, Heidelberg: Springer, 1967; 339–376.
16. Zaias N. The longitudinal nail biopsy. *J Invest Dermatol* 1967;49:406.
17. Zaias N. Psoriasis and the nails. *Arch Dermatol* 1969;99:567.
18. Zaias N. The nail in lichen planus. *Arch Dermatol* 1970;101:264.

Development, structure, and function of the nail

The nail is a plate of hard keratin that overlies the distal dorsal tip of the digits.[1,2] Apart from mechanical protection and an ever-growing aesthetic importance, it has a variety of other functions such as being a most versatile tool, aiding in manual dexterity, being a defense tool, and enhancing the digital tips' extremely elaborate sensory functions. Particularly on the big toe, it provides counterpressure when, during gait, the whole body weight, which is enhanced 2.5 times by the forward thrust, is concentrated on the pulp of the toe, which would otherwise be gradually dislocated dorsally to form a false distal nail wall; in fact, some developmental biologists believe that without our great toe's specific properties human beings would not have evolved. The nail is made up of α-keratin intermediate filaments of approximately 40–70 kDa molecular weight plus a sulfur-rich amorphous interfilament matrix. The keratins of the nail plate belong both to the soft epithelial and the hard hair-nail keratins. The latter were sequenced from their genes and classified into two groups according to their sequence homology: 11 type I or acidic and 9 type II or basic keratins[3–5]; however, apparently not all of these hair and nail keratins are actually expressed in the human nail. The potential different mechanical roles of these hard keratins in the nail are not yet known. The amorphous matrix or interfibrillar component consists of keratin-associated proteins of a molecular weight of 8–30 kDa.[6–8] Over 100 keratin-associated proteins have been identified. Disulfide bonds link them to the 7–10 nm thick intermediate keratin filaments.[9]

Keratin contains about 3% sulfur, 7% hydrogen, 14% oxygen, 15% nitrogen, 45% carbon,[10] and 8%–10% inorganic components, which are mostly polyphosphates with carbonate. Sulfur and nitrogen occur predominantly in amino acids of the nail plate.[11,12] The water content is between 10% and 30% depending on ambient humidity.[13]

1.1 EMBRYOLOGY

Under the influence of transforming growth factor-β (TGF-β), digit formation starts. Activin β A initiates chondrogenesis and activin β B is necessary for the formation of the distal phalanx (Figure 1.1a). Fingers and toes are discernible at week 8 of gestation.[14–16] The development of the human nail starts at around the ninth gestational week[17,18] as a condensation of epithelial cells on the dorsal aspect of the distal phalanx, the so-called apical ectodermal ridge, which develops into the nail anlage; both are dependent on the bone anlage. The anterior-posterior polarity requires sonic hedgehog signaled protein. Probably the number of progenitor cells of the nail plate at each digit is only about 3 as estimated from lyonization studies of female

nails.[19] The cell condensation develops into the placode, a plaque of cells that grow proximally and finally form an invagination (Figure 1.1b).[20] At 10 weeks, the nail field is seen as a continuous shallow groove that is first ovoidal in shape and extends beyond the tip of the finger.[21] Later it becomes flat as in the adult nail with well developed proximal, lateral, and distal nail grooves, the latter being very prominent due to the distal ridge. The nail field grows into a proximal direction with a continuously enlarging area of germinative matrix cells. By week 13, the proximal nail fold overlies part of the matrix and by week 14, a nail plate is seen emerging from under the proximal nail fold. It covers most of the nail field by week 17. The distal ridge has flattened to become the hyponychium. The nail bed stops producing keratohyalin granules and appears parakeratotic. The distal groove gradually disappears and at birth, the nail plate has usually overgrown the tip of the digit.[22] The nail continues to grow for the rest of the life.

In the late embryogenesis when the nail organ resembles that of an adult, the transcription factor B lymphocyte induced maturation protein 1 (Blimp-1), which is expressed in terminally differentiated keratinocytes, appears in the keratogenous cells of the matrix and superficial cells.[23]

The nail plate is the terminally differentiated structure formed by the germinative matrix. It is composed of keratin, which is physico-chemically identical to hair keratin.[24] Its production starts with the embryonal nail anlage, and both soft epithelial as well as hard hair and nail keratins are produced. Keratin 2e is observed in the nail bed as early as from the 10th to the 13th gestational week and then shifts to the nail fold;[25] its exact function is not understood. For correct nail formation, the transcription factor FOXN1 is necessary.[26]

The matrix is the sole structure to form the nail plate[14,16,27–29] although this was disputed based on nail plate thickness measurements.[30,31] Magnetic resonance imaging has shown that the length of the matrix is correlated with the nail plate thickness. Using an antibody to the proliferation marker Ki-67, the matrix was found to have a proliferation index of 20% compared to 1% in the nail bed.[32] However, in nail bed diseases like psoriasis and onychomycosis, 29% nail bed labeling was found. The proliferation index, measured with antibodies to the proliferating cell nuclear antigen and the AgNOR technique, proportionally decreases with age.[33] In adults, no hard keratins are found in the nail bed[22,30,34–37] and only matrix fibroblasts are able to induce hard keratin production by nonmatrical keratinocytes.[38] It was also shown that matrix fibroblasts are CD10+[39] and CD34+; these specialized cells were therefore termed onychofibroblasts. CD10 represents a surface

(a)

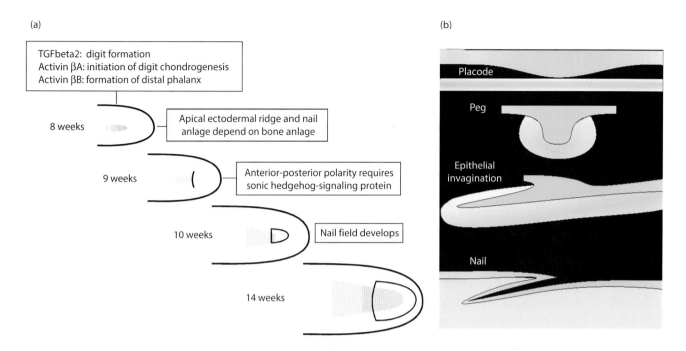

(b)

Figure 1.1 Development of the nail. (a) Time of evolution of the nail and factors necessary to form the nail unit. (b) The nail develops from a cellular densification called placode to an epithelial peg until this develops into a proximally directed invagination to finally form the nail.

metalloproteinase, which is known as the neutral endopeptidase and is also expressed by perifollicular fibroblasts. The CD10+ onychofibroblasts are restricted to the dermis of the matrix and proximal nail bed and not present in the distal nail bed, hyponychium, and proximal nail fold.[40–42]

1.2 MACROSCOPICAL ANATOMY

The nail apparatus consists of epithelial and connective tissue structures (Figure 1.2).[43–46]

Its main epithelial components are

- The matrix, which forms the nail plate,
- The nail bed, which firmly attaches the nail plate to the underlying dermis and terminal phalanx bone,

- The hyponychium, which is the transition between the nail bed and the skin of the digital pulp, and
- The ventral surface of the proximal nail fold, which overlies most of the matrix and forms the true and the false eponychium with the cuticle at its distal margin.

The connective tissue makes up the matrix and nail bed dermis, the dermis of the proximal and the paired lateral nail walls as well as the adjacent digital pulp dermis and hypodermis. In addition, the ligaments and tendons of the distal interphalangeal joints are integral parts of the nail apparatus and indispensable for the nails' mechanical functions; hence, the nail was recently termed a musculoskeletal appendage.[47,48] Both the flexor

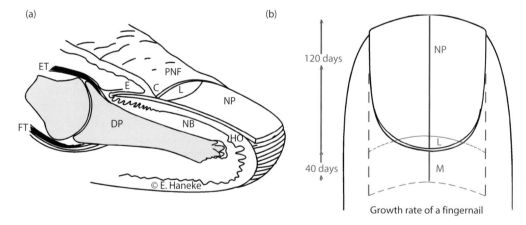

Figure 1.2 (a) Schematic illustration of the anatomy of the nail. (b) Idealized growth pattern of a fingernail. C cuticle, DP distal phalangeal bone, E eponychium, ET extensor tendon, FT flexor tendon, HO hyponychium, L lunula, M matrix, NB nail bed, NP nail plate, PNF proximal nail fold.

and extensor tendons, via volar and dorsal aponeuroses, not only insert at the volar and dorsal base of the terminal phalanx, respectively, but give lateral branches that form together with the lateral ligaments an aponeurosis and ensheath the entire distal interphalangeal joint. Furthermore, fibers from the extensor tendon radiate into the proximal nail fold thus being like a frame or holster for the matrix in between.[49,50] The entire nail apparatus is fixed to the underlying terminal phalanx, the size and shape of which greatly determine those of the nail organ.[51] The distance between the apex of the matrix and the extensor tendon insertion is between 1 mm[44] and 1.4 mm.[45,52–54] In the great toe, the extensor hallucis longus tendon inserts all along the dorsal surface of the bone from the base to the tip of the distal phalanx and is thus in-between the matrix and the bone.[55]

A dorsal view on the nail shows the proximal nail fold with its concave free margin and the cuticle at its end, the whitish lunula as the most distal portion of the matrix, which is, however, normally only seen in the thumb, index, and middle fingers as well as the big toe, but may be made visible by manicuring such as pushing the cuticle and the proximal nail fold back. A long proximal nail fold protects the underlying matrix rendering it less susceptible to trauma and various forms of irritation.[56] Pushing the nail fold back makes the lunula appear longer, which is apparently more attractive for many people, but it often leads to transverse ridges and furrows. In extreme cases, the proximal nail fold is pushed so far back that the cul-de-sac disappears completely in its central part, the nail plate gets a central depression due to innumerable short transverse furrows, and the nail shine gets lost.[57] Another consequence of such a repeated trauma is median canaliform dystrophy of Heller. The bulk of the visible nail is the pink colored nail bed, the color of which is said to be the result of the unique arrangement of its rete ridges and its capillaries. The most distal portion of the nail bed exhibits a deeper pink in light-skinned individuals, is darker brown in Afro-Carribeans, and is called the onychodermal band, which is about 1–1.5 mm wide.[58] Magnification reveals further details: A proximal pink portion, a central white band, and a distal pink zone.[59] Distal of the onychodermal band is the hyponychium, which lies under the free nail margin and is bordered by the distal groove, which demarcates the transition to the digital pulp skin.

The nail plate has parallel proximal and distal margins, being convex in the distal direction. It is gently curved in longitudinal direction and more markedly curved in the transverse direction. Whereas the latter curvature is defined by the shape of the distal phalanx, the former is due to the faster proliferation rate of the proximal as compared to the distal matrix. The nail plate exhibits characteristic longitudinal ridges, which increase and intensify with age. They are characteristic enough to allow distinction even of monozygotic twins.[60] When a nail is torn, the crack is always diverted transversely, parallel to the free margin of the nail. Cutting energy in transverse direction is only half of that in the longitudinal direction: 3 kJ/m^2 versus 6 kJ/m^2, respectively. This is probably due to the thick anisotropic intermediate layer that is composed of long narrow cells oriented transversely whereas the tile-like cells of the thinner dorsal and ventral layers exhibit isotropic behavior. It is assumed that they increase the bending strength of the nail. As they wrap around the nail edge they also prevent cracks from forming.[61]

1.3 NORMAL MICROSCOPIC ANATOMY OF THE NAIL

Virtually all macroscopically different parts of the nail apparatus have their characteristic microscopic appearance, which may vary in disease. To be able to evaluate pathological alterations, the normal microscopic anatomy has to be known.

1.3.1 Nail matrix

The matrix is the structure that produces the nail plate. Its visible part is called the lunula but this is microscopically identical with the major portion that is covered by the proximal nail fold. More than 80% of the nail cells are produced by the proximal 50% of the matrix.[62]

The matrix has a specialized epithelium, the basal compartment of which is basophilic and the superficial compartment eosinophilic (Figure 1.3a). The latter remains adherent to the nail plate when this is avulsed. The basal cells are slightly elongated changing to a cuboid shape and later both enlarging and flattening in the higher epithelial layers while becoming more eosinophilic. The mid-layer is usually lighter with more pronounced cell walls, which then transits to the uniformly eosinophilic keratogenous zone, which is the "onychotization" zone. The cell nuclei become smaller and darker and disappear when the eosinophilic superficial cells turn into nail cells (onychocytes), which are barely stained and thus appear light in normal hematoxylin and eosin (H&E) stained sections. A granular layer is not formed. Often some nuclear remnants remain visible (Figure 1.3b and c); they are called pertinax bodies.[14] In the central part, the matrix has the thickest epithelium. A periodic acid-Schiff (PAS) stain shows the glycocalyx of the onychocytes, which is often barely discernable in H&E sections.

The so-called dorsal matrix is still a matter of debate. Apparently, there is a tiny portion of the most proximal part of the proximal nail fold's ventral surface that is similar to the adjacent matrix epithelium in its staining and keratinization pattern. However, on high magnification it can be seen that these cells are different at their border to the underlying nail as compared with the true onychotizing matrix cells and rather resemble nail bed cells (Figure 1.3b). They may give rise to the so-called true eponychium.

The distal border of the matrix is characterized by a thinning of the epithelium that is visible in most sections of normal nails. Here, the matrix epithelium appears to overlie the basal layer of the most proximal nail bed in an oblique manner.

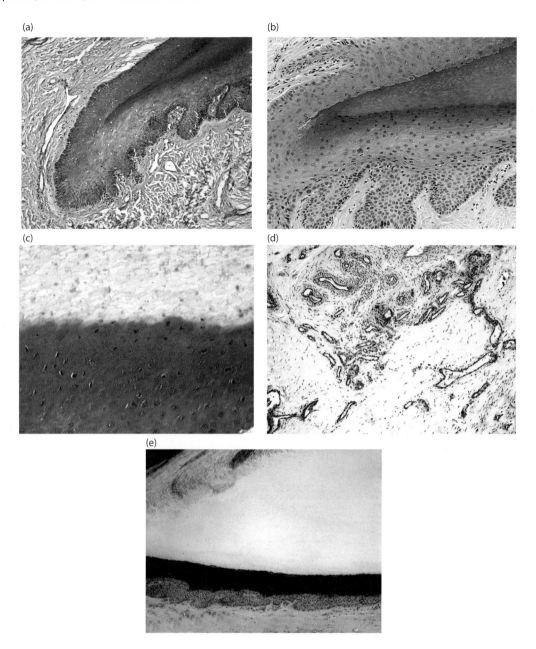

Figure 1.3 Normal nail matrix. (a) Proximal half of the matrix. (b) Close-up of the apical matrix demonstrating that the dorsal cells of the apical matrix do not exhibit the same morphology like the ventral matrix cells; the dorsal cells resemble more those of the nail bed. These are the cells that form the so-called true eponychium. (c) Mid- to distal matrix with a basophilic basal compartment and an eosinophilic keratogenous zone. (d) The connective tissue of the distal matrix contains many blood vessels and glomus bodies. Immunohistochemical demonstration of β_2-microglobulin. (e) Involucrin demonstration of the matrix shows sharply demarcated, intense positivity in the upper half of the matrix epithelium, which represents the prekeratogenous and keratogenous zone.

The matrix expresses cytokeratins 1, 5, 10, and 14 as well as the hard keratin hHa1.[63,64] The upper two thirds of the matrix epithelium are strongly positive for involucrin (Figure 1.3e),[63,65,66] but matrix cells also express actin strongly in their cell membranes and weakly in the cytoplasm as shown by the monoclonal antibody HHF35. Filaggrin is not found in normal nail matrix, neither immunohistochemically[63] nor by electron microscopy[32] but was shown to appear in FOXN1 deficient (nu-/nu-) mice[24] and in the dorsal matrix of monkey nails together with trichohyalin.[67] Others found filaggrin in the human dorsal matrix[68] where we have never seen keratohyalin- or trichohyalin-like structures under normal circumstances. The hair-nail keratin hHb5, but not its type II partner hHa5, is expressed in the entire keratogenous zone of the apical and ventral matrix and also in the uppermost cell layers of the basal compartment of the ventral matrix, where it is co-expressed with K5 and K17. Similar to their sequential expression in the hair follicle cortex, hair keratins hHa1, hHb1, hHb6, and hHa4 are consecutively expressed in the keratogenous zone of both the ventral and, albeit less distinctly, apical matrix, with hHa1 initiating in the lowermost cell layers. The expression of hHa8 in only single cortex cells of the hair follicle is also seen in some cells of the keratogenous zone. Retinoic acid-inducible gene-1 originally identified as an orphan G-protein coupled receptor induced by retinoic acid has been found in the keratogenous zone; it is associated with hard keratin production.[69] In the region of the so-called dorsal matrix, two histologically and histochemically distinct types of epithelia are observed: a dominant type, histologically similar to the eponychium with an associated K5, K17, and K10 keratin pattern, which extends into the apical matrix, and a minor type, histologically resembling the postulated dorsal matrix without a granular layer and a cuticle, and exhibiting extended K5 expression as well as hair keratin expression in superficial cells; this was seen as proof that the so-called dorsal matrix is a transition zone between the matrix and the eponychium.[37] When the matrix develops a granular layer under pathological conditions, keratins 1 and 10 are expressed.[70]

Using the label retaining cell method with bromodeoxyuridine and an antibody to LIM homeobox protein 2 (Lhx2) in mouse nails, stem cells were detected in the basal cell layer of the matrix adjacent to the nail bed.[71] The label retaining cells are controlled by R-spondin family member 4 (RSPO4), which is responsible for an autosomal dominant type of anonychia.[72,73] In adult human nails, stem cells were demonstrated in a zone roughly in the middle between the apical and distal matrix;[74] however, in contrast to the human hair follicle,[75] no cytokeratin 15 antibodies were used for that study. In a later investigation on fetal nails, using a panel of stem cell markers such as two different clones for CK15, CK 19, PHDLA1, CD200, nestin as well as Ki67, the stem cell niche of the developing embryonal and fetal nail was found to be in the ventral part of the proximal nail fold close to the matrix.[76] This was confirmed in a mouse model using label-retaining cells.[77]

CD200 is an immunoprotective membranous molecule rendering an immune privilege to the follicular bulge.[78] Given the overall weak staining for CD8 clone C8/144B and for CD200 in the fetal hair follicle and the lack of staining in the developing nail unit, it is probable that the immunosurveillance during embryogenesis has not yet attained a postnatal level.

Ultrastructurally, the basal compartment of the matrix epithelium is very similar to normal epidermis.[25,79–81] The keratinocytes are rich in ribosomes and contain microfibrils that are arranged haphazardly in the basal compartment and become aligned along the nail growth axis in the transitional zone. In this area, membrane coated granules are secreted into the intercellular space where they enforce the cell membrane thickness and play a role in cell adhesion.[82] They are supposed to be responsible for the membrane glycoproteins of the nail cells.[83]

1.3.2 Nail bed

The nail bed exhibits an epithelium of regular thickness when sectioned longitudinally, but has very pronounced slender rete ridges of equal length and in close vicinity. Their pattern is unique as this is the sole structure where longitudinal ridges run parallel to each other from the matrix until the hyponychium. In the papillary dermis ridges, longitudinally running capillaries are arranged one above the other in 4–6 rows, but almost vertically in the matrix.[84,85] It is believed that this particular pattern of capillary arrangement is responsible for the pink color of the nail bed, and it is the reason of the so-called splinter hemorrhages. The longitudinal nail bed ridges end at the hyponychium. The dermis of the nail bed contains virtually no fat and is firmly anchored to the bone. However, there are many nerves and blood vessels including glomus bodies. Skin appendages do not normally occur although sweat ducts may be seen at its distal margin.[86]

Glomus bodies are small, specialized organs that occur in great number in the nail bed and matrix dermis; in the nail bed, between 90 and 500 glomus bodies are found per mm^3. Normally, they are encapsulated and about 0.3 mm in diameter. They consist of glomus cells and a tortuous vessel linking the arterial with the venous side of the circulation. They are arranged parallel to the capillaries that they are able to bypass. They are important for thermoregulation.[87]

The nail bed epithelium exhibits a great similarity to the epithelium of the catagen follicle with small basal cells that gradually enlarge while migrating upward and abruptly keratinize without forming a granular layer (Figure 1.4). The nail bed epithelium is thinner in its central portion and thicker laterally. Often, single cells appear to protrude into the orthokeratin layer formed by the nail bed epithelium. High magnification reveals that these uppermost cells have very fine indentations that anchor the nail bed cells to the subungual keratin.

Immunohistochemistry shows that the nail bed epithelium expresses K6, K16, and K17 and no hard nail keratins.[37] mK6hf was found in correlation with K17 in the nail bed.[88] Keratin 17 was found by McGowan and Coulombe in the matrix and nail bed;[89] by de Berker et al. in the nail bed, apex of the matrix, and pulp of the digit;[62] in the matrix, nail bed, eponychium, and hyponychium by Perrin et al.,[37] but Lee et al. only found it in the nail bed.[90] Trichohyalin was described in the ventral matrix of the nail, which for some authors is synonymous with the nail bed;[91] however, we have never seen a morphological structure like trichohyalin or keratohyalin in the normal nail bed.

Under normal circumstances, only about 1% of the nail bed cells are labeled with antibodies to proliferation markers such as Ki-67, but this may rise to nearly 30% in nail bed psoriasis and onychomycosis.[32] This is, however, no proof of nail production, but simply reflects the tendency to produce a subungual hyperkeratosis.

Electron microscopy shows interdigitations of the uppermost nail bed cells with the overlying nail plate.[81]

(a)

(b)

(c)

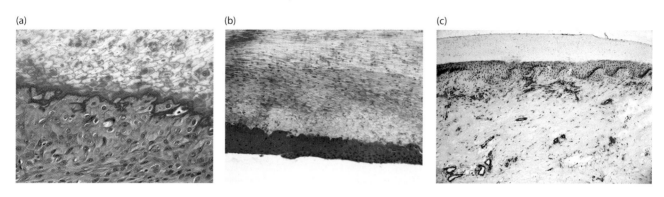

Figure 1.4 Normal nail bed. (a) Proximal nail bed epithelium showing the characteristic cell border to the nail plate. (b) Transition of the matrix to the nail bed epithelium demonstrating that the strongly eosinophilic keratogenous zone grows distally over the deeper portion of the basal cells of the nail bed. (c) Longitudinal section of the mid-nail bed demonstrating an epithelium without granular layer. β_2-Microglobulin demonstration shows vessels in the nail bed dermis.

1.3.3 Hyponychium

The hyponychium area comprises the onychodermal band to the distal ridge. It is the structure where the nail physiologically dissolves from the nail bed without leaving a space. The overhanging free nail margin forms a crevice that may harbor both dirt as well as microorganisms, such as *Staphylococcus epidermidis*, which is very difficult to eradicate,[92] and even *Helicobacter pylori* in subjects with oral colonization.[93]

Recently, the proximal portion of the hyponychium was termed the nail isthmus (Figure 1.5).[94–96]

Keratins K5, K17 (basal), and K10 (suprabasal) are expressed in the orthokeratinizing eponychium and hyponychium,[37] but the presence of K17 is disputed.

1.3.4 Nail plate

The nail plate is produced by the matrix. It consists of onychocytes that are flattened cells mostly containing keratin fibers. Seen under polarized light, they appear to form continuous birefringent fibers. Their arrangement slightly pointing downward distally allows the growth direction of a nail plate to be determined and also explains the split direction seen in a nail regrowing after a considerable trauma.

In histological sections, the most superficial nail plate cells that are produced by the proximal matrix are the flattest and very densely packed (Figure 1.6). With age, the superficial nail cells increase in size whereas they are smaller in fast growing nails. In babies, adults, and aged persons, the onychocyte surface of the thumb in males was 597 versus 920 versus 1008 μ^2, respectively.[97] The height of the corneocytes increases with the depth of the nail plate

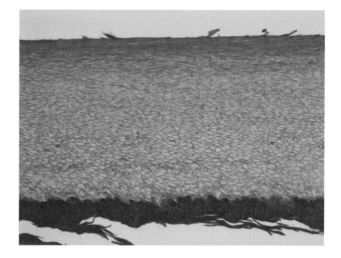

Figure 1.6 Nail plate with very flat cells superficially and higher cells in the deeper layers. The nail bed keratosis is strongly eosinophilic in contrast to the light-appearing nail cells.

from 2 μ to up to 15 μ.[81] The macroscopically evident longitudinal ridges at the nail's undersurface are not seen on longitudinal sections but often appear as prominent almost saw-tooth-like structures on transverse sections fitting into the wavy surface of the nail bed epithelium; this feature is even more pronounced in most cases of subungual hyperkeratosis and particularly in overcurvature of the nails. The dorsal surface of the nail plate is smooth in youngsters but tends to develop longitudinal ridging with age. The fingernail ridges can be best examined using polarized light.[98]

As measured in surgical avulsion specimens, the nail plate becomes slightly thicker over the nail bed, which was taken as proof that the nail bed produces nail plate substance.[30,31] However, histological and in vivo ultrasound examinations have shown a considerable reduction in thickness,[99–101] and both normal histology as well as polarization microscopy demonstrate a completely different staining pattern of the nail plate and the thin orthokeratotic layer produced by the nail bed. Ultrasound also suggests a lamellar structure of the nail plate with

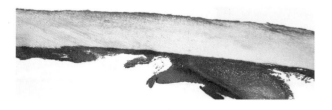

Figure 1.5 Hyponychium of an avulsed normal nail.

the superficial layer being dry and the deep compartment being humid.[102] The longer the matrix, the thicker the nail plate will be. When the nail cannot grow forward, for example, due to a distal nail wall, it usually becomes thicker, more yellow and often loses its transparency.

Histochemically, the superficial layer of the nail is rich in phospholipids, sulfhydryl groups, and calcium, but the latter is mainly due to adsorption from the environment.[103] High acid phosphatase activity and many disulfide bonds characterize the intermediate layer.[104] Synchroton X-ray microdiffraction also shows a layered nail plate structure that gives the nail its high mechanical rigidity and hardness both in the growth direction as well as the curvature.[105]

Scanning electron microscopy of cut surfaces in normal human nails have confirmed the layered nail structure, that is, the hard dorsal nail plate supported by the plastic intermediate nail plate.[106–108]

Transmission electron microscopy shows well-developed cell membranes and intercellular junctions. Ampullar dilatations are apparently part of these junction structures that are, however, mainly seen in the superficial layers whereas anchoring knots are characteristic for the deeper layers. Complete desmosomes are no longer seen,[81] but so-called spot desmosomes may be present.[109] The dorsal nail cells are flatter and become gradually thicker toward the deeper layers. At the junction of the nail plate with the subungual keratinocytes of the nail plate, there are many interdigitations firmly anchoring them to each other.

The nail plate contains DNA fragments, both of nuclear and mitochondrial origin. These DNA fragments are considerably shorter than those of living cells as it is the nail matrix' function to produce large amounts of protein—the keratins. Nuclear fragmentation is aimed at being complete in the fully matured onychocytes.[110]

The nail plate completely blocks ultraviolet B light and only allows a minimum of UV A light, around 0.6%–2.4% (mean 1.65%), to penetrate.[111]

1.3.5 Nail folds

The nail folds are like a frame on the proximal and lateral sides of the nail giving it strong support. The distal nail margin remains free and is used as a versatile tool.

The lateral nail folds are connective tissue rims covered with skin; in their distal portion, this is very similar to the digital pulp whereas it is more like normal skin in the proximal area although hair follicles and sebaceous glands are absent. In the depth of the nail groove, there may be more hyperkeratosis; however, this depends on the digit, the shape of the nail, and where the histological section was taken from.

The proximal nail fold covers the matrix and only in some digits is the lunula as the most distal part of the matrix visible (Figure 1.7).[112] It is made up of three compartments. The dorsal aspect is transitory skin with unremarkable epidermis except that there are no pilosebaceous follicles. Its free margin forms the cuticle (Figure 1.8), which is an extension of the horny layer of both the dorsal as well as the ventral skin of the proximal nail fold. It firmly adheres to the underlying nail plate sealing the nail pocket or cul-de-sac. For a proper cuticle formation, the nail must grow thus pulling the stratum corneum of the ventral surface of the proximal nail fold out, and the free margin of the proximal nail fold must have an acute angle; when this rounds up, for example, in the case of (chronic) paronychia, the cuticle disappears spontaneously; this is also seen when the nail stops growing as seen in the yellow nail syndrome. The undersurface or ventral surface of the proximal nail fold is covered by a flat epidermis with a well-developed stratum granulosum. The distal two-thirds produce the so-called false eponychium, which continues into the cuticle. The proximal third gives rise to the true eponychium, which remains adherent to the underlying nail plate. This is also seen after routine histological processing. The true eponychium may be visible during surgical detachment of the proximal nail fold from the underlying nail plate. The problem of the so-called

(a)

(b)

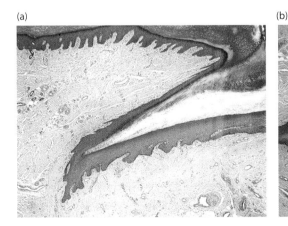
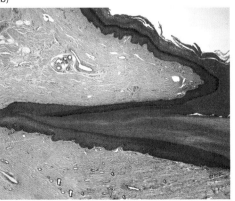

Figure 1.7 Proximal nail fold with dorsal and ventral epidermis as well as the matrix. The dorsal part of the apical matrix has no granular layer in contrast to most of the ventral surface of the proximal fold (a,b), which produces the orthokeratotic so-called false eponychium that often shows a split formation between it and the true eponychium with the nail plate.

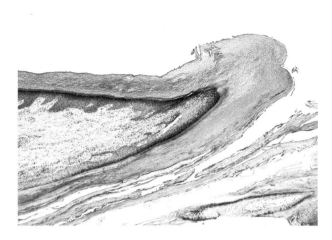

Figure 1.8 Cuticle and so-called false eponychium.

dorsal matrix has already been addressed. The integrity of the proximal nail fold is important for a healthy nail.

The proximal nail fold is assumed to have five different functions:[92]

- The dorsal matrix was recently found to harbor the nail stem cells.[76]
- The dorsal matrix may contribute to the nail plate, particularly to the shiny dorsal surface.
- As it is overlying the matrix it may be responsible for the nail growing out and not up.
- Nail fold capillaries exert patterns more or less specific for certain diseases, which can be reproduced by nail fold capillary microscopy.
- A diseased or traumatized nail fold may profoundly alter the clinical appearance of the nail plate.

In the nail folds like in the eponychium and hyponychium, keratins K5, K17 (basal), and K10 (suprabasal) are found.[37]

1.4 IMMUNOLOGY OF THE NAIL

An interesting investigation has shown that the nail, and in particular the matrix, is a site of relative immune priviledge.[113] Human leukocyte antigen A, B, and C expression is significantly downregulated in the keratinocytes and melanocytes of the proximal matrix whereas it is strongly positive in the periungual epidermis[96] as is β_2-microglobulin.[63] HLA-G+ CD4+ cells are abundant in the proximal nail fold and hyponychium but rare in the proximal matrix. Only a few CD8+ lymphocytes are found in the nail fold and hyponychium and they are even less frequent in the matrix. Langerhans cells in the nail bed and hyponychium are similar to epidermis,[114] but are very rare in the proximal matrix.[96] They exhibit very low HLA-DP, -DQ, and –DR reactivity suggesting that they are weak in antigen presentation in contrast to Langerhans cells and macrophages in the proximal nail fold. Their CD209 (human dendritic cell-specific adhesion receptor DC-SIGN) activity is weak suggesting that the ability of dendritic cells and macrophages to activate resting

lymphocytes is impaired in the matrix due to insufficient CD209 expression. Mast cells and NK cells as markers of innate immunity are scarce in the matrix. However, the antimicrobial peptide cathelicidin (LL37) is expressed in the proximal nail fold including the cuticle and the nail bed.[115] MHC class I antigen (HLA-A, -B, -C) is expressed on all nucleated cells except for immunoprivileged tissues such as the brain, cornea, anterior eye chamber, testis, liver, fetotrophoblast, and hair matrix.[116–124] The nail apparatus is assumed to share part of its embryonal and evolutionary origin as well as many structural and functional features with the hair follicle.[106,125,126] Examination of defined compartments of the nail apparatus demonstrated a downregulation of MHC class I as a key feature of immunoprivileged tissue sites[100,101,104] also in the nail matrix epithelium, and most prominently the proximal nail matrix compared to the proximal nail fold, nail bed, and hyponychium. This low to absent MHC class I expression in nail matrix epithelium is mirrored in the immediately adjacent nail mesenchyme. The functionally important MHC class I-associated molecule, β_2-microglobulin, which stabilizes MHC class I-antigen interactions,[127,128] was found to be either expressed less strongly[96] or was very weak as compared to the endothelial cells in the matrix and nail bed connective tissue and the hyponychial keratinocytes.[63] HLA-G is a nonclassical HLA molecule that is able to downregulate natural killer and CD8+ cytotoxic cells, suppresses NK cell activity against HLA negative cells, and is important to establish fetal immune tolerance.[129] It is upregulated in the nail matrix.[96] The matrix also produces immunosuppressive factors such as the macrophage inhibitory factor that prevents the release of cytotoxic perforin granules from NK cells, transforming growth factor-β1 (TGF-β1), adrenocorticotropic hormone (ACTH), α-melanocyte stimulating hormone (α-MSH), and insulin growth factor-1 (IGF-1).[96] In contrast to cultured human matrix cells,[130] the human nail matrix does not express intercellular adhesion molecule (ICAM, CD54),[131] which upregulates proinflammatory responses. All these data suggest that the nail is indeed an organ of relative immune privilege. However, this may also explain the difficulties in the treatment of a variety of nail infections, such as ungual warts and onychomycoses.

Integrins are expressed in the matrix in a similar way as in the epidermis. The basal membrane zone is strongly positive for the α6 and β4 subunits, the basal layer is positive for α2, α3, α6, αv, β1, and β4, the suprabasal layers of the ventral matrix are positive for α2, α3, weakly positive for αn, and positive for β1, the suprabasal layers of the dorsal matrix are weakly positive for α2, α3, αv, and β1, whereas the keratogenous zone is negative for all integrin subunits.[130]

Pancornulin and sciellin are short proline-rich proteins that act as precursors of the cornified envelope. Pancornulin is expressed in the proximal matrix and nail fold, sciellin in the matrix, nail bed, and nail fold.[66,132] The plasminogen activator inhibitor type 2 is assumed to play a role in regulating and protecting against programmed cell death; it was found both in the matrix as well as the nail bed.[133]

The cysteine protease inhibitor cystatin M/E is a key regulator of a biochemical pathway leading to epidermal terminal differentiation by inhibition of its target proteases cathepsin L, cathepsin V, and legumain. It regulates cross-linking of structural proteins by transglutaminase 3. Cystatin M/E is expressed in the upper granular layer of the epidermis of the proximal nail fold's dorsal and ventral aspect, but it decreases toward the matrix. Here, cystatin M/E expression is faint and only in the uppermost cells of the superficial compartment; it is not present in the nail bed, but markedly expressed at the hyponychium. Cathepsin L is expressed in the whole nail unit and located suprabasally except for the horny layer of the epidermis and hyponychium. Thus, cystatin M/E and cathepsin L are co-localized in the nail organ. Legumain is similarly expressed in the nail whereas cathepsin V appears to be absent in the nail unit except for the epidermis and the hyponychium. Transglutaminase 3 is expressed in all nail regions except for the nail bed, particularly strong in the uppermost cells of the matrix directly before they become onychocytes. Transglutaminase and cathepsin L are co-localized in the granular layer of the epidermis, proximal nail fold, and hyponychium, and very prominent in the matrix.[134] The matrix shows a gradual transition from cathepsin L to transglutaminase 3 expression suggesting that activation of transglutaminase 3 takes place at a location analogous to the human hair bulb; similar findings are observed in the matrix and hair bulb where cystatin M/E is almost undetectable.[135] Loricrin and involucrin are expressed where transglutaminase is present. Cathepsin V was not expressed in the ventral part of the proximal nail fold, in the matrix, and the nail bed, which is logical as cathepsin V appears to be involved in desquamation.[116] Trichohyalin was not found in this study in contrast to monkey nail and one study that presumed to have found trichohyalin in the ventral matrix (probably nail bed).[74]

Lack of transglutaminase 1 activity leads to structural nail abnormalities.[136,137]

1.5 MELANOCYTES OF THE NAIL UNIT

The normal nail matrix contains up to 300 melanocytes per mm^2.[66,138–140] In fair-skinned persons, they are mostly dormant, that is, functionally inactive, whereas in deeply pigmented individuals they usually produce enough melanin to cause physiological nail pigmentation. They are much more numerous in the matrix than in the nail bed[141–143] and more active in the distal than in the proximal matrix. In the proximal matrix, the quiescent melanocytes are DOPA negative and cannot synthesize melanin under normal conditions, but they can be demonstrated by monoclonal antibodies to tyrosine-related protein 1. The functionally active melanocytes are DOPA positive[122] and can be stained with antibodies recognizing tyrosinase.[124,125] Immunohistochemical studies showed a melanocyte density of 237/mm^2 in the matrix, which is far lower than in the epidermis.[125] Most matrix melanocytes

are found in suprabasal position, which is an important normal finding in respect to exclude or confirm melanocytic dysplasia. This was attributed to the fact that the basal matrix keratinocytes form 2–10 layers.[108] Matrix melanocytes, like fetal melanocytes and melanoma cells, are normally positive for HMB45, another potentially confusing fact.[123] Whereas the matrix melanocytes are HLA negative, those in the nail bed and proximal nail fold are strongly HLA positive.[96] Collapse of this immune privilege may expose matrix melanocytes to autoimmune attacks and provoke nail matrix involvement in alopecia areata.[104–106]

Whereas matrix melanocytes are strongly decorated with antibodies like Melan-A and HMB45, they often do not or only weakly stain with protein S100 and MITF antibodies.[144]

Melanocytes are much less numerous in the nail bed[125] or not even demonstrable with immunohistochemical techniques.[124] They retain their distribution in the basal layer.

Electron microscopy of nail melanocytes showed mainly immature melanosomes in the nail of Japanese subjects whereas those of blacks contain mature melanosomes.[66]

In light-skinned individuals, no melanin is normally seen in the plate. However, when present it derives from matrix melanocytes[16] and is seen as melanin granules, which represent melanosome complexes. This is a normal phenomenon in darkly pigmented individuals, in whom the presence of melanin pigmentation increases with age.[145,146] In the Japanese population, about 10%–20% develop longitudinal melanonychia.[147] Melanin is seen as light brown round granules and stains dark with Fontana-Masson's argentaffin reaction. In contrast, most fungal melanins are soluble and stain the nail a diffuse light yellow; in our experience, they are not argentaffin positive.

1.6 MERKEL CELLS IN THE NAIL

Merkel cells are positive for keratins 8 and 20. They were found in the adult nail matrix[148] and in infantile accessory digits,[149] but others could not confirm these findings.[150]

1.7 BLOOD SUPPLY OF THE NAIL APPARATUS

The nail is supplied by both the paired volar as well as dorsal proper digital arteries, but the volar arteries are the main suppliers. The dorsal arteries form their most distal arcades at the level of the distal interphalangeal joint and then only give anastomoses to the volar arteries that now continue in a more dorsal level, but give deep branches to the finger pulp.[43,151] From the most distal portion of the volar digital arteries, three arterial arcades are formed in the level of the proximal nail fold, the matrix, and the nail bed. The venous drainage is less abundant.[43,152]

In the nail bed and matrix dermis, many arteries are usually seen. A hitherto undescribed observation is the occurrence of blood vessels with thin to medium-thick walls that have a cushion-like thickening of smooth muscle cells in one circumscribed area; this may be in direct relation to the normal muscular layer or directly next to

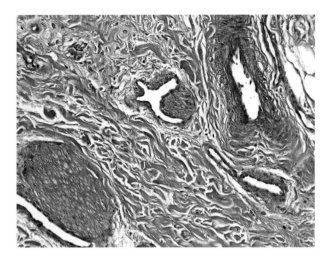

Figure 1.9 Vessels of the matrix dermis with cushions of smooth muscles.

it (Figure 1.9). The function of these muscle pads is not known, but may have something to do with thermoregulation in analogy to the glomus bodies.

1.8 INNERVATION OF THE NAIL

There are paired volar and dorsal proper digital nerves, the dorsal ones probably being responsible for most of the digits;[43] however, some investigators claim that the index, middle, and ring finger nail units get their innervation from the volar nerves. This would explain why these nails can be anesthetized with a transthecal block injecting the anesthetic agent into the sheath of the flexor tendons at the volar metacarpo-phalangeal crease.[153] In the index finger, about 3000 endoneurial tubes enter the finger pulp.[154]

The nail also considerably contributes to tactile sensation[155] and sensibility (Figure 1.10).[156]

1.9 INTERNAL AND FORENSIC MEDICINE AND THE NAIL

Nail keratin has a fixed composition of amino acids. This can be altered by environmental and occupational influences; harmful agents such as alkaline and acidic groups may alter the amount of disulfide bonds and lower the sulfur content.[12] Elemental analyses of the nails may give information about the general health status[157] though very sensitive methods are often not able to differentiate endogenous elements from exogenous impurities. Analysis of nails, as well as of hair, can give valuable retrospective information as to ingestion and exposure of foreign material, but also of abnormal metabolites. Higher nail concentrations of D-amino acids were found in nails of diabetic subjects.[158] Nail sample analyses allow steroid sulfatase to be determined for the screening of X-linked ichthyosis.[159] A number of drugs, doping agents, trace elements, heavy metals, and poisons can be retrieved from the slow-growing nails as long as many months to a year after their ingestion or administration, respectively,[160–162] provided they were not washed out. Ingestion and intoxication of arsenic (As) has particularly been investigated by studying As concentrations in the nails.[163,164] The calcium content of the nail is too low to contribute to nail hardness.[165] Nail calcium and magnesium levels do not reflect bone mineral density[166] although bone collagen and nail keratin require sulfation and disulfide bond formation via cysteine for structural integrity and thus appear to be linked to each other.[167] Some drugs, particularly antifungal azoles, are "keratinophilic" and concentrate in the stratum corneum and the nail compared to blood and tissue values.[168,169] Nails of newborns may be screened for drug intake of the mother during pregnancy.

Both nails as well as fingernail debris may yield enough DNA material to identify a decomposed cadaver or a potential aggressor, respectively.[170,171] DNA samples of nails remain remarkably stable in air, but slowly degrade after one month in a moist environment.[172]

1.10 GENETIC STUDIES

The human androgen receptor gene assay performed on DNA extracted from nail plates allows studying the X chromosome inactivation patterns in human nails suggesting a longitudinal linear band pattern, each of the

(a)

(b)

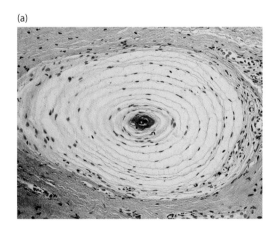 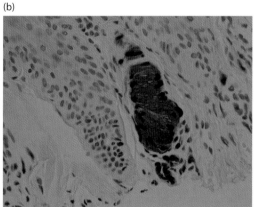

Figure 1.10 (a) Pacini body in the tip of the toe under the hyponychium; original magnification 400×, protein S100 demonstration. (b) Meissner body directly beneath the hyponychium in the papillary dermis of the pulp. S100 demonstration.

bands representing only one active X chromosome. This pattern is stable for at least several regeneration cycles.[18] Thus, the composition of precursor cells in the matrix, where the nail plate is produced continuously,[173] is constant for at least 2 years. The banded pattern may be the reason for the partial involvement of the nail in lichen striatus.

1.11 NAIL AND FINGERTIP REGENERATION

Distal fingertip injuries including amputations to a level distal to the distal interphalangeal joint may heal by complete spontaneous regeneration in a variety of animals as well as in human infants.[174–176] Even complete loss of the distal phalanx, however, with preservation of the nail matrix and its soft tissues, may result in regeneration of the terminal phalanx.[177,178] This has even been observed in an adult.[179] In contrast, active surgical treatment by grafts and flaps prevented digit tip regeneration[180] as did removal of the nail unit.[181,182] Nail transplantation induced bone formation in proximal phalanges.[183] Nail epithelium generates Wnt signaling that attracts nerves to distal sites of amputation inducing blastema formation, bone and digit regrowth.[184] Bone morphogenetic protein (BMP) 7 is another factor needed for nail growth and digit tip regeneration.[77,185] The tissue developing between the stump and the overlying epithelium, the blastema, is thought to contain stem cells with multi-lineage potentials.[186,187] Most recent experiments showed that Lgr 5 and Lgr 6, which are markers of several epithelial stem cell populations and important agonists of the Wnt/b-catenin signaling, are found in the cells of the nail dermis (Lgr 5) just under the matrix cells which are positive for Lgr 6.[188] However, regeneration and nail growth are also dependent on vascular and neurologic factors; thickening and nail hypertrophy develop in toes after spinal cord injury.[189,190]

1.12 IMAGING OF THE NAIL ORGAN

Dermatoscopy and macrophotography of the nail have been aids in diagnosing a variety of nail conditions. "Dry dermatoscopy" allows the inspection of the nail plate surface using immersion oil or a gel to make the surface and in part the nail plate more transparent allowing intraungual and subungual structures to be better visualized.[191–193] Direct intraoperative dermatoscopy of matrix and nail bed melanocytic lesions has been shown to improve diagnostic accuracy.[194,195]

Optical profilometry quantifies surface alterations. It can be used on the nail in vivo, on nail clippings, and on silicone rubber replicas.[196] Different types of surface alterations such as trachyonychia, pitting, grooves, and so on can conveniently be defined by their mean roughness, mean depth of roughness, and the number of peaks and crests.[157]

Reflectance confocal laser scanning microscopy has also been used to investigate nails.[197] It is limited by its relatively superficial penetrance of approximately 200 μ in skin and 400 μ in nails.[198] The nail is "sectioned"

horizontally when it is scanned from the surface to the deeper layers. Due to the limited penetration depth, the nail plate usually cannot be penetrated or only in very thin nails. Reflectance confocal laser scanning microscopy can be employed in vivo and on excised matrix specimens. It gives characteristic images for onychomycosis,[199–201] allows the integrity of corneocytes to be investigated, and was also used for the diagnosis of in situ and early invasive matrix melanoma.[202,203]

Optical coherence tomography (OCT), another noninvasive method, displays the nail plate as a multilayered structure with a varying number of homogeneous horizontal bands of differing intensity and thickness. Compared with 100 MHz ultrasound, OCT has a better resolution.[204] Polarization sensitive (PS) OCT confirms this structure. The refractive index of the nail was 1.47 ± 0.09. Both OCT and PS-OCT had low variation coefficients of 6.31 and 6.53, respectively, whereas high-frequency ultrasound had variation coefficients of 12.70 and calipers 14.03. This method delivers images up to 2 mm in depth thus including the nail plate, the epithelium, and the superficial portions of the matrix and nail bed dermis. The lunula exhibits a horizontal white band at the nail plate's undersurface whereas leukonychia shows a white band within the nail. OCT uses infrared light and therefore has a higher resolution than ultrasound.[205]

Ultrasound has long been used to determine nail thickness and diagnose subungual tumors.[206–210] Measured with 20 MHz ultrasound, the mean nail thickness of healthy persons varies between 0.481 mm (right thumb) and 0.397 mm (left fifth finger).[211] In the last decade, various high-frequency and variable frequency as well as 3-dimensional ultrasound techniques were added to the diagnostic armamentarium of nail conditions.[212,213]

Further, existing imaging methods have been refined such as fine-layer computed tomography and high-resolution magnetic resonance[214–216] adding valuable information to both clinical as well as histopathological examinations.[217–219] MRI also has some value in differentiating nail tumors.[220] Recently, magnetic resonance microscopy was used to study the finger and nail.[221]

Fiber diffraction using special X-ray sources or small angle X-ray beam-lines at synchrotones are said to give specific diffraction patterns allowing the diagnosis of cancers and melanoma to be made from nail samples.[222]

REFERENCES

1. Achten G. L'ongle normal et pathologique. *Dermatologica* 1963;126:229–245.
2. Achten G. Normale Histologie und Histochemie des Nagels. In: Jadassohn J, ed. *Handbuch der Haut- und Geschlechtskrankheiten, Erg-Werk*, Berlin: Springer, 1968; 1:339–376.
3. Langbein L, Rogers MA, Winter H, Praetzel S, Beckhaus U, Rackwitz HR, Schweizer J. The catalog of human hair keratins. I. Expression of the nine type I members in the hair follicle. *J Biol Chem* 1999;274:19874–19884.

4. Langbein L, Rogers MA, Winter H, Praetzel S, Schweizer J. The catalog of human hair keratins. II. Expression of the six type II members in the hair follicle and the combined catalog of human type I and II keratins. *J Biol Chem* 2001;276:35123–35132.

5. Langbein L, Schweizer J. Keratins of the human hair follicle. *Int Rev Cytol* 2005;243:1–78.

6. Gillespie JM. The structural proteins of hair: Isolation, characterization and regulation of biosynthesis. In: Goldsmith LA, ed. *Physiology, Biochemistry and Molecular Biology of the Skin*, Oxford: Oxford University Press, 1991; 625–659.

7. Powell B, Rogers G. Differentiation in hard keratin tissues: Hair and related structure. In: Leigh I, Lane B, Watt F, eds. *The Keratinocyte Handbook*, Cambridge: Cambridge University Press, 1994; 401–436.

8. Rogers MA, Langbein L, Praetzel-Wunder S, Winter H, Schweizer J. Human hair keratin-associated proteins (KAPs). *Int Rev Cytol* 2006;251:209–263.

9. Alibardi L, Dalla Valle L, Nardi A, Toni M. Evolution of hard proteins in the sauropsid integument in relation to the cornification of skin derivatives in amniotes. *J Anat* 2009;114:560–586.

10. Dittmar M, Dindorf W, Banerjee A. Organic elemental composition in fingernail plates varies between sexes and changes with increasing age in healthy humans. *Gerontol/ Int J Exp Clin Behav Gerontol* 2008;54:100–105.

11. Fleckman P. Basic science of the nail unit. In: Scher R, Daniel CIII, eds. *Nails: Therapy Diagnosis Surgery*, 2nd edn. Philadelphia: WB Saunders Company, 1997; 37–54.

12. Schumacher E, Dindorf W, Dittmar M. Exposure to toxic agents alters organic elemental composition in human fingernails. *Sci Total Environm* 2009;407:2151–2157.

13. Baden HP, Goldsmith LA, Fleming B. A comparative study of the physicochemical properties of human keratinized tissues. *Biochim Biophys Acta* 1973;322:269–278.

14. Lewis BL. Microscopic studies of fetal and mature nail and surrounding soft tissue. *AMA Arch Dermatol Syphilol* 1954;70:733–747.

15. Sanchez Conejo-Mir J, Ambrosiani J, Dorado M. Análisis de la morfogénesis ungueal. Estudio con microscopía electrónica de barrido en el embrión humano. *Acad Espan Dermatol Sifiliografía* 1985.

16. Sanchez Conejo-Mir J, Camacho FM. Biología de la uña. Embriología. Anatomía, Fisiología. In: Baran R, Camacho FM, Mascaró JM, eds. *Oncología. Biología y alteraciones de la unidad ungueal*, Madrid: Aula Medica, 2006; 1–18.

17. Zaias N. The embryology of the human nail. *Arch Dermatol* 1963;87:37–53.

18. Achten MG. De l'embryologie et de l'histochimie de l'ongle normal à la pathologie unguéale. *J Méd Lyon* 1968;49(141):705–726.

19. Okada M, Nishimukai H, Okiura T, Sugino Y. Lyonization pattern of normal human nails. *Cells Genes* 2008;13:421–428.

20. Chapman RE. Hair, wool, quill, nail, claw, hoof and horn. In: Bereiter-Hahn J, Matoltsy AG, Richards KS, eds. *Biology of the Integument, Vol. 2, Vertebrates*, New York: Springer-Verlag, 1986; 293–312.

21. Mazzarello V, Dessi AL. Ontogenesis of the human fetal nails. I. Observations using the scanning electron microscope (Italian). *Boll Soc Ital Biol Sper* 1990;66:441–448.

22. Brademas ME. Embryology. In Scher RK, Daniel CRIII, eds. *Nails: Therapy, Diagnosis, Surgery*, Philadelphia: Saunders, 1990; 31–35.

23. Sellheyer K, Krahl D. Blimp-1: A marker of terminal differentiation but not of sebocytic progenitor cells. *J Cut Pathol* 2010;37:362–370.

24. Moll I, Heid HW, Franke WW, Moll R. Patterns of expression of trichocytic and epithelial cytokeratins in mammalian tissues. *Differentation* 1988;39:167–184.

25. Smith LT, Underwood RA, McLean WH. Ontogeny and regional variability of keratin 2e (K2e) in developing human fetal skin: A unique spatial and temporal pattern of keratin expression in development. *Br J Dermatol* 1999;140:582–591.

26. Mecklenburg L, Paus R, Halata Z, Bechtold LS, Fleckman P, Sundberg JP. FOXN1 is critical for onycholemmal terminal differentiation in nude (Foxn1nu) mice. *J Invest Dermatol* 2004;123:1001–1011.

27. Hashimoto K, Gross BG, Nelson R, Lever WF. The ultrastructure of the skin of human emryos. III. The formation of the nail in 16–18 week old embryos. *J Invest Dermatol* 1966;47:205–207.

28. Zaias N, Alvarez J. The formation of the primate nail plate. An autoradiographic study in the squirrel monkey. *J Invest Dermatol* 1968;51:120–136.

29. Norton LA. Incorporation of thymidine-methyl-H3 and glycine-2-H3 in the nail matrix and bed of humans. *J Invest Dermatol* 1971;56:61–68.

30. Johnson M, Comaish JS, Shuster S. Nail is produced by the normal nail bed: A controversy resolved. *Br J Dermatol* 1991;125:27–29.

31. Johnson M, Shuster S. Continuous formation of nail along the nail bed. *Br J Dermatol* 1993;128:277–280.

32. de Berker D, Angus B. Proliferative compartments in the normal nail unit. *Br J Dermatol* 1996;135: 555–559.

33. Raguz JM, Haneke E. Analyse der Proliferationsaktivität der Nagelmatrixzellen mit der AgNOR-Methode. *Hautarzt* 1997;48(Suppl. 1):S62.

34. Heid HW, Moll I, Franke WW. Patterns of trichocytic and epithelial cytokeratins in mammalian tissues. II. Concomitant and mutually exclusive synthesis of trichocytic and epithelial cytokeratins in diverse human and bovine tissues. *Differentation* 1988;27:215–230.

35. de Berker DAR, Leight I, Wojnarowska F. Patterns of keratin expression in the nail unit—An indicator of regional differentiation. *Br J Dermatol* 1992; 127:423.

36. Westgate GE, Tidman N, de Berker D, Blount MA, Phjilpott MP, Leigh IM. Characterisation of LH Tric 1, a new monospecific monoclonal antibody to hair keratin Ha1. *Br J Dermatol* 1997;127:24–31.

37. Perrin C, Langbein L, Schweizer J. Expression of hair keratins in the adult nail unit: An immunohistochemical analysis of the onychogenesis in the proximal nail fold, matrix and nail bed. *Br J Dermatol* 2004;151:362–371.

38. Okazaki M, Yoshimura K, Fujiwara H, Suzuki Y, Harii K. Induction of hard keratin expression in non-nail-matrical keratinocytes by nail-matrical fibroblasts through epithelial–mesenchymal interactions. *Plast Reconstr Surg* 2003;111:286–290.

39. Lee KJ, Kim WS, Lee JH, Yang J-M, Lee E-S, Lee D-Y, Mun G-H, Jang T-K. CD10, a marker for specialized mesenchymal cells (onychofibroblasts) in the nail unit. *J Dermatol Sci* 2006;42:65–67.

40. Lee KJ, Kim WS, Lee JH, Yang J-M. Presence of specialized mesenchymal cells (onychofibroblasts) in the nail unit: Implications for ingrown nail surgery. *J Eur Acad Dermatol Venereol* 2006;21:575–576.

41. Lee DY, Park JH, Shin HT, Yang JM, Jang KT, Kwon GY, Lee KH, Shim JS. The presence and localization of onychodermis (specialized nail mesenchyme) containing onychofibroblasts in the nail unit: A morphological and immunohistochemical study. *Histopathology* 2012;61:123–130.

42. Lee DY, Yang JM, Mun GH, Jang KT, Cho KH. Immunohistochemical study of specialized nail mesenchyme containing onychofibroblasts in transverse sections of the nail unit. *Am J Dermatopathol* 2011;33:266–270.

43. Morgan AM, Baran R, Haneke E. Anatomy of the nail unit in relation to the distal digit. In: Krull E, Zook E, Baran R, Haneke E, eds. *Nail Surgery: A Text and Atlas*, Philadelphia: Lippincott Williams & Wilkins, 2001; 1–28.

44. Fleckman P, Allan C. Surgical anatomy of the nail unit. *Dermatol Surg* 2001;27:257–260.

45. Haneke E. Surgical anatomy of the nail apparatus. *Dermatol Clin* 2006;24:291–296.

46. de Berker DAR, André J, Baran R. Nail biology and nail science. *Int J Cosm Sci* 2007;29:241–275.

47. McGonagle D, Tan AL, Benjamin M. The nail as a musculoskeletal appendage—Implications for a better understanding of the link between psoriasis and arthritis. *Dermatology* 2009;218:97–102.

48. McGonagle D, Fontana NP, Tan AL, Benjamin M. Nailing down the genetic and immunological basis for psoriatic disease. *Dermatology* 2010;221(Suppl.): 15–22.

49. Hoch J, Fritsch H, Frenz C. Gibt es einen knöchernen Strecksehnenab- oder -ausriß? Plastinationshistologische Untersuchungen zur Insertion der Streckaponeurose und deren Bedeutung für die operative Therapie. *Chirurg* 1999;70:705–712.

50. Frenz C, Fritsch H, Hoch J. Plastination histologic investigations on the inserting pars terminalis aponeurosis dorsalis of three-sectioned fingers. *Anat Anz* 2000;182:69–73.

51. Baran R, Juhlin L. Bone dependent nail formation. *Br J Dermatol* 1986;114:371–375.

52. Shum C, Bruno RJ, Ristic S, Rosenwasser MP, Strauch RJ. Examination of the anatomic relationship of the proximal germinal nail matrix to the extensor tendon insertion. *J Hand Surg [Am]* 2000;25:1114–1117.

53. Schweitzer TP, Rayan GM. The terminal tendon of the digital extensor mechanism: Part I, anatomic study. *J Hand Surg [Am]* 2004;29:898–902.

54. Kim JY, Jung HJ, Lee WJ, Kim do W, Yoon GS, Kim DS, Park MJ, Lee SJ. Is the distance enough to eradicate in situ or early invasive subungual melanoma by wide local excision? From the point of view of matrix-to-bone distance for safe inferior surgical margin in Koreans. *Dermatology* 2011;223:122–123.

55. López PP, Becerro de Bengoa Vallejo R, López López D, Prados Frutos JC, Murillo González JA, Losa Iglesias ME. Anatomic relationship of the proximal nail matrix to the extensor hallucis longus tendon insertion. *J Eur Acad Dermatol Venereol* 2015;29:1967–1971.

56. Muto H, Yoshioka I. Relationship between the degree of coverage of the nail root by the posterior nail wall and the length of the visible part of the nail in human toes. *Kaibogaku Zasshi* 1977;52:269–276.

57. Haneke E. Autoaggressive nail disorders. Trastornos de autoagresión hacia las uñas (Engl & Span). *Dermatol Rev Mex* 2013;57:225–234.

58. Terry RB. The onychodermal band in health and disease. *Lancet* 1955;1:179–181.

59. Sonnex TS, Griffiths WA, Nicol WJ. The nature and significance of the transverse white band of human nails. *Sem Dermatol* 1991;10:12–16.

60. Diaz AA, Boehm AF, Rowe WF. Comparison of fingernail ridge patterns of monozygotic twins. *J Forens Sci CA* 1990;35:97–102.

61. Farren L, Shayler S, Ennos AR. The fracture properties and mechanical design of human fingernails. *J Exp Biol* 2004;207:735–741.

62. de Berker DAR, MaWhinney B, Sviland L. Quantification of regional matrix nail production. *Br J Dermatol* 1996;134:1083–1086.

63. Haneke E. The human nail matrix—Flow cytometric and immunohistochemical studies. *Clin Dermatol Year* 2000, Abstr.

64. De Berker D, Wojnarowska F, Sviland L, Westgate GE, Dawber RP, Leigh IM. Keratin expression in the normal nail unit: Markers of regional differentiation. *Br J Dermatol* 2000;142:89–96.

65. Haneke E. Histology, immunohistochemistry and histopathology of the nail. Abstract, VIII. International Congress of Dermatologic Surgery, Barcelona, Oct 10–13, 1987.

66. Baden H. Common transglutaminase substrates shared by hair, epidermis and nail and their function. *J Dermatol Sci* 1994;7(Suppl.):S20–S26.

67. Manabe M, O'Guin WM. Existence of trichohyalin keratohyalin hybrid granules: Co-localisation of 2 major intermediate filament-associated proteins in non-follicular epithelia. *Differentiation* 1994;58:65–75.

68. Kitahara T, Ogawa H. Cellular features of differentiation in the nail. *Microsc Res Tech* 1997;38:436–442.

69. Inoue S, Nambu T, Shimomura T. The RAIG family member, GPRC5D, is associated with hard-keratinized structures. *J Invest Dermatol* 2004;122:565–573.

70. Fanti PA, Tosti A, Cameli N, Varotti C. Nail matrix hypergranulosis. *Am J Dermatopathol* 1994; 16:607–610.

71. Nakamura M, Ishikawa O. The localization of label-retaining cells in mouse nails. *J Invest Dermatol* 2008;128:728–730.

72. Bergmann C, Senderek J, Anhuf D, Thiel CT, Ekici AB, Poblete-Gutiérrez P, van Steensel M et al. Mutations in the gene encoding the Wnt-signaling component Respondin 4 (RSPO4) cause autosomal recessive anonychia. *Am J Hum Genet* 2006;79:1105–1109.

73. Blaydon DC, Ishii Y, O'Toole EA, Unsworth HC, Teh MT, Rüschendorf F, Sinclair C et al. The gene encoding R-spondin 4 (RSPO4), a secreted protein implicated in Wnt signaling, is mutated in inherited anonychia. *Nat Genet* 2006;21:18–31.

74. Körver J. Quantitative visualization of epidermal cell populations. A study in healthy and psriatic skin and its appendages. *PhD thesis*, Univ Nijmegen, The Netherlands, 2009.

75. Kloepper JE, Tiede S, Brinckmann J, Reinhardt DP, Meyer W, Faessler R, Paus R. Immunophenotyping of the human bulge region: The quest to define useful in situ markers for human epithelial hair follicle stem cells and their niche. *Exp Dermatol* 2008;17:592–599.

76. Sellheyer K, Nelson P. The ventral proximal nail fold: Stem cell niche of the nail and equivalent to the follicular bulge—A study on developing human skin. *J Cutan Pathol* 2012;39:835–843.

77. Leung Y, Kandyba E, Chen Y-B, Ruffins S, Chuong C-M, Kobielak K. Bifunctional ectodermal stem cells around the nail display dual fate homeostasis and adaptive wounding response toward nail regeneration. *Proc Natl Acad Sci USA* 2014;111:15114–15119.

78. Meyer KC, Klatte JE, Dinh HV, Harries MJ, Reithmayer K, Meyer W, Sinclair R, Paus R. Evidence that the bulge region is a site of relative immune privilege in human hair follicles. *Br J Dermatol* 2008;159:1077–1085.

79. Hashimoto K. Ultrastructure of the human toenail. Cell migration, keratinization and formation of the intercellular cement. *Arch Dermatol Forsch* 1970;240:1–22.

80. Hashimoto K. Ultrastructure of the human toenail. II. *J Ultrastruct Res* 1971;36:391–410.

81. Hashimoto K. Ultrastructure of the human toenail. I. Proximal nail matrix. *J Invest Dermatol* 1971;56:235–246.

82. Parent D, Achten G, Stouffs-Vamhoof F. Ultrastructure of the normal human nail. *Am J Dermatopathol* 1985;7:529–535.

83. Allen AK, Ellis J, Rivett DE. The presence of glycoprotins in the cell membrane complex of a variety of keratin fibres. *Biochim Biophys Acta* 1991;1074:331–333.

84. Inoue H. Three-dimensional observations of microvasculature of human finger skin. *Hand* 1978;10:144–149.

85. Sangiorgi S, Manelli A, Congiu T, Bini A, Pilato G, Reguzzoni M, Raspanti M. Microvascularization of the human digit as studied by corrosion casting. *J Anat* 2004;204:123–131.

86. Maricq HR. Observation and photography of sweat ducts of the fingers in vivo. *J Invest Dermatol* 1967;48:399–401.

87. Masson P. *Les Glomus Neurovasculaires*, Paris: Hermann et Cie, 1937.

88. Wang Z, Wong P, Langbein L, Schweizer J, Coulombe PA. Type II epithelial keratin 6hf (K6hf) is expressed in the companion layer, matrix, and medulla in anagen-stage hair follicles. *J Invest Dermatol* 2003;121:1276–1282.

89. McGowan KM, Coulombe PA. Keratin 17 expression in the hard epithelial context of the hair and nail, and its relevance for the pachyonychia congenita phenotype. *J Invest Dermatol* 2000;114:1101–1107.

90. Tong X, Coulombe PA. A novel mouse type I intermediate filament gene, keratin 17n (K17n), exhibits preferred expression in nail tissue. *J Invest Dermatol* 2004;122:965–970.

91. O'Keefe EJ, Hamilton EH, Lee SC, Steiner P. Trichohyalin: A structural protein of hair, tongue, nail and epidermis. *J Invest Dermatol* 1993;101:65s–71s.

92. Rayan GM, Flournoy DJ. Microbiologic flora of human fingernails. *J Hand Surg* 1987;12A:605–607.

93. Dowsett SA, Archila L, Segreto VA, Gonzalez CR, Silva A, Vastola KA, Bartizek RD, Kowolik MJ. *Helicobacter pylori* infection in indiginous families of Central America: Serostatus and oral fingernail carriage. *J Clin Microbiol* 1999;37:2456–2460.

94. Perrin C. Peculiar zone of the distal nail unit: The nail isthmus. *Am J Dermatopathol* 2007;29:108–109.

95. Perrin C. Expression of follicular sheath keratins in the normal nail with special reference to the morphological analysis of the distal nail unit. *Am J Dermatopathol* 2007;29:543–550.

96. Perrin C. The 2 clinical subbands of the distal nail unit and the nail isthmus. Anatomical explanation and new physiological observations in relation to the nail growth. *Am J Dermatopathol* 2008;30:216–221.

97. Germann H, Barran W, Plewig G. Morphology of corneocytes from human nail plates. *J Invest Dermatol* 1980;74:115–118.

98. Apolinar E, Rowe WF. Examination of human fingernail ridges by means of polarized light. *J Forens Sci CA* 1980;25:154–161.

99. Heikkilä H, Stubb S, Kiistala U. Nail growth measurement employing nail indentation: An experimental follow-up study of nail growth in situ. *Clin Exp Dermatol* 1996;121:96–99.

100. de Berker D. Nail growth measurement by indentation. *Clin Exp Dermatol* 1997;22:109.

101. Finlay AY, Moseley H, Duggan TC. Ultrasound transmission time: An in vivo guide to nail thickness. *Br J Dermatol* 1987;117:765–770.

102. Jemec GBE, Serup J. Ultrasound structure of the human nail plate. *Arch Dermatol* 1989;125:643–646.

103. Forslind B, Wroblewski R, Afzelius BA. Calcium and sulfur location in human nail. *J Invest Dermatol* 1976;67:273–275.

104. Jarrett A, Spearman JIC. The histochemistry of the human nail. *Arch Dermatol* 1966;94:652–657.

105. Garson C, Baltenneck F, Leroy F, Riekel C, Muller M. Histological structure of human nail as studied by synchrotron X-ray microdiffraction. *Cell Mol Biol (Noisy-le-grand)* 2000;46:1025–1034.

106. Forslind B, Thyresson N. On the structure of the normal nail. A scanning electron microscope study. *Arch Dermatol Forsch* 1975;251:199–204.

107. Dawber RPR. The ultrastructure and growth of human nails. *Arch Dermatol Res* 1980;269:197–204.

108. Meyer JC, Grundmann HP. Scanning electron microscopic investigation of the healthy nail and its surrounding tissue. *J Cutan Pathol* 1984;11:74–79.

109. Arnn Y, Stoehelin IA. The structure and function of spot desmosomes. *Int J Dermatol* 1981;20:331–339.

110. Bengtsson CF, Olsen ME, Brandt LØ, Bertelsen MF, Willerslev E, Tobin DJ, Wilson AS, Gilber MT. DNA from keratinous tissue, Part I: Hair and nail. *Ann Anat* 2010;194:17–25.

111. Stern DK, Creasey AA, Quijije J, Lebwohl MG. UV-A and UV-B penetration of normal human cadaveric fingernail plate. *Arch Dermatol* 2011;147:439–441.

112. Reardon CM, McArthur PA, Survana SK, Brotherston TM. The surface anatomy of the germinal matrix of the nail bed in the finger. *J Hand Surg [Br]* 1999;24:531–533.

113. Ito T, Ito N, Saathoff M, Stampachiacchiere B, Bettermann A, Bulfone-Paus S, Takigawa M, Nickoloff B, Paus R. Immunology of the human nail apparatus: The nail matrix is a site of relative immune privilege. *J Invest Dermatol* 2005;125:1139–1148.

114. Tosti A, Piraccini BM. Biology of nails. In: Freedberg IM, Eisen AZ, Wolff K, Frank Austen K, Goldsmith LA, Stephen K, eds. *Fitspatrick's Dermatology in General Medicine*, New York: McGraw-Hill, 2003; 159–183.

115. Dorschner RA, Lopez-Garcia B, Massie J, Kim C, Gallo RL. Innate immune defense of the nail unit by antimicrobial peptides. *J Am Acad Dermatol* 2004;50:343–348.

116. Head JR, Billingham RE. Immunologically privileged sites in transplantation immunology and oncology. *Perspect Biol Med* 1985;29:115–131.

117. Streilein JW. Immune privilege as the result of local tissue barriers and immunosuppressive microenvironments. *Curr Opin Immunol* 1993;5:428–432.

118. Streilein JW. Ocular immune privilege: Therapeutic opportunities from an experiment of nature. *Nat Rev Immunol* 2003;3:879–889.

119. Mellor AL, Munn DH. Immunology at the maternal-fetal interface: Lessons for T cell tolerance and suppression. *Annu Rev Immunol* 2000;18:367–391.

120. Erlebacher A. Why isn't the fetus rejected? *Curr Opin Immunol* 2001;13:590–593.

121. Niederkorn JY. Mechanisms of immune privilege in the eye and hair follicle. *J Investig Dermatol Symp Proc* 2002;8:168–172.

122. Paus R, Peker S. Biology of hair and nail. In Bolognia JL, Jorizzo JL, Rapini RP, eds. *Dermatology*, London: Mosby, 2003; 1007–1032.

123. Paus R, Ito N, Takigawa M, Ito T. The hair follicle and immune privilege. *J Invest Dermatol Symp Proc* 2003;8:188–194.

124. Paus R, Nickoloff BJ, Ito T. A "hairy" privilege. *Trends Immunol* 2005;26:32–40.

125. Chuong CM, Noveen A. Phenotypic determination of epithelial appendages: Genes, developmental pathways, and evolution. *J Invest Dermatol Symp Proc* 1999;4:307–311.

126. Wu P, Hou L, Plikus M, Hughes M, Scehnet J, Suksaweang S, Widelitz R, Jiang TX, Chuong CM. Evo-Devo of amniote integuments and appendages. *Int J Dev Biol* 2004;48:249–270.

127. Janeway CA, Travers P, Walport M, Shlomchik M, eds. *Immunobiology*, New York: Garland Publishing, 2001.

128. Bos JD, ed. *Skin Immune System—Cutaneous Immunology and Clinical Immunodermatology*, Boca Raton, FL: CRC Press, 2005; 1–494.

129. Fuzzi B, Rizzo R, Criscuoli L, Noci I, Melchiorri L, Scarselli B, Bencini E, Menicucci A, Baricordi OR. HLA-G expression in early embryos is a fundamental prerequisite for the obtainment of pregnancy. *Eur J Immunol* 2002;32:311–315.

130. Picardo M, Tosti A, Marchese C, Zompetta C, Torrisi MR, Faggioni A, Cameli N. Characterization of cultured nail matrix cells. *J Am Acad Dermatol* 1994;30:434–440.

131. Cameli N, Picardo M, Tosti A, Perrin C, Pisani A, Ortonne JP. Expression of integrins in human nail matrix. *Br J Dermatol* 1994;130:583–588.

132. Baden HP, Kvedar JC. Epithelial cornified envelope precursors are in the hair follicle and nail. *J Invest Dermatol* 1993;101(1 Suppl.):72S–74S.

133. Lavker RM, Risse B, Brown H, Ginsburg D, Pearson J, Baker MS, Jensen PJ. Localisation of plasminogen activator inhibitor type 2 (PAI-2) in hair and nail: Implications for terminal differentiation. *J Invest Dermatol* 1998;110:917–922.

134. Cheng T, van Vlijmens-Willems YMJJ, Hitomi K, Pasch MC, van Erp PEJ, Schalkwijk J, Zeeuwen PLJM. Colocalization of cystatin M/E and its target proteases suggests a role in terminal differentiation of human hair follicle and nail. *Int J Dermatol* 2009;129:1232–1242.

135. Zeeuwen PL, van Vlijmen-Willems IM, Olthuis D, Johansen HT, Hitomi K, Hara-Nishimura I, Powers JC et al. Evidence that unrestricted legumain activity is involved in disturbed epidermal cornification in cystatin M/E deficient mice. *Hum Mol Genet* 2004;13:1069–1079.

136. Rice RH, Crumrine D, Hohl D, Munro CS, Elias PM. Cross-linked envelopes in nail plate in lamellar ichthyosis. *Br J Dermatol* 2003;149:1050–1054.

137. Rice RH, Crumrine D, Uchida Y, Gruber R, Elias PM. Structural changes in epidermal scale and appendages as indicators of defective TGM1 activity. *Arch Dermatol Res* 2005;297:127–133.

138. Higashi N. Melanocytes of nail matrix and nail pigmentation. *Arch Dermatol* 1968;97:570–574.

139. Higashi N, Saito T. Horizontal distribution of the DOPA-positive melanocytes in the nail matrix. *J Invest Dermatol* 1969;53:163–165.

140. Tosti A, Cameli N, Piraccini BM, Fanti PA, Ortonne JP. Characterization of nail melanocytes with anti-PEP1, anti-PEP8, TMH-1, and HMB-45 antibodies. *J Am Acad Dermatol* 1994;31:193–196.

141. De Berker D, Dawber RPR, Thody A, Graham A. Melanocytes are absent from normal nail bed; the basis of a clinical dictum. *Br J Dermatol* 1996;134:564.

142. Perrin C, Michiels JF, Pisani A, Ortonne JP. Anatomic distribution of melanocytes in normal nail unit: An immunohistochemical investigation. *Am J Dermatopathol* 1997;19:462–467.

143. Amin B, Nehal KS, Jungbluth AA, Zaidi B, Brady MS, Coit DC, Zhou Q, Busam KJ. Histologic distinction between subungual lentigo and melanoma. *Am J Surg Pathol* 2008;32:835–843.

144. Theunis A, Richert B, Sass U, Lateur N, Sales F, André J. Immunohistochemical study of 40 cases of longitudinal melanonychia. *Am J Dermatopathol* 2011;33:27–34.

145. Monash S. Normal pigmentation in the nails of Negroes. *Arch Dermatol* 1932;25:876–881.

146. Leyden JJ, Spot DA, Goldsmith H. Diffuse banded melanin pigmentation in nails. *Arch Dermatol* 1972;105:548–550.

147. Kopf AW, Waldo F. Melanonychia striata. *Australas J Dermatol* 1980;21:70.

148. Lacour JP, Dubois D, Pisani A, Ortonne JP. Anatomical mapping of Merkel cells in normal human adult epidermis. *Br J Dermatol* 1991;125:535–542.

149. de Berker D, Wojnarowska F, Sviland L, Westgate GE, Dawber RP, Leigh IM. Keratin expression in the normal nail unit: Markers of regional differentiation. *Br J Dermatol* 2000;142:89–96.

150. Boot PM, Rowden G, Walsh N. The distribution of Merkel cells in human fetal and adult skin. *Am J Dermatopathol* 1992;14:391–396.

151. Smith DO, Oura C, Kimura C, Toshimori K. Artery anatomy and tortuosity of the finger. *J Hand Surg* 1991;16A:297–302.

152. Smith DO, Oura C, Kimura C, Toshimori K. The distal venous anatomy of the finger. *J Hand Surg* 1991;16A:303–307.

153. Chiu DTW. Transthecal digital block: Flexor tendon sheath used for anasthetic infusion. *JU Hand Surg* 1990;15A:471–473.

154. Wallace WA, Coupland RE. Variations in the nerves of the thumb and index finger. *J Bone Joint Surg Br* 1975;57:491–494.

155. Wu JZ, Dong RG, Rakheja S, Schopper AW, Smutz WP. A structural fingertip model for simulating of the biomechanics of tactile sensation. *Med Eng Phys* 2004;26:165–175.

156. Dumontier C. Distal replantation, nail bed, and nail problems in musicians. *Hand Clin* 2003;19: 259–272, vi.

157. Olabanji SO, Ajose OA, Makinde NO, Buoso MC, Ceccato D, De Poli M, Moschini G. Characterization of human fingernail elements using PIXE technique. *Nucl Instr Meth Phys Res* 2005;B240:895–907.

158. Min JZ, Hatanaka S, Yu H-F, Higashi T, Inagaki S, Toyo'oka T. Determination of DL-amino acids, derivatized with $R(-)$-4-(3-isothiocyanatopyrrolidin-1-yl)-7-$(N,N$-dimethylaminosulfonyl)-2,1,3-benzoxadiazole, in nail of diabetic patients by UPLC-ESI-TOF-MS. *J Chromatography B Analyt Technol Biomed Life Sci* 2011;879:3220–3228.

159. Matsumoto T, Sakura N, Ueda K. Steroid sulfatase activity in nails: Screening for X-linked ichthyosis. *Pediatr Dermatol* 1990;7:266–269.

160. Daniel CR 3rd, Piraccini BM, Tosti A. The nail and hair in forensic science. *J Am Acad Dermatol* 2004;50:258–261.

161. Ohno T, Sakamoto M, Kurosawa T, Dakeishi M, Iwata T, Murata K. Total mercury levels in hair, toenail, and urine among women free from occupational exposure and their relations to renal tubular function. *Environm Res* 2007;103:191–197.

162. Reddy K, Lowenstein EJ. Forensics in dermatology. Part II. *J Am Acad Dermatol* 2011;64:811–824.

163. Mandal BK, Ogra Y, Suzuki KT. Speciation of arsenic in human nail and hair from arsenic-affected area by HPLC-inductively coupled argon plasma mass spectrometry. *Toxicology and Applied Pharmacology* 2003;189:73–83.

164. Adair BM, Hudgens EE, Schmitt MT, Calderon RL, Thomas DJ. Total arsenic concentrations in toenails quantified by two techniques provide a useful

biomarker of chronic arsenic exposure in drinking water. *Environmental Research* 2006;101:213–220.

165. Forslind B. X-ray microanalysis in dermatology. *Scan Electron Microsc* 1982;4:1715–1724.

166. Vecht-Hart CM, Bode P, Trouerbach WT, Collette HJA. Calcium and magnesium in human toenails do not reflect bone mineral density. *Clin Chim Acta* 1995;236:1–6.

167. Pillay I, Lyons D, German MJ, Lawson NS, Pollock HM, Saunders J, Chowdhury S, Moran P, Towler MR. The use of fingernails as a means of assessing bone health: A pilot study. *J Womens Health (Larchmt)* 2005;14:339–344.

168. Haneke E. Ketoconazol-Verweildauer in der Haut nach oraler Therapie. *Hautarzt* 1987;38:93–96.

169. Haneke E. Fluconazole levels in human epidermis and blister fluid. *Br J Dermatol* 1990;123:273–274.

170. Allouche M, Hamdoum M, Mangin P, Castella V. Genetic identification of decomposed cadavers using nails as DNA source. *Forens Sci Int Genet* 2008;3:46–49.

171. Fernández-Rodríguez A, Iturralde MJ, Fernández de Simón L, Capilla J, Sancho M. Genetic analysis of fingernail debris: Application to forensic casework. *International Congress Series* 2003;1239:921–924.

172. Nakanishi A, Moriya F, Hashimoto Y. Effects of environmental conditions to which nails are exposed on DNA analysis of them. *Leg Med (Tokyo)* 2003;5(Suppl. 1):S194–S197.

173. Runne U, Orfanos CE. The human nail: Structure, growth and pathological changes. *Curr Probl Dermatol* 1981;9:102–149.

174. Douglas BS. Conservative management of guillotine amputation of the finger in children. *Aust Paediatr J* 1972;8:86–89.

175. Illingworth CM. Trapped fingers and amputated finger tips in children. *J Pediatr Surg* 1974;9:853–858.

176. Das SK, Brown HG. Management of lost finger tips in children. *Hand* 1978;10:16–27.

177. Vidal P, Dickson MG. Regeneration of the distal phalanx. A case report. *J Hand Surg Br* 1993;18:230–233.

178. Rinkevich Y, Maan ZN, Walmsley GG, Sen SK. Injuries to appendage extremities and digit tips: A clinical and cellular update. *Develop Dyn* 215;244:641–650.

179. McKim LH. Regeneration of the distal phalanx. *Can Med Assoc J* 1932;26:549–550.

180. Altizer AM, Stewart SG, Albertson BK, Borgens RB. Skin flaps inhibit both the current of injury at the amputation surface and regeneration of that limb in newts. *J Exp Zool* 2002;293:467–447.

181. Neufeld DA, Zhao W. Phalangeal regrowth in rodents: Postamputational bone regrowth depends upon the level of amputation. *Prog Clin Biol Res* 1993;383A:243–252.

182. Neufeld DA, Zhao W. Bone regrowth after digit tip amputation in mice is equivalent in adults and neonates. *Wound Repair Regen* 1995;3:461–466.

183. Mohammad KS, Day FA, Neufeld DA. Bone growth is induced by nail transplantation in amputated proximal phalanges. *Calcif Tissue Int* 1999;65:408–410.

184. Takeo M, Chou WC, Sun Q, Lee W, Rabbani P, Loomis C, Taketo MM, Ito M. Wnt activation in nail epithelium couples nail growth to digit regeneration. *Nature* 2013;499:228–232.

185. Ide H. Bone pattern formation in mouse limbs after amputation at the forearm level. *Dev Dyn* 2012;241:435–441.

186. Tsonis PA. Stem cells and blastema cells. *Curr Stem Cell Res Ther* 2008;3:53–54.

187. Tamura K, Ohgo S, Yokoyama H. Limb blastema cell: A stem cell for morphological regeneration. *Dev Growth Differ* 2010;52:89–99.

188. Lehoczky JA, Tabin CJ. Lgr6 marks nail stem cells and is required for digit tip regeneration. *PNAS* 2015;12:13249–13254.

189. Stover SL, Hale AM, Buell AB. Skin complications other than pressure ulcers following spinal cord injury. *Arch Phys Med Rehab* 1994;75:987–993.

190. Stover SL, Omura EF, Buell AB. Clinical skin thickening following spinal cord injury studied by histopathology. *J Am Paraplegia Soc* 1994;17:44–49.

191. Braun RP, Baran R, Saurat JH, Thomas L. Surgical Pearl: Dermoscopy of the free edge of the nail to determine the level of nail plate pigmentation and the location of its probable origin in the proximal or distal nail matrix. *J Am Acad Dermatol* 2006;55:512–513.

192. Braun RP, Baran R, Le Gal FA, Dalle S, Ronger S, Pandolfi R, Gaide O et al. Diagnosis and management of nail pigmentations. *J Am Acad Dermatol* 2007;56:835–847.

193. Braun RP, Oliviero M, Kolm I, French LE, Marghoob AA, Rabinovitz H. Dermoscopy: What's new? *Clin Dermatol* 2009;27:26–34.

194. Hirata SH, Yamada S, Almeida FA, Tomomori-Yamashita J, Enokihara MY, Paschoal FM, Enokihara MM, Outi CM, Michalany NS. Dermoscopy of the nail bed and matrix to assess melanonychia striata. *J Am Acad Dermatol* 2005;53:884–886.

195. Hirata SH, Yamada S, Almeida FA, Enokihara MY, Rosa IP, Enokihara MMS, Michalany NS. Dermoscopic examination of the nail bed and matrix. *Int J Dermatol* 2006;45:28–30.

196. Nikkels-Tassoudji N, Piérard-Franchimont C, De Doncker P, Piérard GE. Optical profilometry of nail dystrophies. *Dermatology* 1995;190:301–304.

197. Kaufman SC, Beuerman RW, Greer DL. Confocal microscopy: A new tool for the study of the nail unit. *J Am Acad Dermatol* 1995;32:668–670.

198. Sattler E, Kaestle R, Rothmund G, Welzel J. Confocal laser scanning microscopy, optical coherence tomography and transonychial water loss for in vivo investigation of nails. *Br J Dermatol* 2012;166:740–746.

199. Hongcharu W, Dwyer P, Gonzalez S, Anderson RR. Confirmation of onychomycosis by in vivo confocal microscopy. *J Am Acad Dermatol* 2000;42:214–216.

200. Arrese JE, Quatresooz P, Piérard-Franchimont C, Piérard GE. [Nail histomycology. Protean aspects of a human fungal bed]. *Ann Dermatol Venereol* 2003;130:1254–1259.

201. Gupta AK, Ryder JE, Summerbell RC. Onychomycosis: Classification and diagnosis. *J Drugs Dermatol* 2004;3:51–56.

202. Debarbieux S, Hospod V, Depaepe L, Balme B, Poulalhon N, Thomas L. Perioperative confocal microscopy of the nail matrix in the management of in situ or minimally invasive subungual melanomas. *Br J Dermatol* 2012;167:828–836.

203. Cinotti E, Fouilloux B, Perrot JL, Labelle B, Douchet C, Cambazard F. Confocal microscopy for healthy and pathological nail. *J Eur Acad Dermatol Venereol* 2014;28:853–858.

204. Vogt M, Knuttel A, Hoffmann K, Altmeyer P, Ermert H. Comparison of high frequency ultrasound and optical coherence tomography as modalities for high resolution and non invasive skin imaging. *Biomed Tech (Berl)* 2003;48:116–121.

205. Mogensen M, Thomsen JB, Skovgaard LT, Jemec GBE. Nail thickness measurements using optical coherence tomography and 20-MHz ultrasonography. *Br J Dermatol* 2007;157:894–900.

206. Jemec GB, Serup J. Ultrasound structure of the human nail plate. *Arch Dermatol* 1989;125:643–646.

207. Finlay AY, Western B, Edwards C. Ultrasound velocity in human fingernail and effects of hydration: Validation of in vivo nail thickness measurement techniques. *Br J Dermatol* 1990;123:365–373.

208. Chen SH, Chen YL, Cheng MH, Yeow KM, Chen HC, Wei FC. The use of ultrasonography in preoperative localization of digital glomus tumors. *Plast Reconstr Surg* 2003;112:115–119.

209. Jemec G. Measurement of nail thickness. In: Serup J, Jemec J, Grove G, eds. *Handbook of Non-Invasive Methods and the Skin*, 2nd edn. Boca Raton, FL: CRC Press, 2006; 923–925.

210. de Berker D. Methods for nail assessment: An overview. In: Serup J, Jemec J, Grove G, eds. *Handbook of Non-Invasive Methods and the Skin*, 2nd edn. Boca Raton, FL: CRC Press, 2006; 911–918.

211. Wollina U, Berger M, Karte K. Calculation of nail plate and nail matrix parameters by 20 MHz ultrasound in healthy volunteers and patients with skin disease. *Skin Res Technol* 2001;7:60–64.

212. Wortsman X, Jemec GB. Ultrasound imaging of nails. *Dermatol Clin* 2006;24:323–328.

213. Gutierrez M, Wortsman X, Filippucci E, De Angelis R, Filosa G, Grassi W. High-frequency sonography in the evaluation of psoriasis. Nail and skin involvement. *J Ultrasound Med* 2009;28:1569–1574.

214. Drapé JL, Wolfram-Gabel W, Idy-Peretti I, Baran R, Goettmann S, Sick H, Guerin-Surville H, Bittoun J. The lunula: A magnetic resonance imaining approach to the subnail matrix area. *J Invest Dermatol* 1996;106:1081–1085.

215. Drapé JL, Chevrolet A, Bittoun J. Ungual and subungual disease. In: Guglielmi G, Van Kuijk C, Genant HK, eds. *Fundamentals of Hand and Wrist Imaging*. Berlin: Springer, 2001; 481–505.

216. Soscia E, Scarpa R, Cimmino MA, Atteno M, Peluso R, Sirignano C, Costa L et al. Magnetic resonance imaging of nail unit in psoriatic arthritis. *J Rheumatol* 2009;36(Suppl. 83):42–45.

217. Goettmann S, Drapé JL, Baran R, Perrin C, Haneke E, Bélaïch S. Onychomatricome: Deux nouveaux cas, intérêt de la résonance magnétique. *Ann Dermatol Vénéréol* 1994;121(Suppl.):S145.

218. Goettmann S, Drapé JL, Idy-Peretti I, Bittoun J, Thelen P, Arrive L, Bélaïch S. Magnetic resonance imaging: A new tool in the diagnosis of tumours of the nail apparatus. *Br J Dermatol* 1994;130:701–710.

219. Baran R, Haneke E, Drapé J-L, Zook EG. Tumours of the nail apparatus and adjacent tissues. In Baran R, Dawber RPR, de Berker DAR, Haneke E, Tosti A, eds. *Baran and Dawber's Diseases of the Nails and Their Management*, 3rd edn. Oxford: Blackwell, 2001; 515–630.

220. Richert B, Baghaie M. Medical imaging and MRI in nail disorders: Report of 119 cases and review of the literature. *Dermatol Ther* 2002;15:159–164.

221. Langner I, Krüger P-C, Evert K, Zach A, Hadlich S, Ekkernkamp A, Eisenschenk A, Hosten A, Langner S. MR microscopy of the human finger and correlation with histology—A proof-of-principle study. *Clin Anat* 2013;26:719–727.

222. James VJ. Fiber diffraction of skin and nails provides an accurate diagnosis of malignancies. *Int J Cancer* 2009;125:133–138.

Technical aspects

Nail biopsies, handling, processing, sectioning, staining, and reading the slides

2

In order to be able to read a nail biopsy slide correctly, a good specimen of nail tissue has to be obtained. It has to be large enough to allow processing of the tissue, proper orientation, embedding, and cutting to finally yield sections of the site needed to make the diagnosis. This is not always easy to achieve. The proximal nail fold or nail plate covers the very lesion preventing its direct observation. It is therefore of paramount importance to estimate where the pathological lesion is indeed located within the nail apparatus. Here, at the origin of the nail change, has the biopsy to be taken. There is a general rule that longitudinal streaks of whatever color when visible in the lunula and growing to the free margin of the nail come from the matrix. Surface changes of the nail plate must originate from the most proximal or apical matrix. In contrast, nail bed lesions will not be incorporated into the nail and will not grow with the nail plate or only extremely slowly (Figure 2.1).

Examining the nail with margin-on dermatoscopy sometimes shows pigment in the lower or upper layer of the nail plate; this is more clearly seen in histopathology with adequate pigment stains. Pigment in the upper layer must origin from the most proximal matrix, that in the middle layer in the middle portion of the matrix, and pigment in the deep layer of the plate in the distal matrix (Figure 2.1).

2.1 BIOPSY TECHNIQUES

A variety of different nail biopsy techniques has been described, most of which are useful for certain purposes (Figure 2.2).[1-5]

2.1.1 Nail plate biopsy

Nail plate biopsy is in fact clipping of as much of the altered nail as possible **with** its adjacent subungual keratosis and debris. This is easy when the distal lateral nail plate is involved and onycholytic. When the central distal portion is needed, a V-shaped piece of nail may be clipped off with either a straight or a slightly curved nail clipper. This material can directly be sent to the histopathology lab without fixation, as the keratin does not virtually decompose (see Section 2.3). The main indications for nail plate biopsy are onychomycoses and their differentiation from nail psoriasis.[6-10] However, also melanin and sometimes intraungual melanocytes as a sign of a subungual melanoma, blood inclusions, and bacterial biofilms as well as nail cosmetics can be seen.[11] Nail clippings are also sufficient to make the diagnosis of onychomatricoma.[12] It is important that at least 2–3 mm of nail clipping be available as too small a nail piece may not be enough for processing and cutting it.

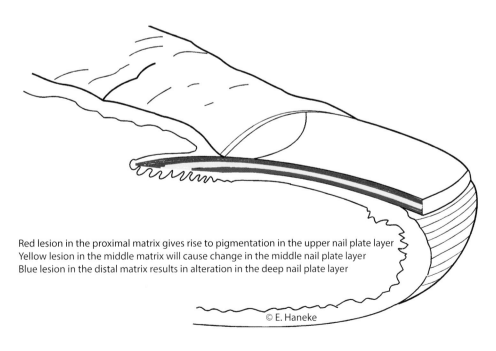

Red lesion in the proximal matrix gives rise to pigmentation in the upper nail plate layer
Yellow lesion in the middle matrix will cause change in the middle nail plate layer
Blue lesion in the distal matrix results in alteration in the deep nail plate layer

© E. Haneke

Figure 2.1 Schematic illustration of the origin of pigmentation in the nail.

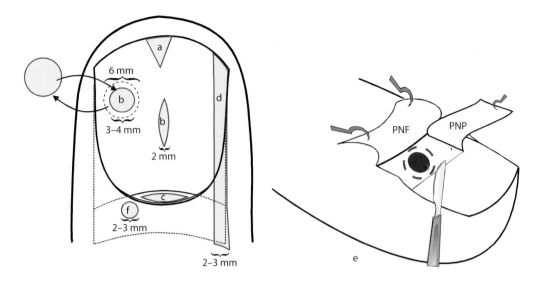

Figure 2.2 Nail biopsy techniques. (a) Nail clipping. (b) Nail bed biopsies: punch, longitudinal fusiform. (c) Matrix biopsy: transverse fusiform. (d) Lateral longitudinal nail biopsy. (e) Tangential matrix and nail bed biopsy. (f) Biopsy of the proximal nail fold. PNF, proximal nail fold; PNP, proximal nail plate.

2.1.2 Biopsy of subungual material

Occasionally, there is plenty of subungual keratotic debris loosely covered by an onycholytic nail. This debris may be cut tangentially with a #15 scalpel blade and submitted for histopathologic examination, again without fixation. It allows the differential diagnosis of onychomycosis and nail psoriasis to be made.[13]

2.1.3 Punch biopsy

Punch biopsies may be taken for different reasons: Small biopsy of the nail bed or matrix or of the nail plate in more proximal location, for example, when a proximal subungual white onychomycosis is suspected.

For matrix biopsies, the punch should not have a diameter wider than 3 mm in order to prevent a post-biopsy split nail deformity.[14] However, even a 3-mm punch may result in a split nail.[15] For the nail bed, the punch may be 4 mm in diameter. For the diagnosis of an onychomycosis, a wider punch of the nail plate is possible.

The nail is very hard and a punch is difficult to run through the nail. The plate should therefore be softened by a 10-min warm hand- or footbath, which allows about 18% water to be taken up by the nail rendering it considerably softer.

A matrix punch biopsy is performed by firmly pressing the punch onto the nail and rotating it clockwise and counterclockwise until one feels that the plate has been cut. The soft tissue is easily cut down to the bone. The punch is withdrawn usually showing the surface of the matrix, as the small disc of nail plate will be stuck in the punch. It can be taken out by a small injection needle, the tip of which has been bent approximately 90–100°. The soft tissue cylinder is cut from the bone with sharp-tipped curved iris scissors without squeezing the tissue with a forceps. No suture is necessary. When the nail plate is deemed unnecessary for the histopathologic diagnosis it is laid back as it gives the best physiologic dressing for the matrix. There

may, however, be one problem: When the lesion to be biopsied is proximal to the visible lunula, the proximal nail fold has to be incised on both sides, separated from the underlying nail plate, and reflected. After the biopsy, it is sutured back in place. The proximal portion of the nail plate may be separated from the nail matrix to allow the lesion to be visualized prior to the biopsy.

A nail bed punch biopsy is made in an analogous way. Care has to be taken as the nail plate is even harder here than over the matrix.

In order to facilitate removal of the soft tissue, a 6-mm punch may be taken from the nail plate. This nail disc is taken apart and then a 4-mm punch is taken from the nail bed.[16] The larger nail disc is put back as a dressing. Simple pressure or a collagen foam is sufficient for hemostasis.[17]

The tissue cylinders are fixed as usual in 4% formalin solution or an alternative (see Section 2.3).

2.1.4 Fusiform biopsy of the nail bed

Due to the unique longitudinal structure of the nail bed rete ridges (see Chapter 1), nail bed biopsies should be oriented longitudinally. The nail plate is difficult to cut together with the nail bed soft tissue and is therefore usually avulsed; however, care has to be taken not to tear the nail bed epithelium off its dermis. Alternatively, one may try to cut the spindle together with the overlying nail plate after having softened it with a 10-min lukewarm bath. The spindle can be very narrow, but should be long enough to deliver a representative piece of tissue. Whether the wound is sutured depends on the width of the biopsy. In case two or three stitches are necessary, the adjacent attached nail is separated from the nail bed epithelium, the nail bed dermis dissected from the bone to mobilize it, and then it is sutured.

It is important to indicate that all fusiform and crescentic nail biopsies have to be cut longitudinally in the laboratory.

2.1.5 Fusiform and crescentic biopsy of the matrix

Matrix biopsies should not be performed as a longitudinal, but always as a transversely arranged spindle or crescent. Usually, the overlying proximal nail fold is detached from the underlying nail, incised on both sides to allow it to be reflected, and the biopsy is performed. It is done as a very narrow one through the nail as this is very soft under the proximal nail fold. A defect of less than 2 mm width does not require a suture; a wider defect is stitched with 6-0 or 7-0 absorbable sutures after gentle undermining of the matrix in both proximal and distal direction. Care has to be taken not to tie the stitches too tight as they may cut through the fragile matrix. The proximal nail fold is laid back and fixed with two stitches or suture strips (e.g., Steristrips®).

2.1.6 Lateral longitudinal nail biopsy

The lateral longitudinal nail biopsy is the biopsy that provides the most information of the nail pathology. It is carried out starting at the distal dorsal crease of the distal interphalangeal joint and carried straight through the proximal nail fold, all along the lateral nail plate to the hyponychium; the second incision starts again at the distal dorsal crease and runs straight through the proximal nail fold and in the depth of the lateral sulcus to the hyponychium. The proximal incision ends are slightly slanted laterally in order not to leave remnants of the lateral matrix horn. The entire longitudinal tissue block is then gently dissected from the bone with fine pointed curved scissors and transmitted into the fixative. The defect is closed with 5-0 sutures that run through the proximal nail fold and do not take the matrix; in the nail bed region, backstitches may be performed that raise and recreate the lateral fold.[18]

2.1.7 Median longitudinal biopsy

The median longitudinal nail biopsy is performed analogous to the lateral one;[19,20] however, we do not recommend it because it leaves a longitudinal scar in the matrix, over which no nail is formed and therefore a split nail may result. Whether matrix flap techniques are of real advantage[21] remains to be seen.

2.1.8 Oblique nail biopsy

An obliquely oriented longitudinal nail biopsy has been described. It is said to combine the advantages of the median and lateral longitudinal nail biopsy without the risk of a split nail.[22]

2.1.9 Tangential (horizontal) matrix biopsy ("matrix shave biopsy")

The systematic examination of many cases of longitudinal melanonychia has shown that most cases are due to melanocyte activation, a lentigo or a junctional nevus; both compound nevi as well as in situ and early invasive melanomas are rare.[23–27] This is particularly the case in children.[28,29] We have therefore developed a tangential biopsy and excision technique that allows large superficial matrix and nail bed lesions to be excised without the risk of postoperative nail dystrophy.[30–33] Many authors have now successfully applied this technique.[34–36] The specimens are thick enough to contain the entire matrix and nail bed epithelium as well as about 5–8 times more of the superficial dermis.[30,37] Tangential excisions are thus therapeutic for benign lesions, but deeper excisions are favored for in situ melanoma and early invasive melanomas (see Chapter 15 for controversies).[38]

The horizontal biopsy is indicated for superficial lesions of the matrix and nail bed. It is technically not very demanding when the lesion is not too big and in median location, but may be difficult in case (almost) the entire matrix has to be superficially removed. The origin of the melanonychia, erythronychia, or longitudinal leukonychia is followed and when under the proximal nail fold, this is incised on both sides, separated from the underlying nail plate and reflected to permit visualization of the entire lesion through the nail. In case of a melanonychia, the nail plate is gently separated from the underlying matrix until about one-third of the plate is freed. It is then cut from one side to allow the proximal third to be lifted like a trap door now exhibiting the melanocyte focus. A shallow incision is carried around it with an adequate safety margin. A #15 scalpel blade, preferably a coated one, is placed on the adjacent matrix and gently pressed on it, slightly bulging the neighboring lesion. With sawing motions, the lesion is cut tangentially from the underlying dermis. The specimen is just so thick as to allow the scalpel blade to be seen shining through. This surgical specimen is transferred upside down to wet gauze, spread out, and from here to a piece of filter paper where it usually remains stuck on. It may be put between another piece of paper or cardboard to keep it spread out without folds.[39] It is transferred to the fixative jar and fixed within 1 to 2 hours. When it is left on the paper it remains perfectly spread out yielding an excellent histological specimen.[36,40]

Re-excision of the nail organ after complete tangential matrix excision has shown that the matrix fully recovers and a normal nail can grow again.

2.1.10 Biopsy of the proximal nail fold

The proximal nail fold may be involved in collagen vascular diseases, some tumors and systemic diseases, such as multicentric reticulohistiocytosis.

For very superficial lesions, a razor blade can be used to yield the epidermis with a bit of the most superficial dermis.[41,42]

A 2-mm punch may be used to perform a full-thickness biopsy of the nail fold down to the underlying nail plate.[16] The free margin of the proximal nail fold should remain intact with this technique.

When the free margin of the nail fold is involved, a narrow wedge may be cut with its base toward the cuticle. After freeing both sides from the underlying nail, primary suture is usually possible. If the defect is larger, for example, after tumor removal, relaxing incisions on both sides allow the two narrow flaps to be brought together and

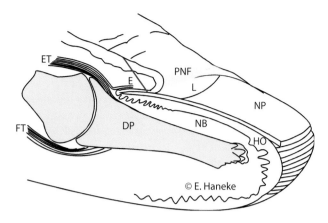

Figure 2.3 Diagnostic and therapeutic biopsy of a chronic paronychia. DP distal phalangeal bone, E eponychium, ET extensor tendon, FT flexor tendon, HO hyponychium, L lunula, NB nail bed, NP nail plate, PNF proximal nail fold.

sutured. The secondary defects heal very fast by second-intention healing.[43]

A thickened proximal nail fold may be partially removed by a beveled excision (Figure 2.3).[44–46]

2.2 BIOPSY HANDLING

Nail biopsies are fragile and require careful handling. The specimen should immediately be transferred into the fixative and not allowed to dry out. If the nail plate and the soft tissue are not in one piece they are submitted in two different jars in order to be mounted on different slides. If they come in one jar, they risk being mounted on the same slide and in case deeper sections are needed tissue of both pieces will be sacrificed.[34]

A drawing of the nail apparatus with marking the biopsy site and how the specimen should be sectioned is very useful both for the dermatopathologist as well as the clinician (Figure 2.4).

2.3 FIXATION

Nail clippings and subungual hyperkeratosis do not require fixation. Formalin fixation is known to increase nail hardness and makes cutting even more difficult. However, if there is microbial contamination, formalin fixation may

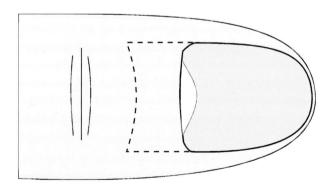

Figure 2.4 Pattern to submit a nail biopsy or excision specimen.

be done after sectioning and deparaffination. The mounted and deparaffinized sections are dipped into 4% buffered formalin for about 30 sec, washed again and then stained.

Biopsies of the soft tissue of the nail apparatus without nail plate are fixed as usual in formalin.

Nail biopsies containing both nail plate and soft tissue are more difficult to process in the laboratory. Many different techniques have been proposed to soften the nail plate without destroying the soft tissue or the elements contained in the nail.

2.4 SOFTENING OF THE NAIL

Older techniques of processing nail specimens used a mixture of potassium bichromate, sodium sulfate, and water to make the nail softer, then decalcification with nitric acid and collodium embedding; however, the nail contains extremely little calcium so the method is entirely empirical.

A mixture of 5% trichloroacetic acid and 10% formalin* for the first 24 h followed by embedding in a mixture of polyethylene glycol and pyroxylin, then cutting 4-μ sections was proposed to preserve the histological details of the nail plate.[47]

Another method is to keep the nail fragment in 10% potassium thioglycollate for 5 days or in 20%–30% hydrogen peroxide for 5–6 days, boiling it in formalin for 1 min and then cutting 10–15 μ thick sections.[48]

An alternative is to soak the nail clippings in 10%–20% urea solution for 24 h before embedding.[49] Phenol 3% is also a good fixative and is said not to harden the nail as formalin.

Fixation in a mixture of mercuric chloride, chromic acid, nitric acid, and 95% alcohol for 2 days and then dehydrating the nail clippings in absolute alcohol before transferring them to xylene and finally embedding them in paraffin is another alternative.[50]

Nail biopsies containing nail plate and soft tissue do not withstand harsh treatment. Soaking the biopsy in distilled water for some hours before formalin fixation was said to make the nail softer.[51] Another option is to cut the block and apply thioglycollate or 10% hydrogen peroxide to the cut surface every two or three sections. Also 1% aqueous polysorbate 40 solution was applied on the cut surface of the block for 1 h at 4°C.[52]

Of all the described techniques, cedarwood oil treatment appears the best to soften the nail. The nail specimen is placed in formalin, transported to the laboratory, immersed in cedar oil for 3 days, rinsed with water, and deposited in a cassette with formalin for 2 h. The nail is processed as usual, cut with a microtome, and stained with hematoxylin and eosin, PAS, or other stains. Cedar oil softens the nail plate, thereby enabling the microtome to cut the tissue "like butter."[53] Cedar oil was originally used as a clearing agent before the introduction of xylene and can be easily ordered.[54]

Comparing the different methods, we found cedarwood oil to be by far the best and the most reliable. It can also

---

* There is often some confusion between 4% and 10% formalin: Those who use "4% formalin" mean its absolute concentration whereas those saying "10% formalin" use a 10% solution of the 40% formaldehyde stock solution. Thus, the formaldehyde concentration is the same.

be used for nail biopsies with soft tissue. There is virtually no shatter, and the nail and the soft tissue are apparently cut with the same ease so that in many cases even the artificial split between the basal compartment and the superficial compartment of the matrix with the adherent nail is avoided. Fixation with 3% phenol makes the nail also better sectionable, but not to the degree of cedar oil treatment, and the entire material stains more eosinophilic. The method used in many laboratories of "decalcification" and treating the nail piece like bone does not really improve the quality of nail biopsy specimens. It remains to be demonstrated whether the cedar oil softening technique is applicable for all special stains and immunohistochemistry reactions.

2.5 MOUNTING NAIL SECTIONS

Whereas sections of nail biopsies with soft tissue adhere to the glass slide, those of the nail plate alone tend to curl and detach when they dry. The use of pretreated slides is often necessary. The slide may be covered with a very thin layer of gelatin or with 3-aminopropyltriethoxysilane. The latter does not stain itself, whereas gelatin may give a certain hue to the slide.

2.6 STAINING

Hematoxylin and eosin (H&E) staining is adequate in most instances (Figure 2.5). Special stains should be indicated whenever anticipated by the clinician/surgeon performing the biopsy although this is usually done in the laboratory. Toluidine blue was claimed to allow better observation of nail plate details.[55,56] PAS is the preferred routine stain for the detection of fungi although Grocott silver methene amine (Gomori) was claimed to be superior, which was, however, disputed.[9,57,58] Because of the glycoproteins in plasma, PAS stains serum inclusions, which may be a source of error when they are very small. Fluorescence microscopy using blancophore is also feasible as it exclusively stains the fungal cell wall.[46] Fontana-Masson's argentaffin reaction demonstrates melanin granules.

Blood is stained with a peroxidase reaction; as there are no macrophages to form hemosiderin in subungual hematomas the Prussian blue and Perls stain remain negative.[44,59,60] Patent blue is an alternative to stain blood in the nail and keratin.[61] However, blood is easily demonstrated by the peroxidase/pseudocatalase reaction: A tiny amount of the dried blood is collected in a small test tube, a few drops of distilled water are added, stirred, and left for a few minutes. A commercial hemostix or hemoccult test stripe as is used for the demonstration of blood in urine or feces is then dipped into the test tube. Even a few erythrocytes cause the characteristic color change.[62–64] Giemsa demonstrates slight changes in the physico-chemical behavior of the nail plate. Polarization microscopy shows the regular arrangement of the keratin fibers in the nail plate and the three layers of the plate,[65] but also in the matrix. Loss of birefringence is seen in leukonychia. Immunofluorescence and immunohistochemical methods are employed for research and the diagnosis of immunodermatoses as well as specific infiltrates and many tumors.[66–68]

2.7 READING OF NAIL SLIDES

There are no principal differences between reading a nail slide or another skin slide. However, it may be of importance in longitudinal nail sections to know in which direction the nail grows and it is important to note which specific region of the nail apparatus—matrix, nail bed, nail fold, hyponychium—is being observed as there are fundamental differences between the various nail parts and their reactions to pathogenic stimuli (Figure 2.6).

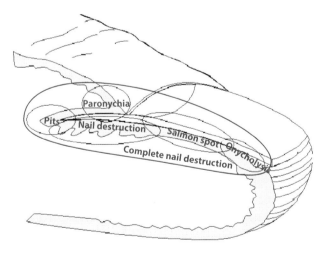

Figure 2.6 The nail structure involved determines the clinical and histological alterations as exemplified in a schematic illustration of nail psoriasis: Pits are caused when the apical matrix is affected, paronychia is the result of psoriasis of the proximal nail fold, extensive matrix involvement leads to nail destruction, nail bed affection causes salmon (oil) spots, and psoriasis of the distal nail bed and hyponychium results in onycholysis. Similarly, involvement of the different nail structures in lichen planus and some other dermatoses will cause analogous changes.

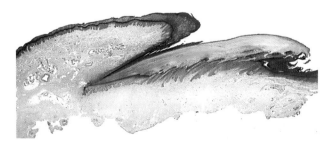

Figure 2.5 Hematoxylin and eosin stained lateral longitudinal nail biopsy. All components of the nail apparatus are shown: proximal nail fold with some eccrine sweat glands, pronounced cuticle, true eponychium as the eosinophilic layer directly on the nail plate reaching until the free end of the cuticle, nail plate, matrix, a slightly papillomatous and acanthotic nail bed, hyponychium as well as nail bed, and matrix dermis without fat.

Table 2.1 Differences in the reactions of skin and nails to a variety of stimuli

	Skin	Nail
Irritation	Parakeratosis	Granular layer and hyperorthokeratosis with onycholysis
Intraepithelial edema	Usually no spongiosis in lichen planus and psoriasis	Often spongiosis in lichen planus and psoriasis
Time course of lesions	Traces of short-living epidermal alterations rapidly shed with the horny layer	Traces of pathologic alterations often included in nail plate or trapped in the subungual keratosis for many months
Pain	Rarely a symptom of skin lesions	May be very pronounced in a number of nail tumors such as glomus tumor, keratoacanthoma, neuroma

The nail apparatus often reacts in a different way from skin (Table 2.1).[69] Irritation that causes parakeratosis in the epidermis often results in the formation of a granular layer and orthokeratin similar to that of epidermis. Conditions that are not characterized by spongiosis in the epidermis, like lichen planus or psoriasis, may be accompanied by spongiosis of the matrix and nail bed. Changes of the nail surface come from the most proximal portion of the matrix, whereas those in the medium layers originate from changes of the intermediate matrix; these alterations tend to grow out with the nail. Nail bed changes are covered by the nail plate and only very slowly move distally.

2.8 NAIL GLOSSARY

There are a number of terms specific to the nails and their pathology. Some of them are often used incorrectly, which may make understanding difficult. What follows is a list of the most important terms used in nail science and pathology.

Anonychia	Lack of nail
Brachyonychia	Disproportionately short (and wide) nail
Chloronychia	Green nail(s)
Clubbing	Swelling of the digital tip with characteristic bidimensional overcurvature and enlargement of the nail; also called hippocratic nail
Dolichonychia	Disproportionately long (and narrow) nail
Elkonyxis	Circumscribed surface defects (bigger than pits)
Erythronychia	Red nail(s)
Hangnail	Small loose skin flap on the nail folds, also called agnail
Hapalonychia	Soft nail (= onychomalacia)
Koilonychia	Spoon nail
Leukonychia	White nail(s)
Melanonychia	Brown to black nail(s)
Nail bed	Structure distal of the matrix that firmly attaches the nail plate to the bone (in the surgical literature also called sterile matrix as it does not produce nail plate substance). Nail bed and matrix *must not* be used interchangeably
Nail matrix	Structure producing the nail plate
Onych-, onycho-	Prefix meaning nail
Onychauxis	Thick(ened) nail
Onychocryptosis	Overgrowing of the nail by (hypertrophic) nail folds
Onychodaknomania	Lustful biting on nails in order to produce pain, psychopathologic behavior
Onychogryphosis	Horn-like thickening of the nail that usually also grows up instead of out (the correct spelling would be onychogryposis as grypos [Greek] means horn and gryphos is a fairy animal)
Onycholysis	Distal detachment of the nail plate from its bed
Onychomadesis	Proximal onycholysis from the matrix
Onychophagia	Chewing of the nails
Onychorrhexis	Longitudinal fissuring of the free nail margin; type of brittle nails
Onychoschizia	Lamellar splitting of the nail; type of brittle nails
Onychoteiromania	Habitual filing or rubbing of the nails leading to nail defects
Onychotemnomania	Habitual cutting of the nail or destroying it with sharp instruments
Onychotillomania	Pulling out (parts of) the nail
Onychotization	Specific form of keratinization of the matrix leading to the formation of nail plate substance
Pachyonychia	Thick nails
Paronychia	Inflammation of the periungual soft tissue, sometimes called perionyxis (mainly in the French literature)
Perionychotillomania	Habit tic of picking and manipulating on the nail folds
Pits	Small depressions in the nail plate surface; most common in psoriasis, but may occur in other nail conditions. Their size is often characteristic for certain conditions

Pterygium	Obstruction of the nail pocket (cul-de-sac)
Pterygium inversum	(Painful) Elongation of the nail bed into the hyponychium
Trachyonychia	Rough nails
Unguis (Latin)	Nail
Unguis incarnatus	Ingrown nail
Xanthonychia	Yellow nail(s)

REFERENCES

1. Baran R, Sayag J. Nail biopsy; where, when, how. *J Dermatol Surg* 1976;2:322–324.
2. André J, Achten G. Techniques de la biopsie unguéale. *Ann Dermatol Vénéréol* 1987;114:889–892.
3. Goettmann S, Grossin M. La biopsie unguéale. *Techniques et indications diagnostiques. Ann Pathol* 1992;12:295–302.
4. Haneke E. Diagnostische Biopsien am Nagelorgan. *Z Hautkr* 1999;74:493–494.
5. Richert B, Di Chiacchio N, Haneke E. *Nail Surgery.* London: Informa Health Care, 2011.
6. Scher RK, Ackerman AB. Subtle clues to diagnosis from biopsies of nails. The value of nail biopsy for demonstrating fungi not demonstrable by microbiologic techniques. *Am J Dermatopathol* 1980;2:55–57.
7. Haneke E. Nail biopsies in onychomycosis. *Mykosen* 1985;28:473–480.
8. Haneke E. Bedeutung der Nagelhistologie für die Diagnostik und Therapie der Onychomykosen. *Ärztl Kosmetol* 1988;18:248–254.
9. Lawry M, Haneke E, Storbeck K, Martin S, Zimmer B, Romano P. Methods for diagnosing onychomycosis: A comparative study and review of the literature. *Arch Dermatol* 2000;136:1112–1126.
10. Baran R, Hay R, Haneke E, Tosti A. *Onychomycosis*, 2nd edn. Oxon: Taylor & Francis, 2006.
11. Kerl H, Trau H, Ackerman AB. Differentiation of melanocytic nevi from malignant melanomas in palms, soles, and nail beds solely by signs in the cornified layer of the epidermis. *Am J Dermatopathol* 1984;(Suppl 6):159–160.
12. Stephen S, Tosti A, Rubin AI. Diagnostic applications of nail clippings. *Dermatol Clin* 2015;33:289–301.
13. Scher RK, Ackerman AB. Subtle clues to diagnosis from biopsies of nails. Histologic differential diagnosis of onychomycosis, psoriasis of the nail unit from cornified cells of the nail bed alone. *Am J Dermatopathol* 1980;2:255–256.
14. Higashi N. On the effect of the matrix and nail bed biopsy on the regeneration of the nail plate (Jap). *Hifu* 1970;12:78–80.
15. Zook EG, Baran R, Haneke E, Dawber RPR, Brauner GJ. Nail surgery and traumatic abnormalities. In: Baran R, Dawber RPR, de Berker DAR, Haneke E, Tosti A, eds. *Baran and Dawber's Diseases of the Nails and their Management*, 3rd edn. Oxford: Blackwell Science, 2001; 437.
16. Siegle RJ, Swanson NA. Nail surgery: A review. *J Dermatol Surg Oncol* 1982;8:659–666.
17. Stone OJ, Bart RJ, Herten RJ. Biopsy of the nail area. *Cutis* 1978;21:257–260.
18. Haneke E. Reconstruction of the lateral nail fold after lateral longitudinal nail biopsy. In: Robins P, ed. *Surgical Gems in Dermatology*. New York, NY: Journal Publ Group, 1988; 91–93.
19. Zaias N. The longitudinal nail biopsy. *J Invest Dermatol* 1967;49:406–408.
20. Scher RK. Longitudinal resection of nails for purposes of biopsy and treatment. *J Dermatol Surg Oncol* 1980;6:805–807.
21. Collins SC, Cordova KB, Jellinek NJ. Midline/paramedian longitudinal matrix excision with flap reconstruction: Alternative surgical techniques for evaluation of longitudinal melanonychia. *J Am Acad Dermatol* 2010;62:627–636.
22. De Berker DR. The oblique nail unit biopsy. *Br J Dermatol* 1994;131(Suppl 44):44–48.
23. Goettmann-Bonvallot S, André J, Belaich S. Longitudinal melanonychia in children: A clinical and histopathologic study of 40 cases. *J Am Acad Dermatol* 1999;41:17–22.
24. Goettmann S. Lésions pigmentées de l'appareil unguéal. *Rev Prat* 2000;50:2246–2250.
25. André J, Goettmann-Bonvallot S. Longitudinal melanonychia. *J Am Acad Dermatol* 2003;49:776.
26. André J, Lateur N. Pigmented nail disorders. *Dermatol Clin* 2006;24:329–339.
27. Theunis A, Richert B, Sass U, Lateur N, Sales F, André J. Immunohistochemical study of 40 cases of longitudinal melanonychia. *Am J Dermatopathol* 2011;33:27–34.
28. Léauté-Labrèze C, Bioulac-Sage P, Taïeb A. Longitudinal melanonychia in children. A study of eight cases. *Arch Dermatol* 1996;132:167–169.
29. Goettmann S. Pathologie unguéale de l'enfant. *Rev Prat* 2000;50:2256–2261.
30. Haneke E. Operative Therapie akraler und subungualer Melanome. In: Rompel R, Petres J, eds. *Operative und onkologische Dermatologie. Fortschritte der operativen und onkologischen Dermatologie*, Berlin: Springer, 1999;15:210–214.
31. Haneke E. Melanonychia longitudinalis und andere braune Nagelpigmentierungen. In: Koller J, Hintner H, eds. *Fortschritte der operativen und onkologischen Dermatologie*. Berlin Wien: Blackwell Wissenschaftsverlag, 2000;16:19–26.

32. Haneke E, Baran R. Longitudinal melanonychia. *Dermatol Surg* 2001;27:580–584.

33. Haneke E. Advanced nail surgery. *J Cutan Aesthet Surg* 2011;4:167–175.

34. Pasch MC, Haneke E, Körver JEM. Shave excisie van de nagelmatrix bij longitudinale melanonychia. *Ned T Dermatol Venereol* 2007;17:10–13.

35. Jellinek NJ. Nail matrix biopsy of longitudinal melanonychia: Diagnostic algorithm including the matrix shave biopsy. *J Am Acad Dermatol* 2007; 56:803–810.

36. Abimelec P. Tips and tricks in nail surgery. *Semin Cutan Med Surg* 2009;28:55–60.

37. Di Chiacchio N, Refkalefsky Loureiro W, Kezam Gabriel FV, Schwery Michalany N. Tangential biopsy thickness versus lesion depth in longitudinal melanonychia—A pilot study. *Dermatol Res Pract* 2012;2012:353864.

38. Duarte AF, Correia O, Barros AM, Azevedo R, Haneke E. Nail matrix melanoma *in situ*: Conservative surgical management. *Dermatology* 2010;220:173–175.

39. Richert B, Theunis A, Norrenberg S, André J. Tangential excision of pigmented nail matrix lesions responsible for longitudinal melanonychia: Evaluation of the technique on a series of 30 patients. *J Am Acad Dermatol* 2013;69:96–104.

40. Reinig E, Rich P, Thompson CT. How to submit a nail specimen. *Dermatol Clin* 2015;33:303–307.

41. Shelley WB. The razor blade in dermatologic practice. *Cutis* 1975;16:843.

42. Grabski WJ, Salasche SJ, Mulvaney MJ. Razor-blade surgery. *J Dermatol Surg Oncol* 1990;16:1121–1126.

43. Haneke E. Cirugía dermatológica de la región ungueal. *Monografías de Dermatología* 1991;4:408–423.

44. Baran R, Bureau H. Surgical treatment of recalcitrant chronic paronychia. *J Dermatol Surg Oncol* 1981;7:106–107.

45. Grover C, Bansal S, Nanda S. En bloc excision of proximal nail fold for treatment of chronic paronychia. *Dermatol Surg* 2006;32:393–399.

46. Haneke E, Richert B, Di Chiacchio N. Surgery of the proximal nail fold. In: Richert B, Di Chiacchio N, Haneke E, eds. *Nail Surgery*. London: Informa Healthcare, 2011;42–54.

47. Alvarez R, Zaias N. A modified polyethylene glycol–pyroxylin embedding method specially suited for nails. *J Invest Dermatol* 1967;49:409–410.

48. Alkiewicz J, Pfister R. *Atlas der der Nagelkrankheiten.* Stuttgart: Schattauer-Verlag, 1976;8.

49. Haneke E. Fungal infections of the nail. *Sem Dermatol* 1991;10:41–53.

50. Suarez, SM, Silvers DN, Scher RK. Histologic evaluation of nail clippings for diagnosing onychomycosis. *Arch Dermatol* 1991;127:1517–1519.

51. Bennett J. Technique of biopsy of nails. *J Dermatol Surg Oncol* 1976;2:325–326.

52. Lewin K, Dewitt S, Lawson R. Softening techniques for nail biopsy. *Arch Dermatol* 1973;107:223–224.

53. Graham J. Pathology of dermatophytosis. Presented at the 10th Combined Skin Pathology Course, Philadelphia, PA, Sept 19, 1995.

54. Grammer-West NY, Corvette DM, Giandoni MB, Fitzpatrick JE. Clinical pearl: Nail plate biopsy for the diagnosis of psoriatic nails. *J Am Acad Dermatol* 1998;38:260–262.

55. Achten G. L'ongle normal et pathologique. *Dermatologica* 1963;126:229–245.

56. Achten G, André J, Laporte M. Nails in light and electron microscopy. *Sem Dermatol* 1991;10:54–64.

57. D'Hue Z, Perkins SM, Billings SD. GMS is superior to PAS for diagnosis of onychomycosis. *J Cutan Pathol* 2008;35:745–747.

58. Barak O, Asarch A, Horn T. PAS is optimal for diagnosing onychomycosis. *J Cutan Pathol* 2010;37: 1038–1040.

59. Achten G, Wanet J. Pathologie der Nägel. In: Doerr W, Seifert G, Uehlinger E, eds. *Spezielle pathologische Anatomie*. Berlin: Springer, 1973;7:487–528.

60. Baran R, Haneke E. Diagnostik und Therapie der streifenförmigen Nagelpigmentierung. *Hautarzt* 1984;35:359–365.

61. Hafner J, Haenseler E, Ossent P, Burg G, Panizzon RG. Benzidine stain for the histochemical detection of hemoglobin in splinter hemorrhage (subungual hematoma) and black heel. *Am J Dermatopathol* 1995;17:362–367.

62. Haneke E, Baran R. Subunguale Tumoren. *Z Hautkr* 1982;57:355–362.

63. Poudyal S, Elpern DJ. Simple diagnostic tests for subungual pigmentation. *Dermatol Pract Res* 2009;2009:278040.

64. Huang Y-H, Ohara K. Medical pearl: Subungual hematoma: A simple and quick method for diagnosis. *J Am Acad Dermatol* 2006;54:877–878.

65. Port E. Das Auftreten von drei Schichten in der Hornsubstanz des Nagels bei der Betrachtung im polarisierten Lichte und ihre Beziehung zur Nagelmatrix. *Z Zellforsch* 1933;19:110–118.

66. Heid HW, Moll I, Franke WW. Patterns of expression of trichocytic and epithelial cytokeratins in mammalian tissues. II. Concomitant and mutually exclusive synthesis of trichocytic and epithelial cytokeratins in diverse human and bovine tissues (hair follicle, nail bed and matrix, lingual papilla, thymic reticulum). *Differentiation* 1988;37:215–230.

67. Barth JH, Wojnarowska F, Millard PR, Dawber RP. Immunofluorescence of the nail bed in pemphigoid. *Am J Dermatopathol* 1987;9:349–350.

68. Parmentier L, Dürr C, Vassella E, Beltraminelli H, Borradori L, Haneke E. Nail alterations in cutaneous T cell lymphoma: Successful treatment of specific nail infiltration with topical mechlorethamine only. *Arch Dermatol* 2010;146:1287–1291.

69. Haneke E. Pathology of inflammatory nail diseases. 7th Int Dermatopathol Coll, Graz, May 23–25, 1986. *Am J Dermatopathol* 1987;9:170.

Inflammatory dermatoses affecting the nail

3

Many inflammatory dermatoses may also involve the nail. Often the skin lesions are obvious and a nail biopsy is not performed. Therefore, the knowledge of specific nail changes in certain inflammatory conditions is sometimes very limited, and it is risky to draw definite conclusions from a few anecdotal descriptions of nail histopathology.

3.1 NAIL PSORIASIS

Psoriasis is the dermatosis with the most frequent nail involvement. About 2% of the population in Central Europe suffers from psoriasis and worldwide 1%–3%. Approximately 50% of psoriatic persons present with nail changes, but during their lifetime, up to 90% will have had nail changes.[1–3] Isolated nail psoriasis is seen in 1%–5%.[4] Nail involvement is more frequent in psoriatic arthritis than in psoriasis vulgaris—80% as opposed to 50% in psoriasis vulgaris.[5] Nail psoriasis is associated with discomfort and even pain in many patients and leads to significant functional impairment and psychological stress. The unsightly appearance of affected nails exerts negative impact on work and social activities. Importantly, 80% of patients with psoriatic arthritis have nail psoriasis. Nevertheless, it is often overlooked or neglected as is evidenced by the lack of inclusion of nail psoriasis into the psoriasis guidelines in many countries. Psoriasis has a strong genetic background, but environmental factors appear to play an important role. However, whereas nail psoriasis is more frequently familiar it is less often positive for the allele Cw*602.[6,7]

The nail organ is an integral part of the functional and sensory fingertip unit.[8,9] It is formed by the nail apparatus itself, all constituents of the distal phalanx, the distal interphalangeal joints with their capsule, tendons, and ligaments. The bone insertions of ligaments and tendons called entheses play an important role for the functional and esthetic integrity of the nail. They have recently been found to be of utmost importance in psoriatic arthritis and nail psoriasis.[10,11] The proximal tip of the matrix is just 0.8 to 1 mm from the bone of the terminal phalanx and also very close to the distal interphalangeal joint.[12,13] The joint capsule is enforced by the flexor and extensor tendons which form the dorsal and volar aponeuroses. They insert mostly at the base of the distal phalanx, but there are also fibers radiating to the more distal dorsal surface of the bone and into the connective tissue of the proximal nail fold.[14] This led some authors to call the nail a musculoskeletal appendage (see Chapter 1).[15,16] These authors believe that the nail involvement in psoriasis is rather a Koebner phenomenon and thus mechanically induced rather than an autoimmune disease. The complex blood supply of the distal joint and nail as well as the anatomic vicinity of matrix and joint are supposed to give an explanation why nail involvement is so frequent in psoriatic arthritis patients.[15] The finding of a mutation in the gene for the interleukin 36 receptor antagonist (IL6RN) leading to a defect in interleukin 36 antagonist (DITRA) in generalized pustular psoriasis and acrodermatitis continua suppurativa supports the assumption of these conditions belonging to the group of autoinflammatory diseases.[17,18]

3.1.1 Clinical features of nail psoriasis

Psoriasis can cause a large variety of nail changes, which may overlap with those caused by other nail disorders. Pits and tiny whitish to ivory spots on the nail plate, salmon or oil spots, onycholysis, subungual hyperkeratosis, nail plate abnormalities, and splinter hemorrhages are the most frequent clinical signs of psoriasis. Pits and spots, leukonychia, nail plate thickening, and destruction as well as red spots in the lunula are signs of matrix involvement whereas salmon spots, subungual hyperkeratosis, onycholysis, and splinter hemorrhages are due to nail bed involvement. Often, both are affected (see Figure 2.6).

3.1.2 Histopathology

The main criteria of cutaneous psoriasis also apply to nail psoriasis; however, there are some differences and some changes not seen in skin elsewhere.[9] Psoriasis may affect any part of the nail.[19]

Pits and whitish to ivory colored spots are due to tiny psoriatic foci in the apical matrix.[1,9] The proximal matrix epithelium develops a slight spongiosis and parakeratosis, but neutrophil exocytosis is rare. Pits are small, mostly superficial depressions that develop from parakeratotic mounds in the surface of the nail plate, which break out when the plate emerges from under the proximal nail fold. When the parakeratosis remains part of the nail plate it is clinically seen as a small whitish to yellowish dot. The parakeratosis fills a shallow saucer-like depression. The more proximal the pit the more parakeratosis is usually still present (Figure 3.1).[20]

A lesion in the middle of the matrix causes a leukonychia.[21,22] This is either due to interspersed parakeratotic cells in the nail plate, then usually also with leukocytes, or to orthokeratosis with an eosinophilic cytoplasm of the onychocytes without leukocytes (Figure 3.2). Red spots in the lunula are very small psoriasis lesions with spongiosis, parakeratosis, and leukocyte exocytosis,[20] but may also be due to dilated tortuous capillaries and suprapapillary plate thinning.[23]

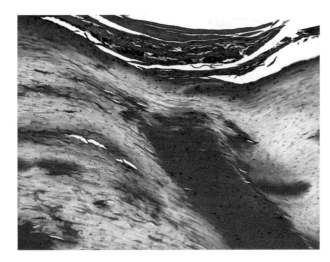

Figure 3.1 Psoriatic pit. This pit is unusual in that it contains neutrophils in the parakeratotic mound.

Salmon spots represent psoriatic spots of the nail bed. The nail bed epithelium develops a spongiosis with mononuclear exocytosis and often a spotty granular layer. There is a moderate to pronounced acanthosis (Figure 3.3). Parakeratosis usually develops and forms columns obliquely ascending distally. Various amounts of leukocytes are usually seen in the form of Munro's microabscesses, often in the summits of the parakeratotic mounds.[24]

Subungual hyperkeratosis is represented by several layers of hyperkeratosis that consists mostly of parakeratosis with interspersed orthokeratosis. Pycnotic neutrophils are arranged in layers. PAS stain very clearly shows the neutrophils and is important for the differential diagnosis of subungual onychomycosis.

Onycholysis is similar to subungual hyperkeratosis. As the overlying nail plate usually shears off a differentiation is commonly impossible. In fact, salmon or oil spots, subungual hyperkeratosis, and onycholysis are due to the same

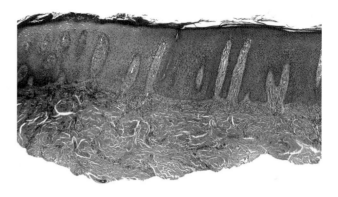

Figure 3.3 Salmon spot. The biopsy does not show the overlying nail plate; thus, it resembles plaque psoriasis of the skin.

fundamental process, a subungual psoriasis lesion, which in the case of onycholysis has reached the hyponychium.

Subungual splinter hemorrhages are seen as small intracorneal blood inclusions at the tip of a subungual keratosis directly under the nail plate.[20]

Psoriasis of the proximal nail fold is identical to chronic psoriasis of the skin elsewhere. The epidermis is acanthotic with club-shaped or rectangular rete ridges and parakeratosis, and there is a lack of the granular layer. Leukocyte exocytosis is sparse. The capillaries are dilated and go high up to the thinned suprapapillary epidermal plate. When the free margin is involved it is rounded up and the cuticle is lost (Figure 3.4). Involvement of the undersurface of the proximal nail fold is commonly associated with slight to moderate spongiosis. When both the dorsal and the ventral surface are affected, the clinical picture of chronic paronychia is seen; this is common in psoriatic arthritis of the distal interphalangeal joint.

A recent study of nail clipping histopathology in psoriasis demonstrated that psoriatic nails have 4.5 layers of subungual corneocytes as compared to normal nails with

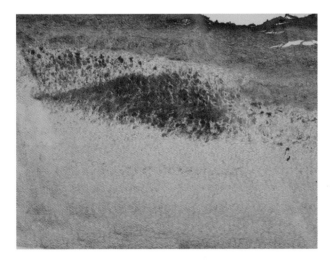

Figure 3.2 Psoriatic leukonychia due to onychocytes displaying an eosinophilic cytoplasm. On top, a shallow pit is seen.

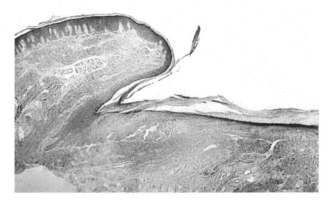

Figure 3.4 Psoriatic paronychia. The proximal nail fold is thickened, its free margin rounded, the cuticle is lacking, the matrix is hyperplastic with columnar orthokeratosis and granular layer, both the matrix and nail bed produce mainly parakeratotic horn.

only 2.4 layers (p = 0.0004). Bacteria, serous lakes, fungi (mostly spores), blood collections, onychokaryosis, and hypereosinophilic nuclear shadows were more frequent in the psoriasis than the control group, but this was not statistically significant.[25]

3.1.2.1 Pustular psoriasis

Nail involvement in pustular psoriasis is very common, both in the localized form of Barber-Königsbeck as well as the generalized form of von Zumbusch. It is the main feature of acrodermatitis continua suppurativa of Hallopeau, once thought to be a different entity but now generally accepted as being a variant of pustular psoriasis with insidious onset and recalcitrant course finally leading to complete nail destruction. Histopathologically, the pustular psoriasis types and Reiter's disease are indistinguishable.

Clinically, palmoplantar pustular psoriasis is characterized by erythematous scaly plaques with variable amounts of scales and pustules. The nails show just a few yellow spots as sign of subungual pustules and the pits are often larger or there are even surface defects called elkonyxis. Generalized pustular psoriasis exhibits many flat yellow pustules of the entire skin including the periungual skin as well as matrix and nail bed. Acrodermatitis continua suppurativa of Hallopeau usually begins as an insidious inflammation of a single finger or toe tip with crusting and pustulation and finally atrophy of the distal phalanx and osteolysis.[26] Young to middle-aged persons, even children, are preferentially affected.[27] One case of acral lentiginous melanoma clinically mimicked acrodermatitis continua suppurativa.[28]

Pustular psoriasis is characterized by the development of large spongiform pustules in the matrix and nail bed, often also in the periungual skin, particularly in acrodermatitis continua suppurativa. These lakes of pus are seen as yellow spots under the nail plate. There is often considerable spongiosis. With time, the nail becomes destroyed and a clinical diagnosis is difficult to be made. When a biopsy is taken at this time, psoriatic alterations are still seen.

Acrodermatitis continua suppurativa has three histological appearances: the classical spongiform pustule, a spongiotic variant, and a mixed form with spongiform pustules and spongiosis. Spongiform pustule formation is very pronounced and leads to necrosis of the superficial layers of the nail bed and matrix epithelium, which may be the reason for the progressive and permanent nail atrophy (Figure 3.5).

Whereas many authors believe that they are the same,[29] in our opinion, palmar plantar pustulosis, also called pustular bacterid of Andrews,[30] is different from palmar plantar psoriasis, both clinically, histologically, as well as immunogenetically.[31–33] Histopathologically, it is not characterized by spongiform pustules but has round to oval, well circumscribed unilocular pustules with sometimes a spongiform shoulder.[34] Nail involvement is very rare.[35,36]

In Reiter's disease, the nail lesions are virtually indistinguishable from pustular psoriasis but there are more extravasated erythrocytes giving the lesions clinically a more brownish aspect, and the pits may be deep.[37] The nail fold may be swollen and red.[38] This is, however, not sufficient to make the differential diagnosis, which requires inspection of the entire skin, mucous membranes including eyes, search for gastrointestinal symptoms, and a series of laboratory abnormalities.

3.1.3 Differential diagnosis

Clinically and histopathologically, a number of diseases have to be considered in the differential diagnosis of nail psoriasis. The acropustuloses and Reiter's disease have already been described in the context of pustular psoriasis.

(a)

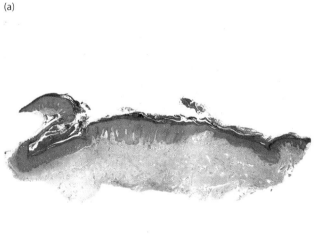

(b)

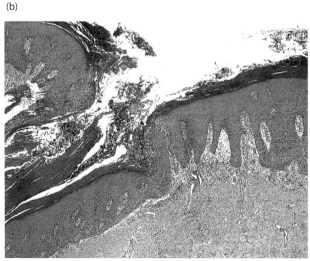

Figure 3.5 Acrodermatitis continua suppurativa of Hallopeau. Lateral longitudinal nail biopsy showing all constituents of the nail apparatus. (a) Scanning magnification. (b) This medium-power magnification shows the matrix and proximal nail bed area with marked spongiform pustule formation. No regular nail plate is formed anymore.

Parakeratosis pustulosa of Hjorth is a rare disease mainly of young girls.[39,40] Pustules are rare and only seen in the beginning. Hyperorthokeratosis, parakeratosis, acanthosis, pustulation, crust formation, mild exocytosis, and a dense perivascular lymphocytic infiltrate are typical signs.[41,42] Dyskeratoses may be observed in the mid-epidermis.[43]

Pityriasis rubra pilaris may be associated with subungual hyperkeratosis, particularly when the palms and soles are affected. Distal subungual hyperkeratosis, splinter hemorrhages, and patchy parakeratosis may occur in the nail plate.[44]

Acrokeratosis paraneoplastica of Bazex is a paraneoplastic dermatosis mainly due to cancers of, and metastases to, the upper aero-digestive tract. The skin of the tips of the digits, of the ears, and of the nose develops a violaceous hue and psoriasiform hyperkeratosis.[45,46] The nails are the first to show alterations with thinning and fragility.[47] Later the nails become flaky, whitened, and develop subungual hyperkeratosis. Finally, the nail may be replaced by epidermis. The histopathological alterations are nonspecific with a lymphocytic perivascular infiltrate in the upper dermis, mild acanthosis, and hyperkeratosis with some parakeratosis.[48]

Crusted (Norwegian) scabies bears some clinical similarity with nail psoriasis. Histologically, there is papillomatosis and marked hyperkeratosis of the distal nail bed and hyponychium with burrows, in which both abundant mites as well as eggs can be seen.[49,50]

Subungual hyperkeratosis is a common consequence of nail overcurvature. The hyperkeratosis is compact, orthokeratotic, and there are no inflammatory changes. Nail clippings with adherent subungual hyperkeratosis show that this is extremely papillomatous. Often, columns of serous lakes are seen in the keratin layers.

Hyponychial dermatitis is a term coined for a condition looking like allergic contact dermatitis, but no patch test is positive. Histology does not show psoriasiform features, but PAS positive serum-like inclusions in the keratotic material.[51]

Psoriasiform acral dermatitis is clinically very similar to psoriasis of the tip of the fingers including the distal nail bed.[52] Onycholysis and finally shortening of the nail bed occur.[53] The cuticles are very long and cover parts of the nail. Histologically, there is marked spongiosis with lymphocytic exocytosis, parakeratosis, and scale formation.[54] No neutrophils are seen in the epithelium and parakeratosis. However, it was also speculated that this condition might be a particular form of acral psoriasis in children.[55] The most recent report proposes to call the condition psoriatic acral dermatitis as the condition is now definitely thought to be a particular variant of acral psoriasis.[56]

Acral psoriasiform hemispherical papulosis is probably just a variant of psoriasis. It is characterized by small erythematous plaques with adherent scales. Histology shows a broad psoriasiform acanthosis with slight spongiosis and marked parakeratosis.[57]

All conditions able to cause *rough nails* or *trachyonychia* have to be included in the differential diagnosis. Eczema and alopecia areata are essentially spongiotic dermatitides. Irritant contact dermatitis may mimic psoriasis or psoriasiform acral dermatitis.[58]

Onychomycosis is by far the most important differential diagnosis, both clinically as well as histologically.[9,59] Distal subungual onychomycosis resembles distal nail bed psoriasis, proximal subungual onychomycosis looks similar to matrix psoriasis, total dystrophic onychomycosis may mimic extensive matrix and nail bed psoriasis.[9] Not only may onychomycosis and nail psoriasis have the clinical signs of onycholysis, subungual hyperkeratosis, nail discoloration, loss of transparency, and pits in common though to a different degree, also the histological signs of hyperkeratosis and collections of neutrophils in the subungual hyperkeratosis are found in both diseases. The problem is confounded by the fact that one may have a secondary fungal colonization of a psoriatic nail and even have a true onychomycosis plus nail psoriasis (Figure 3.6).[60,61] A PAS or Grocott stain will reveal fungi and their

(a)

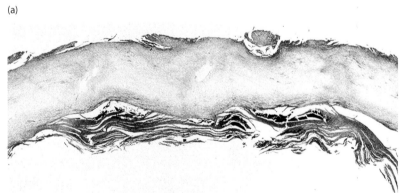

(b)

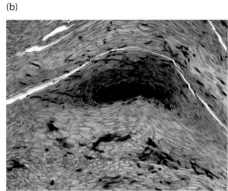

Figure 3.6 Onychomycosis in a psoriatic nail. (a) Scanning magnification of a biopsy of a nail displaying psoriatic features such as pits, subungual columnar parakeratosis, and Munro's microabscesses as well as dermatophytes in the lowermost nail plate layers and subungual keratin. (b) High magnification of a nail biopsy of a patient with nail psoriasis whose other nails had cleared under the treatment with a biological. The PAS stain demonstrates an intraungual Munro's abscess and large masses of fungal elements with variable diameter, culture revealed *Fusarium solani*.

mode of invasion enabling one to differentiate between colonization by a fungus or true infection.[62] Even with the demonstration of fungi in the nail, it may be difficult to rule out ungual psoriasis.

Drug reactions may also look like psoriasis. This has been observed to a variety of different chemical compound classes of which β-blockers are probably the longest known ones. Recently, paradoxical reactions with psoriatic lesions of the nails during treatment with TNF-α blockers, such as infliximab and adalimumab,[63] as well as with the selective inhibitor of T cell costimulation abatacept were observed that were virtually identical to psoriasis of the nails.[64]

3.2 PARAKERATOSIS PUSTULOSA

Parakeratosis pustulosa was first described by Sabouraud in 1931 and again by Hjorth and Thomsen in 1967.[37,38] It is a rare condition and it is still under debate whether it is an entity or a variant of psoriasis or eczema, or distal digital psoriasis in a subject with atopic dermatitis. *Parakeratosis pustulosa* of Hjorth is mainly observed in young girls and the fingers are more often affected than the toes.[38–40] The skin changes start right distal to the nail bed with some small pustules that soon disappear and give way to redness and scaling so that the fingertip looks like chronic eczema. Extension to the dorsal aspect of the distal phalanx is possible. Pustules are no longer seen. Then a marked hyperkeratosis under the free edge of the nail develops, lifting up the nail margin. Sometimes pitting occurs.

3.2.1 Histopathology

The pathological findings resemble more eczema than psoriasis. Hyperorthokeratosis and parakeratosis with marked acanthosis are characteristic. Pustulation is rarely seen as it is present only in the initial phase. A crust containing keratin and serous exudate develops. There is mild to moderate mononuclear exocytosis, and a dense perivascular lymphocytic infiltrate usually fills the papillary dermis.[40,65] Dyskeratoses may be observed in the mid-epidermis.[41]

3.2.2 Differential diagnosis

The most important conditions to be ruled out are nail psoriasis and eczema, but also pustular psoriasis, acrodermatitis continua suppurativa of Hallopeau, contact dermatitis, atopic dermatitis, tinea pedis, paronychia, and dry fissured eczematoid dermatitis.[63]

3.3 PITYRIASIS RUBRA PILARIS

Pityriasis rubra pilaris is a fairly common erythematosquamous skin disorder. It is characterized by follicular keratotic papules, general mild hyperkeratosis, and a particular red color with an orange-yellow hue. It may involve large skin areas and characteristically leaves out islands of normal appearing skin, called nappes claires or Leredde's sign. Palms and soles develop diffuse hyperkeratoses, again with an orange hue, frequently with painful cracking.[66] Five different clinical types were outlined, but without type-specific nail changes although most nail changes were described in type I.[67] The nails develop longitudinal ridging and splinter hemorrhages, lose their shine, and hyperkeratosis of the distal nail bed may lift the nails. Distal yellow-brown discoloration is also seen. Trachyonychia is not a clinical feature of pityriasis rubra pilaris. The clinical differential diagnoses are erythroderma, drug eruption, Sézary's syndrome, and other cutaneous lymphomas with nail changes.

3.3.1 Histopathology

Histopathology of pityriasis rubra pilaris of the nail is not very specific. There is hyperkeratosis of the nail bed containing parakeratotic foci, and a mild inflammatory infiltrate around the vessels of the superficial dermis. Focal hydropic basal cell degeneration was described.[66] Neutrophils are not seen in pityriasis rubra pilaris. The nail plate changes may be explained by matrix involvement with parakeratotic onychotization.

3.3.2 Differential diagnosis

Nail changes in several chronic, particularly erythrodermic disorders are similar.[68] The nail changes are clearly different from those of ungual psoriasis; however, old lesions may be extremely difficult to differentiate.

3.4 ECZEMA

Eczema is commonly divided into contact dermatitis, nummular eczema, seborrheic dermatitis, and atopic eczema. In many countries, the terms eczema and dermatitis are used synonymously. Contact eczema can be divided into allergic and nonallergic (toxic/traumiterative) contact eczema.

Allergic contact dermatitis (eczema): Whereas allergic and nonallergic contact dermatitides are common diseases of the hands, they are less common on the feet, and occur much less frequently in the nail unit. Most allergic contact dermatitis cases involve the proximal nail fold. However, toluene sulfonamide/formaldehyde resin, nail hardeners,[69] cyanoacrylate glue,[70,71] acrylic nails,[72,73] and some other substances[74] may cause allergic contact dermatitis of the nail bed and matrix,[75,76] and they are also often responsible for ectopic allergic dermatitis of the eyelids[77] and neck. Chronic contact eczema with nail involvement is seen in housewives, tulip growers, and many other professions, but may also be due to sculptured nails. Some authors claim that chronic and chronic relapsing paronychia, particularly in housewives, chefs, and other people handling food have to be seen as a particular type of allergic contact dermatitis, mainly of the immediate type.[78] Nail pitting leading to trachyonychia is often a feature of nail eczema.[79] Subungual allergic eczema causes subungual hyperkeratosis and onycholysis.[71]

Nonallergic or irritant contact dermatitis is often due to harsh environmental factors such as repeated maceration and dehydration of the skin, to alkaline substances, detergents, mineral oils, but also to mechanical strain and chronic friction. It is mainly observed on the finger pulps and nail folds, but nailbed affection with onycholysis and subungual hyperkeratosis is also seen.[80]

Nummular eczema may be seen on the proximal nail fold.

Seborrheic dermatitis does not occur in the nonhairy skin of the nail unit.

Atopic dermatitis often involves the hands with thickening of the skin, coarse surface relief also called lichenification, accentuated velvety to warty hyperkeratoses over the finger joints, and mild nail affection.[81] The cuticles may be thick and ragged. The nails are often shiny as the patients use the dorsa of the fingers to rub their itchy skin thus polishing the nail surface. Pits may also be observed in atopic eczema.[82] Pulpitis sicca and atopic winter feet are often associated with painful dry cracking and fissuring of the periungual skin. Further, the subungual space of atopics often harbors *Staphylococcus aureus*.[83,84]

Any eczema involving the proximal nail fold usually leads to thickening and rounding of its free margin with spontaneous loss of the cuticle, in the long run also separation of the nail plate from the overlying ventral surface of the proximal nail fold; the resulting space may be colonized with different yeasts or bacteria that are not necessarily pathogenic. From affection of the undersurface of the proximal nail fold, the eczema may extend to the matrix resulting first in surface irregularities and later in spongiotic matrix dermatitis with inspissation of plasma into the nail plate, pitting, loss of nail shine, and loss of nail transparency.

3.4.1 Histopathology

All eczemas are histologically characterized by the development of spongiosis, lymphocytic exocytosis, and spongiotic vesicles though to a widely varying degree. Depending on which nail structure is involved, the matrix, nail bed, proximal nail fold epidermis or hyponychium, and/or digital pulp become slightly acanthotic, the intercellular spaces of the epithelia widen so that the intercellular connections may be seen as spiny extensions of the keratinocytes. The serum collections increase to form small spongiotic vesicles often containing lymphocytes. When this happens in the nail matrix, the plasma and lymphocytes are transported up through the keratogenous zone, which often disappears, and are included into the nail plate. Often, a granular layer develops in the matrix.[85] The nail cells take on a wavy appearance. The nail becomes thicker, brittle, loses its transparency, and in most cases also its surface shine looking dull and lusterless. Involvement of the most proximal matrix causes a superficial localization of these serum inclusions that break out of the nail and leave small depressions, the characteristic pits of nail eczema. When the eczema is localized in the nail bed it leads to subungual hyperkeratosis, which contains many serum inclusions and also lymphocytes. Long-standing serum inclusions may look foamy. The hyperkeratosis is mostly orthokeratotic in contrast to skin.

In chronic allergic contact dermatitis of the matrix and nail bed, there may be a very dense lichenoid lymphocytic epidermotropic infiltrate, particularly in patients with persistent allergen exposure as in sculptured nails. The matrix and nail bed may develop papillomatosis and a granular layer with irregular hyperorthokeratosis (Figure 3.7).

Chronic contact dermatitis of the hyponychium and the immediately adjacent pulp skin may lead to considerable hyperkeratosis, sometimes up to 1 to 2 cm thick that is cracked and contains dried globules of plasma. When it is more rhagadiform, split-like fissures extend from the surface to the basal layer with eosinophilic homogenous necrosis of the keratinocytes neighboring it.

Nummular eczema is characterized by small red plaques on the proximal nail fold that exhibit tiny small papules topped with a minute serous crust. This may sometimes contain a few neutrophils.

(a) (b)

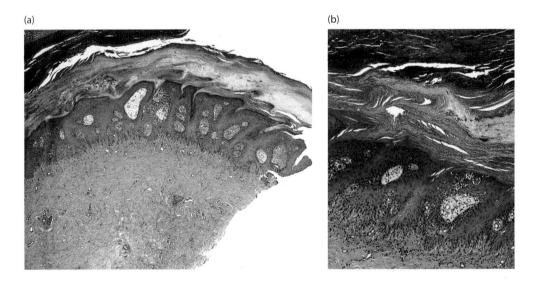

Figure 3.7 Eczematous alterations of the nail due to artificial nails. (a) Low magnification showing an almost lichenoid dense lymphocytic infiltrate with massive acanthosis of the nail bed and an irregular overlying nail plate. (b) High magnification from the matrix area with spongiosis, lymphocytic exocytosis, and spongiotic vesicles as well as irregular nail substance formation.

Nail changes due to atopic eczema are often indirect: brilliant shine from rubbing of the nail surface and distal phalanges on itchy skin, and the topicals used by the atopic subject may act as a polishing cream. Histologically no apparent changes are seen although pits are occasionally present. Chronic rubbing may, however, cause thickening of the epidermis with slight papillomatosis and hyperkeratosis as well as dense collagen in the upper dermis, features also seen in knuckle pads.

Atopic subjects may develop twenty-nail syndrome that is clinically characterized by rough, gray, intransparent nails. Histopathologically, a dense infiltrate is seen in the upper dermis with epitheliotropism. Immunophenotyping shows that almost all lymphocytes are CD3+ with the majority also being CD4+ and about one-third CD8+ whereas CD20+ B cells are very rare (Figure 3.8).[86]

Chronic paronychia whatever its etiology usually causes thickening of the proximal nail fold with rounding up of its free margin and spontaneous loss of the cuticle. The eponychium, which is normally closely attached to the underlying nail, is split off the nail. Spongiosis and spongiotic vesicles may be seen in the epidermis of both the dorsal and the ventral surface of the proximal nail fold.

3.4.2 Differential diagnosis

Chronic allergic contact dermatitis may be difficult to differentiate from nail lichen planus as there is a dense band-like epidermotropic infiltrate; this, however, does not cause liquefaction degeneration of the basal cells in eczema as opposed to lichen planus. Alopecia areata of the nails is essentially a spongiotic dermatitis. Sometimes, no differentiation is possible on histologic grounds alone. Paronychia due to yeasts or molds may look similar to chronic eczema and a PAS stain may be necessary to make the correct diagnosis. Psoriasis may rarely cause difficulties in the clinical differential diagnosis but is usually diagnostic enough to make the correct diagnosis. Onychomycoses also lead to spongiosis, sometimes even spongiotic vesicles, hyperkeratosis, and serum inclusions as well as Munro microabscess-like accumulations of neutrophils; a PAS or Grocott stain may be necessary. Nevertheless, onychomycoses poor in fungal elements may be overlooked.

Parakeratosis pustulosa is said to demonstrate both eczematoid and psoriasiform characteristics.

3.5 ALOPECIA AREATA

Alopecia areata is a relatively common autoimmune disorder characterized by the appearance of round bald spots on the scalp and potentially all areas of glabrous skin.[87–89] It is speculated to be due to the collapse of immune privilege of the hair and nail.[90] Roughly one-fifth are familiar cases.[91] Males predominate with almost two-thirds of the cases. Patients in the third to fifth decade are most frequently affected. Association with other dermatological disorders, particularly autoimmune, is common.[92,93] Nail involvement is frequent, correlates with the severity of alopecia areata,[94] and is said to be a sign of poor prognosis.[95] Children appear to have their nails affected more frequently.[96,97] Apparently, alopecia areata of the nails can occur isolated without hair loss. Pitting is by far the most common sign of nail alopecia areata.[89] Sometimes the pits are arranged in rows. When the entire nail is pitted this is called trachyonychia, which means rough nail. The nails may lose their shine and their transparency. When all or almost all nails are affected, the condition is called twenty-nail dystrophy. The nails look like they have been treated with coarse sandpaper.[98] Leukonychia is less frequent. Red lunulae appear to be a sign of sudden onset.[99]

3.5.1 Histopathology

In contrast to scalp histopathology, the nail in alopecia areata demonstrates a spongiotic dermatitis with a lymphocytic epitheliotropic infiltrate in the dermis of the matrix, spongiosis of the matrix epithelium, lymphocytic exocytosis, and often small spongiotic vesicles.[100] These are transported into the higher epithelial layers and may be included into the newly formed nails. This proteinaceous exudate is seen as homogenously stained, slightly eosinophilic, but PAS positive inclusions in the nail plate and sometimes in the subungual keratin. They make the nail lose their shine and transparency and may also be responsible for the thickening and friability of the nail. The nail keratin arrangement is irregularly wavy with shallow surface depressions, which, however, do not contain parakeratosis in contrast to psoriatic pits (Figure 3.9).[101–103] The proximal matrix, which is responsible for the production of the superficial nail layers, is more severely affected than the middle and distal matrix; this explains why the superficial nail layers exhibit more pronounced changes in ungual lichen planus.

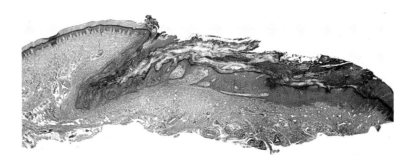

Figure 3.8 Trachyonychia in an 11-year-old boy with atopic dermatitis, scanning power of a lateral longitudinal nail biopsy.

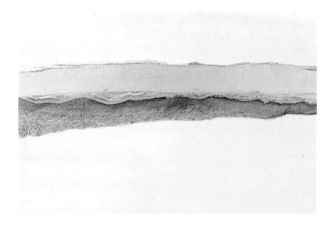

Figure 3.9 Alopecia areata of the nail. Distal matrix and proximal to mid-nail bed area.

3.5.2 Differential diagnosis

The clinical differential diagnosis comprises all conditions that may cause an irregular or rough nail surface, that is, psoriasis, lichen planus, eczema, and so on. Histologically, the spongiotic dermatitis may be indistinguishable from a mild to moderate eczematous dermatitis. This often shows involvement of the eponychium and nail folds, which is not seen in alopecia areata.[90,94]

3.6 NAIL LICHEN PLANUS

Lichen planus is a relatively common skin and mucous membrane disease characterized by small flat red papules on skin and net-like white lesions on the oral and genital mucosa. About 10% of lichen planus patients have nail lesions.[104] Isolated nail lichen planus is seen in 1%–4%.[105–107] Nail alterations are also observed in lichen plano-pilaris.[108] It may cause twenty-nail dystrophy[109] and "idiopathic atrophy of the nails."[103,110,111] Most patients are between 40 and 60 years of age.[112] The most common clinical features are thinning, longitudinal ridges, loss of nail shine, and distal splitting. Trachyonychia is seen in about one-fifth of the cases. Onycholysis and subungual hyperkeratosis are signs of nail bed involvement. Pterygium formation highlights irreversible scarring of the matrix. Red lunula spots as well as yellow nails are rare.[113,114] In children, atypical clinical features seem to be more common.[115] The etiology of lichen planus is not known, but there appears to be a higher susceptibility for persons that are positive for HLA-A3 and B7.[116,117] Nail lichen planus is treated with moderate to good success with oral corticosteroids,[118] steroid injections,[119] potent topical steroids, tacrolimus,[120] various retinoids,[121] and TNF-α blockers.[122] The close clinical and histopathological similarity between nail changes in lichen planus and in graft-versus-host disease[123,124] also suggests an immunological mechanism, probably an autoimmune disorder. There are also associations with other autoimmune diseases like alopecia areata, vitiligo, Sjögren's syndrome, Castleman's syndrome, and chronic liver disease.[125,126] Lichenoid drug reactions involving the nail may be indistinguishable. Lichen planus results in permanent

dystrophy of one to several nails due to irreversible scarring in about 4%–18% of the patients.[109,110]

3.6.1 Histopathology

Histopathology of lichen planus is usually typical and diagnostic (Figure 3.10), but the alterations may be very mild in long-standing lichen planus, which is sometimes called postlichen status (Figure 3.11), and extremely pronounced in hyperplastic lichen.[109,127,128] Involvement of the skin of the proximal nail fold shows a thickened orthokeratotic horny layer with focal hypergranulosis. The rete ridges are saw-tooth like due to a dense lymphocytic epidermotropic infiltrate leading to vacuolar degeneration of the basal

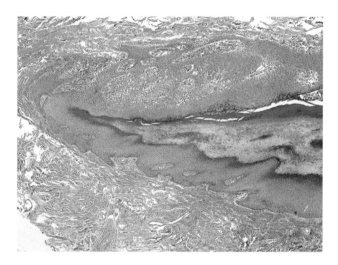

Figure 3.10 Lichen planus of the nail. This lateral longitudinal nail biopsy demonstrates severe involvement of the dorsal aspect of the apical matrix with a dense lymphohocytic epitheliotropic infiltrate causing vacuolar degneration of the basal cells.

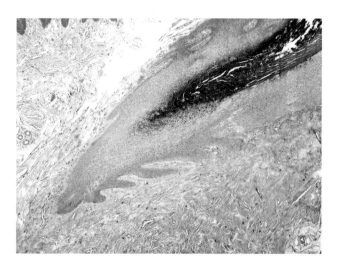

Figure 3.11 Nail postlichen status. Lateral longitudinal nail biopsy of a 54-year-old woman with very thin and fragile nails. The Giemsa stain reveals thickening of the apical matrix epithelium with a broad stratum granulosum and with no regular nail formation anymore.

layer with a variable amount of apoptotic cells. In contrast to skin, spongiosis is very often present and sometimes so pronounced that an eczema may be suspected. The most common histological appearance of nail lichen planus is proximal and dorsal nail matrix involvement. There is a dense band-like epidermotropic lymphocytic infiltrate from the middle of the ventral surface of the proximal nail fold to the matrix and toward the nail bed. It causes marked hydropic degeneration of the basal cell layer, particularly of the proximal matrix, and a granular layer as well as ortho-hyperkeratosis instead of a normal nail plate. This is the reason for the longitudinal ridging and loss of nail shine as the proximal matrix is responsible for the latter. In dark-skinned persons, pigmentary incontinence as well as longitudinal melanonychia are frequent.[129] This is often overlooked as it is not obvious in histological sections. When the more distal matrix and nail bed are involved, subungual hyperkeratosis is a leading feature. The epidermotropic infiltrate that virtually eats up the epithelium causes progressive obliteration of the nail pocket or cul-de-sac until finally it is completely obstructed resulting in a cicatricial pterygium. An even more severe matrix involvement may lead to ulcerative nail lichen planus.[130,131] Severe hydropic degeneration of the basal layer of the matrix and nail bed with a band-like lymphocytic infiltrate is seen in bullous lichen planus of the nail.[132] The infiltrating lymphocytes were shown to be strongly positive for OKT 6 (CD1) in the dermis and matrix epithelium and positive for OKT 8 (CD8) in the epithelium and strongly positive in the dermis.[133] The irreversible scarring may be a result of the involvement of the most proximal to dorsal matrix where the nail stem cells were located.[134]

3.6.2 Differential diagnosis

Differential diagnosis comprises lichen striatus, drug-induced lichenoid eruption with nail involvement, graft-versus-host disease, amyloidosis, disseminated lichenoid papular dermatosis with nail changes in AIDS,[135] subungual tumor when only one nail is affected,[136] yellow nail syndrome,[119] and lichen sclerosus et atrophicans.[137] Postlichen nail dystrophy is difficult to differentiate from nail dystrophy after Stevens–Johnson syndrome, Lyell syndrome, impaired peripheral circulation, radiodermatitis, after bacterial infections, bleomycin injection, and mechanical trauma to the matrix[138] as there are usually no diagnostic features anymore. β-blockers may induce lichenoid-psoriasiform changes.

3.7 NAIL LICHEN STRIATUS

Lichen striatus is a rare self-limiting skin disease mainly affecting children and adolescents. Approximately 3% of the cases show nail involvement.[139] It is characterized by an abrupt onset of linearly arranged scaly erythematous papules often involving an entire extremity. When the proximal nail fold is affected, there is usually also segmental nail involvement. This appears as longitudinal striation of a part of the nail, splitting, fraying, leukonychia, and partial or even total nail loss.[140] There may also be isolated nail involvement.[141,142] Usually, the disease clears spontaneously[143] with the nail lesions lagging behind, but nail plate alterations may persist for a period of several years.[144] Its etiology is not known, but many authors believe that it may be a manifestation of mosaicism, which is characterized by the presence of genetically abnormal keratinocyte clones. These are recognized by the immune system through a precipitating event and induce an inflammatory T-cell response mediated in the affected skin along the Blaschko lines.[145,146] A viral trigger has also been suggested.[137] Lichen striatus is assumed to be identical with adult blaschkitis.[147–149]

3.7.1 Histopathology

Histopathology of lichen striatus shows a superficial perivascular mainly lymphocytic infiltrate with an admixture of histiocytes. In the papillary dermis, there is a focal band-like lymphocytic infiltrate with epidermotropism and some spongiosis of the proximal nail fold, the matrix, and the nail bed. The basal cell layer shows variable vacuolar degeneration and necrotic epidermal cells in the spinous layer. The matrix epithelium may show some apoptotic cells.[150] There may also be focal parakeratosis, but usually the differentiation from ungual lichen planus is only possible in the context with the clinical picture.[151] Immunohistochemically, the epidermotropic infiltrate was shown to be made up of CD8+ and CD7+ T lymphocytes.[152,153]

3.7.2 Differential diagnosis

The clinical differential diagnoses are linear lichen planus, lichenoid linear drug eruption,[154] linear epidermal nevus, inflammatory linear verrucous epidermal nevus,[155–157] and linear porokeratosis.[158] Histologically, mainly nail lichen planus has to be excluded, but other interface dermatitides also have to be considered.

3.8 LICHEN AUREUS

Lichen aureus is a localized chronic variant of pigmented purpuric dermatitis mainly affecting the lower extremity. It occurs as one or a few plaques that are composed of densely aggregated flat papules of an orange, red, or rust color.[159] Involvement of the proximal nail folds of fingers and toes was described.[160]

3.8.1 Histopathology

Histopathology of lichen aureus exhibits a relatively dense band-like and perivascular lymphocytic infiltrate limited to the upper dermis. Extravasated erythrocytes are always seen and often hemosiderin is observed extracellularly and in macrophages. Iron stains are positive. Sometimes there is a band-like infiltrate in addition with slight spongiosis and even intraepidermal erythrocytes may be seen. One case showed Birbeck granules in large histiocytes suggesting that they were Langerhans cells.[161]

3.8.2 Differential diagnosis

The clinical differential diagnoses are other pigmented purpuric dermatoses, lichen planus, purpuric drug eruption, and localized vasculitis.[162]

3.9 LICHEN NITIDUS

Lichen nitidus is a rare skin disease mainly affecting children and young adults. It is characterized by the development of multiple, very small, flat-topped, mostly skin colored papules sometimes occurring in groups, but not coalescing. It usually remains asymptomatic. Nail involvement is rare and mainly seen as longitudinal ridging, pitting, or fine rippling.[163,164] The nails tend to become fragile. Also the proximal nail fold may develop small papules.

3.9.1 Histopathology

Histopathology of lichen striatus of the nail fold shows small granulomas that are located in a dermal papilla, which becomes widened and finally gives the impression of the epidermal rete ridges embracing the granuloma. The granulomas consist of lymphocytes, histiocytes, and some giant cells. The overlying epidermis is thinned and parakeratotic. Often vacuolar changes of the basal layer and small areas of clefting are seen on top of the granuloma. Lesions in the matrix and nail bed mimic lichen planus with giant cells.[165]

3.9.2 Differential diagnosis

The clinical differential diagnoses are lichen planus, lichenoid drug eruption, id reactions, and keratosis follicularis.[166] Histologically, mainly nail lichen planus has to be excluded.

3.10 ERYTHEMA MULTIFORME, STEVENS–JOHNSON SYNDROME, AND TOXIC EPIDERMAL NECROLYSIS OF LYELL

Erythema multiforme (EM) is a relatively common, self-limited skin disease with symmetrical round red lesions, many of which evolve into typical target lesions with a central bulla. Bullous erythema multiforme is a more severe yet localized form. Stevens–Johnson syndrome (SJS) is a severe disease with similar cutaneous lesions but more extensive skin and mucous membrane involvement, fever, and malaise. Toxic epidermal necrolysis (TEN), also called Lyell's syndrome, involves more than 30% of the body surface and is characterized by full-thickness epidermal necrosis. This evolves from tender diffuse erythema that develops into large flaccid bullae denuding the skin and leaving a raw surface. Stevens–Johnson syndrome/toxic epidermolysis overlap is when between 10% and 30% of the body surface are affected. Drugs (allergic EM, SJS, or TEN),[167,168] recurrent herpes simplex (postherpetic EM, SJS, or TEN), and infections (postinfectious EM, SJS, or TEN) are thought to be the cause. Whether they are a continuum of the same pathological process or different entities is still not clear.[169,170] Nail involvement in erythema multiforme and SJS is usually seen as blisters whereas in TEN denudement of the surrounding skin is typical. After some time, the nail may fall out[171] leaving dystrophic nails[172] or the entire nail organ may be shed, a process called nail degloving.[173] Particularly after TEN, the nail loss may lead to permanent scarring, pterygium formation, and cicatricial anonychia.[162,174,175]

3.10.1 Histopathology

The histopathology of EM varies according to the structure involved. The most common localization is periungual skin. Biopsy shows a vacuolar interface dermatitis. In the early phase, the basal cells appear vacuolar through lymphocytes that are aligned at the dermo-epidermal junction. There is a mild spongiosis in the lower epidermis. The superficial perivascular infiltrate is usually sparse. Some papillary edema and extravasated erythrocytes are often found. Necrotic keratinocytes are present. The stratum corneum is usually orthokeratotic as the process is acute. With time, the infiltrate is more lichenoid band-like with more apoptotic cells both in the infiltrate as well as the epidermis. In pronounced cases, the epidermis splits from the dermis and a bulla is formed. The blister roof may become completely necrotic.

In the SJS/TEN overlap syndrome, there are more necrotic keratinocytes from the beginning. With time, they increase in number and there may be focal full-thickness epidermal necrosis.

TEN is characterized by extensive full-thickness epidermal necrosis. There is almost no inflammatory infiltrate.

It is common to make a quick diagnosis from the blister roof: full-thickness necrotic epidermis is in favor of TEN whereas when only a horny layer is seen with a few neutrophils this hints at staphylococcal scalded skin syndrome or bulla repens around the nails (runaround).

3.10.2 Differential diagnosis

The clinical differential diagnoses are all conditions lead to blisters, for example, drug eruptions, fixed drug eruption, bullous pemphigoid, epidermolysis bullosa acquisita, hereditary epidermolyses, pemphigus vulgaris, but also graft-versus-host disease.[176] EM and SJS cannot be distinguished histologically.

3.11 KERATOSIS LICHENOIDES CHRONICA

Keratosis lichenoides chronica is a rare condition characterized by an extensive eruption of linear, net-like, lichenoid and warty hyperkeratoses, yellowish keratotic papules and plaques mostly on the dorsal aspect of the extremities and the trunk. First described as lichen ruber moniliformis by Kaposi in 1886[177] and again in 1895 under the term of lichen ruber acuminatus verrucosus et reticularis,[178] it was later termed porokeratosis striata lichenoides by Nékam, then lichenoid tri-keratosis,[179] and keratosis lichenoides striata.[180] Because of its chronic course, the term keratosis lichenoides chronica was finally introduced.[181,182] Most patients are between 20 and 50 years old although also children were observed. Roughly one-third have nail affection.[183] Nail alterations comprise involvement of the nail folds with typical plaques and patches covered with a firm, often verrucous hyperkeratosis.[184,185] One patient developed skin, mucosal, and nail lesions at the age of 1 year and a mantle cell lymphoma in adulthood; his skin and mucosal lesions improved with the lymphoma treatment.[186]

3.11.1 Histopathology

Histopathology of keratosis lichenoides chronica shows a dense lichenoid infiltrate of lymphocytes, histiocytes, and often also plasma cells obscuring the dermo-epidermal junction. Hydropic degeneration of the basal cell layer is pronounced and necrotic keratinocytes are abundant. There is alternating focal epidermal acanthosis and atrophy with a thickened irregular horny layer often containing ortho- and parakeratotic areas (Figure 3.12). Follicular plugging is not a feature around the nails but common in other localizations.

3.11.2 Differential diagnosis

Clinically, hypertrophic and verrucous variants of lichen planus, lupus erythematosus, and acral psoriasis as well as widespread prurigo nodularis and lichen simplex chronicus have to be considered. Histologically, irritated hypertrophic lichen planus but also hyperkeratotic variants of lupus erythematosus have to be ruled out. The presence of parakeratosis, alternating areas of hypotrophy and acanthosis, and the very dense and heavy infiltrate with many plasma cells help to distinguish it from lichen planus.

3.12 GRANULOMA ANNULARE

Granuloma annulare (GA) is a fairly common granulomatous disorder of the skin of unknown etiology. Clinically, rings of small, flat, flesh-colored nodules, approximately 3 to 5 mm in diameter, are seen mainly on the extremities of young persons. Apart from the typical form, other variants of granuloma annulare exist, for example, generalized granuloma annulare, perforating GA, and subcutaneous GA. The distal digits are very rarely affected.[187] Nail fold involvement may occur.

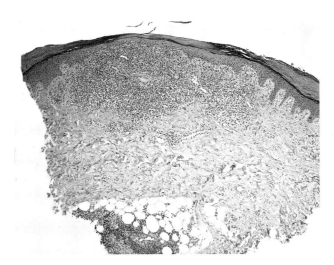

Figure 3.12 Keratosis lichenoides chronica of the nail fold. The overlying epidermis is thinned with para- and orthokeratosis whereas the adjacent epidermis is acanthotic. The infiltrate is mainly composed of lymphocytes and many of them are epidermotropic resulting in some liquefaction degeneration.

3.12.1 Histopathology

Granuloma annulare is characterized histopathologically by an infiltrate composed of histiocytes and few lymphocytes. In the center, there may be necrobiotic material, which sometimes stains moderately eosinophilic. The granulomatous features may be minor, but in the center of the lesion there is often some mucin. The histiocytes may be in irregular arrangement or be palisaded. The inflammatory infiltrate is usually sparse with only slight perivascular lymphocytic infiltrates. The long axis of the granulomas tends to be horizontal. Perforating GA is located superficially in the dermis leading to disruption of the epidermis.

3.12.2 Differential diagnosis

Clinically, lichen planus and lichen nitidus of the periungual skin have to be considered. Histologically, other necrobiotic granulomas, for example, necrobiosis lipoidica, have to be ruled out; however, there is no report of necrobiosis lipoidica in the nail apparatus.

3.13 ERYTHEMA ELEVATUM DIUTINUM

Erythema elevatum diutinum (EED) is a rare skin disorder clinically characterized by red to violaceous, later brown, persistent plaques and nodules in symmetrical arrangement on the extensor surfaces of the extremities. The lesions are usually asymptomatic, but pruritus, pain, and arthralgia of involved joints have been reported. Whether immunoglobulin A plays a role in the pathomechanism is not yet clear.[188-190] Periungual lesions exhibit small plaques and nodules.[191] Nail involvement with subungual hemorrhage, onycholysis, and paronychia has been described.[192]

3.13.1 Histopathology

Erythema elevatum diutinum was initially classified as a neutrophilic disorder, but is now seen as a rare type of chronic fibrosing leucocytoclastic vasculitis.[193] It starts with a so-called lymphocytic perivasculitis, which soon develops into a dense diffuse mixed infiltrate, sometimes granulomatous, with abundant neutrophils and often signs of karyorrhexis.[194] The capillaries may be thickened with fibrinoid material and there is often a concentric lamellar perivascular fibrosis. The grenz zone may or may not be spared. Old lesions become fibrotic with an orderly array of spindle cells and collagen fibers that may run parallel to the skin surface.

3.13.2 Differential diagnosis

Clinically, a variety of other chronic vascular disorders have to be considered. Histopathologically, granuloma faciale (GF) has to be ruled out.[195] High density of the infiltrate was noted in 97% of cases of GF but only in 56% of cases of EED. Eosinophils were the predominant cell type in 59% of cases of GF but in none of the cases of EED. Plasma cells were more frequent in GF (64%) than in EED (22%), and granulomas were never found in GF but in 22% of EED. A zone of perijunctional sparing (Grenz zone) was observed in about three quarters of the cases in both groups. The bullous variant may look like dermatitis herpetiformis with collections of neutrophils and nuclear dust in the tips of the papillae.[196]

3.14 DERMATOMYOSITIS

Dermatomyositis is an uncommon autoimmune disease characterized by both muscle and skin inflammation. It is usually a serious condition and up to one quarter to one half of the cases are thought to be paraneoplastic.[197] Clinically, there is an edematous livid-red discoloration of the face, particularly around the eyes, called heliotropic edema. There is severe muscle weakness, which is easily tested when asking the patient to raise both arms together or to bend their knees to go down and then raise again without the help of their arms. Gottron's nodules are characteristic and seen as whitish flat papules on the dorsa of the fingers, particularly on the distal phalanges. The capillaries of the proximal nail fold may be altered.[198] The cuticles are often hyperkeratotic and ragged.[199,200] The lunulae may be red[201] and the nail beds show splinter hemorrhages.[202] Pterygium inversum occurs at the hyponychium.[203] Nail thickening and hardness were observed. A case of loss of toenails was also described.[204]

3.14.1 Histopathology

Although dermatomyositis is often diagnosed histopathologically, there are few reports on microscopic alterations of the nail. Periungual erythema usually shows mild inflammatory changes not distinguishable from those of systemic lupus erythematosus. Epidermal atrophy, vacuolar degeneration of basal cells, basal membrane degeneration, and a sparse to moderate perivascular lymphocytic infiltrate are seen (Figure 3.13). Microhemorrhage may lead to hemosiderin deposits in the cuticle.[205] No immune complexes are observed along the basement membrane, but fibrin deposition may be present in severe inflammation. Vasculitic changes were repeatedly described.

Biopsy of the proximal nail fold shows capillary dilatation, numerous epidermal and dermal colloid bodies, basal lamina thickening as well as immunoglobulin deposits. These are found not only in dermatomyositis, but also in lupus erythematosus, scleroderma, and Raynaud's phenomenon.[206]

Gottron papules are characterized by acanthosis or epidermal atrophy with orthokeratosis, vacuolar changes in the basal cell layer, cytoid bodies, melanophages in dark-skinned individuals, a mild perivascular mononuclear infiltrate, and mucin deposition in the upper dermis.

3.14.2 Differential diagnosis

Systemic lupus erythematosus (SLE) may not be differentiated histopathologically, but the lupus band test is always negative in about one-half of the SLE cases. Hydroxyurea can induce a clinical condition virtually identical to that of amyopathic dermatomyositis, and even Gottron-like papules are present with the same histopathologic criteria.[207]

3.15 LUPUS ERYTHEMATOSUS

Lupus erythematosus is an autoimmune disease with various clinical variants. It may rarely affect the nail, both in the chronic cutaneous (discoid) (CDLE) as well as the systemic forms (SLE).[208,209] The nails may exhibit longitudinal ridging[210] and splitting, subungual hyperkeratosis may develop, and finally even total nail loss may occur.[211,212] A Koebner phenomenon was observed to lead to partial nail loss.[213] Longitudinal leukonychia was seen in an African patient who had scarring discoid lupus erythematosus with complete loss of pigment in many of his LE scars in the face and on the scalp. Often the nail lesions are not specific.[214]

Systemic lupus erythematosus shows periungual erythema due to dilated and tortuous loops of capillaries and prominent dermal venous plexus, nailfold telangiectasiae, splinter hemorrhages, red lunulae,[215] sometimes bluish nail pigmentation,[216] onycholysis, focal nail fold necroses, vasculitis, thrombosis of dermal vessels as well as digital ulcers and gangrene.[217] Further nonspecific skin lesions associated with active SLE are cuticle abnormalities such

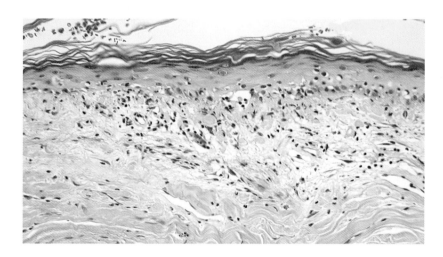

Figure 3.13 Periungual erythema in dermatomyositis. The epidermis is thinned and displays severe basal liquefaction degeneration whereas the subepidermal infiltrate is sparse.

as ragged cuticles.[218,219] Splinter hemorrhages may be a hint at antiphospholipid syndrome. Cuticular abnormalities and nailfold telangiectasiae are often encountered in other autoimmune disorders, in particular dermatomyositis, the differential diagnosis of which with SLE can be very difficult, in particular in early disease manifestations.[220]

In chilblain lupus,[221] being the form to involve the nails most frequently, the tip of the digit—mostly toes—turns livid red, is tender, and the nail becomes more and more destroyed.[222] Ulceration may be seen.[223] Familial chilblain lupus is due to a mutation in the TREX1 gene that encodes a 3′-5′ DNA exonuclease, which inhibits initiation of autoimmunity.[224]

3.15.1 Histopathology

Histology greatly depends on the clinical type of lesion. Many are nonspecific and would not allow the diagnosis of lupus erythematosus to be made without the clinical context as well as laboratory and immunological investigations. In the periungual skin, there is mild to moderate epidermal atrophy, hyperkeratosis, hydropic degeneration of the basal cells, thickening of the PAS positive basal membrane, an epidermotropic and perivascular lymphocytic infiltrate, edema, and dilatation of the papillary capillaries (Figure 3.14).[225] Nail bed involvement causes hyperkeratosis, development of a granular layer, atrophy of the prickle cell layer, and an interface dermatitis with liquefaction degeneration of basal cells due to the epidermotropic lymphocytic infiltrate. Some hyaline bodies may be seen in the upper dermis as remnants of necrotic keratinocytes.[201,226]

The histopathological alterations in early chilblain lupus are very subtle. There may be some ectatic capillaries in the upper dermis and perivascular lymphocytic infiltrates in the middle to deep dermis reminding one faintly of perniosis. In full-blown chilblain lupus, the histological features of chronic cutaneous lupus erythematosus are usually very well developed allowing the diagnosis to be made. There is severe nail dystrophy due to matrix and nail bed involvement. A band-like lymphocytic infiltrate leading to atrophy

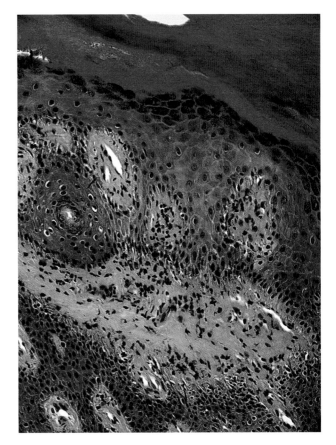

Figure 3.14 Lupus erythematosus of the nail in a black patient. The punch biopsy contains the dorsal and ventral surface of the proximal nail fold with hydropic degeneration of the basal cells, a sparse lymphocytic infiltrate, and many melanophages.

of the matrix and nail bed epithelium, sometimes even to shallow ulceration, is seen with liquefaction degeneration of the basal cells, necrotic keratinocytes, Civatte bodies in the upper dermis, and marked irregular thickening of the PAS positive basal membrane (Figure 3.15). Mucin stain may reveal increased amounts of mucin.

(a)

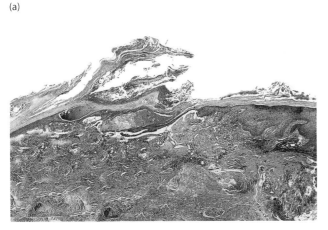

(b)

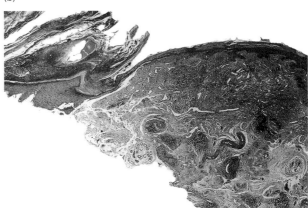

Figure 3.15 Chilblain lupus in an elderly woman. There is no regular nail plate formation; the matrix is markedly thinned and partially necrotic whereas the nail bed epithelium is acanthotic. (a) Nail bed and (b) proximal nail fold and matrix region.

3.15.2 Differential diagnosis

The clinical differential diagnoses are lichen planus, drug eruptions, id reactions, and erythema multiforme. Histologically, mainly nail lichen planus has to be excluded. Hypertrophic lupus erythematosus may mimic squamous cell carcinoma[227] but elastic fiber trapping is rare in LE.[228] The clinical and histopathological skin changes in the rare Aicardi-Goutières syndrome that is associated with a mutation of the TREX1 gene are identical with chilblain lupus.[229]

3.16 PEMPHIGUS VULGARIS AND PEMPHIGUS FOLIACEUS

Pemphigus represents a group of autoimmune blistering diseases characterized by autoantibodies to desmogleins 3 and 1, which are constituents of the keratinocyte adhesion structures desmosomes. This leads to acantholysis, which is the histopathological hallmark of the pemphigus diseases. Autoantibodies are demonstrable in more than 80% of the patients both by direct and indirect immunofluorescence and their titer correlates with disease activity. Five pemphigus types are generally accepted: pemphigus vulgaris including pemphigus vegetans, pemphigus foliaceus including pemphigus erythematosus and fogo selvagem (endemic Brazilian pemphigus), drug-induced pemphigus, IgA pemphigus, and paraneoplastic pemphigus. Except for IgA pemphigus, IgG is the main immunoreactant. Most patients are between 30 and 60 years of age, but in principle any age may be affected.[230] Nails are mainly involved by pemphigus vulgaris,[231] rarely in Brazilian type of pemphigus foliaceus.[232] Apparently, nail involvement correlates with the severity of (muco)cutaneous lesions and the duration of the disease.[233,234] In general, nail involvement appears to be rare[235,236]—roughly one-third—however, some authors found it in more than 70% of the patients with about half of them presenting initially with cutaneous and mucosal lesions, one-third having nail lesions first,[237] and one-fifth exhibiting nail lesions as the only sign of their pemphigus.[238] It was assumed that high antidesmoglein 3 titers may be responsible for paronychia in pemphigus vulgaris.[239] In contrast to lesions on other body sites, acute or chronic paronychia and onychomadesis caused by blisters in the immediate vicinity of the nail organ are the most common clinical presentation of nail pemphigus vulgaris. Secondary infection with *Staphylococcus aureus* and *Candida albicans* may exacerbate the paronychia.[240] Beau's lines and onychomadesis are likely the consequence of matrix involvement.[241] Less commonly, subungual hemorrhage, discoloration of the nail plate, subungual hyperkeratosis, trachyonychia, nail pitting, onycholysis, onychodystrophies, and nail loss are seen.[236,237,242–246] Hemorrhagic nail lesions were associated with poor prognosis.[247–250]

Paraneoplastic pemphigus, also called paraneoplastic autoimmune multiorgan syndrome, is characterized by intractable erosive lesions and blisters, sometimes with severe erosive nail lesions.[251] It is mostly due to malignant lymphomas, chronic lymphocytic leukemia, Castleman's syndrome, thymoma, and a number of other less common malignancies.[252]

3.16.1 Histopathology

Usually the diagnosis is made with a biopsy from another localization, but when only the nail is involved a biopsy of the nail fold or the affected matrix or nail bed is indicated. A Tzanck test is easily performed from a fresh bulla, an erosive lesion, or in paronychia by gently squeezing the nail fold and collecting the exudate on a slide. A Tzanck cell is a rounded keratinocyte with a round nucleus, light perinuclear cytoplasm, and a condensation of the peripheral cytoplasm in Giemsa stain; this is the result of the acantholysis by the pathogenic autoantibodies. An early lesion, whether a full-blown lesion or just a red spot, should be selected for biopsy. Punch biopsies are not recommended as the blister roof is most often torn off. The earliest change is spongiosis, sometimes eosinophilic spongiosis. Acantholysis is seen as suprabasal clefting with the basal cells standing in line on the basement membrane like a "row of tombstones," but often also some acantholytic cells are seen above them and look like Tzanck cells. In noninfected blisters, the inflammatory infiltrate is mild (Figure 3.16), but in case of eosinophilic spongiosis it contains many eosinophils, a finding also seen in early bullous pemphigoid.

Pemphigus vegetans is a pemphigus vulgaris variant usually occurring in intertriginous folds. When occurring on the nails, it may clinically mimic acrodermatitis continua suppurativa of Hallopeau.[253] Histologically, there are spongiform pustules with neutrophilic cell infiltration in a hyperplastic epithelium. The dermal inflammatory cell infiltration is dense and mainly consists of neutrophil granulocytes and an increase in eosinophils. Acantholysis may not be obvious and further sections or biopsies may

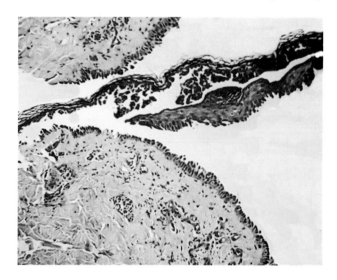

Figure 3.16 Pemphigus of the nail fold. There is extensive acantholysis splitting the epidermis off the basal layer, which is made up of cells in row-like tombstones. (Courtesy of Dr. Patricia Chang, Guatemala.)

be necessary.[254] Immunofluorescence shows intercellular antibodies.

In the Brazilian type of pemphigus foliaceus, fogo selvagem, which is believed to be, at least in part, due to stings of the black fly *Simulium pruinosum*, plus sunlight,[255] there is subtle acantholysis in or just beneath the granular layer. This may easily escape notice if there is no clinical information.

Whenever possible the diagnosis of pemphigus vulgaris should be confirmed by immunofluorescence. This shows a lacelike intercellular fluorescence pattern of the epidermis with immunoglobulin G and complement 3 both in the matrix[235] and nail bed[242,256] and also allows the distinction between pemphigus vegetans and acrodermatitis continua suppurativa.[243]

Histology of paraneoplastic pemphigus is variable according to the polymorphous clinical lesions. Three main patterns are observed: suprabasal intraepithelial acantholysis similar to pemphigus vulgaris, necrosis of single keratinocytes as in a variety of drug reactions, and vacuolar changes of the basal cell layer similar to lichen planus. There is an intercellular fluorescence of the epidermis plus immunoglobulin and/or complement along the basal membrane.[257]

3.16.2 Differential diagnosis

When the biopsy is taken from an early lesion with an intact blister roof there is little inflammation and the changes are pathognomonic. Hailey-Hailey disease of the nail is clinically characterized by multiple whitish longitudinal lines and histologically by modest acantholysis that may easily be overlooked. Darier's disease may look like Hailey-Hailey disease, but exhibits more apoptotic cells in the nail. Abundant eosinophils are a feature of pemphigus vegetans and early bullous pemphigoid.

3.17 BULLOUS PEMPHIGOID AND CICATRICIAL PEMPHIGOID

Bullous pemphigoid was differentiated from pemphigus vulgaris in 1953.[258] It is mainly seen in elderly patients and is characterized by tense bullae on a urticarial erythematous base. A nonspecific initial pruritic phase may persist for several months. Nail involvement was infrequently described. Usually, clear blisters are seen around the nail with consecutive paronychia, onycholysis, Beau's lines, onychomadesis, onychodystrophy, and nail loss.[259–265] Pterygium formation was recently observed.[266]

3.17.1 Histopathology

Histologically, there is a subepidermal blister formation usually with abundant eosinophils (Figure 3.17). Immunofluorescence demonstrates a linear immunoglobulin G and complement deposition. The targets are mainly bullous pemphigoid antigen (BPAg) 1 (BP230) and BPAg2 (BP180).

Cicatricial pemphigoid involving the nail is very rare.[267] No histopathological examinations of the nail have been performed.

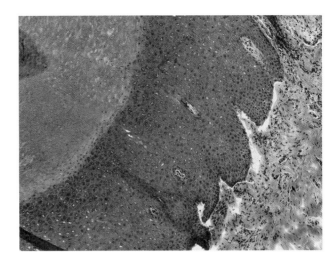

Figure 3.17 Bullous pemphigoid of the proximal matrix with detachment of the epithelium from the underlying connective tissue and development of a broad granular layer. Frozen section from Mohs surgery of an adjacent *in situ* carcinoma.

Immunofluorescence of the nail bed in bullous pemphigoid shows the typical linear fluorescence along the basement membrane,[254] which is to be expected as the basement membrane zone of the nail apparatus contains all constituents of the surrounding skin.[268]

3.17.2 Differential diagnosis

The differential diagnosis comprises all blistering disorders like erythema multiforme, Stevens–Johnson syndrome, dyshidrotic eczema, bullous crusted scabies,[269] hereditary bullous epidermolyses, cicatricial pemphigoid,[258] and epidermolysis bullosa acquisita.[270,271] For the differentiation of the latter, immunofluorescence and/or immunoblotting methods are necessary.

3.18 SCLERODERMA

Scleroderma is considered to be a connective tissue disease, which is characterized by a progressive hardening of the skin, and in systemic sclerosis, of fibrosis of lungs and other internal organs. There are several variants with acrosclerosis and CREST syndrome being of great importance for nail pathology. The digits are particularly affected with volume reduction of the fingertips, flattening and small ulcerations of the finger pulps, shortening of the terminal phalanx bone with increased longitudinal curvature eventually leading to a parrot-beak nail, nail fold capillary changes and bleeding,[272] nail fold infarctions,[273] thickened and ragged cuticles, disappearance of the lunula, shiny nails[274] or loss of nail plate shine, thinning and ridging of the nail, onycholysis, but also pterygium inversum.[203] Gangrene of the fingertips is occasionally observed.[275] Increased transverse curvature was associated with disease activity.[276] Capillaroscopic changes are also found in systemic scleroderma induced by the injection of foreign substances.[277]

3.18.1 Histopathology

The histologic alterations of diffuse scleroderma and morphea are virtually identical but show differences depending on the severity and depth of the changes. In early lesions, there is a dense perivascular lymphocytic infiltrate. With time, the collagen bundles change to large, eosinophilic, hyaline, swollen ones. In nail pathology, proximal nail fold biopsies have been used for diagnostic purposes.[278] They show perivascular lymphocytic infiltrates, splitting of the basal lamina, broadening of the perivascular connective tissue, and immunoglobulin deposits.[279] The latter are usually easily identified by PAS stain.[280] Although it can be assumed that the sclerodermatous changes of the digital tips will also show thick collagen bundles, this is not the site for a biopsy as healing is extremely poor. This is also the case for ulcerations in scleroderma and Raynaud's phenomenon.

Pterygium inversum unguis shows a hyperkeratosis of the hyponychium reaching farther distal and adhering to the nail plate. The isthmus appears to extend to the medial third of the nail bed.[281–283]

3.18.2 Differential diagnosis

A number of clinically different conditions can cause sclerodermatous changes: genetic diseases such as Rothmund–Thomson, Werner's, Huriez syndrome, progeria, and phenylkeronuria; metabolic disorders like porphyria cutanea tarda, Hashimoto's disease, primary systemic amyloidosis, and childhood diabetes mellitus; and professional risks like vibration, jackhammer and chainsaw working, exposition to silica, epoxy resin, polyvinyl chloride, adulterated oils, chronic graft-versus-host disease, and some chemotherapeutic agents, particularly bleomycin. However, the digit tip will not be the site of biopsy. Lichen sclerosus et atrophicans may occur in association with scleroderma/morphea, but its occurrence in the nail unit is disputed.

Lichen sclerosus et atrophicans of the nail area is a very rare condition. It may affect the nail fold[284] but nail involvement is exceptional.[285–287] One case was examined histopathologically and the diagnosis of lichen sclerosus et atrophicans was confirmed.[276] Lichen sclerosus et atrophicans of the nail region shows compact hyperkeratosis, vacuolar degeneration of the basal cell layer and a homogenized edematous, light appearing papillary dermis. With time, the spinous layer may become atrophic. This in turn leads to nail dystrophy.

Lichen sclerosus et atrophicans may overly morphea, but this has not been described in the nail.

3.19 CUTANEOUS VASCULITIS

Of the many different types of cutaneous vascular lesions, leukocytoclastic vasculitis is sometimes seen on the nail folds and rarely as dark red to black spots under the nail. It may be immune complex mediated, drug induced, due to infections, or autoimmune.[288] Between one-quarter and one-third of the patients present with extracutaneous lesions, such as hematuria, and joint and abdominal pain.[289] Large vessel vasculitis of the nail unit has not specifically been described.

3.19.1 Histopathology

Leukocytoclastic vasculitis is a reaction pattern involving mainly the superficial dermal postcapillary venules. An infiltrate around these vessels predominantly consisting of neutrophils, which penetrate the vessel walls, is seen. There is fibrinoid change of the vessel wall, endothelial cell swelling, and fragmentation of the neutrophil nuclei called karyorrhexis. Depending on the severity of vessel damage, extravasated erythrocytes may almost obscure the neutrophils. Severe vessel injury will also cause circumscribed necroses, occasionally with small ulcerations. Sometimes, there are so many neutrophils that the aspect of a pustular vasculitis develops. Severe edema may cause a blister-like appearance.

In fresh lesions, complement factor 3 can be demonstrated in the vessel walls by immunofluorescence.[290] Immunoglobulin A is found in Henoch-Schönlein purpura.[291]

3.19.2 Differential diagnosis

Depending on the timing of the biopsy, the diagnosis may be difficult. Early biopsy is mandatory for a reliable diagnosis. In case of general symptoms or sepsis, special stains such as Gram in case of suspected meningococcal or staphylococcal sepsis, Fite-Faraco in Lucio's phenomenon as well as direct immunofluorescence with specific antibodies to bacteria or fungi in a variety of other infections, and PAS or Grocott for suspected mycologic etiology may be necessary. Leukocytoclastic vasculitis of superficial vessels is also seen in SLE and mixed cryoglobulinemia, which clinically results in palpable purpura.[292] Septic vasculitis shows intravascular fibrin thrombi with variable intensity of inflammation. Different types of cryoglobulinemia also cause intravascular protein deposits, particularly in acral regions where it is cooler. When there is an extensive neutrophilic infiltrate, Sweet's syndrome has to be considered.[293,294] Atrophie blanche, which commonly involves the ankles and dorsa of the feet, may rarely be seen on the dorsa of the toes. Histologically, the vessel walls are hyaline with fibrinoid material in them and often some erythrocytes both in the remaining lumina and around them. The lumina may also be obliterated by fibrinoid material or by thickened intima. As this may lead to necrosis, cicatricial tissue may be seen in that area.

3.20 PYODERMA GANGRENOSUM

Pyoderma gangrenosum is considered a rare neutrophilic dermatosis of unkown etiology. Gastrointestinal, rheumatic, and other diseases are often associated linking it to the group of autoinflammatory disorders.[295] It is characterized by progressive cutaneous ulceration that may start with a tiny tender papule or pustule, which rapidly enlarges. Differentiation from an infection is crucial and may sometimes be difficult.[296,297] The pathogenesis is assumed to include immune complexes mediating neutrophilic vascular lesions. Trauma and Koebner phenomenon may elicit new lesions. Nail involvement was observed in association with cyclosporin A treatment.[298,299]

3.20.1 Histopathology

It is generally held that the histopathology of pyoderma gangrenosum is nonspecific and requires clinical data. In the beginning, there is an infiltrate mainly composed of neutrophils. This develops into a necrotizing and suppurative lesion with a lymphocytic margin with perivascular and intramural lymphocytes. Around these, cuffs of neutrophils may be seen. Sometimes a Sweet-like aspect is present. Later, scarring may predominate.

3.20.2 Differential diagnosis

Pyoderma gangrenosum can only be diagnosed when there is no leukocytoclastic vasculitis and an infection has reliably been ruled out.[287,300] In early lesions, Sweet's syndrome may histologically be identical, but it does not exhibit collagen lysis and vessel wall necrosis in areas of dense neutrophilic infiltrates. Pyoderma gangrenosum may be vegetating and even resemble pemphigus vegetans.[301,302] Pustular vasculitis of the hands limited to the dorsal aspect of the fingers and hands[303] has now been reclassified as neutrophilic dermatosis of the dorsal hands as it does not show true vasculitis with direct vessel wall damage.[304]

3.21 INFLAMMATORY LINEAR VERRUCOUS EPIDERMAL NEVUS (ILVEN)

This is a rare condition presenting with linear, pruritic, persistent lesions most commonly on the limbs, mainly the legs. In most cases, it starts in childhood,[155] but adult-onset cases were also reported.[305] Psoriasiform lesions with cuticle loss and onycholysis around the nail without nail pitting were observed. Nail involvement, however, is rare.[157]

3.21.1 Histopathology

The histopathology is fairly typical. Hyperkeratosis with focal parakeratosis, moderate acanthosis, elongated and thickened rete pegs, and occasional spongiosis with lymphocytic exocytosis are seen. Sometimes, alternating ortho- and parakeratosis with sharp delimitation are present. Then, the parakeratosis is slightly elevated, the orthokeratosis slightly depressed. Despite its name, the inflammatory infiltrate is usually mild to moderate.

Immunohistochemistry has shown a difference between ILVEN and linear psoriasis. Keratin 10 is increased and T lymphocytes important in the pathogenesis of psoriasis are significantly reduced as is the number of proliferating Ki67+ keratinocytes.[306,307]

3.21.2 Differential diagnosis

The differential diagnosis comprises all linear hyperkeratotic and lichenoid lesions, such as lichen striatus,[156] linear psoriasis,[155,305] linear porokeratosis,[308] or linear lichen planus.

REFERENCES

1. Zaias N. Psoriasis of the nail. A clinical-pathologic study. *Arch Dermatol* 1969;99:567–579.
2. Scher RK. Psoriasis of the nail. *Dermatol Clin* 1985;3:387–394.
3. Augustin M, Reich K, Blome C, Schäfer I, Laass A, Radtke MA. Nail psoriasis in Germany: Epidemiology and burden of disease. *Br J Dermatol* 2010;163:580–585.
4. Lavaroni G, Kokelj F, Pauluzzi P, Trevisan G. The nails in psoriatic arthritis. *Acta Derm Venereol (Suppl) (Stockh)* 1994;186:113.
5. Wittkowski KM, Leonardi C, Gottlieb A, Menter A, Krueger GG, Tebbey PW, Belasco J et al. Clinical symptoms of skin, nails and joints manifest independently in patients with concomitant psoriasis and psoriatic arthritis. *PLoS ONE* 2011;6(6):e20279.
6. Gudjonsson JE, Karason A, Runarsdottir EH, Antonsdottir AA, Hauksson VB, Jónsson HH, Gulcher J, Stefansson K, Valdimarsson H. Distinct clinical differences between HLA-Cw*0602 positive and negative psoriasis patients—An analysis of 1019 HLA-C and HLA-B typed patients. *J Invest Dermatol* 2006;126:740–745.
7. Armesto S, Esteve A, Coto-Segura P, Drake M, Galache C, Martínez-Borra J, Santos-Juanes J. Nail psoriasis in individuals with psoriasis vulgaris: A study of 661 patients. *Actas Dermosifiliogr* 2011;102:365–372.
8. Morgan AM, Baran R, Haneke E. Anatomy of the nail unit in relation to the distal digit. In: Krull EA, Zook EG, Baran R, Haneke E, eds. *Nail Surgery. A Text and Atlas*. Philadelphia: Lippincott Williams & Wilkins. 2001; 1–28.
9. Haneke E. Nail psoriasis. In: Soung J, ed. *Psoriasis*. Rijeka: Intech. 2011.
10. McGonagle D, Ash Z, Dickie L, McDermott M, Aydin S Z. The early phase of psoriatic arthritis. *Ann Rheum Dis* 2011; 70(Suppl 1):i71–6.
11. McGonagle D, Palmou Fontana N, Tan AL, Benjamin M. Nailing down the genetic and immunological basis for psoriatic disease. *Dermatology* 2010;221(Suppl 1):15–22.
12. Haneke E. Surgical anatomy of the nail apparatus. *Dermatol Clin* 2006;24:291–296.
13. Kim JY, Jung HJ, Lee WJ, Kim DW, Yoon GS, Kim D-S, Park MJ, Seok-Jong Lee S-J. Is the distance enough to eradicate in situ or early invasive subungual melanoma by wide local excision? From the point of view of matrix-to-bone distance for safe inferior surgical margin in Koreans. *Dermatology* 2011;223:122–123.
14. Frenz C, Fritsch H, Hoch J. Plastination histologic investigations on the inserting pars terminalis aponeurosis dorsalis of three-sectioned fingers (in German). *Ann Anat* 2000;182:69–73.
15. McGonagle D, Tan AL, Benjamin M. The nail as a musculoskeletal appendage—Implications for an

improved understanding of the link between psoriasis and arthritis. *Dermatology* 2009;218:97–102.

16. McGonagle D. Enthesitis: An autoinflammatory lesion linking nail and joint involvement in psoriatic disease. *J Eur Acad Dermatol Venereol* 2009; 23(Suppl 1):9–13.

17. Marrakchi S, Guigue P, Renshaw BR, Puel A, Pei XY, Fraitag S, Zribi J et al. Interleukin-36-receptor antagonist deficiency and generalized pustular psoriasis. *N Engl J Med* 2011;365:620–628.

18. Abbas O, Itani S, Ghosn S, Kibbi AG, Fidawi G, Farooq M, Shimomura Y, Kurban M. Acrodermatitis continua of Hallopeau is a clinical phenotype of DITRA: Evidence that it is a variant of pustular psoriasis. *Dermatology* 2013;226:28–31.

19. Lewin K, Dewit S, Ferrington RA. Pathology of the fingernail in psoriasis. A clinicopathological study. *Br J Dermatol* 1972;86:555–563.

20. Haneke E. Pathology. In: Rigopoulos D, Tosti A, eds. *Nail Psoriasis. From A to Z.* Berlin: Springer. 2014; 15–21.

21. Alkiewicz J. Psoriasis of the nails. *Br J Dermatol* 1948;60:195–200.

22. Alkiewicz J, Pfister R. *Atlas der Nagelkrankheiten: Pathohistologie, Klinik und Differentialdiagnose.* Stuttgart: FK Schattauer. 1976.

23. Peña-Romero A, Toussaint-Caire S, Judith Domínguez-Cherit J. Mottled lunulae in nail psoriasis: Report of three cases. *Skin Appendage Disord* 2016;2:70–71.

24. Ackerman AB. Subtle clues to diagnosis by conventional microscopy. Neutrophils within the cornified layer as clues to infection by superficial fungi. *Am J Dermatopathol* 1979;1:69–75.

25. Werner B, Fonseca GP, Seidel G. Microscopic nail clipping findings in patients with psoriasis. *Am J Dermatopathol* 2015;37:429–439.

26. Mahowald ML, Parrish RM. Severe osteolytic arthritis mutilans pustular psoriasis. *Arch Dermatol* 1982;18:434–437.

27. Piraccini BM, Fanti PA, Morelli R, Tosti A. Hallopeau's acrodermatitis continua of the nail apparatus: A clinical and pathological study of 20 patients. *Acta Derm-Venereol* 1994;74:65–67.

28. Heppt M, Beheshti M, Berking C. Akrolentiginöses Melanom unter dem Bild einer Acrodermatitis continua suppurativa. Dia-Klinik, 24. Fortbildungswoche für praktische Dermatologie und Venerologie, Munich, 19–25 July 2014:34–36.

29. Enfors W, Molin L. Pustulosis palmaris et plantaris. A follow up study of ten-year material. *Acta Derm-Venereol* 1971;51:284–289.

30. Andrews G, Machacek G. Pustular bacterids of the hands and feet. *Arch Dermatol* 1935;32:835–837.

31. Djawari D, Deinlein E, Hornstein OP. I Immune responses. *Dermatol Monatsschr* 1980;166:297–304.

32. Djawari D, Deinlein E. Immunology of the pustular bacterid of Andrews. II. HLA-typing. *Dermatol Monatsschr* 1980;166:305–308.

33. Ammoury A, El Sayed F, Dhaybi R, Bazex J. Palmoplantar pustulosis should not be considered as a variant of psoriasis. *J Eur Acad Dermatol Venereol* 2008;22:392–393.

34. Hornstein OP, Haneke E. Pustular psoriasis (palms and soles) vs. recalcitrant pustular eruption (palms and soles). Histological Differential Diagnosis of Skin Diseases. International Dermatopathology Symposium, Munich, 16–18 June 1978; *Skin & Allergy News* 10, 1978.

35. Ward JM, Barnes RMR. HLA antigens in persistent palmoplantar pustulosis and its relationship to psoriasis. *Br J Dermatol* 1978;99:477–483.

36. Burden AD, Kemmert D. The spectrum of nail involvement in palmoplantar pustulosis. *Br J Dermatol* 1996;134:1079–1082.

37. Samman P. *The Nails in Disease.* 3rd ed. London: Heinemann. 1978.

38. Zandieh F, Loghmani M. Reiter's syndrome in a patient with polyarthritis and nail involvement. *Iran J Allergy Asthma Immunol* 2008;7:185–186.

39. Sabouraud R. Les parakératoses microbiennes du bout des doigts. *Ann Dermatol Syph* 1931;11:206–210.

40. Hjorth N, Thomsen K. Parakeratosis pustulosa. *Br J Dermatol* 1967;79:527–532.

41. Botella R, Martinez C, Albero P, Mascaró JM. *Parakeratosis pustulosa* de Hjorth. Discusión nosológica a proposito de tres casos. *Actas Dermato-Sif* 1973; 101:1–2.

42. De Dulanto F, Armijo-Moreno M, Camacho Martínez F. Parakeratosis pustulosa: Histological findings. *Acta Derm-Venereol* 1974;54:365–367.

43. Avci O, Günes AT. Parakeratosis pustulosa with dyskeratotic cells. *Dermatology* 1994;189:413–414.

44. Sonnex TS, Dawber RPR, Zachary CB, Millard PR, Griffiths AD. The nails in adult type I pityriasis rubra pilaris. A comparison with Sezary syndrome and psoriasis. *J Am Acad Dermatol* 1986;15:956–960.

45. Bazex A, Salvator R, Dupré A, Christol B. Syndrome paranéoplasique à type d'hyperkératose des extrémités. Guérison après traitement de l'épithélioma laryngé. *Bull Soc Franc Dermatol Syphiligr* 1965;72:182.

46. Bazex A, Dupré A, Christol B, Combes P. Onychose paranéoplasique, forme localisée d'acrokératose paranéoplasique. *Bull Soc Franc Dermatol Syphilogr* 1973;80:117–118.

47. Baran R. Paraneoplastic acrokeratosis of Bazex. *Arch Dermatol* 1977;113:1613.

48. Bazex A, Griffiths A. Acrokeratosis paraneoplastica. A new cutaneous marker of malignancy. *Br J Dermatol* 1980;102:301–306.

49. Schiff BL, Ronchese F. Norwegian scabies. *Arch Dermatol* 1964;89:236–238.

50. Scher RK. Biopsies of nails: Subungual scabies. *Am J Dermatopathol* 1983;5:187–189.

51. De Berker DAR, Baran R, Dawber RPR. The nail in dermatological disease. In: Baran R, Dawber RPR, de Berker DAR, Haneke E, Tosti A, eds. *Baran and*

Dawber's Diseases of the Nails and their Management. 3rd ed. Oxford: Blackwell Science. 2001:183.

52. Zaias N. *The Nail in Health and Disease.* 2nd ed. Norwalk, CT: Appleton & Lange. 1990.

53. Caputo R, Gelmetti C, Grimault R, Gianotti R. Psoriasiform and sclerodermoid dermatitis of the fingers with apparent shortening of the nail plate: A distinct entity? *Br J Dermatol* 1994;134:126–129.

54. Tosti A, Fanti PA, Morelli R, Badazzi F. Psoriasiform acral dermatitis: Report of three cases. *Acta Derm-Venereol* 1992;72:206–207.

55. Patrizi A, Bardazzi F, Neri I, Fanti PA. Psoriasiform acral dermatitis: A peculiar clinical presentation of psoriasis in children. *Ped Dermatol* 1999;16:439–443.

56. Patrizi A, Medri M, Neri I. Psoriasiform acral dermatitis: Long-term follow-up of 10 cases. *Acta Derm Venereol* 2009;89:179–180.

57. Osawa H. Acral psoriasiform hemispherical papulosis, a new entity? *Dermatology* 1994;189:159–161.

58. Takeuchi S, Matsuzaki Y, Ikenaga S, Nishikawa Y, Kimura K, Nakano H, Sawamura D. Garlic-induced irritant contact dermatitis mimicking nail psoriasis. *J Dermatol* 2011;38:280–282.

59. Haneke E. Onychomycosis and psoriasis restricted to the nails—Distinguishable? 50th Ann Meeting Am Acad Dermatol, Dallas TX, 7–12 Dec 1991.

60. Baran R, Haneke E. *The Nail in Differential Diagnosis.* Abingdon, Oxon: Informa Healthcare. 2007:129–135.

61. Natarajan V, Nath AK, Thappa DM, Singh R, Verma SK. Coexistence of onychomycosis in psoriatic nails: A descriptive study. *Indian J Dermatol Venereol Leprol* 2010;76:723.

62. Haneke E. Fungal infections of the nail. *Sem Dermatol* 1991;10:41–53.

63. Sfikakis PP, Iliopoulos A, Elezoglou A, Kittas C, Stratigos A. Psoriasis induced by antitumor necrosis factor therapy: A paradoxical adverse reaction. *Arthritis Rheum* 2005;52;2513–2518.

64. Konsta M, Rallis E, Karameris A, Strigos A, Sfikakis PP, Iliopoulos A. Psoriasiform lesions appearing in three patients with rheumatoid arthritis during therapeutic administration of abatacept, a selective inhibitor of T-cell costimulation. *J Eur Acad Dermatol Venereol* 2012;26:257–258.

65. Pandhi D, Chowdhry S, Grover C, Reddy BS. Parakeratosis pustulosa—A distinct but less familiar disease. *Indian J Dermatol Venereol Leprol* 2003;69:48–50.

66. Haneke E. Papulosquamous and related disorders including psoriasis. In: Ruszczak Z, ed. *Skin Diseases. Clinical Pediatrics.* New York: Springer. 2011.

67. Griffiths WA. Pityriasis rubra pilaris: The problem of its classification. *J Am Acad Dermatol* 1992;26:140–142.

68. Sonnex TS, Dawber RPR, Zachary CB, Millard PR, Griffiths AWD. The importance of nail morphology in the differential diagnosis of pityriasis rubra pilaris, psoriasis and chronic erythroderma *Br J Dermatol* 1984;111(Suppl s26):16–17.

69. Jawny L, Spada FJ. Contact dermatitis to a new nail hardener. *Arch Dermatol* 1967;95:199.

70. Belsito DV. Contact dermatitis to ethyl-cyanoacrylate containing glue. *Contact Dermatitis* 1987;17:234–236.

71. Guin JD, Baas K, Nelson-Adesokan P. Contact sensitization to cyanoacrylate adhesive as a cause of severe onychodystrophy. *Int J Dermatol* 1998;37:31–36.

72. Lazarov A. Sensitization to acrylates is a common adverse reaction to artificial fingernails. *J Eur Acad Dermatol Venereol* 2007;21:169–174.

73. Hemmer W, Focke M, Wantke F, Götz M, Jarisch R. Allergic contact dermatitis to artificial fingernails prepared from UV light-cured acrylates. *J Am Acad Dermatol* 1996;35:377–380.

74. Militello G. Contact and primary irritant dermatitis of the nail unit diagnosis and treatment. *Dermatol Ther* 2007;20:47–53.

75. Goossens A, Beck M, Haneke E, McFadden JP, Nolting S. Cutaneous reactions to cosmetic products, a retrospective survey in 5 European dermatological centres. *Contact Dermatitis* 1999;40:112–113.

76. Ortiz KJ, Yiannias JA. Contact dermatitis to cosmetics, fragrances, and botanicals. *Dermatol Ther* 2004;17:264–271.

77. Guin JD. Eyelid dermatitis: A report of 215 patients. *Contact Dermatitis* 2004;50:87–90.

78. Tosti Piraccini BM, Ghetti E, Colombo MD. Topical steroids versus systemic antifungals in the treatment of chronic paronychia: An open, randomized double-blind and double dummy study. *J Am Acad Dermatol* 2002;47:73–76.

79. Scheinfeld NS. Trachyonychia: A case report and review of manifestations, associations, and treatments. *Cutis* 2003;71:299–302.

80. Dahdah MJ, Scher RK. Nail diseases related to nail cosmetics. *Dermatol Clin* 2006;24:233–239.

81. Simpson EL, Thompson MM, Hanifin JM. Prevalence and morphology of hand eczema in patients with atopic dermatitis. *Dermatitis* 2006;17:123–127.

82. Nnoruka EN. Current epidemiology of atopic dermatitis in south-eastern Nigeria. *Int J Dermatol* 2004;43:739–744.

83. Namura S, Nishijima S, Higashida T, Asada Y. Staphylococcus aureus isolated from nostril anteriors and subungual spaces of the hand: Comparative study of medical staff, patients, and normal controls. *J Dermatol* 1995;22:175–180.

84. Nishijima S, Namura S, Higashida T, Kawai S. *Staphylococcus aureus* in the anterior nares and subungual spaces of the hands in atopic dermatitis. *J Int Med Res* 1997;25:155–158.

85. Fanti PA, Tosti A, Cameli N, Varotti C. Nail matrix hypergranulosis. *Am J Dermatopathol* 1994;16:607–610.

86. El-Kehdy J, Perruchoud DL, Haneke E. *Trachyonychia.* Zürich: Swiss Cong Dermatol. 2015.

87. Paus R, Ito N, Takigawa M, Ito T. The hair follicle and immune privilege. *J Investig Dermatol Symp Proc* 2003;8:188–194.

88. Alexis AF, Dudda-Subramanya R, Sinha AA. Alopecia areata: Autoimmune basis of hair loss. *Eur J Dermatol* 2004;14:364–370.

89. Wasserman D, Guzman-Sanchez DA, Scott K, McMichael A. Alopecia areata. *Int J Dermatol* 2007;46:121–131.

90. Ito T, Meyer KC, Ito N, Paus R. Immune privilege and the skin. *Curr Dir Autoimmun* 2008;10:27–52.

91. Al-Mutairi N, Eldin ON. Clinical profile and impact on quality of life: Seven years experience with patients of alopecia areata. *Indian J Dermatol Venereol Leprol* 2011;77:489–93.

92. Alkhalifah A, Alsantali A, Wang E, McElwee KJ, Shapiro J. Alopecia areata update: Part I. Clinical picture, histopathology, and pathogenesis. *J Am Acad Dermatol* 2010;62:177–188, quiz 189–190.

93. Brenner W, Diem E, Gschnait F. Coincidence of vitiligo, alopecia areata, onychodystrophie, localized scleroderma and lichen planus. *Dermatologica* 1979;159:356–360.

94. Haneke E. Non-infectious inflammatory disorders of the nail apparatus. *J Dtsch Dermatol Ges* 2009;7:787–797.

95. Cho HH, Jo SJ, Paik SH, Jeon HC, Kim KH, Eun HC, Kwon OS. Clinical characteristics and prognostic factors in early-onset alopecia totalis and alopecia universalis. *J Korean Med Sci* 2012;27:799–802.

96. Tosti A, Morelli R, Bardazzi F, Peluso AM. Prevalence of nail abnormalities in children with alopecia areata. *Ped Dermatol* 1994;11:112–115.

97. Sharma VK, Kumar B, Dawn G. A clinical study of childhood alopecia areata in Chandigarh, India. *Ped Dermatol* 1996;13:372–377.

98. Baran R, Dupré A, Christol B, Bonafé JL, Sayag J, Ferrère J. L'ongle grésé peladique. *Ann Dermatol Vénéréol* 1978;105:387–392.

99. Bergner T, Donhauser G, Ruzicka T. Red lunulae in severe alopecia aereata. *Acta Derm Venereol* 1992;72:203–205.

100. Haneke E. Pathology of inflammatory nail diseases. 7th Coll Int Soc Dermatopathol, Graz 1984.

101. Alkiewicz J. Pathologische Reaktionen an den epithelialen Anhangsgebilden. Nagel. In: *Jadassohns Handbuch der Haut- und Geschlechtskrankheiten*, Berlin: ErgWerk, Springer. 1964; Vol I/2:299–343.

102. Laporte M, André J, Stouffs-Vanhoof F, Achten G. Nail changes in alopecia areata, light and electron microscopy. *Arch Dermatol Res* 1988;280(Suppl):585–589.

103. Achten G, André J, Laporte M. Nails in light and electron microscopy. *Sem Dermatol* 1991;10:54–64.

104. Samman P. The nails in lichen planus. *Br J Dermatol* 1961;73:288–292.

105. Marks R, Samman PD. Isolated nail dystrophy due to lichen planus. *Transact St John Hosp Dermatol Soc* 1972;58:93–97.

106. Scott MJ Jr, Scott MJ Sr. Ungual lichen planus. *Arch Dermatol* 1979;115:1197–1199.

107. Tosti A, de Padova MP, Tuffarelli M, Passarini B, Varotti C. Lichen planus limited to the nails. *Cutis* 1987;40:25–26.

108. Mehregan DA, Van Hale HM, Muller SA. Lichen planopilaris: Clinical and pathologic study of forty-five patients. *J Am Acad Dermatol* 1992;27:935–942.

109. Scher RK, Fischbein R, Ackerman AB. Twenty-nail dystrophy. A variant of lichen planus. *Arch Dermatol* 1978;114:612–613.

110. Samman PD. Idiopathic atrophy of the nails. *Br J Dermatol* 1969;81:746–749.

111. Colver GB, Dawber RPR. Is childhood idiopathic atrophy of the nails due to lichen planus? *Br J Dermatol* 1987;116:709–712.

112. Goettmann S, Zaraa I, Moulonguet I. Nail lichen planus: Epidemiological, clinical, pathological, therapeutic and prognosis study of 67 cases. *J Eur Acad Dermatol Venereol* 2012;26:1304–1309.

113. Tosti A, Piraccini BM, Cameli N. Nail changes in lichen planus may resemble those of yellow nail syndrome. *Br J Dermatol* 2000;142:848–849.

114. Baran R. Lichen planus of the nails mimicking the yellow nail syndrome. *Br J Dermatol* 2000;143:1117–1118.

115. Tosti A, Piraccini BM, Cambiaghi S, Jorizzo M. Nail lichen plansu in children: Clinical features, response to treatment, and long-term follow-up. *Arch Dermatol* 2001;137:1027–1032.

116. Lowe NJ, Cudworth AG, Woodrow JC. HL-A antigens in lichen planus. *Br J Dermatol* 1976;95:169–171.

117. Copeman PWM, Tan RSH, Timlin D, Samman PD. Familial lichen planus. Another disease or a distinct people? *Br J Dermatol* 1978;98:573.

118. Evans AV, Roest MA, Fletcher CL, Lister CL, Hay RJ. Isolated lichen planus of the toe nails treated with oral prednisolone. *Clin Exp Dermatol* 2001;26:412–414.

119. Piraccini BM, Saccani E, Starace M, Balestri R, Tosti A. Nail lichen planus: Response to treatment and long-term follow-up. *Eur J Dermatol* 2010;20:489–496.

120. Ujiie H, Shabki A, Akiyama M, Shimizu H. Successful treatment of nail lichen ruber planus with topical tacrolimus. *Acta Derm Venereol* 2010;90:218–219.

121. Pinter A, Pätzold S, Kaufmann R. Lichen planus of nails—Successful treatment with alitretinoin. *J German Soc Dermatol* 2011;9:1033–1034.

122. Irla N, Schneiter T, Haneke E, Yawalkar N. Nail lichen planus: Successful treatment with etanercept. *Case Rep Dermatol* 2010;2:173–176.

123. Saurat JH, Gluckman E. Lichen planus-like eruption following bone marrow transplantation, a manifestation of the graft-versus-host disease. *Clin Exp Dermatol* 1977;2:335–344.

124. Liddle BJ, Cowan MA. Lichen planus-like eruption and nail changes in a patient with graft-versus-host-disease. *Br J Dermatol* 1990;122:841–843.

125. Aloi FG, Colonna SM, Manzoni R. Associazione di lichen ruber planus, alopecia areata, vitiligine. *G Ital Dermatol Venereol* 1987;122:197–200.

126. Kanwar AJ, Ghosh S, Thami GP, Kasur S. Twenty nail dystrophy due to lichen planus in a patient with alopecia areata. *Clin Exp Dermatol* 1993;18:293–294.

127. Zaias N. The nail in lichen planus. *Arch Dermatol* 1970;101:264–271.

128. Tosti A, Peluso AM, Fanti PA, Piraccini BM. Nail lichen planus. Clinical and pathological study of 24 patients. *J Am Acad Dermatol* 1993;28:724–730.

129. Juhlin L, Baran R. Longitudinal melanonychia after healing of lichen planus. *Acta Derm-Venereol* 1989;69:338–339.

130. Oberste-Lehn H, Kühl M. Lichen planus pemphigoides mit Ulzerationen und Anonychie. *Z Haut GeschlKr* 1954;17:195–199.

131. Weidner F, Ummenhofer B. Lichen ruber ulcerosus (dystrophicans). *Z Hautkr* 1979;54:1008–1017.

132. Haneke E. Isolated bullous lichen planus of the nails mimicking yellow nail syndrome. *Clin Exp Dermatol* 1983;8:425–428.

133. Brun P, Baran R, Desbas C, Czernielewski J. Dystrophie lichénienne isolée des 20 ongles. Etude en immunofluorescence par les anticorps monoclonaux. Conséquences pathologiques. *Ann Dermatol Vénéréol* 1985;112:215.

134. Sellheyer K, Nelson P. The ventral proximal nail fold: Stem cell niche of the nail and equivalent to the follicular bulge—A study on developing human skin. *J Cutan Pathol* 2012;39:835–843.

135. Büchner SA, Itin P, Rufli T, Hungerbühler U. Disseminated lichenoid papular dermatosis with nail changes in acquired immunodeficiency syndrome: Clinical, histological and immunohistochemical considerations. *Dermatologica* 1989;179:99–101.

136. Lambert DR, Siegle RJ, Camisa C. Lichen planus of the nail presenting as a tumor. *J Dermatol Surg Oncol* 1988;14:1245–1247.

137. Kossard S, Cornish N. Localized lichen sclerosus with nail loss. *Australas J Dermatol* 1998;39:119–120.

138. Norton LA. Diseases of the nails. In: Conn HF, ed. *Current Therapy.* Philadelphia: WB Saunders. 1982:664.

139. Patrizi A, Neri I, Fiorentini C, Bonci A, Ricci G. Lichen striatus: Clinical and laboratory features of 115 children. *Pediat Dermatol* 2004;21:197–204.

140. Baran R, Dupré A, Lauret P, Puissant A. Le lichen striatus onychodystrophique. A propos de 4 cas avec revue de la littérature. *Ann Dermatol Vénéréol* 1979;106:885–891.

141. Karp DL, Cohen BA. Onychodystrophy in lichen striatus. *Ped Dermatol* 1993;10:359–362.

142. Al-Niaimi FA, Cox NH. Unilateral lichen striatus with bilateral onychodystrophy. *Eur J Dermatol* 2009;19:511.

143. Sandreva T, Bygum A. Lichen striatus with nail abnormality is a self-limiting condition. *(Dan) Ugeskr Læger* 2012;174:652–653.

144. Niren NM, Waldman GD, Barski S. Lichen striatus with onychodystrophy. *Cutis* 1981;27:610–613.

145. Taieb A, El Youbi A, Grosshans E, Maleville J. Lichen striatus: A Blaschko linear acquired inflammatory skin eruption. *J Am Acad Dermatol* 1991;25:637–642.

146. Keegan BR, Kamino H, Fangman W, Shin HT, Orlow SJ, Schaffer JV. "Pediatric Blaschkitis": Expanding the spectrum of childhood acquired Blaschko-linear dermatoses. *Pediatr Dermatol.* 2007;24:621–627.

147. Grosshans EM. Acquired blaschkolinear dermatoses. *Am J Med Genet* 1999;85:334–337.

148. Monteagudo B, Cabanillas M, Suárez-Amor O, Ramírez-Santos A, Alvarez JC, de Las Heras C. Adult blaschkitis (lichen striatus) in a patient treated with adalimumab. *Actas Dermosifiliogr* 2010;101:891–892.

149. Johnson M, Walker D, Galloway W, Gardner JM, Shalin SC. Interface dermatitis along Blaschko's lines. *J Cutan Pathol* 2014;41:950–954.

150. Tosti A, Peluso AM, Misciali C, Cameli N. Nail lichen striatus: Clinical features and long term follow up. *J Am Acad Dermatol* 1997;36:906–913.

151. Herd RM, McLaren KM, Aldridge RD. Linear lichen planus and lichen striatus—Opposite ends of a spectrum. *Clin Exp Dermatol* 1993;18:335–337.

152. Gianotti R, Restano L, Grimalt R, Berti E, Alessi E, Caputo R. Lichen striatus—Chameleon: A histopathological and immunohistological study of forty-one cases. *J Cutan Pathol* 1995;22:18–22.

153. Zhang Y, McNutt NS. Lichen striatus. Histological, immunohistochemical and ultrastructural study of 37 cases. *J Cutan Pathol* 2001;28:65–71.

154. Muñoz MA, Pérez-Bernal AM, Camacho FM. Lichenoid drug eruption following the Blaschko lines. *Dermatology* 1996;193:66–67.

155. Altman J, Mehregan AH. Inflammatory linear verrusose epidermal nevus. *Arch Dermal* 1971; 104:385–389.

156. Laugier P, Olmos L. Naevus linéaire inflammatoire et lichen striatus. Deux aspects d'une même affection. *Bull Soc Franc Dermatol Syph* 1976;83:48–53.

157. Landwehr AJ, Starink TM. Inflammatory linear verrucous epidermal naevus, report of a case with bilateral distribution and nail involvement. *Dermatologica* 1983;166:107–109.

158. Rahbari H, Cordero AA, Mehregan AH. Linear porokeratosis. *Arch Dermatol* 1974;109:526–528.

159. Waisman M, Waisman M. Lichen aureus. *Arch Dermatol* 1976;112:696–697.

160. Palleschi GM, Giacomelli A, Falcos D. Lichen aureus acrale bilaterale. *G Ital Dermatol Venereol* 1995;130:271–274.

161. Aoki M, Kawana S. Lichen aureus. *Cutis* 2002;69:145–148.

162. Watts RA, Carruthers DM, Scott DGI. Isolated nail fold vasculitis in rheumatoid arthritis. *Ann Rheum Dis* 1995;54:927–929.

163. Munro CS, Cox NH, Marks JM, Natarajan S. Lichen nitidus presenting as palmoplantar hyperkeratosis and nail dystrophy. *Clin Exp Dermatol* 1993;18:381–383.

164. Bettoli V, De Padova MP, Corazza M, Virgili A. Generalized lichen nitidus with oral and nail involvement in a child. *Dermatology* 1997;194:367–369.

165. Fanti PA, Tosti A, Morelli R, Bardazzi F. Lichen planus of the nails with giant cells: Lichen nitidus? *Br J Dermatol* 1991;125:194–195.

166. Fritsch P. Lichen nitidus (Pinkus). *Z Haut Geschlechtskr* 1967;42:649–666.

167. Wanscher B, Thormann J. Permanent anonychia after Stevens–Johnson syndrome. *Arch Dermatol* 1977;113:970.

168. Moisidis C, Möbius V. Erythema multiforme major following docetaxel. *Arch Gynec Obstet* 2005;271:267–269.

169. Assier H, Bastuji-Garin S, Revuz J, Roujeau JC. Erythema multiforme with mucous membrane involvement and Stevens–Johnson syndrome are clinically different disorders with distinct causes. *Arch Dermatol* 1995;131:539–543.

170. Sotozono C, Ueta M, Koizumu N, Inatomi T, Shirakata Y, Ikezawa Z, Hashimoto K, Kinoshita S. Diagnosis and treatment of Stevens–Johnson syndrome and toxic epidermal necrolysis with ocular complications. *Ophthalmology* 2009;116:685–690.

171. Fellahi A, Zouhair K, Amraoui A, Benchikhi H. Sequelles cutanéo-muqueuses et oculaires des SJS et de Lyell. *Ann Dermatol Venereol* 2011;138:88–92.

172. Magina S, Lisboa C, Leal V, Palmares J, Mesquita-Guimarães J. Dermatological and ophthalmological sequels in toxic epidermal necrolysis. *Dermatology* 2003;207:33–36.

173. Baran R, Perrin C. Nail degloving, a polyetiologic condition with 3 main patterns: A new syndrome. *J Am Acad Dermatol* 2008;58:232–237.

174. Lyell A. A review of toxic epidermal necrolysis in Britain. *Br J Dermatol* 1967;79:662–672.

175. Hansen RC. Blindness, anonychia and mucosal scarring as sequelae of the Stevens–Johnson syndrome. *Ped Dermatol* 1984;1:298–300.

176. Kim SJ, Choi JM, Kim JE, Cho BK, Kim DW, Park HJ. Clinicopathologic characteristics of cutaneous chronic graft-versus-host diseases: A retrospective study in Korean patients. *In J Dermatol* 2010;49:1386–1392.

177. Kaposi M. Lichen ruber moniliformis. *Vjsch Dermatol* 1886;13:571–582.

178. Kaposi M. Lichen ruber acuminatus und Lichen ruber planus. *Arch Dermatol* 1895;31:1–32.

179. Piñol Aguadé J, De Asprer J, Ferrando J. Lichenoid tri-keratosis (Kaposi-Bureau-Barrière-Grupper). *Dermatologica* 1974;148:179–188.

180. Duperrat B, Carton FX, Denoeux JP, Locquet MC, Miller M. Kératose lichénoide striée. *Ann Dermatol Vénéréol* 1977;104:564–566.

181. Margolis MG, Cooper GA, Johnson SAM. Keratosis lichenoides chronica. *Arch Dermatol* 1972;105:739–743.

182. Böer A. Keratosis lichenoides chronica: Proposal of a concept. *Am J Dermatopathol* 2006;28:260–275.

183. Baran R. Nail changes in keratosis lichenoides chronica are not a variant of lichen planus. *Br J Dermatol* 1983;109:43–46.

184. Panizzon R, Baran R. Keratosis lichenoides chronica. *Akt Dermatol* 1981;7:6–9.

185. Baran R, Panizzon R, Goldberg LH. Nails in keratosis lichenoides chronica, characteristics and response to treatment. *Arch Dermatol* 1984;120:1471–1474.

186. Lombardo GA, Annessi G, Baliva G, Monopoli A, Girolomoni G. Keratosis lichenoides chronica. Report of a case associated with B-cell lymphoma and leg panniculitis. *Dermatology* 2000;201:261–264.

187. Samlaska CP, Sandberg GD, Maggio KL, Sakas EL. Generalized perforating granuloma annulare. *J Am Acad Dermatol* 1992;27:319–322.

188. Ayoub N, Charuel JL, Diemert MC, Barete S, André M, Fermand JP, Piette JC, Francès C. Antineutrophil cytoplasmic antibodies of IgA class in neutrophilic dermatoses with emphasis on erythema elevatum diutinum. *Arch Dermatol* 2004;140:931–936.

189. Shimizu S, Nakamura Y, Togawa Y, Kamada N, Kambe N, Matsue H. Erythema elevatum diutinum with primary Sjögren syndrome associated with IgA antineutrophil cytoplasmic antibody. *Br J Dermatol* 2008;159:733–735.

190. Crichlow SM, Alexandroff AB, Simpson RC, Saldanha G, Walker S, Harman KE. Is IgA antineutrophil cytoplasmic antibody a marker for patients with erythema elevatum diutinum. A further three cases demonstrating this association. *Br J Dermatol* 2011;164:675–677.

191. Soubeiran E, Wacker J, Hausser I, Hartschuh W. Erythema elevatum diutinum with unusual clinical appearance. *J German Soc Dermatol* 2008;6:303–305.

192. Futei Y, Knohara I. A case of erythema elevatum diutinum associated with B-cell lymphoma: A rare distribution involving palms, soles and nails. *Br J Dermatol* 2000;142:116–119.

193. El Fekih N, Belgith I, Fazaa B, Remmah S, Zéglaoui F, Zermani R, Kamoun MR. Erythema elevatum diutinum: An "idiopathic" case. *Dermatol Online J* 2011;17(7):7.

194. Navarro R, de Argila D, Fraga J, García-Diez A. Erythema elevatum diutinum or extrafacial granuloma faciale? *Actas Dermosifiliogr* 2010;101:814–815.

195. Ziemer M, Koehler MJ, Weyers W. Erythema elevatum diutinum—A chronic leukocytoclastic vasculitis microscopically indistinguishable from granuloma faciale? *J Cutan Pathol* 2011;38:876–883.

196. Tomasini C, Zeia S, Dapovo P, Soro E, Addese C, Pippione M. Infantile erythema elevatum diutinum: Report of a vesiculo-bullous case. *Eur J Dermatol* 2006;16:683–686.

197. Fardet L, Dupuy A, Gain M, Kettaneh A, Chérin P, Bachelez H, Dubertret L, Lebbe C, Morel P, Rybojad M. Factors associated with underlying malignancy in a retrospective cohort of 121 patients with dermatomyositis. *Medicine (Baltimore)* 2009;88:91–97.

198. De Angelis R, Cutolo M, Gutierrez M, Bertolazzi C, Salaffi F, Grassi W. Different microvascular involvement in dermatomyositis and systemic sclerosis. A preliminary study by a tight videocapillaroscopic assessment. *Clin Exp Rheumatol* 2012;30(Suppl 71) S67–70.

199. Samitz MH. Cuticular changes in dermatomyositis. *Arch Dermatol* 1974;110:866–867.

200. Ekmekci TR, Ucak S, Aslan K, Koslu A, Altuntas Y. Exaggerated changes in a patient with dermatomyositis. *J Eur Acad Dermatol* 2005;19:135–136.

201. Jorizzo JL, Gonzalez EB, Daniels JC. Red lunulae in a patient with rheumatoid arthritis. *J Am Acad Dermatol* 1983:711–714.

202. Tunc SE, Ertam I, Pirildar T, Turk T, Ozturk M, Doganavsargil E. Nail changes in connective tissue diseases: Do nail changes provide clues for the diagnosis? *J Eur Acad Dermatol Venereol* 2007;21:497–503.

203. Caputo R, Cappio F, Rigoni C, Scarabelli G, Toffolo P, Spinelli G, Crosti C. Pterygium inversum unguis. Report of 19 cases and review of the literature. *Arch Dermatol* 1993;129:1307–1309.

204. Tosti A, De Padova MP, Fanti P, Bonelli U, Taffurelli M. Unusual severe nail involvement in dermatomyositis. *Cutis* 1987;40:261–262.

205. McBride JD, Sontheimer RD. Proximal nailfold microhemorrhage events are manifested as distal cuticular (eponychial) hemosiderin-containing deposits (CEHD) (syn. Maricq sign) and can aid in the diagnosis of dermatomyositis and systemic sclerosis. *Dermatol Online J* 2016;22(2).

206. Schnitzler L, Baran R, Verret JL. La biopsy du repli sus-unguéal dans les maladies dites du collagène. Etude histologique, ultrastructurale et en immunofluorecence. *Ann Dermatol Vénéréol* 1980;107:777–785.

207. Agrawal OPG, Mahajan SA, Khopkar US, Kharkar V. Gottron-like papules induced by hydroxyurea. *Indian J Dermato Venereol Leprol* 2012;78:775.

208. Urowitz MB, Gladman DD, Chalmers A, Ogryzlo MA. Nail lesions in systemic lupus erythematosus. *J Rheumatol* 1978;5:441–447.

209. Obermoser G, Sontheimer RD, Zelger B. Overview of common, rare and atypical manifestations of cutaneous lupus erythematosus and histopathological correlates. *Lupus* 2010;19:1050–1070.

210. Matsumura M, Suzuki Y, Yamagishi M, Kawano M. Prominent ridged nail deformity in systemic lupus erythematosus. *Intern Med* 2012;51:1283–1284.

211. Kint A, Van Herpe L. Ungual anomalies in lupus erythematosus discoides. *Dermatologica* 1976;153:298–302.

212. Heller J. Lupus erythematodes der Nägel. *Dermatol Z* 1906;13:613–615.

213. Berger E, Robinson M, Patel R, Franks Jr AG. Koebner phenomenon to heat in cutaneous (discoid) lupus erythematosus (lupus ab-igne). *Dermatol Online J* 2012;18(12):17.

214. Trüeb RM. Involvement of scalp and nails in lupus erythmatosus. *Lupus* 2010;19:1078–1086.

215. Wollina U, Barta U, Uhlemann C, Oelzner P. Lupus erythematosus-associated red lunula. *J Am Acad Dermatol* 1999;41:419–421.

216. Kapadia N, Haroon TA. Cutaneous manifestations of SLE. *Int J Dermatol* 1996;35:408–409.

217. Hashimoto H, Tsuda H, Takasaki Y. Digital ulcers/gangrene and immunoglobulin classes complement fixation of anti-dsDNA in systemic lupus erythematosus. *J Rheumatol* 1983;10:727–732.

218. Cardinali C, Caproni M, Bernacchi E, Amato L, Fabbri P. The spectrum of cutaneous manifestations in lupus erythematosus—The Italian experience. *Lupus* 2000;9:417–423.

219. Kuhn A, Sticherling M, Bonsmann G. Clinical manifestations of cutaneous lupus erythematosus. *J Dtsch Dermatol Ges* 2007;5:1124–1137.

220. Bouaziz JD, Barete S, Le Pelletier F, Amoura Z, Piette JC, Francès C. Cutaneous lesions of the digits in systemic lupus erythematosus: 50 cases. *Lupus* 2007;16:163–167.

221. Hutchinson J. Harveian lectures on lupus: The varieties of common lupus. *BMJ* 1888;1:58–63.

222. Millard LG, Rowell NR. Chilblain lupus erythematosus (Hutchinson). *Br J Dermatol* 1978;98:497–506.

223. Sifuentes Giraldo WA, Ahijón Lana M, García Villanueva MJ, González García C, Vázquez Diaz M. Chilblain lupus induced by TNF-α antagonists: A case report and literature review. *Clin Rheumatol* 2012;31:563–568.

224. Günther C, Meurer M, Stein A, Viehweg A, Lee-Kirsch MA. Familial chilblain lupus—A monogenic form of cutaneous lupus erythematosus due to a heterozygous mutation in TREX1. *Dermatology* 2009;219:162–166.

225. Mackie RM. Lupus erythematosus associated with finger clubbing. *Br J Dermatol* 1973;89:533–535.

226. Sannicandro F. Contributo alla conoscenza clinica ed istologica del lupus eritematoso cronico del complesso ungueale. *Min Dermatol* 1960;35:32–34.

227. Giacomel J, Zalaudek I, Argenziano G, Lallas A. Dermoscopy of hypertrophic lupus erythematosus and differentiation from squamous cell carcinoma. *J Am Acad Dermatol* 2015;72(1 Suppl):S33–36.

228. Shah K, Kazlouskaya V, Lal K, Molina D, Elston DM. Perforating elastic fibers ('elastic fiber trapping') in the differentiation of keratoacanthoma, conventional squamous cell carcinoma and pseudocarcinomatous epithelial hyperplasia. *J Cutan Pathol* 2014;41:108–112.

229. Kolivras A, Aeby A, Crow YJ, Rice GI, Sass U, André J. Cutaneous histopathological findings of Aicardi-Goutières syndrome, overlap with chilblain lupus. *J Cutan Pathol* 2008;35:774–778.

230. Martins CR, Squiquera HL, Diaz LA. Pemphigus vulgaris and pemphigus foliaceus. *Curr Probl Dermatol* 1989;1:33–61.

231. Serratos BD, Rashid RM. Nail disease in pemphigus vulgaris. *Dermatol Online J* 2009;15:2.

232. Azulay RD. Brazilian pemphigus foliaceus. *Int J Dermatol* 1982;21:122–124.

233. Habibi M, Mortazavi H, Shadianloo S, Balighi K, Ghodsi SZ, Daneshpazhooh M, Valikhani M, Ghassabian A, Pooli AH, Chams-Davatchi C. Nail changes in pemphigus vulgaris. *Int J Dermatol* 2008;47:1141–1144.

234. Schlesinger N, Katz M, Ingber A. Nail involvement in pemphigus vulgaris. *Br J Dermatol* 2002;146:836–839.

235. Engineer L, Norton LA, Ahmed AR. Nail involvement in pemphigus vulgaris. *J Am Acad Dermatol* 2000;43:529–535.

236. Lieb J, Levitt J, Sapadin AN. Nail findings in pemphigus vulgaris. *Int J Dermatol* 2006;45:172–174.

237. Apalla Z, Chaidemenos G, Karakatsanis G. Nail unit involvement during severe initial pemphigus vulgaris development. *Eur J Dermatol* 2009;19:290–291.

238. Cahali JB JB, Kakuda EY, Santi CG, Maruta CW. Nail manifestations in pemphigus vulgaris. *Rev Hosp Clin Fac Med São Paulo* 2002;57:229–234.

239. Laffitte E, Panizzon RG, Borradori L. Orodigital pemphigus vulgaris: A pathogenic role of anti-desmoglein-3 autoantibodies in pemphigus paronychia? *Dermatology* 2008;217:337–339.

240. Lee HE, Wong WR, Lee MC, Hong HS. Acute paronychia heralding the exacerbation of pemphigus vulgaris. *Int J Clin Pract* 2004;58:1174–1176.

241. Patsatsi A, Sotiriou E, Devliotou-Panagiotidou D, Sotiriadis D. Pemphigus vulgaris affecting 19 nails. *Clin Exp Dermatol* 2009;34:202–205.

242. Baumal A, Robinson MJ. Nail bed involvement in pemphigus vulgaris. *Arch Dermatol* 1973;107:751.

243. De Berker D, Dolziel K, Dawber RPR, Wojnarowski F. Pemphigus associated with nail dystrophy. *Br J Dermatol* 1993;129:461–464.

244. Rivera Diaz R, Alonso Llamazares J, Rodriguez Peralto JL, Sebastian Vanaclocha F, Iglesias Diez L. Nail involvement in pemphigus vulgaris. *Int J Dermatol* 1996;35:581–582.

245. Kolivras A, Gheeraert P, André J. Nail destruction in pemphigus vulgaris. *Dermatology* 2003;206:351–352.

246. Mascarenhas R, Fernandes B, Reis JP, Tellechea O, Figueiredo A. Pemphigus vulgaris with nail involvement presenting with vegetating and verrucous lesions. *Dermatology Online Journal* 2003; 9 (5): 14.

247. Böckers M, Bork K. Multiple gleichzeitige Hämatome der Finger- und Zehennägel mit nachfolgender Onychomadesis bei Pemphigus vulgaris. *Hautarzt* 1987;38:477–478.

248. Szepietowski JC, Różycka B, Baran E. Subungual haemorrhages in fatal pemphigus vulgaris. *J Eur Acad Dermatol Venereol* 2001;15:87–88.

249. Reich A, Wisnicka B, Szepietowski JC. Haemorrhagic nails in pemphigus vulgaris. *Acta Derm Venereol* 2008;88:542.

250. Tosti A, André M, Murrell DF. Nail involvement in autoimmune bullous disorders. *Dermatol Clin* 2011;29:511–512.

251. Jansen T, Plewig G, Anhalt GJ. Paraneoplastic pemphigus with clinical features of erosive lichen planus asociated with Castleman's tumor. *Dermatology* 1995;190:245–250.

252. Czernik A, Camilleri M, Pittelkow MR, Grando SA. Paraneoplastic autoimmune multiorgan syndrome: 20 years after. *Int J Dermatol* 2011;50:905–914.

253. Leroy D, Lebrun J, Maillard V, Mandard JC, Deschamps P. Pemphigus végétant à type clinique de dermatite pustuleuse chronique de Hallopeau. *Ann Dermatol Venereol* 1982;109:549–555.

254. Török L, Husz S, Ócsai H, Krischner Á, Kiss M. Pemphigus vegetans presenting as acrodermatitis continua suppurativa. *Eur J Dermytol* 2003;13:579–581.

255. Lombardi C, Borges PC, Chaul A, Sampaio SA, Rivitti EA, Friedman H, Martins CR, Sanches Júnior JA, Cunha PR, Hoffman RG, Diaz LA. Environmental risk factors in endemic pemphigus foliaceus (fogo selvagem). *J Invest Dermatol* 1992;98:847–850.

256. Fulton RA, Campbell L, Carlyle D, Simpson NB. Nail bed immunofluorescence in pemphigus vulgaris. *Acta Derm-Venereol* 1983;63:170–172.

257. Anhalt GJ, Kim SC, Stanley JR, Korman NJ, Jabs DA, Kory M, Izumi H, Ratrie H 3rd, Mutasim D, Ariss-Abdo L, Labib RS. Paraneoplastic pemphigus: An autoimmune mucocutaneous disease associated with neoplasia. *N Engl J Med* 1990;320:1729–1735.

258. Lever WF. Pemphigus. *Mecidine (Baltimore)* 1953;32:1.

259. De Berker D, Nayar M, Dawber R, Wojnarowska F. Beau's lines in immunobullous disorders. *Clin Exp Dermatol* 1995;20:358–361.

260. Esterly NB, Gotoff SP, Lolekha S, Moore ES, Smith RD, Medenica M, Furey NL. Bullous pemphigoid and membranous glomerulonephropathy in a child. *J Ped* 1973;83:466.

261. Barth JH, Wojnarowska F, Millard PR, Dawber RP. Immunofluorescence of the nail bed in pemphigoid. *Am J Dermatopathol* 1987;9:349–350.

262. Delaporte E, Piette F, Janin A, Cozzani E, Joly P, Thomine E, Nicolas JF, Bergoend H. Pemphigoïde simulant une épidermolyse bulleuse acquise. *Ann Dermatol Venereol* 1995;122:19–22.

263. Namba Y, Koizumi H, Kumakiri M, Hashimoto T, Muramatsu T, Ohkawara A. Bullous pemphigoid with permanent loss of the nails. *Acta Derm Venereol* 1999;79:480–481.

264. Tomita M, Tanei R, Hamada Y, Fujimura T, Katsuoka K. A case of localized pemphigoid with loss of toenails. *Dermatology* 2002;204:155.

265. Gualco F, Cozzani E, Parodi A. Bullous pemphigoid with nail loss. *Int J Dermatol* 2005;44:967–968.

266. Haneke E, Borradori L. Pterygium in bullous pemphigoid. Submitted.

267. Burge SM, Powell SM, Ryan TJ. Cicatricial pemphigoid with nail dystrophy. *Clin Exp Dermatol* 1985;10:472–475.

268. Sinclair RD, Wojnarowska F, Leigh IM, Dawber RP. The basement membrane zone of the nail. *Br J Dermatol* 1994;131:499–505.

269. Nakamura E, Taniguchi H, Ohtaki N. A case of crusted scabies with a bullous pemphigoid-like eruption and nail involvement. *J Dermatol* 2006;33:196–201.

270. Meissner C, Hoefeld-Fegeler M, Vetter R, Bellutti M, Vorobyev A, Gollnick H, Leverkus M. Severe acral contractures and nail loss in a patient with mechano-bullous epidermolysis bullosa acquisita. *Eur J Dermatol* 2010;20:543–544.

271. Gupta R, Woodley DT, Chen M. Epidermolysis bullosa acquisita. *Clin Dermatol* 2012;30:60–69.

272. Ohtsuka T. The relation between nailfold bleeding and capillary microscopic abnormalities in patients with connective tissue diseases. *Int J Dermatol* 1998;37:23–26.

273. Maeda M, Kachi H, Tagaki H, Kitajima Y. Hemorrhagic patterns in the cuticles distal to the proximal nail folds in the fingers of patients with systemic scleroderma. *Eur J Dermatol* 1997;7:191–196.

274. Ghosh SK, Bandyopadhyay D, Saha I, Barua JK. Mucocutaneous and demographic features of systemic sclerosis: A profile of 46 patients from Eastern India. *Indian J Dermatol* 2012;57:201–205.

275. Barr WG, Robinson JA. Systemic sclerosis and digital gangrene without scleroderma. *J Rheumatol* 1988;15:875–877.

276. Tunc SE, Ertam I, Pirildar T, Türk T, Öztürk M, Doganavsargil E. Nail changes in connective tissue diseases: Do nail changes provide clues for the diagnosis? *J Eur Acad Dermatol Venereol* 2007;21:497–503.

277. Andreu-Barsoain M, Pinedo-Moraleda F, Gómez de la Fuente E, Almódovar-González R, Pampin-Franco A, López-Estebaranz JL. Systemic sclerosis after silicone injections for facial cosmetic surgery. *J Eur Acad Dermatol Venereol* 2015;29:1644–1645.

278. Von Bierbrauer AF, Mennel HD, Schmidt JA, von Wichert P. Intravital microscopy and capillaroscopically guided nail fold biopsy in scleroderma. *Ann Rheuma Dis* 1996;55:305–310.

279. Maeda M, Matubara K, Kachi H, Mori S, Kitajima Y. Histopathological and capillaroscopical features of the cuticles and bleeding clots in ring or middle fingers of systemic scleroderma patients. *J Dermatol Sci* 1995;10:35–41.

280. Scher RK, Tom DW, Lally EV, Bogaars HA. The clinical significance of periodic acid-Schiff-positive deposits in cuticle-proximal nailfold biopsy specimens. *Arch Dermatol* 1985;121:1406–1409.

281. Oiso N, Kurokawa I, Tsuruta D, Narita T, Chikugo T, Tsubura A, Kimura M, Baran R, Kawada A. The histopathological feature of the nail isthmus in an ectopic nail. *Am J Dermatopathol* 2011;33:841–844.

282. Oiso N, Narita T, Tsuruta D, Kawara S, Kawada A. Pterygium inversum unguis: Aberrantly regulated keratinization in the nail isthmus. *Clin Exp Dermatol* 2009;34:e514–e515.

283. Oiso N, Kurokawa I, Kawada A. Nail isthmus: A distinct region of the nail apparatus. *Dermatol Res Pract* 2012;2012:925023.

284. Steff M, Toulemonde A, Croue A, Lemerle E, Le Corre Y, Verret JL. Lichen scléreux acral. *Ann Dermatol Venereol* 2008;135:201–204.

285. Kossard S, Cornish N. Localized lichen sclerosus with nail loss. *Australas J Dermatol* 1998;39:119–120.

286. Ramrakha-Jones VS, Paul M, McHenry P, Burden AD. Nail dystrophy due to lichen sclerosus? *Clin Exp Dermatol* 2001;26:507–509.

287. Noda Cabrera A, Sáez Rodríguez M, García-Bustínduy M, Guimerá Martín-Neda F, Dorta Alom S, Escoda García M, Fagundo González E, Rodríguez García F, Sánchez González R, García Montelongo R. Localized lichen sclerosus et atrophicus of the finger without nail dystrophy. *Dermatology* 2002;205:303–304.

288. Carlson JA, Ng BT, Chen KR. Cutaneous vasculitis update: Diagnostic criteria, classification, epidemiology, etiology, pathogenesis, evaluation and prognosis. *Am J Dermatopathol* 2005;27:504–528.

289. Nandeesh BN, Tirumalae R. Direct immunofluorescence in cutaneous vasculitis: Experience from a referral hospital in India. *Indian J Dermatol* 2013;58:22–25.

290. Grunwald MH, Avinoach I, Amichai B, Halevy S. Leukocytoclastic vasculitis—Correlation between different histologic s tages and direct immunofluorescence results. *Int J Dermatol* 1997;36:349–352.

291. Magro CM, Crowson AN. A clinical and histologic study of 37 cases of immunoglobulin A-associated vasculitis. *Am J Dermatopathol* 1999;21:234–240.

292. Westers-Attema A, van Tubergen A, Plasschaert H, van Marion AM, Frank J, Poblete-Gutiérrez P. Nodular vasculitis in systemic lupus erythematosus. *Int J Dermatol* 2008;47(Suppl 1):3–6.

293. Viseux V, Boulenger A, Jestin B, Plantin P. Transient subungual erythema in a patient with idiopathic Sweet's syndrome. *J Am Acad Dermatol* 2003;49:554–555.

294. Rech G, Balestri R, La Placa M, Magnano M, Girardelli CR. Single nail involvement as first sign of Sweet's syndrome. *Sin Appendage Disord* 2016;2:61–62.

295. Crowson AN, Mihm MC Jr, Magro C. Pyoderma gangrenosum: A review. *J Cutan Pathol* 2003;30:97–107.

296. Weenig RH, Davis MDP, Dahl PR. Skin ulcers misdiagnosed as pyoderma gangrenosum. *N Engl J Med* 2002;347:1412–1418.

297. El-Kehdy J, Haneke E, Karam P. Pyoderma gangrenosum: A misdiagnosis. *J Drugs Dermatol* 2013;12:228–230.

298. Reich A, Maj J, Cisło M, Szepietowski JC. Periungual lesions in pyoderma gangrenosum. *Clin Exp Dermatol* 2009;34:e81–84.

299. Bashir SJ, McGibbon D. Subungual pyoderma gangrensoum complicated by myopathy induced by ciclosporin and tacrolimus. *Clin Exp Dermatol* 2009;530–532.

300. Su DWP, Davis MDP, Weenig RH. Pyoderma gangrenosum: Clinicopathologic correlation and proposed diagnostic criteria. *Int J Dermatol* 2004;43:790–800.

301. Schnetter D, Haneke E. Pyoderma gangraenosum vegetans. Eine zusammenfassende Betrachtung chronisch vegetierender Pyodermien und des Pyoderma gangraenosum. *Hautarzt* 1994;45:635–638.

302. Schnetter D, Haneke E. Pyoderma gangraenosum vegetans. Neue Aspekte in der Differentialdiagnose des Pemphigus vegetans Hallopeau (Pyodermite végétante Hallopeau) und Vorschlag einer neuen Klassifizierung. *Z Hautkr* 1994;69:605–612.

303. Strutton C, Weedon D, Robertson I. Pustular vasculitis of the hands. *J Am Acad Dermatol* 1995;32:192–198.

304. Galaria NA, Junkins-Hopkins JM, Kligman D, James WD. Neutrophic dermatosis of the dorsal hands: Pustular vasculitis revisited. *J Am Acad Dermatol* 2000;43:870–874.

305. Goldman K, Don PC. Adult onset of inflammatory linear verrucous nevus in a mother and her daughter. *Dermatology* 12994;189:170.

306. De Jong EMJG, Rulo HFC, van de Kerkhof PCM. Inflammatory linear verrucous epidermal nevus (ILVEN) versus linear psoriasis: A clinical, histological and immunohistochemical study. *Acta Derm Venereol* 1991;71:343.

307. Chu G-Y, Hu SC-S, Lan C-CE. Unusual presentation of inflammatory linear verrucous epidermal naevus mimicking linear psoriasis successfully treated with oral retinoid. *J Eur Acad Dermatol Venereol* 2015;29:2255–2257.

308. Rahbari H, Cordero AA, Mehregan AH. Linear porokeratosis. *Arch Dermatol* 1974;109:526–528.

Infections and infestations affecting the nail

4

Many of the infections and infestations of the skin are also seen in and around the nail apparatus though to a very variable degree. Their clinical and histopathologic features may be similar or be specific for the nail unit.

4.1 VIRAL INFECTIONS

4.1.1 Herpes simplex

Infections due to herpes simplex virus (HSV) types 1 and 2 are extremely frequent. Whereas HSV1 (human herpes virus 1 or HHV1) is mainly seen in the face, HSV2 (HHV2) is usually called the genital type. In and around the nail apparatus, both types are said to occur in approximately the same frequency in adults whereas in children it is mainly due to HSV 1.[1,2] This hints at a probable orodigital or genitodigital transmission. Thumb and index fingers are most frequently involved, but any finger may be infected; herpes simplex of the toenail unit is exceedingly rare. Even blisters around all fingernails were described.[3] The first episode is usually very painful. After an incubation period of 3 to 7 days and an early visible lymphangitis, a group of clear blisters develops that soon become putrid and are very often mistaken for a bacterial infection; the patients are given antibiotics, the hand is splinted, even the nail may be avulsed.[4,5] This is often repeated for many episodes until the physician recognizes that this is something else and refers the patient to a dermatologist.[6] Healing takes between one and three weeks. Aciclovir shortens the course.[7] Herpetic whitlow is also a professional hazard for physicians[8] and dentists[9] with the risk of spreading herpes simplex to their patients.

4.1.1.1 Histopathology

Biopsies are not performed when the clinical diagnosis is obvious. However, a Tzanck test from the base or margin of an early blister is easily done showing the characteristic multinucleated keratinocytes with "steel-blue to slate-gray" homogenous nuclei.[10] Fluorescence microscopy is also positive for HSV.

Histopathologically, nuclear swelling of the keratinocytes is seen in the beginning. They stain homogeneously gray with some marginal condensation. With further evolution of the lesion, acantholysis and unilocular vesicles appear, mainly in the basal layers. The keratinocytes swell to form balloon cells with homogeneous eosinophilic cytoplasm and loss of desmosomes. Some are multinuclear. When balloon cells rupture, reticular degeneration is seen, predominantly in the periphery and higher epidermal layers forming multilocular vesicles. With time the walls of the ruptured cells disappear and the blister again becomes unilocular. Eosinophilic inclusion bodies, 3–8 μ in diameter and surrounded by a clear halo, are observed in the center of the nuclei of balloon cells. Particularly in herpetic whitlow, neutrophils are present. In the upper dermis, an inflammatory infiltrate is seen, sometimes with vessel wall damage. The thick and resistant horny layer of the periungual skin often prevents the erosion seen early in labial herpes simplex, but the underlying epidermis may finally show full thickness necrosis (Figure 4.1).

In severely immunocompromised patients, ulcerative chronic herpetic whitlow develops.[11] A biopsy from the margin may show an occasional cytopathic effect but a

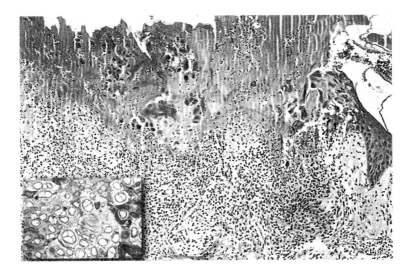

Figure 4.1 Necrotizing digital herpes simplex in an immunocompromised patient exhibiting abundant large keratinocyte nuclei, serous crust formation, and a dense inflammatory infiltrate. (Inset: Semithin section showing multinucleated keratinocytes.)

high degree of suspicion is necessary to make the diagnosis and ask for further investigations such as direct immunofluorescence test, *in situ* hybridization, viral cultures, HSV-specific immunohistochemistry, and PCR, some of which allow the specific HSV type to be determined.

4.1.1.2 Differential diagnosis

The differentiation of HSV from varicella zoster (VZV, HHV3) is not possible by Tzanck smear and histopathology; molecular methods may be necessary. Reticular degeneration may be seen in the vesicles of contact dermatitis. Other types of blistering dactylitis lack the cytopathic effects of viral infections.

4.1.2 Varicella and herpes zoster

Chickenpox and shingles are caused by the varicella zoster virus (VZV) also called HHV3. Varicella is very contagious and characterized by a typical generalized rash of small, often umbilicated blisters in nonimmune persons whereas herpes zoster is due to reactivation of VZV in a cranial or spinal ganglion from where it spreads in the characteristic dermatomal distribution. Some vesicles around the nail may be observed in varicella but this is often overlooked. One case with severe toe involvement was observed.[12] Postvaricella onychomadesis was recently described.[13]

Although herpes zoster may involve the limbs, the vesicle groups rarely extend to the tip of the digits and the nail apparatus. Small vesicles, usually with a hemorrhagic tinge, are seen on the proximal nail fold. Nail bed involvement is particularly painful showing small blood spots under the nail and finally causing transverse leukonychia.[14] In elderly and severely immunocompromised patients, generalized herpes zoster may develop mimicking varicella that are often hemorrhagic and may even become verrucous.[15]

4.1.2.1 Histopathology

Usually biopsies are not performed as the diagnosis is obvious in most cases. A Tzanck test from the base or margin of an early blister characteristically shows multinucleated keratinocytes as in herpes simplex.[9] Fluorescence microscopy is positive for VZV.

Histopathology of herpes simplex, varicella, and herpes zoster is virtually identical. There is an intraepidermal blister featuring keratinocyte necrosis and homogenization of the nuclei with margination of the nucleoplasm. Vacuolization of the cytoplasm, first in the basal cells, then in the entire epidermis, occurs. However, in herpes zoster, there are often more hemorrhage, vessel damage, and microthrombi. A vasculitic pattern is seen in severe herpes zoster. Inclusion bodies may be seen in the endothelial cells in generalized herpes zoster and in neurilemmal cells in localized herpes zoster. A specific antibody against VZV may help to distinguish it from HSV.[16,17] It is also positive in nerve structures of herpes zoster.[18,19]

In severely immunocompromised patients, gangrenous herpes zoster may develop. Without the characteristic epidermal changes, a hemorrhagic vasculitis may be seen.[11] Again,

a high degree of suspicion is necessary to make the correct diagnosis. Direct immunofluorescence test, *in situ* hybridization, viral cultures, VZV-specific immunohistochemistry, and PCR often allow the pathogen to be identified.[20]

4.1.2.2 Differential diagnosis

The differentiation of varicella zoster (VZV, HHV3) from HSV is not possible by Tzanck smear. Histopathology of the epidermal changes is virtually identical, but there is much more inflammation and vessel damage in herpes zoster.

4.1.3 Cytomegalovirus infection

Cytomegalovirus (CMV, HHV5) infection occurs transplacentally in about 1% and another 5% at birth.[21] The prevalence increases with age. Most patients only get a flu-like episode, but the virus remains latent and persistent in many tissues. In immunosuppression, reactivation may occur causing a severe systemic infection.[22] Skin lesions vary considerably from a mild rash to urticarial, vesiculobullous, and keratotic lesions and ulcers.[23] In HIV infected individuals, CMV cytopathic effects may be seen as a chance observation not directly linked to primary pathology. No specific nail changes have been described.

4.1.3.1 Histopathology

Dilated vessels in the dermis may show some enlarged endothelial cells exhibiting a very large eosinophilic inclusion body of about 10 µ in diameter. Commonly a mild perivascular lymphocytic infiltrate is present.[20]

In chronic ulcerative CMV infection, multinucleate cells and chromatolysis occur very similar to other ulcerating herpetic infections.[24]

4.1.3.2 Differential diagnosis

The type of viral inclusion body is unique for CMV. A polyclonal antibody can reveal the viral protein. PCR further helps to make the diagnosis.[25,26]

4.1.4 Kaposi sarcoma–associated virus

Kaposi sarcoma is associated with HHV8. It is dealt with in Chapter 10 on vascular tumors.

4.1.5 Variola

Smallpox was officially declared eradicated in 1977 by the World Health Organization (WHO). However, in the old literature, nail involvement in smallpox was described clinically and histopathologically. Heller[27] cited Virchow who mentioned that a yellowish spot develops when a pustule involves the nail bed whereas the proximal nail fold affection leads to a sharply circumscribed nail defect several weeks later. Complete nail fold destruction permanently disturbs nail formation. The nail is shed when pustules appear in the matrix and nail bed. Onychogryposis was observed as a sequel.

4.1.5.1 Histopathology

Reticular degeneration of the epithelium is prominent whereas ballooning is less pronounced. Balloon cells are few in number, small, and rarely multinucleated.[28] Guarnieri bodies, aggregations of variola virus particles, may be seen in the cytoplasm.

Pustules in the nail matrix were differentiated from the epithelium by a sharp red line of strongly eosinophilic cells tending to develop like epidermal cells until they degenerated.[29]

4.1.5.2 Differential diagnosis

Fortunately, smallpox is no longer seen and certainly nail biopsies would not be performed. A variety of other viral infections also causes ballooning and reticular degeneration, particularly herpes virus infections. The eosinophilic intracytoplasmic Feulgen-positive inclusion bodies are not seen in herpes virus infections, but are a feature of vaccinia, cow pox, and milker's nodule.

4.1.6 Vaccinia

The vaccinia virus was used to vaccinate the population against smallpox with fantastic success. The skin was gently cut superficially to inoculate the virus. Within 4 to 5 days, a papule developed that became vesicular and finally developed into an umbilicated blister healing in approximately 3 weeks with a scab and a characteristic pockmark-like scar. Inadvertent inoculation, usually from a vaccinated person, was rarely seen around the nail.

4.1.6.1 Histopathology

There is a great similarity with herpes simplex and early varicella; however, eosinophilic Feulgen-positive intracytoplasmic inclusions are seen in vaccinia and not in herpes simplex.

4.1.6.2 Differential diagnosis

As vaccination is no longer a clinical routine, one may probably not see a single case in a lifetime.

4.1.7 Cowpox infection

Rodents represent the reservoir of cowpox virus from where the virus may spread to domestic and zoo animals. Infection of humans by this orthopox virus is usually due to inoculation from infected teats during milking, or from pets, particularly cats.[30,31] Hence, face and hands are the main localizations.[30] Clinically, a painful hemorrhagic pustule, ulcer, or eschar develops with surrounding edema, lymphadenopathy, and systemic symptoms. The infection is usually self-limiting; however, in atopic subjects, Darier disease, and immunodeficiency, it may run a fatal course.[32]

4.1.7.1 Histopathology

The histopathological alterations are similar to smallpox with prominent reticular degeneration, but there is more epidermal hyperplasia and less cell necrosis. Neutrophil infiltration and numerous large eosinophilic intracytoplasmic inclusions are seen, consistent with a poxvirus infection. PCR can confirm the diagnosis.[33]

Negative contrast of smear material shows the characteristic brick-shaped morphology under the electron microscope.[34]

4.1.7.2 Differential diagnosis

Based on the presence of reticular degeneration and eosinophilic inclusion bodies in the cytoplasm, the differential diagnosis includes catpox,[35] smallpox, vaccinia (orthopoxvirus infections), orf, and pseudocowpox (both parapoxvirus infections). PCR and serologic tests are necessary to make an exact diagnosis.

4.1.8 Milker's nodule and orf (ecthyma contagiosum)

These two parapoxvirus infections are virtually indistinguishable. Milker's nodule (pseudocowpox virus) is acquired from infected udders, orf (orf virus) from sheep or goats. Whereas milker's nodules often present as multiple lesions, orf is usually solitary. The incubation period is 3–7 days until one or more painful nodular lesions develop that attain a diameter of 1–2 cm. Six clinical stages are seen each lasting approximately 1 week: maculopapular, target, acute weeping, nodular, papillomatous, and finally regressive stage. Involution is without scarring.

4.1.8.1 Histopathology

The parapoxviruses of both conditions are very closely related and their histological differentiation is not possible. There is an acanthotic proliferation of the epidermis with loss of the horny layer, very marked spongiosis and exocytosis of inflammatory cells, necrotic keratinocytes, and also acantholysis. Some ballooning may be seen. Round to oval cytoplasmic inclusion bodies are surrounded by a clear halo; they are called Guarnieri's bodies.[36,37] The inflammatory infiltrate is mixed and contains many erythrocytes.

Systematic studies have shown the different stages of the conditions. Vacuolization in the upper third of the spinous layer is seen in the first stage leading to a multilocular vesicle. Eosinophilic inclusions are present. In the second stage, they are only seen in the surrounding pale ring. Then ballooning with rupture of keratinocytes and acanthosis develops. In the acute weeping stage, the entire epidermis is necrotic and a dense inflammatory infiltrate, which is sometimes lichenoid, is seen sublesionally. The lymphocytes may be very large. Finally, there is re-epidermization with acanthosis of the epithelium, chronic inflammation, and vasodilatation.

4.1.8.2 Differential diagnosis

Ballooning and basophilic intracytoplasmic inclusion bodies in surface and infundibular epidermal keratinocytes are a clue to these barnyard pox infections. Orf and milker's nodules cannot be distinguished histopathologically, but on a molecular biologic basis.[38] Herpes virus infections do not show intracytoplasmic inclusion bodies. When the inflammatory infiltrate is very pronounced and there are large lymphocytes, a lymphoma has to be excluded; this does not show the cytoplasmic viral inclusions.

4.1.9 Molluscum contagiosum

Molluscum contagiosum (MC) is due to an infection of molluscipoxvirus (MCV), which belongs to the poxviridae. The infection is characterized by small round papules, each forming a central crater filled with a waxy plug of cell debris mixed with large numbers of virus particles. MC is most common in young children and teenagers, particularly in atopics. MC in immunocompromised patients results in more numerous and extensive, sometimes tumorous lesions. In immunocompetent patients, a lesion may persist for up to 12 months; however, new lesions may appear during this period, again particularly in atopic subjects. Spontaneous regression of MC lesions is commonly preceded by clinical signs of inflammation, indicating a strong immune response. Localization at the nail is rare.

4.1.9.1 Histopathology

Histopathologically, MC causes a benign epidermal hyperproliferation. This acanthoma has an oval shape with a central superficial indentation, which soon opens to the skin surface. When the basal cells mature they become larger and larger and contain more and more eosinophilic to violet stained inclusion bodies that are also PAS positive. Mature mollusca exhibit very large cells completely filled with these inclusion bodies making the cells rupture. Normally, there is hardly an inflammatory infiltrate. Around the nail with its relatively resistant thick horny layer, opening to the surface of the epidermis may occur late—if at all—giving the molluscum a cystic aspect. With resolution, a dense lymphocytic infiltrate appears at the base of the lesion invading the epidermis and destroying the molluscum, which then heals without a scar.

4.1.9.2 Differential diagnosis

Fully developed mollusca contagiosa are so typical that the diagnosis is obvious; however, tangential sections or early lesions may not show the characteristic inclusions but just a small acanthoma.

4.1.10 Human papillomavirus infections

Human papillomavirus (HPV) infections are extremely common. Approximately 200 different types of HPV are known, of which the types 1, 2, 4, and 7 cause common warts.[39] These are hyperkeratotic acanthopapillomas with a rough grayish surface that tends to split in certain localizations such as around the nail. On the lateral nail folds, they are often oval in shape. Under the nail plate they may mimic a subungual corn, and along the hyponychium they may only present as a hyperkeratotic rim that tends to swell and become white when the digit is immersed in water for 5 or more minutes. Bone erosion causes intense pain.[40,41] The clinical differential diagnosis depends on the age: from 30 years onward, Bowen's disease and squamous cell carcinoma have to be considered;[42] in younger individuals, an exostosis may be similar. Amelanotic melanoma is another serious differential diagnosis. This is the reason why a biopsy or even curettage material should always be submitted for histopathologic examination. In elderly women with hyperextension of the distal phalanx of the hallux, a painful subungual wart-like lesion may be a subungual corn.[43]

4.1.10.1 Histopathology

Most ungual warts are acanthopapillomas with hyperkeratosis that exhibit a fan-like architecture with the superficial portions spreading out (Figure 4.2).[44,45] Parakeratotic columns extend from the tips of the papillomatous surface. They may contain blood inclusions as a consequence of microthromboses in the capillaries that extend high up in the connective tissue papillae. In the upper epidermis, particularly in the granular layer, vacuolar cells are seen with small round nuclei, perinuclear halo, and pale cytoplasm; they are called koilocytes. On the crests of the papillomatous projections, vertical tiers of parakeratotic cells are seen that contain deeply basophilic, round to oval nuclei. Depending on the type of wart, keratohyalin clumping and inclusion bodies may abound. With the duration of the warts, these cytopathic effects decrease and may finally be completely absent in inveterated warts. Particularly between the papillomatous projections, the epidermal cells may enlarge toward the surface and show a trichilemmal type of keratinization.

Myrmecia warts, mainly due to HPV 1, also occur around the nails. They are very rich in inclusion bodies that can be seen throughout the epidermis where they increase in size from the suprabasal to the granular layer. Here they merge, forming inclusion bodies of regular staining but a very irregular shape and surrounding the nuclei with or without a narrow clear perinuclear halo. Often these changes can be followed into the horny layer.

Subungual warts have another architecture. There are koilocytes and some large keratohyaline granules that are round in most cases and of a very different size.

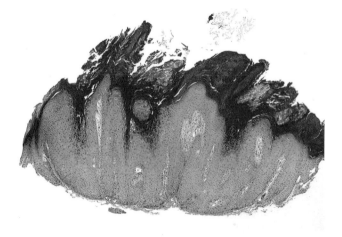

Figure 4.2 Viral wart of the nail fold with the typical fan-like architecture of the papillomatous epidermal projections.

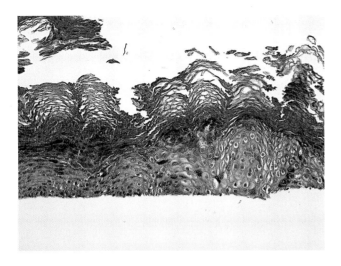

Figure 4.3 Flat wart in a case of epidermodysplasia verruciformis. There are many koilocytes and some large pale keratinocytes.

Hyperkeratosis is not pronounced. The overlying nail plate apparently prevents papillomatosis.

Juvenile plane warts do not occur in the nail region; however, epidermodysplasia verruciformis (EDV) may cause histologically similar changes.[46] The lesions represent flat acanthomas without the papillomatous component of common warts. The granular layer is thickened and the cells are larger with small, mostly centrally located basophilic dense nuclei. Vacuolization of cells in the spinous to the horny layer is characteristic, often the cells are very large and appear swollen with a light blue cytoplasm (Figure 4.3).[47] At least 20 different HPV types have been isolated from EDV patients.[48]

Benign warts share a common HPV antigen that can be demonstrated immunohistochemically[49] and by *in situ* hybridization.[50] PCR allows the HPV types to be further identified;[51] however, in old warts it may be negative.[52]

Infections with high-risk HPVs are dealt with in Chapter 8 on malignant epidermal nail tumors (see Section 8.2).

4.1.10.2 Differential diagnosis

Verrucous hyperplasia is typically seen on an amputation stump and was also observed on three toes of a 62-year-old diabetic subject. There was digitate epidermal hyperplasia with dilated tortuous capillaries in thin dermal papilla without invasive features, mitotic figures, or acanthotic downgrowth. Polymerase chain reaction ruled out a human papilloma virus infection.[53] Epithelioma cuniculatum is a variant of verrucous carcinoma and may occur under the nail. It is usually a bland looking epidermoid lesion with epithelial hyperplasia and deep burrows; virus-characteristic cytopathic effects are not seen.[54] An EDV-like dermatosis was described with similar clinical and histopathologic criteria, but without demonstration of a viral etiology.[55] EDV-associated subungual carcinoma with melanonychia was observed in an African-American patient.[56]

4.1.11 Hand-foot-mouth disease

Hand-foot-mouth disease (HFM) is a relatively common viral infection. Most cases are due to Coxsackie A16 but other enterovirus types may also cause the same disease. Whether some specific types cause a more severe infection is not yet clear. Clinically, there are small blisters on the palms and soles, the long axis of which is arranged parallel to the dermatoglyphics. Similar vesicles with a grayish blister roof and a narrow red margin occur around the nails. The oral lesions of small aphthoid ulcers are similar to those of herpangina, but their distribution is different. The disease occurs in small outbreaks mainly in spring and autumn. Roughly 6 weeks after the vesicular rash, an onychomadesis may be seen in several nails.[57]

4.1.11.1 Histopathology

The blisters are intraepidermal with large pale cells and ballooning in the upper epidermal layers (Figure 4.4). With time, pronounced reticular degeneration develops in the entire epidermis. Giant cells and inclusion bodies are rare. There is edema of the upper dermis and a perivascular lymphocytic infiltrate.[58]

4.1.11.2 Differential diagnosis

All other viral diseases with blistering have to be considered.

4.1.12 Parvovirus infection

Both erythema infectiosum and purpuric gloves and socks syndrome are due to parvovirus infections. Nail involvement is usually not noted by the clinician, particularly in the former. The purpuric gloves and socks syndrome due to parvovirus B 19 shows red palms and soles with some redness around the nails. A variety of other, mainly drug-induced syndromes with red palms and soles have been described. Red palms are also seen in patients with HIV infection. Others may have a periungual erythema[59] or red lunulae.[60]

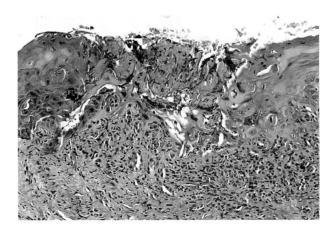

Figure 4.4 Older lesion of an eroded blister in hand-foot-mouth disease with some multinucleated keratinocytes.

4.1.12.1 Histopathology

There is spongiosis in the epidermis with some parakeratotic foci. A discrete perivascular inflammatory infiltrate is seen in the superficial dermis with some extravasated erythrocytes. Immunohistochemically, parvovirus B 19 may be demonstrated in some endothelial cells of the superficial vessels.[20]

4.1.12.2 Differential diagnosis

The pattern of epidermal spongiosis with some parakeratosis and discrete perivascular lymphocytic infiltrate around the superficial vessels is not diagnostic for a single condition and more details are required to reach the correct diagnosis.

4.2 BACTERIAL INFECTIONS

A great number of different bacteria can cause skin and nail infections. Most of them are diagnosed microbiologically as an infection is often thought to be a contraindication for a nail biopsy. Lesions of the nail unit may be direct to the bacterial infection, due to toxin production, immunologically mediated or vasculitic.

Most bacterial infections of the nail apparatus are due to pyogenic cocci, mostly *Staphylococcus aureus* and β-hemolytic streptococci. Enterobacteria may cause both severe infections as well as colonize the nail surface. Bacterial infections of the nail unit may also give rise to severe general infections including sepsis.[61]

4.2.1 Pyogenic infections

Impetigo contagiosa is the most frequent superficial skin infection and mainly seen in children between 2 and 5 years although, in principle, any age may be affected. Heat and humidity favor its outbreak.[62] Approximately 30% of impetigo cases are bullous, which is due to staphylococcal exfoliatin toxins. *Staphylococcus aureus* and, more rarely, β-hemolytic streptococci, are the most common causes of putrid infections of the nail. Around the nail, they give rise to bulla repens (bulla rodens), also called runaround. This starts as a clear blister of the proximal to lateral nail fold, which soon becomes cloudy and yellow. Removal of the blister roof and disinfective baths are usually sufficient for treatment; systemic antibiotics are rarely needed for this superficial infection. The clinical differential diagnoses are burns and congelations as well as other blistering dermatoses.

In staphylococcal scalded syndrome, periungual skin and subungual structures may be involved and lead to complete nail loss.

4.2.1.1 Histopathology

The blister roof may be submitted for histopathologic examination. In contrast to normal bullous impetigo, it shows a relatively thick horny layer, which is the cause for the blister remaining intact for many days. Under it, the superficial epidermis is attached, which is necrotic, a feature also seen in staphylococcal scalded skin. Thus, when

in doubt, the clinician may send in the blister roof for cryostat sections or may even perform a Tzanck smear, which is said to be highly specific and very sensitive. Both at the top and the bottom of the blister, acantholytic necrotic cells are seen. Cytology also reveals acantholytic cells and clusters of gram-positive cocci in bullous impetigo[63] whereas no cocci are seen in staphylococcal scalded skin syndrome as the epidermal necrosis is due to systemic action of the staphylococcal exfoliative toxin.[36] In bulla repens, there is usually a perivascular infiltrate in the upper dermis. Subungual abscesses may develop from secondary infection of subungual blisters (see Chapter 7).

4.2.1.2 Differential diagnosis

Whereas bullous impetigo and pemphigus foliaceus may be difficult to differentiate at other skin sites as both have desmoglein-1 as their target,[64,65] the latter is virtually not seen in the nail unit. In toxic epidermal necrolysis, many digits are involved and the entire epidermis forms the blister roof. There is almost no inflammatory infiltrate in the dermis. Subcorneal pustulosis shows no gram-positive cocci. Herpes simplex exhibits the characteristic keratinocytic giant cells with steel-blue homogenous nuclei.

4.2.2 Blistering distal dactylitis

Blistering distal dactylitis is a rarely diagnosed condition involving the tips of the fingers or toes in children.[66] It can coexist with and may be secondary to clinically imperceptible infections of the nasopharynx, conjunctiva, or anus underlining the need for systemic antibiotic treatment. The blisters appear as whitish-grayish oval areas of 10–30 mm in diameter[67] that soon desquamate and leave a red surface. This soon becomes keratinized again with superficial fissures. Group A beta-hemolytic streptococci are thought to be the cause.[68] It was also observed in association with an ingrown nail.[69] In recent years, several cases were described in adults[70,71] that were due to group B hemolytic streptococci[72] and staphylococci.[73,74] The relation of blistering distal dactylitis to bullous impetigo is not entirely clear.[75]

4.2.2.1 Histopathology

The condition has not been systematically examined by histopathology. The blister is very superficial and its roof consists almost exclusively of the stratum corneum.

4.2.2.2 Differential diagnosis

Bullous impetigo is histologically indistinguishable.

4.2.3 Ecthyma

This is a chronic ulcerative infection due to group A streptococci. It is almost invariably observed on the lower extremities and may rarely involve the dorsum of a toe.

4.2.3.1 Histopathology

There is a punched-out ulcer with sero-putrid exudate containing abundant neutrophils. Under and around the ulcer, the dermis is densely invaded by neutrophils.

4.2.3.2 Differential diagnosis

In ulcerating pyoderma gangrenosum, there are usually overhanging epidermal margins, a central suppurative inflammation with leukocytoclasia, and a peripheral lymphocytic infiltrate.

4.2.4 Erysipelas

Erysipelas is an acute superficial infection of the lymph vessels by group A streptococci. It is predominantly observed on the legs as a slightly indurated red plaque with flame-like extensions proximally thought to represent the lymph vessels. It is often recurring in the same area. In the feet and lower legs, interdigital mycosis or onychomycosis may be the portal of entry for the streptococci. Complications are superficial skin necrosis and progression to deeper tissue with the development of necrotizing fasciitis. Although occurring on the toes, nail involvement of erysipelas is rare.

4.2.4.1 Histopathology

The lymphatic and capillary vessels in the edematous dermis are markedly dilated and there is a diffuse infiltrate of mainly neutrophil leukocytes. Gram and Giemsa stains often show streptococci in the tissue and the lymphatics.

4.2.4.2 Differential diagnosis

All diffuse neutrophilic infiltrates in an edematous tissue have to be considered, but they are negative for cocci.

4.2.5 Erysipeloid

Erysipeloid, also known under the term of swine erysipelas or rouget de porc, is an acute infection caused by the gram-positive bacillus *Erysipelothrix rhusiopathiae*. It is mainly seen as a professional infection in individuals handling meat and fish and is due to an inoculation through a tiny wound or prick by contaminated bones or splinters. Severe systemic symptoms are lacking. Fingers and hands are the primary site of infection in the majority of cases, particularly the index finger and thumb.[76] Periungual localization is frequent and mimics acute to subacute paronychia. Endocarditis[77,78] and septicemia[79] are rare. The treatment of choice is penicillin or cephalosporin.[80]

4.2.5.1 Histopathology

As the synonym swine erysipelas suggests, this infection presents as a subacute mild cellulitis starting as a tender purplish-red nodule that slowly spreads to involve larger skin areas while becoming paler in the center. There is a superficial and deep perivascular dermatitis with edema of the papillary dermis. The pathogen can usually be cultured from a biopsy.

4.2.5.2 Differential diagnosis

Erysipelas is the main differential diagnosis. Seal finger is a mycoplasma infection seen in aquarium workers, veterinarians, and professionals working with seals; it is more painful than erysipeloid, but the erythema is less pronounced.[81–84] Histopathology reveals perivascular infiltration with lymphocytes and plasma cells in the subcutaneous adipose tissue, and a few granulocytes without pus or necrosis. Fibrosis eventually takes place.[85] Involved joints demonstrate a severe inflammatory reaction with chronic granulation tissue and scarring with destruction of the articular cartilage.[86] *Vibrio vulnificus* infection is commonly more acute and characterized by rapid spread of the infection with progressive necrosis of the tendon sheath, subcutaneous tissues, and the skin.[87] A case of cutaneous diphtheria clinically similar to blistering erysipeloid involved the right fourth toe in a 50-year-old woman; the infection by nontoxin producing *Corynebacterium diphtheriae* was acquired in South Asia.[88] Leishmaniasis of the finger was seen to resemble erysipeloid.[89] Subacute parathion intoxication caused a red finger like in erysipeloid.[90]

4.2.6 Pseudomonas infections

Pseudomonas may both colonize and infect the nail organ. The former is seen as a green to greenish-black discoloration of the lateral nail plate portion, often coming out from under the proximal nail fold and with a mild accompanying localized paronychia of the lateral aspect of the proximal nail fold with circumscribed loss of the cuticle. Also oncholytic areas may be colonized with *Pseudomonas aeruginosa*.[91] A true subungual infection looking like a subungual yellowish-green spot may develop. When treated successfully, an onychomadesis or even temporary total loss of the nail plate develops.

4.2.6.1 Histopathology

In green nails, a bacterial biofilm can be seen as a basophilic layer on the undersurface of the nail. In very faintly stained sections, a greenish tinge may be detectable. It is not rare to see an additional fungal infection of the nail in PAS or Grocott stained sections, which is an important aspect for treatment of the condition (Figure 4.5).[92]

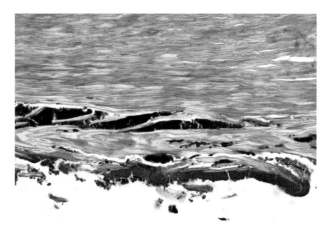

Figure 4.5 A dense agglomerate of bacteria forms a biofilm at the undersurface of the nail plate. In addition to the *Pseudomonas aeruginosa* biofilm, the PAS stain also shows fungal elements.

A subungual *Pseudomonas aeruginosa* infection is characterized by a spongiform abscess involving the epithelium and a very dense neutrophilic infiltrate in the upper and mid-dermis of the matrix and nail bed with a lympho-plasmocytic periphery. Some gram-negative slender short rods may be seen. The surface is eroded.

4.2.6.2 Differential diagnosis

Other subungual abscesses cannot safely be differentiated; bacterial cultures are necessary.

4.2.7 Anthrax

This infection is caused by *Bacillus anthracis*, which is usually contracted from infected livestock, wool, hair, animal skin, during slaughter, or even due to accidental injection.[93] It occurs as a gastrointestinal, pulmonary, or cutaneous infection. It is almost not seen in developed countries but still poses a considerable risk in many countries, particularly in Asia.[94,95] Two-thirds to over 90% of the cases are localized on the hand and fingers.[96] The clue to the diagnosis is a hemorrhagic papule rapidly developing to a pustule and then painless ulcer with surrounding edema after contact with infected animals or material. The diagnosis is usually made from smears and with bacteriologic culture growing an aerobic gram-positive spore-forming rod.[97]

Bacillus megatherium (anthracoides), although held not to be pathogenic for humans, was seen to cause a lesion on the hand very similar to anthrax.

4.2.7.1 Histopathology

In the center of the lesion, the epidermis is necrotic and the ulcerated surface is covered with necrotic debris. The upper dermis is markedly edematous. Under this zone, a dense inflammatory infiltrate is seen with vasculitis and hemorrhage. Gram-positive bacilli about 6–10 µ long and shaped like a bamboo cane are present in large numbers in the necrotic material.

4.2.7.2 Differential diagnosis

A variety of necrotizing inflammations including many infections can exhibit very similar features. The demonstration of the bacilli is necessary to make the diagnosis although when the diagnosis is suspected clinically, a biopsy is usually not taken.

4.2.8 Tularemia

This primary infection of rodents may occasionally be contracted by humans having rabbits, through direct contact with other rodents and carcasses or indirectly by arthropod assaults.[98] The ulceroglandular form also affects the skin. Direct inoculation of *Francisella (Pasteurella) tularensis* into the skin is mainly seen on hands and fingers and may be multiple.[99] It starts as a tender or pruritic papule after an incubation period of 1–10 days getting ulcerated and granulating. A black eschar may appear over time.[100] Subcutaneous nodules may develop along the lymph vessels and lymph node swelling often occurs. Occasionally,

paronychia may develop. Treatment is with chloramphenicol, tetracyclines, or gentamycin.

4.2.8.1 Histopathology

An ulcer with a nonspecific inflammatory infiltrate at its base is seen soon demonstrating a granulomatous component with well-developed tuberculoid granulomas with central necrosis and nuclear dust. Late lesions may resemble sarcoidosis with epithelioid cell granulomas and no necrosis.

4.2.8.2 Differential diagnosis

In the late stage, the lesions are similar to sarcoidosis and other sarcoidal granulomas.

4.2.9 Cat scratch disease

This is an uncommon infection mainly due to scratch injuries and bites by domestic animals, mainly pet cats;[101] it is more frequently seen in veterinary personnel.[102] Hence, fingers, hands, and arms are most frequently involved.[103,104] *Bartonella (Rochalimea) henselae* is the common pathogen, but *B quintana* and *claridgeiae* were also described.[105, 106] The latency period is between one week to one month. The disease usually starts with fever and lymphadenopathy before a papule at the inoculation site appears. Reactive arthritis was observed after a cat bite.[107]

4.2.9.1 Histopathology

The histopathology is not really specific but usually allows a suspect diagnosis. There is a diffuse inflammatory infiltrate associated with many neutrophils and histiocytes as well as scattered eosinophils and plasma cells. The lymph nodes usually show a granulomatous reaction with stellate microabscesses containing many neutrophils in the necrotic material. Warthin-Starry stain may show clumps of silver-impregnated bacilli in the necrosis. Gimenez stain reveals the gram-negative bacilli.[108] PAS is negative. Immunohistochemistry may show the pathogens.[109]

4.2.9.2 Differential diagnosis

Whereas Warthin-Starry stain is usually positive,[110] culture and serology may remain negative.[111] PCR is highly specific but not very sensitive.[112] Bacillary angiomatosis is caused by the same *B. henselae*, but is a disease of immunocompromised subjects.[113] Warthin-Starry stain is technically demanding as silver tends to clump out.

4.3 MYCOBACTERIAL INFECTIONS

Mycobacteria are divided into species growing rapidly or slowly in culture with *Mycobacterium leprae* not growing in culture. In dermatopathology, tuberculosis and leprosy are distinguished from the so-called atypical mycobacterioses. *M. tuberculosis* including *M. bovis* and *M. leprae* are intracellular bacilli requiring contact with infected people or animals for transmission. Virtually all mycobacteria are weakly gram positive and resist decoloration by acid. As a whole, mycobacterial infections of the nails are rare.

4.3.1 Tuberculosis

Tuberculosis once thought to be a decreasing problem is again on the rise. Immigration from and travels to endemic countries, poverty, declining health care, insufficient treatment of manifest tuberculosis, and drug resistance, HIV infection, iatrogenic immunosuppression including treatment with TNF-α inhibitors all contribute to the rise of tuberculosis. Direct inoculation, hematogenous spread, and extension from underlying tissue cause different clinical types that are further modified by the host's immune system. A high index of suspicion is needed to diagnose possible cutaneous mycobacteriosis, and appropriate cultures have to be performed to confirm the diagnosis.[114]

Tuberculosis of the nail apparatus is a rare event in the United States and Europe. Many different forms occur that can both involve the skin and the underlying bone.[115]

4.3.1.1 Tuberculosis cutis verrucosa

Tuberculosis cutis verrucosa is also called prosector's wart or butcher's nodule. It is due to direct inoculation of *M. tuberculosis* or *M. bovis* in a subject with a certain degree of immunity, either due to previous organ tuberculosis or after BCG immunization. Hands and finger are primarily involved in adults. Clinically, a verrucous lesion with a red inflammatory margin is seen that slowly extends peripherally and develops surface fissures from which some pus may be expressed. Usually the previously negative skin test converts to positive.[116–120]

Miliary and primary tuberculosis of the skin due to inoculation in a nonimmune individual was not described in the nail apparatus.

4.3.1.1.1 Histopathology

The epidermis is acanthotic and hyperkeratotic. Subepidermally, a dense inflammatory infiltrate is seen, often with small abscesses that may also be seen intraepidermally; often there is the impression of transepidermal elimination of abscesses. In the mid- and deep dermis, tuberculoid granulomas are seen that exhibit some necrosis. *M. tuberculosis* is rarely found in Ziehl-Neelsen stain; thus, an attempt at culturing the organism is indicated.

4.3.1.1.2 Differential diagnosis

All verrucous lesions including common warts, deep mycoses, and Bowen's disease have to be considered. A PPD test may be performed that becomes positive in the previously negative individuals.

4.3.1.2 Tuberculosis cutis luposa

This type of skin tuberculosis is also called lupus vulgaris. Most lesions occur in cool regions of the body, for instance the face, nose, and ears. One or a few well-circumscribed reddish-brown lesions are seen that tend to ulcerate. Pressing on such a lesion with a glass slide makes the blood disappear and an apple jelly color is seen. The chronic lesion tends to ulcerate anew in the old cicatricial areas leading to mutilation (which gave the name to the disease: lupus [Latin] wolf—thus devouring skin disease). Over time, squamous cell carcinoma may develop in long-standing lupus vulgaris. It is apparently very rare in the nail apparatus.[121]

4.3.1.2.1 Histopathology

The hallmark of lupus vulgaris is the presence of tuberculoid granulomas composed of epithelioid and giant cells of the Langhans type. These granulomas are embedded in a dense lymphocytic infiltrate. Caseation necrosis in the granulomas is not pronounced. Healing is seen with fibrosis. Cutaneous adnexa are destroyed by the infiltrate. Depending on the localization, there may be secondary epidermal changes; atrophy is mainly seen in the face whereas acanthosis and hyperkeratosis are characteristic for acral sites.

M. tuberculosis is exceptionally rare in the lesions and PCR may be required. PPD testing is strongly positive as this is usually due to mycobacteria from an internal tuberculosis.

4.3.1.2.2 Differential diagnosis

Syphilitic gumma is characterized by a granulomatous inflammation with central acellular necrosis. In contrast to lupus vulgaris, nodular tertiary syphilis does not reappear in old lesions. Scattered granulomas are seen in the dermis with islands of epithelioid cells, lymphocytes, and plasma cells, but little necrosis and few giant cells.

4.3.1.3 Scrophuloderma

Tuberculosis scrophulosa is the result of direct extension of tuberculosis from the lymph node or bone to the overlying skin. It is first seen as a painless bluish-red swelling, which breaks through the skin to form an ulcer with an irregular border. Once frequent, it is now a rare condition. Scrophuloderma of the nail bed was observed due to osteitis tuberculosa of the terminal phalanx.[60]

4.3.1.3.1 Histopathology

There is an unspecific abscess or ulcer in the center with tuberculoid granulomas at the periphery. The necrosis is extensive. *M. tuberculosis* may be found in Ziehl-Neelsen stained slides.

4.3.1.3.2 Differential diagnosis

Cutaneous tuberculosis can produce a great variety of tissue changes; there may be nonspecific inflammation, non-necrotic and caseating granulomas, abscesses, epidermal hyperplasia, and so on. First and foremost, leprosy and atypical mycobacterial infections have to be ruled out, which often requires cultures and molecular techniques. Sarcoidosis is another classical differential diagnosis. Its granulomas are often "naked," that is, without or with only a few lymphocytes and giant cells may be rare. Necrosis is only seen in the acral location and is fibrinoid instead of caseating. Deep mycoses may cause granulomas that may or may not be suppurating and cause epithelial hyperplasia. Leishmaniasis causes granulomatous infiltrates that harbor intracellular parasites in early lesions and later develop more and more fibrosis and become rich in plasma cells. Tertiary syphilis develops granulomatous infiltrates, which are usually plasma cell rich. Syphilis serology is positive. Immunohistochemistry may also show treponemas.[122–124] However, the antibodies are not highly specific and may show also mycobacteria.[125] Certain foreign body granulomas exhibit central necrosis, such as sea-urchin spines or beryllium.

4.3.2 Leprosy

Leprosy, also called Hansen's disease, is a chronic infection of the skin and nerves due to *Mycobacterium leprae*. It is still found almost worldwide though in Northern and Central Europe most cases are now imported from endemic regions. Depending on host immunity, different types of leprosy develop. For reasons of simplicity, we only differentiate paucibacillary and multibacillary leprosy. It primarily affects the skin and nerves, but nail changes are seen in roughly three-quarters of the patients; however, the vast majority is secondary to neuropathy, repeated trauma, vascular impairment, secondary infections, lepra reactions, and the drugs used to manage the disease.[126] The most commonly observed changes are subungual hematomas, onycholysis, onychauxis, onychogryposis, *pterygium unguis*, nail dystrophy,[127] and onychoheterotopia; most of them can be attributed to nerve damage and trauma. Furthermore, the acro-osteolysis that occurs in the advanced stages of the disease may present with brachyonychia, racquet nails, cutaneous horn-like nail,[128] or even anonychia. Infections of the nail bed, paronychia, and onychomycosis are frequent associations. Longitudinal melanonychia and ridging, pitting, macrolunula, Terry nails,[129] leukonychia, hapalonychia, and Beau's lines are signs of frequent matrix damage.[130] Pterygium inversum is rare.[131] Bilateral fingernail atrophy has also been described and may have been a sign of medial nerve damage.[124] Alternating horizontal bands of whitish and pinkish discoloration of the nail were called the flag sign.[132] In darkly pigmented individuals, melanonychia is extremely frequent. Multibacillary (lepromatous leprosy) cases may have more nail changes[130] though another study found both the frequency and the kind of nail changes not to differ between multibacillary and paucibacillary leprosy except for the flag sign being more frequent in multibacillary leprosy. Factors only associated with lepromatous disease are invasion of the bones of terminal phalanges by lepromatous granulomas and endarteritis occurring during type 2 lepra reactions.[133, 134]

Leprosy research has long been hampered by the lack of adequate means to culture *M. leprae* until it was found to be able to grow in the armadillo. A report of possible *M. leprae* multiplication in the nail bed of a laboratory worker was not confirmed by further observations.[135]

Syringomyelia may cause very similar lesions due to the associated neuropathy.

4.3.2.1 Histopathology

A treatise on nail histopathology is not the place to fully cover all aspects of leprosy. Therefore, the changes seen are only summarily dealt with.

M. leprae is usually demonstrated using a modified Ziehl-Neelsen stain with milder removal of carbol fuchsin called Fite-Faraco stain. Methene amine silver stain is performed to detect fragmented bacilli.

The leprotic skin changes may be very subtle to full blown granulomas. In the earliest and mildest changes (indeterminate leprosy), a predominantly lymphocytic perineurovascular infiltrate is seen. With time, granulomas appear in the mid- and deep dermis, the cells of which characteristically have a foamy cytoplasm and are called Virchow cells. The granulomas are often arranged along cutaneous nerves and thus may show an oval or even longitudinal shape. They have a dense lymphocytic periphery. Giant cells are usually lacking. In lepromatous leprosy, there is a dense diffuse infiltrate composed mainly of epithelioid cells that extends from a narrow free subepidermal zone into the cutaneous fat and destroys the cutaneous adnexa. With time, the macrophages contain more and more bacillary debris. Histoid leprosy has the highest bacillary load and often contains spindled macrophages in a storiform arrangement. To demonstrate the pathogen, immunohistochemistry with antibodies to *M. leprae* and BCG may be used in addition to Fite-Faraco stain.[136] In paucibacillary leprosy, such as tuberculoid leprosy, *M. leprae* is rarely, if ever, found, but in multibacillary leprosy masses of slender pink rods are seen in the granuloma cells and often in cutaneous nerves.

Leprosy reactions are subdivided into types 1 and 2. Type 1 is due to a delayed hypersensitivity to *M. leprae* and may cause severe nerve damage. No nail changes have yet been described. Erythema nodosum leprosum is the type 2 reaction. In this reaction, an obliterative arteritis and endangiitis are observed that lead to circumscribed necrosis in the nail organ, which in turn, causes a pterygium and destruction of the nails.[130] However, by far the most nail changes seen in leprosy are scars due to neural damage with loss of sensibility.

4.3.2.2 Differential diagnosis

Whereas the diagnosis is usually suspected in endemic regions, it may be very difficult to make the correct diagnosis in nonendemic regions and in the paucibacillary forms. The antibodies used for immunohistochemistry are not specific enough to allow the distinction between the various mycobacteria. All other granulomatous infections, particularly those due to acid-fast bacilli, have to be considered. Sarcoidal reactions can also mimic leprosy.

Many of the nonspecific lesions of the nail apparatus are also seen in syringomyelia.

4.3.3 Atypical mycobacteriosis

Infections due to non-tuberculosis (and non-leprosy) mycobacteria are generally called atypical mycobacterioses.

They are relatively rarely observed at the nail organ. Clinically, they usually present as a tender erythematous, sometimes verrucous swelling of the nail fold,[137,138] but may even mimic a herpetic paronychia.[139] Draining may develop and persist for some weeks, sometimes a sporotrichoid pattern of inflammatory nodules along the lymphatic vessels is observed. They are usually acquired while cleaning an aquarium. Treatment often remains unsuccessful, but tetracyclines, minocycline, doxycycline, trimethoprim-sulfamethoxazole, amikacin, and ethambutol plus rifamycin have generally been reported to be successful.[140] Small lesions may be excised.[141] Spontaneous healing has been observed.

An osteomyelitis (osteitis) of the distal phalanx due to *M. avium* complex was described.[142] Other atypical mycobacteria have not yet been described at the nail; however, epidemics of atypical mycobacterial infections of various types had their origin from nail salons.[143–149]

4.3.3.1 Histopathology

The most common atypical mycobacteriosis of the skin around the nail is due to *M. marinum*. It is usually contracted via small lacerations when swimming in a pool or cleaning an aquarium. Histopathology shows an unspecific infiltrate composed of neutrophils, monocytes, and macrophages in the early phase (Figure 4.6). After 3 to 4 months, granulomas with foreign body giant cells, neutrophils, and often some eosinophils are seen, but mycobacteria are often not found in Ziehl-Neelsen stain.[113, 116] Though caseation necrosis is common in the furunculoid lesions of the lower legs from infections in whirlpools of nail salons, this is apparently not the case in *M. marinum* infections.

Culture from biopsy material has to be performed at 30 to 33° and is positive in 3%–30%, PCR in 30%–67%.[150]

Other atypical mycobacterioses have, to our knowledge, not been seen at the nail apparatus.

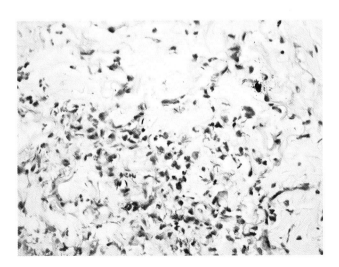

Figure 4.6 *Mycobacterium marinum* infection of the nail fold exhibiting many slender acid-fast rods in the Ziehl-Neelsen stain.

4.3.3.2 Differential diagnosis

The diagnosis requires clinical and histologic suspicion. The various classical and atypical mycobacterial infections cannot be distinguished by histopathology alone but require culture and/or PCR.

4.4 TREPONEMAL DISEASES
4.4.1 Syphilis

Syphilis is caused by *Treponema pallidum*, which belongs to the spirochetes. Syphilis has been observed at the nail unit as a primary chancre, in the second as well as late stages. There are many illustrations of nail involvement in the old literature.

The primary syphilitic chancre develops after direct contact with a contagious lesion, usually through a minor skin break, such as a hangnail. The incubation period is approximately 3 weeks. The ulcer is characteristically painless where enough soft tissue is under it but may be tender or frankly painful when it reaches down to the bone or under the nail plate. When treated adequately it will heal with a barely noticeable scar.

Secondary syphilis under the nail was observed to cause onychomadesis and onychoptosis and later a succulent area over the entire matrix and nail bed.[151,152]

Tertiary syphilis of the nail apparatus is rarely documented.[153]

Nail loss was repeatedly described in congenital syphilis; however, no histopathologic reports are available.[154–157]

4.4.1.1 Histopathology

The syphilitic chancre is a sharply demarcated ulcer with a very plasma cell rich infiltrate in the surrounding dermis. *Treponema pallidum* can usually be found with Warthin-Starry stain and immunohistochemically.

In the second stage, a dense infiltrate mainly of plasmocytes with relatively few lymphocytes is observed. The vessels show endovasculitis obliterans. Leukocytes are migrating into the spongiotic epithelium causing detachment of the nail plate. They may accumulate in the upper epithelium to form a spongiform abscess.[158] These lesions are rich in spirochetes. With time, the proportion of lymphocytes increases and the nail bed exhibits a very marked psoriasiform acanthosis with regular long rete ridges (Figure 4.7).

Tertiary syphilis shows granulomas with central necrosis and many plasma cells in the periphery.

4.4.1.2 Differential diagnosis

Plasma cell rich infiltrates usually raise the suspicion of syphilis or borreliosis. When a spongiform pustule is seen, psoriasis, some other acute bacterial infections as well as acute candidiasis have to be looked for.

4.4.2 Other treponematoses

To our knowledge, no specific nail involvement has been described in frambesia and pinta.

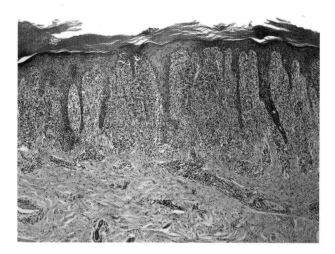

Figure 4.7 Second stage syphilis of the nail bed with psoriasiform acanthosis and a dense plasma cell rich infiltrate. (Courtesy of Dr. A. Ozores, São Paulo, Brazil.)

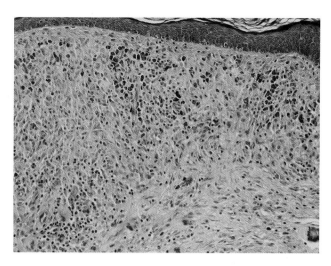

Figure 4.8 Acrodermatitis chronica atrophicans of the distal big toe phalanx of a 67-year-old patient. Giemsa stains the plasma cells a darker blue.

4.4.3 Borreliosis

Borreliosis is a tick-borne infection due to one of the several pathogenic borrelia that belong to the group of treponemas. The main vector in Europe is the tick *Ixodes ricinus*, whereas it is *I. dammini* in North America, but other ticks also harbor borrelias. *Borrelia afzelii* is mainly responsible for the European cases and *B. burgdorferi* is prevalent in North America. The different stages of cutaneous borreliosis have long been known in Europe as erythema chronicum migrans, benign lymphocytoma, or lympadenosis cutis benigna, now also called borrelioma, and acrodermatitis chronica atrophicans. The American type of borreliosis, known as Lyme disease, has a slightly different clinical course and extracutaneous manifestations. Specific nail lesions of borreliosis are not known although one case of painful nail discoloration was thought to be due to a *Borrelia* infection[159] and nail root inflammation was reported in a patient suffering from neuroborreliosis due to *B. garinii*.[160] However, acrodermatitis chronica atrophicans of Herxheimer (ACA) may also involve toes and fingers. An avascular area in the nail fold of a single finger was seen in a patient with ACA.[161] Joint pain and swelling of the distal phalanges may occur.[162] A case of photo-onycholysis induced by doxycycline given for the treatment of erythema chronicum migrans was described.[163]

4.4.3.1 Histopathology

In acrodermatitis chronica atrophicans, usually only one extremity is affected with a bluish-red discoloration and a peculiarly soft skin that gradually turns into atrophy with cigarette-paper like atrophy. The epidermis is atrophic with loss of the rete ridges, a thin granular layer, but nevertheless often a hyperkeratosis is seen. The papillary dermis may be edematous. A band-like lymphocytic infiltrate often containing considerable numbers of plasma cells may develop in the upper dermis that rarely may become lichenoid. In the dermis the infiltrate is seen around vessels, sweat glands, and follicles and typically contains many plasma cells (Figure 4.8). Pseudorosettes defined by histiocytes completely surrounding collagen bundles may be observed.[164] The collagen fibers may be destroyed and elastic fibers disappear. In the late stage, epidermal and dermal atrophy prevail.

4.4.3.2 Differential diagnosis

Morphea and scleroderma have to be considered.[165]

4.5 MYCOSES OF THE NAIL APPARATUS

Mycotic infections of the nails are extremely common and may be due to all pathogenic fungi. Their classification is usually made according to clinical criteria. The International Society for Human and Animal Mycoses proposed another nomenclature: Nail infection by dermatophytes be replaced by the term tinea unguium, yeast infection be called onyxis, *Candida* nail infection ungual candidiasis, and infection by opportunistic molds ungual mycosis.[166]

4.5.1 Superficial mycoses

Superficial fungal infections of the nail including the surrounding skin are very frequent.[167] Onychomycoses make up for approximately 40% of all nail diseases. They are often only clinically diagnosed and treated by general practitioners and dermatologists without laboratory proof of diagnosis. Nevertheless, the diagnostic accuracy is fairly high.[168,169]

4.5.1.1 Onychomycoses

Onychomycoses are a group of fungal nail infections that may be classified according to the responsible pathogen in dermatophyte, yeast, nondermatophyte mold or other onychomycosis, according to the duration in recent-onset or chronic onychomycosis, or according to the way of nail unit invasion into distal-lateral subungual, superficial white and black, proximal white subungual, endonyx, and total

Table 4.1 Clinical classification of onychomycosis

Distal and distal-lateral subungual onychomycosis (DLSO)

Proximal subungual onychomycosis (PSO)

   Without paronychia

      Classical PSO

      Transverse PSO

   Acute (rapid) PSO

      Candida PSO

      PSO in AIDS patients

   With paronychia

      Due to *Candida* spp.

      Due to nondermatophyte molds

      Very rarely due to dermatophytes

Superficial onychomycosis (SO)

   Classical SO limited to the nail plate

   SO under the proximal nail fold

   Acute SO

   Transverse SO

   SO with deep invasion

   Mixture with 3 variants: SO associated with DLSO

      SO associated with PSO

      SO associated with histologically restricted changes on the ventral portion (?)

Endonyx onychomycosis, mostly *T. soudanense* or *T. violaceum*

Total dystrophic onychomycosis (TDO)

   Secondary to any of the aforementioned types

   Primary in chronic mucocutaneous candidiasis (CMCC)

   Acute TDO

Source: Hay RJ, Baran R. Onychomycosis: A proposed revision of the clinical classification. *J Am Acad Dermatol* 2011;65:1219–1227.

dystrophic onychomycosis. The latter may develop from any of the aforementioned types or occur primarily in chronic mucocutaneous candidiasis.[170] Paronychia and onycholysis colonized with fungi may also be classified as onychomycosis in a broader sense (Table 4.1). The list of fungi isolated from diseased nails is long[171] and is getting longer,[172] but it is not always clear whether they are the true pathogen or just a colonizer.[173] On the other hand, direct microscopy after clearing with 20%–40% potassium hydroxide and mycological cultures often remain false negative. Histopathologic examination has proven to be doubly as sensitive as cultures and to be able to distinguish between an invasive fungus and a surface colonizer,[174] but it does not allow species identification. This is possible with culture, PCR,[175,176] and matrix-assisted laser desorption/ionization time-of-flight mass spectrometry (MALDI-ToF MS),[177–179] but these methods cannot differentiate between a colonizer and a true pathogen. Immunohistochemical methods[180,181] and *in situ* hybridization for the identification of pathogenic fungi in onychomycosis are not yet commercially available.

4.5.1.1.1 *Distal subungual onychomycosis*

Distal or distal-lateral subungual onychomycosis is by far the most common type in temperate climates.

Trichophyton rubrum is the most frequent pathogen, but other dermatophytes may also be the cause whereas yeasts and nondermatophyte molds are more commonly found in warm climates. There is a strong, probably autosomal dominant hereditary component in *T. rubrum* onychomycosis as evidenced by family examinations showing a vertical infection chain.[183] Further, predisposing factors such as peripheral arterial disease, neuropathy, edema, diabetes mellitus, and immune incompetence play an important role. Heredity and predisposing factors are probably the reason that onychomycoses are the most difficult to treat of all fungal skin infections and have a very high rate of recurrences. Clinically, there is a subungual hyperkeratosis, yellow discoloration of the nail, and loss of transparency that progress from distal to proximal, breaking of the distal nail and sometimes nail thickening. The most important clinical differential diagnosis is psoriasis, but similar nail dystrophies are seen in chronic venous insufficiency, lower leg edema, and so on.

4.5.1.1.1.1 *Histopathology*

Histopathologic examinations can be performed on nail clippings and deep biopsies; the former are able to confirm the diagnosis, the latter give information on the reaction of the nail unit to the infection. There is a huge variability in the morphology of the infecting fungi.

4.5.1.1.1.2 *Nail clippings*

As with taking material for mycological cultures, the histopathologic changes of nail clippings depend on the correct biopsy taking. It is essential to include as much of the subungual keratotic debris as possible as this is the site where most fungi are seen. The diagnosis requires a PAS (Figure 4.9a) or another stain for fungi although often fungal hyphae are seen in H&E sections (Figure 4.9b). Depending on the severity of the DSLO, variable amounts of fungal elements are seen. In the subungual keratin, their arrangement is moderately irregular, both hyphae as well as arthrospores are seen. Most dermatophyte hyphae are slender and segmented. The arthrospores have a thicker cell wall and sometimes can be discerned even in H&E sections as they have a basophilic central round core (Figure 4.10). The deep nail plate layer often shows hyphae in parallel arrangement to the longitudinal axis of the nail plate. They rarely occupy more than 20% of the nail plate thickness. Occasionally, budding structures are seen in association with hyphal structures in the nail plate (Figure 4.11). They probably represent nondermatophyte molds. Serum inclusion is often found in the subungual keratin.

4.5.1.1.1.3 *Nail biopsies*

Nail biopsies, preferably as lateral longitudinal biopsies, give a profound insight into the fungal invasion and the host's response. In DSLO, one can rarely see a few hyphae in the hyponychium and/or adjacent pulp skin. An inflammatory infiltrate is lacking here. The main alterations are seen in the nail bed and in very advanced cases also in the matrix (Figure 4.12). There is an inflammatory

(a)

(b)

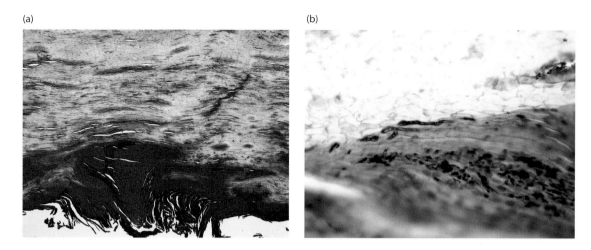

Figure 4.9 Distal-lateral subungual onychomycosis. (a) H&E stain shows small holes in the subungual keratosis and deepest layer of the nail plate. Note that small splits in the nail plate must not be confused with fungi. (b) PAS stain reveals many fungal elements in the nail.

(a)

(b)

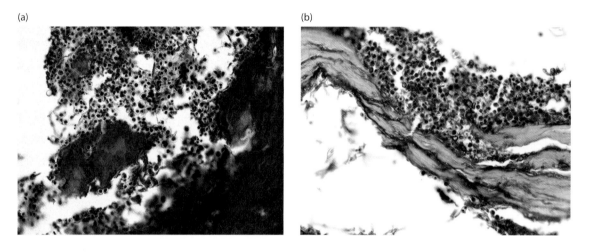

Figure 4.10 Arthrospores in distal-lateral subungual onychomycosis: (a) H&E, (b) PAS stain.

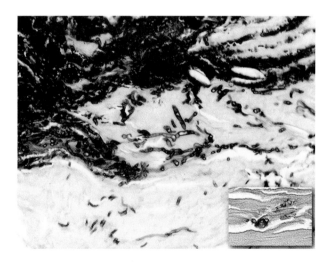

Figure 4.11 Onychomycosis due to nondermatophyte molds. (Inset: Budding structures in the nail of a liver-transplant recipient.)

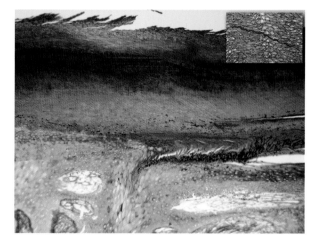

Figure 4.12 Biopsy of an advanced distal-lateral subungual onychomycosis with marked papillary edema in the dermis of the proximal nail bed and distal matrix (Grocott stain). (Inset: Long dermatophyte hypha in the hyperkeratotic distal nail bed.)

perivascular infiltrate in the upper and mid-dermis with migration of lymphocytes toward the nail bed epithelium and spongiosis in more pronounced cases. In the superficial epithelium, some neutrophils are often present. The overlying keratin is mostly orthokeratotic and may contain variable amounts of Munro's microabscesses. When they are seen in the nail plate, this may be a sign of associated psoriasis or that the fungal pathogens have reached the matrix. It is the nail bed keratosis where most of the fungi are present. In mild to moderate cases, hyphae are arranged mostly in parallel, but in severe cases they may show a haphazard arrangement. The overlying nail plate is only invaded in the deepest layers overlying the subungual hyperkeratosis; it appears that the nail plate is rather a barrier for fungal invasion than the main site of infection. Whether there are *Candida*-specific alterations of the nail is not clear.[184]

4.5.1.1.1.4 Differential diagnosis

The most important disease to be differentiated is nail psoriasis (Table 4.2). Both have subungual hyperkeratosis and Munro's microabscesses in common, and the problem can be confounded by fungal colonization or true infection of psoriatic nails. However, the microabscesses in onychomycosis are usually surrounded by orthokeratosis whereas those in psoriasis are found in a parakeratotic area, which often forms an oblique column that is not seen in onychomycosis. When there is spongiosis, whatever the cause, there are usually serum inclusions in the subungual keratosis that are PAS positive and may, particularly when being small, be mistaken for fungal elements. The latter have a cell wall staining whereas serum inclusions are homogenously positive.

4.5.1.1.2 Proximal subungual (white) onychomycosis

Proximal subungual onychomycosis is a rare type of fungal nail infection. In the beginning, a whitish area of the nail plate is seen growing out from under the proximal nail fold without accompanying paronychia. It extends relatively rapidly distally as it profits from the distal movement of the nail plate during growth. It is more frequently seen in immunocompromised persons. The fungus infects the cuticle and then slowly progresses along the eponychium toward the matrix. When it arrives there it will be included in the newly formed nail plate and also invade the lower proximal nail layers. This may be a fast process in AIDS patients. A similar infection due to *Candida albicans* may be seen in the newborn. Another type of PSO is associated with paronychia. These infections are mainly due to nondermatophyte molds and rarely to dermatophytes and in excessively chronic *Candida* infections. A particular form of PSO is seen as repeated transverse white streaks in the nail and is thought to be due to a systemic or lymphatic spread of dermatophytes to the nail.[185,186]

Table 4.2 Differential diagnosis of onychomycosis and psoriasis

	Onychomycosis	Psoriasis
Frequency	High: 30%–40% of all nail diseases Most frequent nail disease	High, most frequent dermatosis with nail involvement
Course	Chronic, often progressive	Chronic, often relapsing
Symptoms	Embarrassing, sometimes pain	Embarrassing, sometimes pain
Signs	Variable, depend on stage and severity	Variable, depend on nail structure affected
Pits	Rare	Frequent
Onycholysis	Frequent	Frequent
Discoloration	Yellow to brown	None to yellow
Spores and hyphae	Very frequent	Rarely spores (except for double pathology)
Transverse furrows	Rare	Rare
Skin lesions elsewhere	Often tinea pedum, tinea manuum	Often psoriasis on other body sites
Trauma	Important predisposing factor	May induce Köbner phenomenon
Heredity	Autosomal dominant susceptibility	High degree
Histopathology	Marked hyperkeratosis with little parakeratosis, neutrophils, and intracorneal PAS-positivie serum inclusions	Marked hyperkeratosis with accumulation of neutrophils and serum globules, sometimes columnar parakeratosis, focal hypergranulosis
	Munro's abscesses	Munro's abscesses
	Sometimes papillomatosis of the nail bed	Sometimes papillomatous hyperplasia of the nail bed
	Spongiosis and mononucelar exocytosis	Spongiosis and mononuclear exocytosis
	Hyphae and spores in nail bed keratosis and deep nail plate layers (distal subungual onychomycosis)	Depressions of the nail surface with parakeratosis: pits
Double pathology	Nail psoriasis may be colonized by fungi or show co-existent onychomycosis	

4.5.1.1.2.1 Histopathology

The histologic diagnosis may be made from the nail plate alone or from a biopsy. For the former, a disc of nail is punched out from the white area of the nail. This can usually be done without anesthesia as the white area is detached from the living matrix. After soaking the nail in lukewarm water for 5–10 min, a 4 mm disc of nail is cut by gently pressing and rotating a punch on the nail. The patient will tell when it starts hurting. The disc of nail can be taken out using a #30 gauge injection needle the tip of which has been bent 90–100°. Histopathology of H&E sections usually shows horizontal splits in the nail whereas PAS exhibits masses of fungi arranged parallel to the nail surface. There may be hyphae as well as spores or both as well as microabscesses; they are the reason for the white color of the nail plate. In longitudinal nail biopsies, fungi may be seen in the hyperkeratotic eponychium at the undersurface of the proximal nail fold as well as in several layers of the nail plate in different levels (Figure 4.13). There is no inflammatory response in the dermis of the matrix as the fungal elements are transported away from the matrix with the nail growth.

4.5.1.1.3 Superficial white and black onychomycosis

Superficial white onychomycosis (SWO) has recently been reclassified into a superficial and deep type.[187] In Central Europe, most cases occur on toenails as chalky-white spots and are due to a particular growth form of *T. mentagrophytes*. Fingernail SWO has a more cloudy aspect with a shiny nail surface; which is due to *T. rubrum* and seen almost exclusively in AIDS patients.[188] In subtropical climates, nondermatophyte molds such as *Acremonium* spp., *Aspergillus* spp., and *Fusarium* spp. are often the cause. When occurring under, or originating from under the proximal nail fold, it may invade a higher proportion of the nail thickness. A few cases of black superficial onychomycosis were due to *T. rubrum*[189]

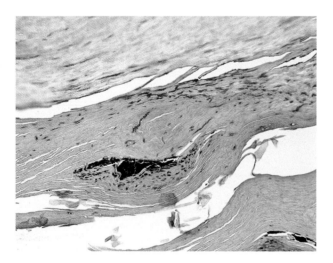

Figure 4.13 Proximal white subungual onychomycosis showing fungal hyphae in all layers of the nail plate and a Munro abscess within the nail plate (PAS stain).

and *Scytalidium dimidiatum*.[190] The localization of SWO is important for its treatment as it cannot be reached by topical antifungals when it is localized under the proximal nail fold.

4.5.1.1.3.1 Histopathology

In the common or "classical" type, a superficial saucer-shaped piece of nail may be taken with a #15 scalpel from the surface and examined with both H&E and PAS stains. In the case of *T. mentagrophytes* SWO, chains of uniformly small spores are seen in the tiny splits of the nail surface (Figure 4.14a–c). A nail biopsy exhibits exactly the same pattern with no inflammatory reaction of the matrix and eponychial dermis.

In the type due to *T. rubrum*, spores and short hyphae prevail in the uppermost layer of the nail plate. In contrast to the *T. mentagrophytes* infection, the localization is slightly deeper explaining why this SWO has a shiny nail surface.

In the deep type of SWO, fungal spores and hyphae are seen in enormous numbers in the uppermost three-quarters of the nail plate (Figure 4.15).

Superficial black onychomycosis can be diagnosed histopathologically from a horizontal nail plate biopsy. In faintly stained H&E sections, the brown pigment is seen whereas PAS shows the typical hyphae.

Mold SWO has usually thicker, shorter, and more irregular hyphae.

4.5.1.1.3.2 Differential diagnosis

The diagnosis of SWO is obvious with PAS, Grocott, and other fungal stains. A certain differentiation of the causative fungi is not possible histologically.

4.5.1.1.4 Endonyx onychomycosis

This is a recently described form, which has, however, been seen before. The nail is dull, intransparent, without surface shine, and the nail tends to show lamellar splitting. There is virtually no inflammation visible. Most cases are due to *T. soudanense*, some to *T. violaceum*;[191] both dermatophytes are known to cause endothrix tinea capitis.[192]

4.5.1.1.4.1 Histopathology

The nail is of normal or only slightly increased thickness. Stains for fungi show mostly slender hyphae in the nail plate, the subungual keratin is free. There is no visible inflammation in the dermis.[193]

4.5.1.1.4.2 Differential diagnosis

Lamellar splitting may be seen in other types of onychomycoses, in dystrophic nails due to peripheral vascular disease and other conditions, but the distribution of the fungal elements is unique.

4.5.1.1.5 Total dystrophic onychomycosis

Total dystrophic onychomycosis is diagnosed when the fungal infection has destroyed the nail and no orderly nail plate is produced anymore. It can develop from any of the

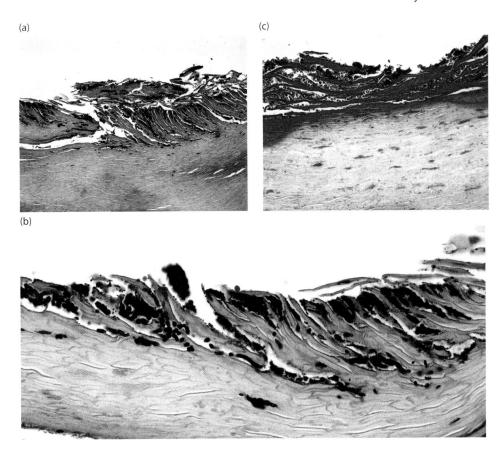

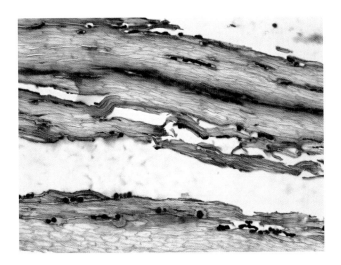

Figure 4.14 (a–c) Superficial white onychomycosis with dense aggregates of fungal spores and short hyphae in the frayed surface of the nail plate (a, b—PAS, c—H&E stain).

onychomycoses discussed above or primarily in chronic mucocutaneous candidiasis (CMCC). The latter is a group of immunodeficiencies that all result in a defect of defense against *Candida albicans*, but may be associated with other conditions.[194]

Figure 4.15 So-called deep type of superficial white onychomycosis with spores and short hyphae in all layers of the nail plate (PAS stain).

4.5.1.1.5.1 Histopathology

The nail is substituted by keratotic debris and no orderly nail plate is seen. This debris contains large masses of fungi. In contrast to DLSO, the fungi are haphazardly arranged and are no longer parallel to the growth direction.

In CMCC, the nail production is even more severely disturbed. Keratotic masses are seen where normally a plate is present. The proximal nail fold is reduced to a small bulge and the nail pocket has virtually disappeared (Figure 4.16a). The matrix and nail bed are markedly acanthotic. There is a diffuse inflammatory infiltrate in the dermis with perivascular accentuation. The matrix and nail bed epithelium are spongiotic and often have developed a thick granular layer. Fungal stains show variable amounts of spores and short filaments. There may be a double infection, predominantly with *T. rubrum*. Semithin sections reveal fungal elements in the keratinocytes of the matrix and nail bed (Figure 4.16b). Electron microscopy shows *Candida* spores (Figure 4.16c) and composite and heterogeneous keratohyalin.[195]

In acute total dystrophic onychomycosis, there is heavy inflammation, acanthosis, and papillomatosis of the matrix and nail bed, a dense infiltrate, abscess-like material between the epithelium and the overlying nail, and masses of fungal elements (Figure 4.17).

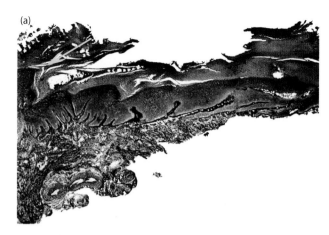

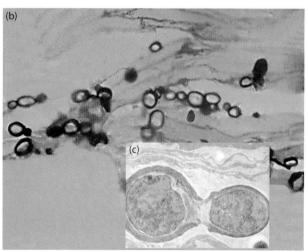

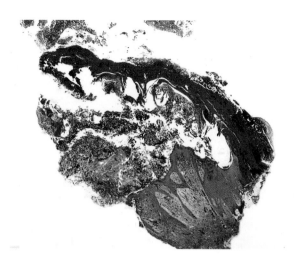

Figure 4.17 Acute type of total dystrophic onychomycosis of the middle finger of an 86-year-old cancer patient. Acrodermatitis continua suppurativa was ruled out by the demonstration of innumerable invasive fungal elements, culture revealed *Trichophyton rubrum* (H&E stain).

Figure 4.16 Total dystrophic onychomycosis in a patient with chronic mucocutaneous candidiasis. (a) Scanning magnification shows keratotic debris instead of a normal nail plate and a very short proximal nail fold (arrow) (Grocott stain). (b) Semithin section stained with Grocott showing *Candida* spores. (c) Electron microscopy demonstrates a budding yeast cell (inset).

possible before starting the therapy, which is best a combination of oral and topical antifungal agents.[204]

4.5.1.1.6.1 Histopathology

Dermatophytoma in onychomycosis is a fairly common phenomenon. It is easily diagnosed from a nail clipping that includes the subungual keratin.[205] The overlying nail plate is indented at its undersurface and short thick-walled hyphae invade the nail substance. Under it, a huge mass of densely packed hyphae and spores is seen (Figure 4.18), sometimes with a peripheral radiating pattern. Their cell walls are very thick, which is another cause why dermatophytomas are so difficult to treat with antifungals. In the neighboring nail and subungual keratin, slender hyphae are seen in the case of a true dermatophyte infection.

4.5.1.1.5.2 Differential diagnosis

All types of severe nail dystrophy have to be considered. PAS stain usually allows the diagnosis to be made.

4.5.1.1.6 Dermatophytoma and other subungual "mycetomas"

The phenomenon of the yellow streak or spike in a toenail has been known for many years. However, less than 20 years ago, it was assumed that the fungi in this yellow streak might behave in another way. As the fungal elements are extremely numerous and compressed to a ball of pathogens similar to aspergilloma, the term of dermatophytoma was coined.[196] It was later hypothesized that they represent a fungal biofilm,[197] which would at least in part explain the recalcitrant behavior of the fungi.[198–202] The presence of dermatophytoma is also highly rated in the onychomycosis severity index.[203] Treatment includes mechanical removal of as much of the dermatophytoma as

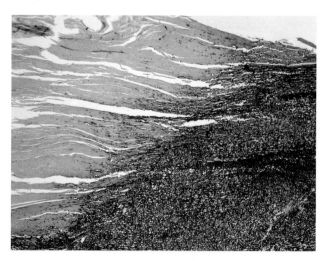

Figure 4.18 Dermatophytoma with huge masses of fungi that invade the nail plate (PAS) clinically seen as a yellow streak under the big toenail.

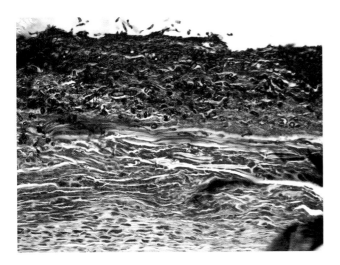

Figure 4.19 Mycetoma by nondermatophyte molds between the nail plate and the underlying parakeratosis. The fungal elements have large and variable calipers, are septate, and exhibit occasional branching.

Large masses of densely compressed fungi with the morphologic criteria of nondermatophyte molds are also occasionally seen. Their hyphae often have a very thick diameter, 6–12 μ, and they branch in an acute angle of approximately 45° in the case of *Aspergillus* spp. and *Fusarium* spp. and at roughly 90° in *zygomycetes* (Figure 4.19). We prefer to call dense agglomerations of non-dermatophyte molds subungual mycetomas and not dermatophytomas.[206]

4.5.1.1.6.2 Differential diagnosis

Dense agglomerations of huge fungal masses are easily seen in PAS and Grocott stained slides. They should not be confused with serum inclusions in subungual keratin, which are PAS positive due to their glycoprotein content and almost always homogeneously positive except in long-standing cases where they may look partially vesicular but nevertheless never attain the cell wall staining of fungal elements.

4.5.1.1.7 Nondermatophyte mold onychomycoses

Several nondermatophyte molds are able to digest keratin and produce onychomycoses. Clinically, they are almost invariably indistinguishable from dermatophyte infections although they often cause paronychia in addition. Distal-lateral, superficial white, proximal subungual, or total dystrophic onychomycoses may develop.[207] They may be the source for a cutaneous-subcutaneous infection with an eventually fatal outcome.[208, 209] However, as they are usually more resistant to the antifungal drugs commonly used for onychomycosis treatment, their identification is strongly recommended. Histopathology may give a hint at a nondermatophyte mold, but culture and more sophisticated techniques as PCR and MALDI-TOF are necessary for genus and species determination, particularly for *Scytalidium dimidiatum*, which also forms long, slender hyphae like many dermatophytes.[210–212] *Aspergillus* spp., *Scopulariopsis brevicaulis,* and *Fusarium* spp. are the most common pathogens.[213]

Nondermatophyte molds are often considered to be contaminants and strict criteria have to be used to confirm that they are really the pathogen of a particular case of onychomycosis: Microscopic identification of the mold by direct microscopy of a potassium hydroxide preparation, isolation by culture or another method able to correctly identify the fungus, repeated isolation by culture, high inoculum count, failure to isolate a dermatophyte, and proof of the onychomycosis by histology.[214] However, this does not solve the problem of double infections with dermatophytes and nondermatophyte molds; histopathology may again help to identify hyphae of different morphology.

4.5.1.1.7.1 Histopathology

Under the microscope, sub- and intraungual nondermatophyte molds often stand out by a large diameter of the fungal filaments or vesicular enlargement of the hyphae, the latter is particularly characteristic for *Fusarium* infections. Further, intraungual sprouting may be seen.

4.5.1.1.7.2 Differential diagnosis

Dermatophyte onychomycoses can only be ruled out with certainty by exact species determination usually requiring a positive culture, PCR, or MALDI-TOF MS.

4.5.1.1.8 Mycotic paronychia

Paronychia is a relatively common condition due to various infections, trauma, and foreign bodies. Whereas the diagnosis of candidal paronychia used to be made in most chronic and repeatedly recurring paronychias until some 20 years ago, it is now believed that most of these cases are primarily due to allergies, predominantly of the immediate type to various foods. However, there are undoubted cases of fungal infections[215] that also respond to pure antimycotic treatment. The nail fold is thickened, its free end is rounded, the cuticle is lacking, and there is a split formation between the proximal nail fold and the underlying nail plate. This allows foreign substances including bacteria and fungi to enter and be trapped. It is possible that the resulting close contact with these substances under the nail fold facilitates sensitization.

4.5.1.1.8.1 Histopathology

The nail fold is swollen and its free margin rounded. There is no cuticle. The eponychium is detached from the underlying nail plate. Fungal elements may be seen in the horny layer of the nail fold's undersurface. There is a chronic lymphocytic perivascular infiltrate in the dermis.

A purulent paronychia was described in association with a *Fusarium oxysporum* onychomycosis.[216]

4.5.1.1.8.2 Differential diagnosis

Nail fold involvement in psoriasis also causes a similar picture although psoriatic criteria are usually seen.

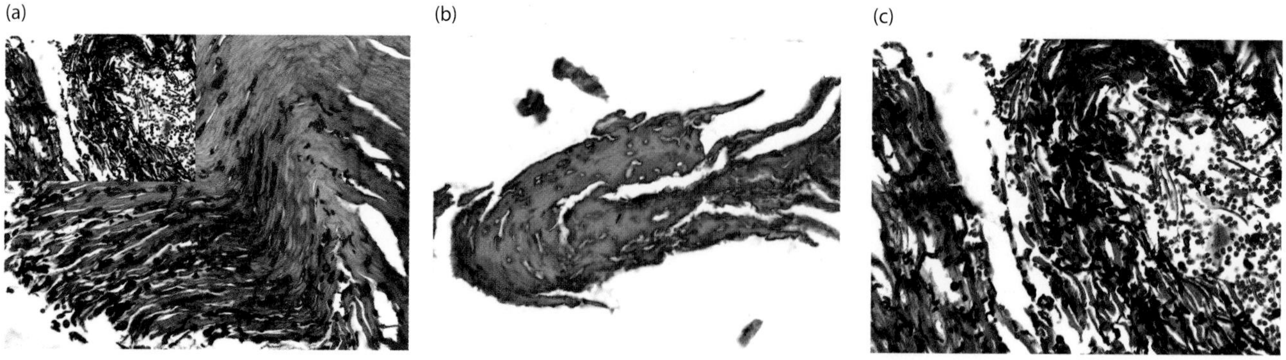

Figure 4.20 Fungal melanonychia. (a) Part of the nail is stained brown as well as some large spores. (b) Dark brown nail due to nondermatophyte mold infection. (c) The spores and short hyphae are deeply pigmented. The erythrocytes may be used for comparison of the color (PAS stain).

4.5.1.1.9 Mycotic onycholysis

Onycholysis is the distal detachment of the nail plate from the nail bed. It is a very common event seen in more nail diseases than not. The nail plate itself appears to be rather normal except that it is whitish or yellowish and intransparent. Under the nail plate, microorganisms and foreign substances can accumulate, among them also fungi. They may colonize the dead space under the nail, form a fungal biofilm and prevent reattachment of the plate.

4.5.1.1.9.1 Histopathology

Nail clippings exhibit a near-normal nail plate with fungal elements, mainly spores, attached to its undersurface. Concomitant bacterial colonization is frequent.

4.5.1.1.9.2 Differential diagnosis

Any type of onycholysis may show some fungal spores and bacteria. This usually does not allow a specific diagnosis to be made without further investigations.

4.5.1.1.10 Fungal melanonychia

A variety of pathogenic and saprophytic fungi are able to produce soluble pigment, mostly melanin.[217] *Trichophyton rubrum* var. *nigricans*, *Candida albicans*,[218] common black molds such as *Aspergillus* and *Alternaria* spp., *Penicillium* spp., *Acremonium* spp., *Scytalidium dimidiatum*,[219] phaeohyphomycetes such as *Wangiella dermatitidis*, *Exophiala* spp.,[220] chromoblastomycosis, but also *Phialophora* spp.[221] were observed to cause black onychomycosis. Clinically, part or all of the mycotically infected portion of the nail is brown to black. This is usually seen as a pigmented wedge with its base at the free margin. Careful inspection and dermatoscopy show in most cases that the subungual keratosis is more intensely stained than the nail itself, a pattern not seen in melanonychia due to human melanin except for pigmented onychopapilloma.

4.5.1.1.10.1 Histopathology

When the fungal nature of melanonychia is suspected and a PAS or Grocott stain is available, the fungi are easily identified. In a pale H&E stain, a faint yellow to light brown diffuse staining of the nail plate is seen in dermatophyte infections (Figure 4.20a,b). No granular melanin is present. In phaehyphomycosis and chromoblastomycosis, the pigmented fungal cell wall is usually recognizable (Figure 4.20c).

4.5.1.1.10.2 Differential diagnosis

Melanonychia due to human melanin stands out by its finely granular nature and is seen in an argentaffin stained section (see Chapters 7 and 15).

4.5.2 Subcutaneous mycoses

4.5.2.1 Sporotrichosis

Sporotrichosis is the most common cutaneous-subcutaneous fungal infection of the hand in North America.[222,223] It is due to *Sporothrix schenckii* complex and results from direct inoculation at a site of minor trauma. From here either a fixed nodule or a lymphocutaneous form develops; dissemination is very rare and only seen in immunodepressed individuals. Most patients are gardeners and florists with an ulcerating nodule from which a chain of lesions may spread along the lymph vessels.[224] Cats as a source of *S. schenckii* infections were observed in Brazil.[225] Nail involvement is rare.[226] It was observed in a veterinarian as an infection of the tip of the thumb elevating the nail and causing bone infection.[227] Another case from Rio de Janeiro presented with a huge granulating lateral paronychia (R. Nakamura, personal observation). Onychomycosis due to *Sporothrix* spp. is rare.[228,229] *Sporothrix pallida* was isolated from under the big toenail of a Chilean woman and the soil of her home garden.[230]

4.5.2.1.1 Histopathology

The nodular lesion starts with a nonspecific inflammatory infiltrate composed of neutrophils, lymphocytes, plasma cells, and histiocytes. With time the epidermis develops acanthosis and often a verrucous hyperkeratosis as well as intraepidermal collections of lymphocytes. Small lympho-plasmocytic infiltrates in the dermis develop abscesses and show eosinophils and giant cells. Initially, small granulomas are seen that may show

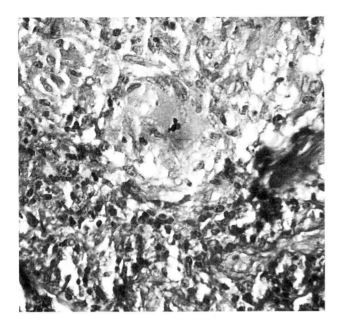

Figure 4.21 Sporotrichosis of the soft tissue of the nail organ, *Sporothrix schenckii* is seen in a giant cell. (Courtesy of Dr. R. Nakamura, Rio de Janeiro, Brazil.)

asteroid bodies. They may coalesce to larger lesions with a characteristic zonal architecture: a suppurative center with neutrophils and tissue debris, a tuberculoid ring of histiocytes and macrophages, and a peripheral ring of lymphoid and plasma cells. In the lymphocutaneous form, granulomas in an inflammatory lympho-plasmocytic infiltrate are seen in the deep dermis and subcutis. They merge to finally form large suppurative granulomas and abscesses. Fungal stains should be employed,[231] but the causative *S. schenckii* is often difficult to find (Figure 4.21).[232] In our experience, Grocott yields better results than PAS, but this is disputed.[233] Immunohistochemical demonstration of *S. schenckii* is doubly as sensitive as common fungal stains.[234] Culture remains the diagnostic gold standard.

4.5.2.1.2 Differential diagnosis

All cutaneous diseases with suppurative granulomas have to be considered, particularly cutaneous leishmaniasis. As the demonstration of the causative organisms is often impossible, a marker list allowing sporotrichosis to be discriminated from American tegumentary leishmaniasis (ATL) was established. It showed that "suppurative granuloma," "stellate granuloma," "different types of giant cells," "granulomas in granulation tissue," and "abscess outside the granuloma" were associated with a diagnosis of sporotrichosis whereas the markers "macrophage concentration," "tuberculoid granuloma," and "extracellular matrix degeneration" were associated with ATL. "Macrophage concentration" and "suppurative granuloma" had the highest reliability with 92.0% accuracy whereas the "intuitive diagnosis" had 82.5% diagnostic accuracy and substantial reliability.[235]

4.5.2.2 Lobomycosis

Lobomycosis, also called lacaziosis, is caused by *Lacazia (Loboa) loboi*. It is an excessively chronic granulomatous mycosis first described in 1930.[236] Most cases were seen in individuals from the Amazon region in tropical Brazil, but some cases were also reported from Central America and Mexico.[237] Sporadic cases seen in the United States, Canada, and Europe occurred in persons who had travelled to endemic regions.[238] The etiological agent is a yeast-like organism that cannot yet be cultured, but has been examined by molecular biologic techniques.[239,240] A lobomycosis-like disease has been observed in two dolphin species, the bottle-nosed dolphin (*Tursiops truncatus*) from the Atlantic coast of Europe and the United States and the Guayana dolphin (*Sotalia guianensis*) living in the Surinam River estuary.[241–243] It is not entirely clear whether extra South American human cases might be due to an infection acquired from dolphins.[244,245]

Most patients come from tropical areas of the Amazon basin and some countries of Central America. These areas are about 200 to 250 m above sea level and characterized by dense vegetation, less than 2000 mm annual rainfall, and an average temperature of about 24°C; the humidity is above 75%.[246] There is no racial predilection. Most cases are diagnosed between 40 and 70 years of age, but the disease most probably starts many years earlier. Whereas generally 90% of the lobomycosis patients are male, there is one indigenous tribe of Caiabi Indians of the Amazon where the female proportion is almost one-third of the cases; these women work mainly in agriculture and the forest. Professional exposure is the main source of infection, usually through minor trauma leading to inoculation of the fungus from rotting vegetation, soil, and water.[247] This also explains why not only earlobes, but also the extremities, are often involved. Clinically, keloid-like growths develop at sites of presumed inoculation. They very slowly extend, may become plaque-like, and may also ulcerate. Involvement of the hands, feet, fingers, and toes may lead to secondary affection of the nail unit.[248]

4.5.2.2.1 Histopathology

The epidermis may be atrophic or exhibit pseudoepitheliomatous hyperplasia. Often a free grenz zone is seen. In the superficial dermis, there is a dense, often granulomatous infiltrate with histiocytes, many foreign body type giant cells, and perivascular lymphocytes. Occasionally microabscesses and pronounced fibrotic areas are seen. The fungi are yeast-like with a diameter of 7–10 μ and seen both intra- as well as extracellularly. In many cases they are abundant and may be arranged in groups of 10–20 yeasts. In H&E stained sections, the cell wall is pale and refractile (Figure 4.22). Grocott and PAS stains clearly demonstrate the fungi. Gridley stain shows a yellow-brown cytoplasm, a black nucleus, and a pink cell wall. The cell wall brightly fluoresces with blancophore staining. There are no inflammatory cells such as lymphocytes and neutrophils. Keloid-like tumors may involve the

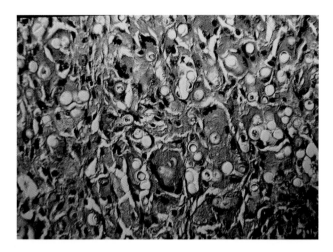

Figure 4.22 Lobomycosis of the distal digit. (Courtesy of Dr. A. C. de Brito, Belém, Brazil.)

periungual tissues. Immunohistochemistry has also been used to demonstrate the fungi.[249] Electron microscopy shows multinucleated yeast cells and vacuolated inclusion bodies.

Fine-needle aspiration may also collect material for diagnosis and inoculation studies.[250, 251]

4.5.2.2.2 Differential diagnosis

Lacaziosis is unique in that it shows large amounts of yeast cells with virtually no inflammatory infiltrate. The fungi have to be differentiated from *Paracoccidoides braziliensis*, *Histoplasma capsulatum* var. *duboisii*, *Cryptococcus neoformans*, and *Leishmania* spp.

4.5.2.3 Chromoblastomycosis

A variety of dematiaceous fungi cause chromomycosis. They have in common that the spores are pigmented. The most common pathogens are *Cladosporium carionii*, *Exophiala jeanselmi*, *E. spinifera*, *Fonsecaea*

pedrosoi, *F. compactum*, *Phialophora verrucosa*, and *Rhinocladiella aquaspersa*. All these pigmented fungi form spores and grow on soil, decaying plants, and rotten wood, mainly in subtropical and tropical regions. Infection is thought to occur after direct inoculation into the skin.[252] Eighty percent of the lesions occur on feet and lower legs. Men are 9 times more frequently affected and most are agricultural workers.[253] Cases in Europe were mainly imported[254] although autochthonous chromoblastomycosis was also observed in Northern Europe.[255,256] Clinically, verrucous lesions develop that may also affect the periungual skin and secondarily lead to nail dystrophy. Longitudinal melanonychia was observed due to *F. pedrosoi*.[257] Medlar bodies, also called fumagoid cells, caused melanonychia in a child.[258] *Cladosporium sphaerospermum* has been recovered from nail scrapings.[259]

4.5.2.3.1 Histopathology

In most cases, there is a granulomatous inflammation with a lichenoid epidermotropic lymphocytic infiltrate. The epidermis shows very marked pseudoepitheliomatous hyperplasia. The infiltrate contains macrophages and giant cells as well as small abscesses that may also be seen intraepidermally. Lymphocytes and plasma cells are the main cell type but eosinophils may be present in variable numbers. Brown fungal spores may be seen in the giant cells, free in the tissue and often in the area of the verrucous epidermis. This is sometimes seen clinically as black dots. They are easily identified in H&E sections due to their brown pigment. In most cases, one, two, or three spores are seen. Their diameter is 6–12 µ. They reproduce by intracellular wall formation and septation and are then seen as fumagoid cells.

We have seen a short chain of dark brown spores in a wooden splinter under the nail of a middle-aged German woman (Figure 4.23). No other fungi were present and there was no inflammation of the nail bed.

(a)

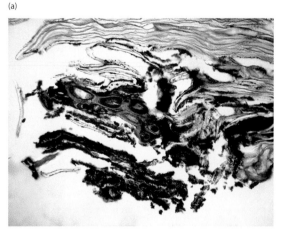

(b)

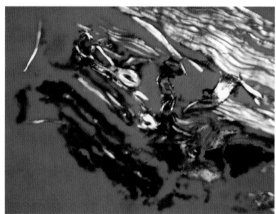

Figure 4.23 (a) Pigmented spores in a subungual wooden splinter and large masses of bacteria; (b) polarization microscopy demonstrates the wooden splinter.

4.5.2.3.2 Differential diagnosis

Pseudoepitheliomatous epidermal hyperplasia with granulomas and lympho-plasmocytic infiltrates is also seen in some other blastomycoses and chronic mycobacterioses such as tuberculosis cutis verrucosa.

4.5.2.4 Alternariosis

Alternaria species are found worldwide as saprophytes and plant pathogens.[260] Some *Alternaria* species are able to infect humans, particularly immunosuppressed individuals.[261, 262] *Alternaria alternata*, but also other species, may be found. The infection has been classified into an epidermal and a dermal type, but virtually all reports on cutaneous alternariosis concern the dermal type.[263] The clinical signs and symptoms are usually not pathognomonic.[264] Probably through minor trauma the fungus is inoculated and causes a chronic infection. Clinically, a papillomatous to verrucous lesion that may ulcerate over time develops. As it may be similar to chronic vegetating pyoderma, it is often primarily treated with antibiotics and then with corticosteroids that markedly favor fungal invasion. In the nail region, there may be "true" alternaria onychomycosis and subcutaneous alternariosis of the periungual skin.

4.5.2.4.1 Histopathology

In the epidermal type, the fungus remains in the epidermis and does not invade the dermis. Hyphae are prevailing. In the dermal type, the epidermis is focally hyperplastic with irregular hyperkeratosis. It may contain intraepidermal abscesses resembling transepidermal elimination of fungal material. From the papillary dermis to the subcutaneous fat, irregularly shaped infiltrates of macrophages, lymphocytes, some plasma cells and neutrophils, giant cells, and an occasional eosinophil are seen. Vessel wall invasion is not rare. In H&E stained sections, spores and short, irregularly shaped hyphae can often be discerned because of their thick refractile cell wall. Fungal stains reveal even more spores and hyphae that again stand out by their thick cell wall. They are seen within the giant cells, in the tissue, and also in vessel walls (Figure 4.24).

4.5.2.4.2 Differential diagnosis

Virtually all other cutaneous-subcutaneous mycoses with epidermal hyperplasia, granuloma, and abscess formation have to be considered. However, fungal morphology allows deep mycoses due to fungi showing spores only to be ruled out.

4.5.2.5 Eumycetoma

Mycetomas are a group of chronic infections of the dermis and subcutaneous tissue due to fungi and filamentous bacteria, the latter are called actinomycetomas. Eumycetomas are due to fungi with thick septate hyphae. *Petriellidium (Allescheria, Pseudoallescheria) boydii, Madurella grisea,* and *M. mycetomatis* are the most common causes. It is an indolent fistulating infection with draining sinuses from indurated plaques. Although insidiously progressing,

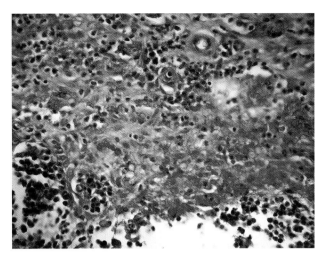

Figure 4.24 Alternariosis of the distal phalanx of the big toe in a farmer with Wegener's granulomatosis. Short chain of thick-walled spores in center left (PAS stain).

there is no systemic spread. Most infections occur on the feet as the infection is by inoculation through a minor trauma. Untreated, the eumycetoma slowly extends to the underlying structures such as bones, tendons, and joints. The foot may be tremendously enlarged (Madura foot). From the sinuses, granules or grains may be discharged; they are black in the case of *M. grisea* and *M. mycetomatis* and colorless in *P. boydii* infections.

Mycetomas due to dermatophytes (*Microsporum audouinii, Microsporum canis, Microsporum ferrugineum, Microsporum langeronii, Trichophyton mentagrophytes, Trichophyton rubrum,* and *Trichophyton verrucosum*) are very rare and mainly occur on the scalp and nape in African or immunosuppressed patients.[265,266]

4.5.2.5.1 Histopathology

Biopsy material from eumycetoma shows pronounced granulation tissue with many abscesses and fistulae. Around the abscesses, lymphocytes, plasma cells, histiocytes, and fibroblasts are seen in the early phase. Fibroblasts prevail in later stages. Sulfur granules may be found in the abscesses and sinuses and these regions must be biopsied for the histologic diagnosis. They measure 0.5–2 mm in diameter and are composed of septate hyphae with a caliber of 4–5 μ. They are positive for PAS and Grocott; however, also the filamentous bacteria of actinomycetomas are positive. They can be differentiated with Gram stain: eumycetoma is gram-negative, actinomycetoma is gram-positive, and the filaments are much thinner.[267]

Sulfur granules can be crushed between two glass slides and stained with lactophenol blue staining the thick septate hyphae.[231]

4.5.3 Deep and systemic mycoses

Whereas superficial mycoses, particularly those due to dermatophytes, are extremely common in the nail apparatus, deep mycoses rarely affect the nail organ. In most cases, personal history, geographic data, and a high index of suspicion are necessary to make the diagnosis.

4.5.3.1 Coccidioidomycosis

Coccidioidomycosis is a systemic mycosis due to the dimorphic fungus *Coccidiodes immitis*, less frequently *C. posadasii*. It results from inhalation of the fungus and may remain asymptomatic, or run a benign, a serious, or a fatal course. It affects immunocompetent as well as immunocompromised subjects as a primary pathogen or an opportunistic agent, respectively. Most cases are seen in California, Arizona, and bordering Mexico with 60% remaining asymptomatic. All persons living or travelling to endemic areas are exposed. Many animals including cats and dogs are infected.[268] All ages and both sexes are affected. In severe cases of disseminated coccidioidomycosis, bones and joints may be involved and thus nail unit and skin lesions secondarily occur in 15%–20% of the cases.[269] Primary skin infection is very rare, mostly resulting from accidental inoculation in laboratories or autopsy rooms,[270,271] rarely as infection resulting from an injury by a thorn or splinter.[272,273] One to three weeks after the inoculation, a tender nodule forms that enlarges to a plaque and ulcerates. Regional lymphangitis and lymphadenitis follow. Healing takes several months. The coccidioidin test aids in making, or confirming, the diagnosis. Treatment of severe cases is with intravenous amphotericin B, which is a relatively toxic regimen. Alternatives are posaconazole, ketoconazole, and the triazoles itraconazole and fluconazole. Trials have been performed with nikkomycin Z, which inhibits chitin synthetase, caspofungin, and voriconazole.

4.5.3.1.1 Histopathology

Primary cutaneous coccidioidomycosis is characterized by a dense inflammatory infiltrate composed of neutrophils, eosinophils, lymphocytes, plasma cells, and a few giant cells. Small abscesses and areas of caseation may develop as well as pseudoepitheliomatous hyperplasia of the epidermis. The latter corresponds to the verrucous lesions. The pathogens are seen both within giant cells as well as in the tissue. In H&E sections, large spores with a diameter of 30–60 (10–80) μ are seen, the walls of which are not stained but strongly refractile, have an inner eosinophilic rim representing their cytoplasm, and a faintly recognizable vacuolar internal structure. Both in PAS as well as Grocott stains, the spherules, also called sporangia, have a thick cell wall and small spores inside; these endospores have a diameter of approximately 2–5 μ. Fluorescence microscopy with blancophore only shows the large spherules without their internal structure. Direct microscopy after clearing with potassium hydroxide allows the spherules to be detected.

Six skin patterns are observed in disseminated coccidioidomycosis.[274]

1. Pseudoepitheliomatous hyperplasia with a dense neutrophilic infiltrate, abscess formation, epithelioid cells, some eosinophils, and masses of spherules. The vessels have enlarged endothelial cells and dense perivascular infiltrates.
2. Pseudoepitheliomatous hyperplasia with ulceration and initial infiltration with lymphocytes and plasma cells in the superficial and mid-dermis with gradual transition to an epithelioid and multinucleated giant cell rich infiltrate with abundant spherules.
3. Ulceration with suppurative granulomas formed of histiocytes and giant cells, neutrophil abscesses with eosinophils, and a few spherules.
4. This may become necrotic and show large areas of caseation.
5. Intense eosinophilia with small granulomas.
6. Sarcoidal reaction with large masses of epithelioid cells mainly in the mid-dermis and surrounding fibrosis.

These patterns are usually not all seen in the nail region.

4.5.3.1.2 Differential diagnosis

The sporangia of *Rhinoporidium seeberi* are 50–350 μ in diameter and contain a large amount of endospores or sporangiospores of 7–12 μ, the sporangia have an eosinophilic cell wall and stain with PAS, Grocott, and Giemsa, the spores only with Giemsa. Further, *Cryptococcus*, *Candida* spp., *Phialophora*, and *Blastomyces dermatitidis* have to be differentiated.

4.5.3.2 Paracoccidioidomycosis

This systemic mycosis is also called South American blastomycosis[275] and has indeed many features in common with the North American blastomycosis. It occurs in Central and South America, from the southern part of Mexico in the north to Uruguay and Argentina in the south, but it is most prevalent in Brazil, particularly its southeast and midwest regions. The causative agent is the dimorphic fungus *Paracoccidioidis brasiliensis*, of which three morphologically indistinguishable subtypes (S1, PS2, and PS3) and *P. lutzii* exist.[276] At 37°C, the yeast form is seen, at 24°C its mycelial form.[277] It mainly occurs in the soil although it was repeatedly found in the nine-banded armadillo, other armadillos, and also in dogs.

Mainly men from rural areas are affected with a male-to-female ratio of 9:1–13:1. This is due to a certain protective effect of estradiol. Smoking appears to be a risk factor.[278] Most cases occur through inhalation, but only a small proportion of the infected individuals develop active disease. Quiescent foci containing viable fungi develop in silent infections, which can only be detected by a paracoccidioidin skin test.[279] The chronic pulmonary-integumentary form is the most common one whereas acute-subacute forms affect young persons[280] and show a tropism for the monocyte-macrophage system developing lymph node swelling and hepatosplenomegaly.[281] Disseminated oral mucous and skin lesions are common in the chronic form as a sign of hematogenous spread of the disease or develop from a neighboring lesion. They start as small papules and nodules tending to ulcerate and subsequently forming large granulomatous and ulcerated lesions. Regional lymphadenopathy is usually present, often with suppuration. Extension to many other lymph nodes and the lower gastrointestinal tract is common. Extensive lung involvement resembles pulmonary tuberculosis.[282] Adrenal involvement leads to adrenal destruction with subsequent adrenal insufficiency.[283] Virtually all organs can be affected.[284] Skin lesions are often seen in the lower extremities. Primary cutaneous paracoccidioidomycosis is rare and results from direct traumatic inoculation to the skin.[285] The incubation period is estimated to be 1–3 weeks.[286] Recently, a case of primary ungual paracoccidioidomycosis was described in a 55-year-old male smoker from a rural area of Brazil who developed an ulcerating granulomatous lesion of the left big toenail after a trauma. Within six months, he experienced complete destruction of the nail organ.[287]

Clinical differential diagnoses depend on the organs involved. Tuberculosis, leprosy, systemic leishmaniasis, and other disseminated infections have to be considered. Skin and mucous membrane lesions may mimic carcinomas.

4.5.3.2.1 Histopathology

Paracoccidioidomycosis is a granulomatous systemic mycosis with histopathologic changes that are virtually the same in all affected organs. In the skin, which is often pseudoepitheliomatous, there is an acute inflammation with granuloma formation, exhibiting epithelioid and giant cells as well as abscess formation. Round spores are seen both in giant cells as well as free in the abscesses (Figure 4.25). They demonstrate a refractile cell wall and stain with PAS, preferably after diastase digestion, as well as silver methene amine according to Grocott. Budding is a frequent phenomenon. Multiple budding is less frequent giving the spores an appearance of a marine pilot's wheel. Single spores have a diameter of 6–20 μ, but spores with multiple buds may measure up to 60 μ. In the ungual

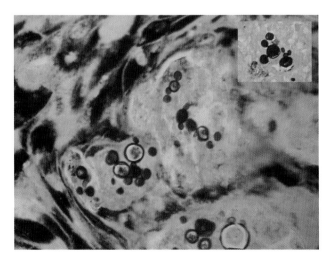

Figure 4.25 Paracoccidiodomycosis of the nail unit. (Inset: Close-up of sporulating spore [Grocott stain].) (Courtesy of Dr. R. Nakamura, Rio de Janeiro, Brazil.)

paracoccidioidomycosis, no nail remnants were left by the pathologic process.

4.5.3.2.2 Differential diagnosis

The tissue reaction to other deep mycoses, particularly *Blastomyces dermatitidis* and *Cryptococcus neoformans*, may be indistinguishable when only single budding yeast cells are present. North American blastomycosis due to *Histoplasma capsulatum* has very thick and strongly refractile cells with broad-based blastospores. *Cryptococcus neoformans* has a mucin capsule that is positive for mucicarmine.

4.5.3.3 Histoplasmosis

Histoplasmosis is a cosmopolitan disease and is considered the most frequent respiratory fungal infection with approximately 40 million patients worldwide and more than 200,000 new cases annually. Endemic areas are found in the Americas, particularly central eastern United States, due to *Histoplasma capsulatum*, and in Africa due to *H. duboisii*. Most primoinfections remain asymptomatic. The most common disease form is pulmonary histoplasmosis caused by inhalation of the fungal spores. This may develop into disseminated histoplasmosis. Primary cutaneous histoplasmosis is caused by inoculation, almost invariably as a laboratory infection.[288] Hence, the hands are most commonly affected. It develops as an ulcerated painless nodule with lymphangitis and regional lymphadenitis.[289] It clears spontaneously in immunocompetent subjects within a few weeks or months. Skin and mucosal lesions are also seen in disseminated histoplasmosis, which is further characterized by weight loss, fever, anemia, persistent cough, lymph node swellings, hepatosplenomegaly, and diarrhea. Papules, nodules, and verrucous, molluscoid, and purpuric lesions, abscesses, ulcers, cellulitis, and panniculitis may occur and in three-quarters of these patients also mucosal lesions.[290–292] Fulminant histoplasmosis is observed in the severely immunocompromised and AIDS patients.[293] *Histoplasma duboisii* may cause relatively benign lesions of the skin, subcutis, lymph nodes, and bones.

4.5.3.3.1 Histopathology

The histopathologic changes depend on the time of evolution and the host's immune system. In the acute stage, abundant yeasts of a diameter of 3 (2–4) μ are found in histiocytes and giant cells and can be seen in H&E, Gram, PAS, Gridley, and Grocott stained sections (Figure 4.26). Giemsa staining shows a clear halo around the yeast cells and gives the impression of a capsule. In addition, the infiltrate contains neutrophils, lymphocytes, and plasma cells. The subacute stage shows epithelioid granulomas with lymphocytes, plasma cells, macrophages, multinucleated giant cells, and neutrophils; fungal spores are considerably less frequent. Tuberculoid granulomas with caseation necrosis, fibrosis, and calcification characteristic for the pulmonary involvement are rare in skin.

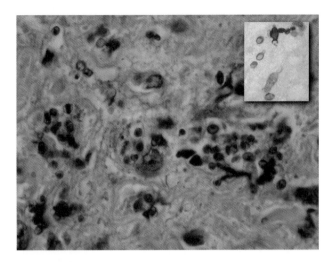

Figure 4.26 Histoplasmosis of the periungual soft tissue (PAS; inset, Grocott stain). (Courtesy of Dr. P. Chang, Guatemala.)

Electron microscopy shows that the clear halo of H&E section is in part the yeast's cell wall and a substance separating it from the cytoplasm of the macrophage.[294]

African histoplasmosis is due to *H. duboisii*; the yeast cells have a diameter of 8–15 μ.

4.5.3.3.2 Differential diagnosis

Rhinoscleroma, cutaneous leishmaniasis, and granuloma inguinale have intracellular parasites of approximately the same size; however, *Histoplasma* can be demonstrated with the usual fungal stains in contrast to the other diseases.

4.5.3.4 North American blastomycosis

North American blastomycosis is endemic in the eastern part of the United States and Mexico as well as in all of Africa. It is caused by *Blastomyces dermatitidis*. Different forms are known: primary pulmonary blastomycosis, disseminated or systemic blastomycosis with 70% of the patients exhibiting skin lesions, primary cutaneous inoculation blastomycosis, and chronic tegumentary blastomycosis with skin and bone involvement. Again, primary inoculation blastomycosis of the skin is very rare and almost exclusively seen in laboratory and autopsy room personnel as a chancre with lymphangitis, often small lesions along the lymph vessel like in sporotrichosis, and regional lymphadenitis. This form usually heals within a few weeks or months. The skin lesions of disseminated blastomycosis are predominantly verrucous or ulcerative.[295,296] Nail changes were seen as paronychias and nail bed polyps.[297]

4.5.3.4.1 Histopathology

A dermal infiltrate with many neutrophils and abundant yeasts characterizes the early stage. The yeasts are 8–15 μ in diameter and often show a double contoured membrane. Only after a few weeks are histiocytes and some giant cells seen, the latter often lying alone. There is also considerable vasodilation. Verrucous changes with pseudoepitheliomatous hyperplasia and intraepidermal microabscesses develop later. At this stage, the organisms are best seen

in the numerous giant cells of the regional lymphadenitis. It can be very difficult to find them in skin biopsies. Although they may be recognized in H&E section as small round to oval holes in the cytoplasm of giant cells, they are better seen with PAS, Grocott, Gridley, and even Congo red, Gram, and Papanicolaou stains. Direct immunofluorescence and immunohistochemistry allow the spores to be more easily found.[298,299]

4.5.3.4.2 Differential diagnosis

As long as the fungal spores are not seen, many other conditions, in particular other deep mycoses, tuberculosis cutis verrucosa, late syphilis, squamous cell carcinoma, or bromoderma and iododerma have to be differentiated. *Cryptococcus neoformans* has a mucin capsule staining with mucicarmine. *B. dermatitidis* has broad-based buds giving it the appearance of a shoe sole in contrast to the narrow based budding of *H. capsulatum*. Verrucous tuberculosis has no fungal elements. Squamous cell carcinoma and the flat form of keratoacanthoma can usually be distinguished as they do not show a mixed infiltrate with giant cells.

Highly sensitive serologic methods such as enzyme immuno assay (EIA), enzyme-linked immunosorbent assay (ELISA), and a sandwich immunoassay help to make the correct diagnosis.

4.5.3.5 Cryptococcosis

Cryptococcus neoformans is a saprophyte basidiomycete found worldwide in soil and pigeon droppings. *Cryptococcus gattii* is mainly found in the tropics. It is an opportunistic yeast causing invasive infections mainly in immunodepressed individuals, such as HIV infection, high-dose corticosteroid therapy and advanced cancer,[300] and after organ transplantation.[301–303] Fever and meningitis not responding to antibacterial antibiotics are the main clinical presentations.[304] However, skin and nail involvement occurs in 10%–15% of patients with systemic cryptococcosis and primary cutaneous cryptococcosis occasionally occurs in solid organ transplant recipients, but also in otherwise healthy individuals, particularly after a minor trauma.[305–307] Cutaneous cryptococcosis of the great toe was observed to precede systemic disease for several months.[308] In the hand, tenosynovitis and osteomyelitis were observed.[309] Skin lesions are usually very variable and nonspecific.[310,311] There was severe ulcerating paronychia in a case of a cryptococcus nail unit infection and a hemorrhagic whitlow in another immunocompetent patient.[312–314]

The diagnosis is established by direct exam of smears, histopathology, fungal culture, and serum tests. Cytologically, *Cryptococcus neoformans* is a round to oval structure with a diameter of 5–10 μ, which is embedded in a gelatinous capsule as easily seen in an India ink preparation.[315]

4.5.3.5.1 Histopathology

Cutaneous cryptococcosis is histopathologically divided into two major reaction types: intense granulomatous inflammatory response with lymphocytes, macrophages, and mutinucleated giant cells with intracellular yeasts; paucireactive pattern with extracellular yeasts and minimal or even absent inflammatory infiltrate but tissue destruction resulting from compression necroses due to large masses of *cryptococci*; this gives a gelatinous tissue aspect.[316–318]

Circumscribed granulomas are composed of aggregated histiocytes and giant cells of both the Langhans and foreign body type with numerous phagocytosed yeasts that are often visible in H&E stained sections as pale round structures surrounded by a clear halo.[319] Central necrosis and marginal fibrosis may occur. The paucireactive type shows large masses of yeasts. Lesions may have both gelatinous and granulomatous components.[320] Mucicarmin stain reveals a pink capsule,[321] whereas Grocott stains the cell walls intensely and budding is seen with a very narrow base. Fontana-Masson's silver technique is positive for the cell walls presumably due to fungal melanin.[322–324] Some strains do not develop a capsule and remain mucicarmine negative; they stain positive with Fontana-Masson allowing their diagnosis to be made.[325,326] The treatment of choice is fluconazole or itraconazole, in case of insufficient effect posaconazole and voriconazole.

4.5.3.5.2 Differential diagnosis

The acapsular cryptococcus variants are particularly difficult to identify as they are also seronegative. Fontana-Masson stain is necessary to make the diagnosis.

4.5.3.5.2.1 Hyaloyphomycoses

Hyalohyphomycetes are fungi with branched hyaline septate hyphae. This group includes *Aspergillus* spp., *Fusarium* spp., *Scedosporium* spp., *Acremonium* spp., *Scopulariopsis* spp., and *Paecilomyces* spp. They are emerging pathogens able to produce severe and disseminated infections mostly in immunocompromised individuals. Their mortality rate is high. Infections of the fingertip and nail unit may occur.

4.5.3.6 Aspergillosis

Fungi of the genus *Aspergillus* are widely distributed in the environment. They grow on soil, decaying vegetation, and foods. *Aspergillus fumigatus, A. flavus,* and *A. niger* but also other *A.* species are able to cause systemic infections in immunocompromised and neutropenic patients,[327–329] but rarely in immunocompetent persons.[330–332] Burn patients are also at risk for aspergillosis. Lung and sinus infections are the most frequent form. Hematogenous spread to the skin, but also primary cutaneous aspergillosis are rare.[333,334] Primary cutaneous aspergillosis is almost invariably due to *A. flavus* whereas *A. fumigatus* is the main pathogen in secondary cutaneous aspergillosis.[335] Nail apparatus involvement may either be due to direct inoculation or by angioinvasive spread from fungal emboli.[336] Periungual lesions may appear as paronychia or deep inflammatory infiltrates, particularly in primary invasive cutaneous aspergillosis. Violaceous macules, purplish papules and nodules, hemorrhagic blisters, pustules,

and subcutaneous abscesses may develop that tend to ulcerate and develop necroses.[337,338]

For *Aspergillus* onychomycosis, see above.

4.5.3.6.1 Histopathology

Biopsies show a dense neutrophilic infiltrate of the dermis and superficial edema. There is often epidermal necrosis and dermal necrobiosis with lymphocytes in the periphery. Epidermal necrosis is more likely to be seen in primary than in secondary cutaneous aspergillosis.[339] Abundant fungal hyphae are demonstrated in PAS and Grocott stains. *Aspergillus* is seen in the tissue as branching septate hyphae in the necrotic tissue. They are often very densely aggregated forming balls of hyphae. Necrosis is due to vascular obstruction by the fungi, endothelial damage, and finally vessel necrosis (Figure 4.27).[340] Plasma cells and granulomas do not occur. In the tissue, the hyphae have a diameter of 4–6 μ, have a bubbly cytoplasm, and show arboreal dichotomous branching with an angle of approximately 30–45°. However, previous antifungal treatment may alter the fungal morphology. Cultures are more sensitive than histopathology in demonstrating *Aspergillus* fungi.

4.5.3.6.2 Differential diagnosis

Invasive fusariosis and *Pseudoallescheria boydii* and *Scedosporium* infections also show septate hyphae branching with an acute angle.[341] *Zygomycetes* branch at an angle of 90° and are aseptate. *Fusarium* spp. typically have vesicular swellings in their hyphae. Thus, culture is necessary to confirm the diagnosis. Embolic lesions are also observed in approximately 12% of patients with systemic candidiasis.[342] A Sweet-like aspect was observed in one case.[343]

4.5.3.7 Fusariosis

Fusariosis is another hyalohyphomycetic infection mainly affecting immunocompromised individuals and *Fusarium* species are the second most common pathogenic molds

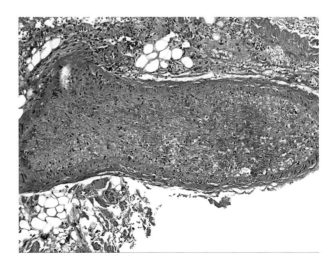

Figure 4.27 *Aspergillus* embolus in a subungual artery. (Courtesy of Dr. O. Sangüeza, Winston-Salem, NC.)

in patients with hematologic malignancies and neutropenia.[344,345] *Fusarium* infections vary from superficial to invasive systemic. In immunocompetent patients, onychomycosis of the toes, rarely the fingers,[346] and keratitis are the most common *Fusarium* infections.[347,348] Superficial fusariosis may remain for years if left untreated even in the immunocompetent host.[349] This is important as *Fusarium* onychomycosis and paronychia may spread to other sites[350] and cause fatal dissemination.[351] Blood cultures are often positive as intravascular adventitious sporulation from necrotic tissue continually releases spores into the bloodstream. *Fusarium* spp. produce dangerous mycotoxins such as trichothecenes and zearalenones.[352] The skin is affected in 70% of systemic disease and thus the most frequently involved organ, but other organs may be affected.[353–357] Skin lesions most frequently occur in the extremities and are usually seen as painful, livid, red infiltrates and nodes that may be disseminated and tend to develop a necrotic eschar and ulcerate. The nail bed was observed to be necrotic after the nail had fallen off.[358] *Fusarium chlamydosporum* was isolated from a patient's toe after ingrown nail surgery.[359] Fusariosis is relatively resistent to many antifungal drugs and the treatment results depend on early therapy and an efficacious antifungal such as amphotericin B, itraconazole, or voriconazole;[360] however, some of these drugs are often not well tolerated.[361]

4.5.3.7.1 Histopathology

Depending on the stage of fusariosis, there may be a marked epidermal necrosis with a dense inflammatory infiltrate mainly composed of neutrophils and lymphocytes. Hyaline branched septate hyphae are usually seen extending from the surface deep into the dermis. They may even be seen in H&E stained sections, but PAS or Grocott stains prove their fungal origin (Figure 4.28).[362] Usually, there are more fungal elements in the superficial portion of the necroses.

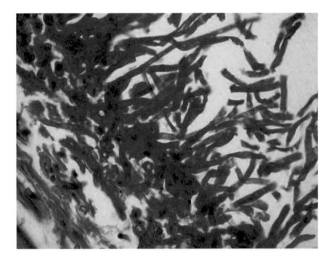

Figure 4.28 *Fusarium oxysporon* conglomerate in the tip of a digit (PAS).

Fusarium onychomycosis is characterized by hyphae and yeast-like elements with variable diameter. Enlargements during the course of fungal filaments are said to be characteristic.

Cultures taken from a biopsy yield colonies of white to creamy color on Sabouraud's dextrose agar without cycloheximide.[363] Slide cultures reveal single or two-celled oval microconidia of 8×2 to 9×3 µ in size that may be grouped in verticilliums produced by elongated phialides, and banana-shaped macroconidia.[364,365] Intercalary chlamydoconidia are characteristic. Further identification is possible with polymerase chain reaction.

4.5.3.7.2 Differential diagnosis

Aspergillosis is the most important differential diagnosis. The fungal morphology is almost identical with hyaline septate hyphae branching at an acute angle, and both diseases are angio-invasive causing thrombosis and tissue infarction. The diagnosis of fusariosis is confirmed by culture showing banana-shaped macroconidia.

4.5.3.8 Zygomycosis (Phycomycosis, Mucormycosis)

Zygomycosis is a collective term for infections by fungi of the orders of *Entomophthorales* including *Basidiobolus* and *Conidiobolus* species, and *mucorales*.[366] The former are primary pathogens whereas the latter are opportunistic fungi. Zygomycoses are rare, but ubiquitous infections. There are about 500 new cases each year in the United States.[367] It is held to be the third most frequent opportunistic fungal infection. The prognosis of the enthomophthoromycoses is often poor because of late diagnosis, the fulminant course of the disease, and lack of efficacious treatment, whereas primary skin mucormyoses have a good prognosis when diagnosed early.[368] Zygomycetes may affect the skin, subcutaneous tissue, and virtually all organs; infections often do not respect tissue and organ boundaries. Rhinocerebral and pulmonary infections are most frequent. Patients with uncontrolled diabetes mellitus and with immunosuppression are most commonly affected with systemic and secondary cutaneous zygomycosis; other predisposing diseases are leukemia, malignant lymphoma, solid organ transplantation, treatment with steroids and deferioxamine, and AIDS. Immunosuppressed patients with a long hospital stay are at a high risk.[369–371] Primary cutaneous and subcutaneous zygomycosis in immunocompetent persons is probably due to minor laceration trauma and makes up for 7%–15% of all zygomycosis cases.[372,373] Skin lesions are variable but most of them are rapidly growing and exhibit a characteristic black necrotic eschar that feels like hard parchment.[374] Systemic spread may occur. The isolation of the pathogen from skin swabs is not reliable and a biopsy may be needed.[375] Even from biopsy material it is difficult to culture the fungus because the aseptate hyphae are often damaged and become nonviable during surgery and tissue grinding in the laboratory. Sabouraud-dextrose agar is used to grow zygomycetes, which may show a woolly culture within a few days that should be examined microscopically after staining with lactophenol

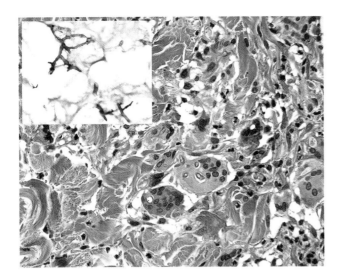

Figure 4.29 Mucor mycosis in a renal transplant recipient. Short fungal segments are visible in giant cells (H&E). (Inset: Giemsa shows branching fungi.)

cotton blue. Real-time PCR allows species identification in virtually all cases.[376,377] Treatment is with itraconazole, voriconazole, or amphotericin B.[378]

4.5.3.8.1 Histopathology

With due suspicion, the diagnosis can usually be made with H&E stain but is more reliable with PAS, Grocott, and/or Giemsa. In early or peripheral lesions, there are small granulomas in the dermis and subcutis that contain a variable amount of multinucleated macrophages and giant cells often with phagocytosed fungal elements (Figure 4.29). Neutrophils are present in variable numbers. Plasma cells and esosinophils may be seen. In the center of fully developed lesions, there are masses of fungi with broad, thin-walled, infrequently septate hyphae with focal bulbous enlargements branching at a wide angle. The fungi invade all tissues including fasciae, muscles, and vessels causing tissue infarction and necrosis. *Entomophthorales* infections often show an eosinophilic sheath around the hyphae, called Splendore-Hoeppli phenomenon. This is not present in infections by *Mucorales* and therefore serves as a differential diagnostic criterion.[379]

4.5.3.8.2 Differential diagnosis

All other cutaneous-subcutaneous mycoses have to be ruled out, which is in part possible due to their morphology in histopathological sections. Cultural fungus identification and/or PCR are necessary to further classify the pathogen. When necrosis is prevalent and fungi are not seen, tuberculosis and other necrotizing diseases have to be considered.

4.6 PROTOTHECOSIS

Although prothecosis is due to algae that are distinct from fungi, this disease is usually dealt with in Chapter 4.6 on fungal infections as the algae grow on Sabouraud agar. *Prototheca* are saprophytes growing in soil, water, and on decaying plants. Occasionally, domestic animals are affected. Prothecosis is seen in immunocompetent and immunosuppressed hosts.[380] It develops when a wound gets in contact with water or even by direct inoculation from a splinter on which algae grew. Skin lesions are uncharacteristic and usually appear as small papules and plaques that tend to become papillomatous and verrucous and may even ulcerate. Subungual prothecosis clinically resembles onychomycosis.[381]

4.6.1 Histopathology

Material for the diagnosis of prothecosis may be scales or serous, bloody or purulent exudate. The identification of the algae is necessary to make the diagnosis. Hence, both microbiological as well as histopathological examinations are recommended.[382,383] Direct microscopy is performed after clearing with 10%–20% potassium hydroxide and staining with lactophenol cotton blue allowing the sporangia to be identified. Endosporulation leads to the characteristic morula aspect of the sporangia.[384] The two species pathogenic to humans can be distinguished by the size of their sporangia: *P. wickerhamii* has a symmetrical morula and *P. zopfii* shows increased segmentation.[385]

If endosporulation is seen, the diagnosis of prothecosis is evident. There is a predominantly granulomatous infiltrate with lymphocytes, plasma cells, neutrophils, eosinophils, macrophages, and giant cells. Pseudoepitheliomatous epithelial hyperplasia and ulceration may be present. The tissue has to be stained with PAS, Grocott, or Gridley for better visualization of the morula.[386]

In subungual prothecosis, there is usually a loose subungual hyperkeratosis with cocci and bacilli as secondary colonizers (Figure 4.30). PAS and Grocott stain show morula-like sporangia ranging from small organisms consisting of a few spores to larger globular structures composed of many spores.[371]

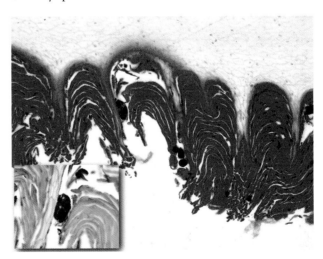

Figure 4.30 Subungual prothecosis. The fungal elements are both visible in H&E as well as PAS stains. (Inset: Higher magnification.)

4.6.2 Differential diagnosis

The presence of sporangia with the morula aspect allows the diagnosis of protothecosis to be made. However, small sporangia may be confused with fumagoid cells and single cells have to be differentiated from *Blastomyces dermatitidis*, *Cryptococcus neoformans*, *Paracoccidiodis brasiliensis*, *Coccidioides immitis,* and *Rhinosporidium seeberi*.[383,387,388]

4.7 PROTOZOAL INFECTIONS

Protozoan diseases of the nail are rarely seen in Europe and North America, but are not uncommon in the tropics.

4.7.1 Leishmaniasis

Depending on the type of *Leishmania* species responsible for the infection and of the immune competence of the host, various forms of leishmaniasis are recognized.[389] The *Leishmania* are transmitted via sandflies that belong to the *Phlebotomus* genus in the Old World and to the *Lutzomia* and *Psychodopygus* genera in the New World. In the intestines of the sandflies, the protozoa are flagellar promastigotes capable of active movement whereas after they have entered the human (or other vertebrates) they become intracellular parasites in histiocytes with internalized flagella.[390] The most common type of leishmaniasis is the acute localized cutaneous form mainly due to *Leishmania major* and *tropica* in Europe, Africa, and Asia and to *Leishmania braziliensis* and *mexicana* with various subspecies in the Americas. On the exposed skin, a nontender reddish papule develops over a period of 1–3 months to a nodule or plaque with a diameter of 1–2 cm. Ulceration may occur. After several months to a year, spontaneous healing resulting in an obvious scar is observed in most cases. In the immunocompromised host, an acute disseminated leishmaniasis can be observed starting with a single papule and spreading over the body. Ulceration is uncommon. Chronic and recurrent (lupoid) leishmaniasis occurs when the lesion does not heal within two years or recurs. Post-kala azar dermal leishmaniasis develops 1–5 years after successful treatment of visceral leishmaniasis and is characterized first by development of hypopigmented macules, then of papules and nodules mostly in the face resulting in a facies leonina aspect. Mucocutaneous leishmaniasis is mainly seen in South America. No nail involvement was reported in visceral and viscerotropic leishmaniasis. Nail lesions may occur in the first four different forms, usually as an ulcerating paronychia or even with bone destruction.[391,392]

4.7.1.1 Histopathology

The histopathologic features depend on the time of biopsy. In fresh lesions, a dense infiltrate of macrophages and histiocytes with some plasma cells is seen, often with thinning or superficial necrosis of the epidermis. Ulceration is accompanied with neutrophils in the infiltrate. In the cytoplasm of the macrophages, small round to oval, blue-gray bodies are seen that have a basophilic round nucleus and exhibit a tiny paranuclear rod-shaped kinetoplast

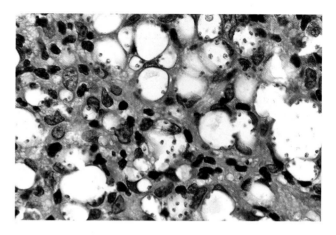

Figure 4.31 Leishmanial paronychia showing masses of leishmania bodies. (Courtesy of Dr. Patricia Chang, Guatemala.)

(Figure 4.31) that stains red with Giemsa; they are called Leishman-Donovan bodies. With time, the number of *leishmania* bodies decreases and that of plasma cells increases. At this stage, *leishmanias* may only be seen in subepidermal histiocytes.

In the acute diffuse leishmaniasis, the protozoa are abundant and the lymphocyte admixture is minimal.

The non-healing type of localized leishmaniasis as well as the recurrent lupoid type exhibit a diffuse dense or a nodular tuberculoid infiltrate with epithelioid cells, Langhans giant cells, lymphocytes, and plasma cells. *Leishmanias* are usually not found.

Immunohistochemistry and polymerase chain reaction help to confirm the diagnosis.[393,394]

4.7.1.2 Differential diagnosis

The leishmania bodies have about the size of *Histoplasma capsulatum* and do not stain with fungal stains such as PAS and Grocott. Small intracellular organisms with a paranuclear kinetoplast are also seen in cutaneous Chagas disease (American trypanosomiasis).[395,396] *Klebsiella rhinoscleromatis* is also an intracellular pathogen with a diameter of 2–3 μ, but the plasma cell number is much higher and there are numerous Russell bodies. Granuloma inguinale is characterized by multiple small abscesses in the infiltrate. Chronic leishmaniasis has to be differentiated from tuberculosis cutis luposa (lupus vulgaris).

4.8 INFESTATIONS

The nail can harbor a great variety of parasites, both as a carrier as well as the target of the pathogen. However, when the clinical diagnosis is made from lesions elsewhere, then a biopsy will be made from there rather than from the nail.[397] On the other hand, fingers and to a certain degree also toes may be characteristic localizations for infestations.

4.8.1 Scabies

Scabies is caused by the human itch mite *Sarcoptes scabiei*. It is transmitted from human to human by direct physical contact, particularly when it is warm. Nail involvement is characteristic for crusted (Norwegian) scabies that usually develops in immunocompromised persons,[398] but has also been seen in seemingly usual scabies,[399–401] particularly in children.[402] The nails are dystrophic and display various degrees of mainly distal subungual hyperkeratosis harboring mites and eggs.[403–405] Longitudinal fissuring may occur.[406] Subungual mites are often the cause of recurrence[407] and "unexplained" spread by insufficiently treated patients. Therapy is by atraumatic partial nail avulsion[408] and long-term application of scabicides under occlusion.[409–411] Whereas ivermectin is usually highly effective, a treatment failure was observed in nail involvement.[412]

4.8.1.1 Histopathology

For the diagnosis of nail scabies, a generous nail clipping is sufficient in most cases. It reveals pronounced subungual hyperkeratosis with huge amounts of mites, eggs, and scyballa in classical burrows.[413] Scrapings of subungual debris also exhibit myriads of mites. In the skin, the mites may be localized with a dermatoscope and extracted from the burrow with a needle or by gently removing the roof, with a #15 scalpel,[414] of the tiny vesicle containing the female mite. Pink pigtail-like structures may be found connected to the horny layer (Figure 4.32); they probably represent parts of eggshells of the mites.[415]

4.8.1.2 Differential diagnosis

A variety of dermatoses can evoke clinically similar alterations, but the histopathology of crusted scabies of the nail is so characteristic that the diagnosis cannot be missed.

4.8.2 Tungiasis

Tungiasis is a relatively common infestation of tropical and subtropical regions. In temperate climates, it is seen as an imported disease. The foot is the common site of the parasite, the fertilized sand flea female, but depending on the body position, for example, lying at an infested beach, other regions may be involved. Subungual location is quite characteristic. The female *Tunga penetrans*

painlessly digs into the epidermis (stage 1), very often of the hyponychium. It grows extremely fast (stage 2) in the epidermis while its proboscis, a specialized suction device, takes blood from the papillary vessels. Within two weeks, the body enlarges by a factor of 2000 to reach the size of a pea. The last three abdominal segments are outside the epidermis to allow the eggs to be laid and feces to be shed (stage 3). When all eggs have been expulsed, the enlarged abdominal segments start to atrophy and the parasite finally dies 3 to 4 weeks after the infestation (stage 4). Its remnants are eliminated via the horny layer and a small residual scar remains (stage 5). The diagnosis is often delayed because the patients only notice the sandflea as a black nodule in stage 3 or 4; this has sometimes even been mistaken for a subungual melanoma. A geographic patient history, characteristic symptoms such as itch, local tenderness and foreign body sensation, the visible abdominal segments under a magnifier lens or with a dermatoscope, the pulsations of the flea body, brownish feces around the dark nodule, and possibly eggs permit the diagnosis to be made clinically. The treatment of choice is surgical enucleation, often with additional antibiotic treatment. As the disease is self-limiting, a systemic antiparasitic therapy is only necessary in case of disseminated lesions.[416,417]

4.8.2.1 Histopathology

A complete lesion of the entire parasite in the skin is rarely obtained. There is a localization-specific thick horny layer with parakeratotic portions and a grossly acanthotic epidermis harboring polycyclic eosinophilic structures corresponding to the chitin wall of the organism. Sectioned inner organs and particularly gut structures are more basophilic. Round to oval bodies probably represent eggs.[418] These structures are negative in PAS stains but fluoresce brightly when stained with calcofluor. The surrounding epidermis forms a colarette around the sand flea and is often slightly spongiotic (Figure 4.33). There is a predominantly perivascular infiltrate in the dermis and eosinophils may be seen.

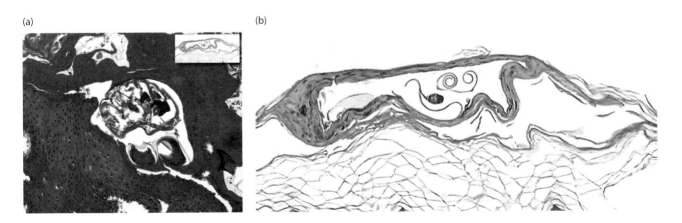

(a)   (b)

Figure 4.32 (a) Subungual scabies with mites in burrows in the subungual hyperkeratosis. (Courtesy of Dr. P. Chang, Guatemala.) (b) Pigtail structures from a mite burrow of the lateral nail fold.

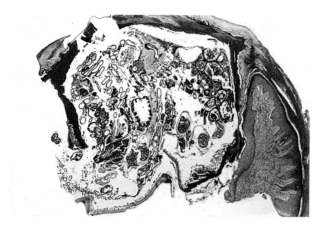

Figure 4.33 Subungual tungiasis. The eggs are seen as oval structures.

4.8.2.2 Differential diagnosis

The diagnosis relies on a good biopsy or excision specimen and the characteristic patient history. When only a few parasite parts are present in the biopsy other intraepithelial parasites have to be differentiated, which is not possible on histologic grounds alone.

4.8.3 Myiasis

Myiasis is caused by fly larvae of different species. Whereas wound myiasis is extremely rare on fingers, it may occur on toes in neglected individuals; many different flies including *Calliphoridae* from Central Europe are responsible.[419] Furuncular myiasis is mainly seen on the head and trunk; it is due to the African tumbu fly *Cordylobia anthropophaga* or by the American botfly *Dermatobia hominis*.[420] This lesion is painful in the nail region. The creeping myiasis, which must not be confused with larva migrans, is caused by larvae of *Gasterophilus* and *Hypoderma* species, flies that parasite in horses and cattle.

4.8.3.1 Histopathology

Wound myiasis of the nail apparatus has not been examined histopathologically as the fly larvae are alive and can be seen with the naked eye.[419]

Furuncular myiasis is also only biopsied when the diagnosis was not made clinically. The botfly larvae are relatively large and have a spiny exoskeleton with characteristic black pigmentation of their chitin spines. An intense inflammatory infiltrate composed of neutrophils, lymphocytes, eosinophils, plasma cells, and occasional Langhans giant cells surrounds the parasite.[421] Bacteria are virtually absent as both larvae secrete a bacteriostatic product.

Creeping myiasis may be seen around the nail. Biopsies show only a minimal infiltrate and are rarely diagnostic.[422]

4.8.3.2 Differential diagnosis

The diagnosis of an infestation requires at least parts of the parasite to be seen. The characteristic black spines of the exoskeleton of the botfly larva are diagnostic. Further, the patient's history is important.

4.8.4 Cutaneous larva migrans

Most cases of cutaneous larva migrans are due to hookworms of cats and dogs. In temperate climates, they represent imported dermatoses, mainly by travellers returning from tropical countries.[423] They get infected by larvae that contaminate the soil.[424] Therefore, the feet are most commonly affected. Once the hookworm has penetrated the skin, it migrates a few millimeters per day forming irregular winding raised burrows, which are 2–3 mm wide. After some weeks, the hookworm dies as the human is not its correct host.

In Africa, many children present lesions also around the nails.

4.8.4.1 Histopathology

The parasite is usually 1–2 cm ahead of the visible burrow and mostly not seen in biopsies.[425] However, the track shows a strong lymphocytic reaction with many eosinophils in a spongiotic epidermis that may contain necrotic keratinocytes. Eosinophils are also seen in the upper dermis. In case the parasite is sectioned, it is seen between the horny and granular layers as small round structures. The tissue reaction is weak.

4.8.4.2 Differential diagnosis

Strong tissue and epidermal eosinophilia are characteristic for many parasitic infestations.

4.8.5 Pediculosis

A case of pediculosis in a patient with onychomycosis[426] and two cases of subungual book louse infestation were described.[427]

4.8.5.1 Histopathology

Removal of the subungual masses with the nail revealed multiple cavities.

4.8.5.2 Differential diagnosis

The cavities are reminiscent of those of subungual scabies but bigger.

REFERENCES

1. Feder HM Jr, Long SS. Herpetic whitlow. Epidemiology, clinical characteristics, diagnosis, and treatment. *Am J Dis Child* 1983;137:861–863.
2. Gill MJ, Arlette J, Tyrrell DL, Buchan KA. Herpes simplex virus infection of the hand. Clinical features and management. *Am J Med* 1988;85:53–56.
3. Ruiter M. Aphthous stomatitis and herpetic paronychia in an adult. *Acta Derm Vener* 1950;30:497–502.
4. Bandlow G, Kohlschutter A. Herpes simplex causing a therapy-resistant panaritium. *Dtsch Med Wochenschr* 1977;102:759–760.
5. McNicholl B. Recurrent herpetic whitlow. *Arch Emerg Med* 1990;7:124–125.
6. Karpathios T, Moustaki M, Yiallouros P, Sarifi F, Tzanakaki G, Fretzayas A. HSV-2 meningitis disseminated from a herpetic whitlow. *Paediatr Int Child Health* 2012;32:121–122.

7. Ishak RS, Abbas O. Recurrent vesicular eruption on the right hand. *J Fam Pract* 2014;63:33–35.

8. Avitzur Y, Amir J. Herpetic whitlow infection in a general pediatrician—An occupational hazard. *Infection* 2002;30:234–236.

9. Merchant VA, Molinari JA, Sabes WR. Herpetic whitlow: Report of a case with multiple recurrences. *Oral Surg Oral Med Oral Pathol* 1983;55:568–571.

10. Durdu M, Ruocco V. Clinical and cytologic features of antibiotic-resistant acute paronychia. *J Am Acad Dermatol* 2014;70:120–6.e1.

11. El Hachem M, Bernardi S, Giraldi L, Diociaiuti A, Palma P, Castelli-Gattinara G. Herpetic whitlow as a harbinger of pediatric HIV-1 infection. *Pediatr Dermatol* 2005;22:119–121.

12. Feichtner K, Goldscheider I, Herzinger T, Ruzicka T. Varizellen unter dem klinischen Bild eines Podopompholyx. Dia-Klinik, 24. Fortbildungswoche für praktische Dermatologie und Venerologie, Munich, 19–25 July 2014:26–29.

13. Kocak AY, Koçak O. Onychomadesis in two sisters induced by varicella infection. *Pediatr Dermatol* 2013;30:e108–109.

14. Zizmor J, Deluty S. Acquired leukonychia striata. *Int J Dermatol* 1980;19:49–50.

15. Mabuchi T, Yamaoka H, Kato M, Ikoma N, Tamiya S, Song HJ, Nakamura N, Ozawa A. Case of disseminated vesicles of herpes zoster developing one day before the onset of local eruption in a hospitalized immunocompromised patient. *Tokai J Exp Clin Med* 2013;38:52–54.

16. Solomon AR, Rasmussen JE, Weiss JS. A comparison of the Tzack smear and viral isolation in varicella and herpes zoster. *Arch Dermatol* 1986;122:282–285.

17. Lenac Roviš T, Bailer SM, Pothineni VR, Ouwendijk WJ, Šimić H, Babić M, Miklić K et al. Comprehensive analysis of varicella-zoster virus proteins using a new monoclonal antibody collection. *J Virol* 2013;87:6943–6954.

18. Worrell JT, Cockerell CJ. Histopathology of peripheral nerves in cutaneous herpesvirus infection. *Am J Dermatopathol* 1997;19:133–137.

19. Muraki R, Baba T, Iwasaki T, Sata T, Kurata T. Immunohistochemical study of skin lesions in herpes zoster. *Virchows Arch A Pathol Anat Histopathol* 1992;420:71–76.

20. Requena L, Requena C. Histopathology of the more common viral skin infections. *Actas Dermosifiliogr* 2010;101:201–216.

21. Lee JY. Cytomegalovirus infection involving the skin in immunocompromised hosts. A clinicopathologic study. *Am J Clin Pathol* 1989;92:96–100.

22. Khoshnevis M, Tyring SK. Cytomegalovirus infections. *Dermatol Clin* 2002;20:291–299, vii.

23. Ryan C, De Gascun CF, Powell C, Sheahan K, Mooney EE, McCormick A, Kirby B. Cytomegalovirus-induced cutaneous vasculopathy and perianal ulceration. *J Am Acad Dermatol* 2011;64:1216–1218.

24. Cachafeiro TH, Escobar GF, Bakos L, Bakos RM. Chronic cutaneous cytomegalovirus infection in a patient with severe combined immunodeficiency syndrome. *Br J Dermatol* 2014;170:223–225.

25. Choi YL, Kim JA, Jang KT, Kim DS, Kim WS, Lee JH, Yang JM, Lee ES, Lee DY. Characteristics of cutaneous cytomegalovirus infection in non-acquired immune deficiency syndrome, immunocompromised patients. *Br J Dermatol* 2006;155:977–982.

26. AbdullGaffar B, Raman LG, Al Muala A. Cutaneous cytomegalovirus infection in a patient with acquired immunodeficiency syndrome. *Int J Dermatol* 2008;47:944–946.

27. Heller J. *Die Krankheiten der Nägel*. Berlin: August Hirschwald, 1900; 174–175.

28. Michelson HE, Ikeda K. Microscopic changes in variola. *Arch Dermatol Syph* 1927;15:1927.

29. Suchard. Modification des cellules de la matrice et du lit de l'ongle. *Arch Physiol* 1882;X:445 (cit by J Heller).

30. Lawn SD, Planche T, Riley P, Holwill S, Silman N, Bewley K, Rice P, Wansbrough-Jones MH. A black necrotic ulcer. *Lancet* 2003;361:1518.

31. Schupp CJ, Nitsche A, Bock-Hensley O, Böhm S, Flechtenmacher C, Kurth A, Saenger K et al. A 14-year-old girl with a vesicle on her finger and lymphadenitis. *J Clin Virol* 2011;50:1–3.

32. Haase O, Moser A, Rose C, Kurth A, Zillikens D, Schmidt E. Gneralized cowpox infection in a patient with Darier disease. *Br J Dermatol* 2011;164:1116–118.

33. Feuerstein B, Jürgens M, Schnetz E, Fartasch M, Simon M Jr. Cowpox and catpox infection. 2 clinical case reports. *Hautarzt* 2000;51:852–856.

34. Slanina H, Schüttler CG, König M, Mayser P. Eschar after a journey to the forest: Cowpox infection. *J Dtsch Ges Dermatol* 2015;13:1045–1047.

35. Vestey JP, Yirrell DL, Aldridge RD. Cowpox/catpox infection. *Br J Dermatol* 1991;124:74–78.

36. Gupta LK, Singhi MK. Tzanck smear: A useful diagnostic tool. *Indian J Dermatol Venereol Leprol* 2005;71:295–299.

37. Durdu M, Seçkin D, Baba M. The Tzanck smear test: Rediscovery of a practical diagnostic tool. *Skinmed* 2011;9:23–32.

38. Friederichs S, Krebs S, Blum H, Wolf E, Lang H, von Buttlar H, Büttner M. Comparative and retrospective molecular analysis of Parapoxvirus (PPV) isolates. *Virus Res* 2014;181:11–21.

39. Tosti A, Piraccini BM. Warts of the nail unit: Surgical and nonsurgical approaches. *Dermatol Surg* 2001;27:235–239.

40. Kattan KR, Babcock DS, Felson B. Solitary phalangeal defect in the hand. Report of 2 rare cases. *Am J Roentgenol Radium Ther Nucl Med* 1975;124:29–31.

41. Thappa DM, Garg BR, Thadeus J, Ratnakar C. Cutaneous horn: A brief review and report of a case. *J Dermatol* 1997;24:34–37.

42. Kaiser JF, Proctor-Shipman L. Squamous cell carcinoma in situ (Bowen's disease) mimicking subungual verruca vulgaris. *J Fam Pract* 1994;39:384–387.

43. De Berker DAR, Wlodek C, Bristow IR. Subungual corn: A tender pigmented subungual lesion in older people. *Br J Dermatol* 2014;171:69–72.

44. Steigleder GK. Histology of benign virus induced tumors of the skin. *J Cutan Pathol* 1978;5:45–52.

45. Bender ME. The protean manifestations of human papillomavirus infection. New facies of an old foe: A clinical perspective. *Arch Dermatol* 1994;130: 1429–1430.

46. Nuovo GJ, Ishag M. The histologic spectrum of epidermodysplasia verruciformis. *Am J Surg Pathol* 2000;24:1400–1406.

47. Majewski S, Jabłońska S. Epidermodysplasia verruciformis as a model of human papillomavirus-induced genetic cancer of the skin. *Arch Dermatol* 1995;131:1312–1318.

48. Rogers HD, Macgregor JL, Nord KM, Tyring S, Rady P, Engler DE, Grossman ME. Acquired epidermodysplasia verruciformis. *J Am Acad Dermatol* 2009;60:315–320.

49. Haneke E. Immunhistochemische Untersuchungen an formalinfixiertem Gewebe in der Dermatologie. *Akt Dermatol* 1985;11:66–72.

50. Ashida M1, Ueda M, Kunisada M, Ichihashi M, Terai M, Sata T, Matsukura T. Protean manifestations of human papillomavirus type 60 infection on the extremities. *Br J Dermatol* 2002;146:885–890.

51. Yanagi T, Shibaki A, Tsuji-Abe Y, Yokota K, Shimizu H. Epidermodysplasia verruciformis and generalized verrucosis: The same disease? *Clin Exp Dermatol* 2006;31:390–393.

52. Ergun SS, Su O, Büyükbabany N. Giant verruca vulgaris. *Dermatol Surg* 2004;30:459–462.

53. Scheinfeld N, Yu T, Lee J. Verrucous hyperplasia of the great toe: A case and a review of the literature. *Dermatol Surg* 2004;30:215–217.

54. Tosti A, Morelli R, Fanti PA, Morselli PG, Catrani S, Landi G. Carcinoma cuniculatum of the nail apparatus: Report of three cases. *Dermatology* 1993;186:217–221.

55. Salamon T, Halepović E, Berberović L, Nikulin A, Lazović-Tepavac O, Cerkez A, Basić V. Epidermodysplasia verruciformis-ähnliche Genodermatose mit Veränderungen der Nägel. *Hautarzt* 1987; 38:525–531.

56. Stetsenko GY, McFarlane RJ, Chien AJ, Fleckman P, Swanson P, George E, Argenyi ZB. Subungual Bowen disease in a patient with epidermodysplasia verruciformis presenting clinically as longitudinal melanonychia. *Am J Dermatopathol* 2008;30:582–585.

57. Haneke E. Onychomadesis and hand, foot and mouth disease—Is there a connection? *Eurosurveillance* 2010 Sept 16; 15(37):pii:19664. Available online: http://www.eurosurveillance.org/ViewArticle.aspx?ArticleId=19664

58. Haneke E. Electron microscopic demonstration of virus particles in hand, foot and mouth disease. *Dermatologica* 1985;171:321–326.

59. Courvoisier S, Grob H, Weisser M, Itin PH, Battegay M. Relationship between erythema of the proximal nailfold in HIV-infected patients and hepatitis C virus infection. *Eur J Clin Microbiol Infect Dis* 1998;17:596–597.

60. Wilkerson MG, Wilkin JK. Red lunulae revisited: A clinical and histopathologic examination. *J Am Acad Dermatol* 1989;20:453–457.

61. Veneman NG, Waalkens HJ, van Raaij JJ, Brouwer RW. Septic polyarthritis due to an infected nail bed around an ingrown toenail in a previously healthy boy. *Ned Tijdschr Geneeskd* 2006;150:973–976.

62. Loffeld A, Davies P, Lewis A, Moss C. Seasonal occurrence of impetigo: A retrospective 8-year review (1996-2003). *Clin Exp Dermatol* 2005;30: 512–514.

63. Durdu M, Baba M, Seçkin D. The value of Tzanck smear test in diagnosis of erosive, vesicular, bullous, and pustular skin lesions. *J Am Acad Dermatol* 2008;59:958–964.

64. Stanley JR, Amagai M. Pemphigus, bullous impetigo, and the staphylococcal scalded-skin syndrome. *N Engl J Med* 2006;355:1800–1810.

65. Amagai M, Stanley JR. Desmoglein as a target in skin disease and beyond. *J Invest Dermatol* 2012;132:776–784.

66. Hays GC, Mullard JE. Blistering distal dactylitis: A clinically recognizable streptococcal infection. *Pediatrics* 1975;56:129–131.

67. McCray MK, Esterly NB. Blistering distal dactylitis. *J Am Acad Dermatol* 1981;5:592–594.

68. Schneider JA, Parlette HL 3rd. Blistering distal dactylitis: A manifestation of group A beta-hemolytic streptococcal infection. *Arch Dermatol* 1982;118:879–880.

69. Telfer NR, Barth JH, Dawber RP. Recurrent blistering distal dactylitis of the great toe associated with an ingrowing toenail. *Clin Exp Dermatol* 1989;14:380–381.

70. Palomo-Arellano A, Jiménez-Reyes J, Martín-Moreno L, de Castro-Torres A. Blistering distal dactylitis in an adult. *Arch Dermatol* 1985;121:1242.

71. Parras F, Ezpeleta C, Ezpeleta C, Romero J, Sendagorta E, Buzón L. Blistering distal dactylitis in an adult. *Cutis* 1988;41:127–128.

72. Frieden IJ. Blistering dactylitis caused by group B streptococci. *Pediatr Dermatol* 1989;6:300–302.

73. Zemtsov A, Veitschegger M. Staphylococcus aureus-induced blistering distal dactylitis in an adult immunosuppressed patient. *J Am Acad Dermatol* 1992;26:784–785.

74. Fretzayas A, Moustaki M, Tsagris V, Brozou T, Nicolaidou P. MRSA blistering distal dactylitis and review of reported cases. *Pediatr Dermatol* 2011;28:433–435.

75. Scheinfeld NS. Is blistering distal dactylitis a variant of bullous impetigo? *Clin Exp Dermatol* 2007;32:314–316.

76. Marinescu-Dinizvor G. On the dermal form of erysipeloid in slaughter house workmen. *Med Klin* 1979;74:1686–1688.

77. Hjetland R, Søgnen E, Våge V. Erysipelothrix rhusiopathiae—A cause of erysipeloid and endocarditis. *Tidsskr Nor Laegeforen* 1995;115:2780–2782.

78. Blaich A, Fasel D, Kaech C, Frei R. Mitral valve endocarditis after Turkish "Festival of Sacrifice". *Internist (Berl)* 2011;52:1109–1110, 1112–1113.

79. Clyti E, Claudel P, Gautier C, Geniaux M. Cutaneous manifestations of erysipeloid septicemia. *Ann Dermatol Venereol* 1998;125:196–198.

80. Veraldi S, Girgenti V, Dassoni F, Gianotti R. Erysipeloid: A review. *Clin Exp Dermatol* 2009;34:859–862.

81. White CP, Jewer DD. Seal finger: A case report and review of the literature. *Can J Plast Surg* 2009;17:133–135.

82. Sundeep S, Cleeve V. Isolation of Bisgaardia hudsonensis from a seal bite. Case report and review of the literature on seal finger. *J Infect* 2011;63:86–88.

83. Jansen LC, Justesen US, Roos SM, Dargis R, Jensen JS, Christensen JJ, Kemp M. Seal finger in Denmark diagnosed by PCR-technique. *Ugeskr Laeger* 2012; 174:426–427.

84. Lewin MR, Knott P, Lo M. Seal finger. *Lancet* 2004;364:448.

85. Bergholt A, Christensen RB, Cordtz T. Seal finger— Diagnosis, prevention and treatment. *Arctic Med Res* 1989;48:3–5.

86. Mass D, Newmeyer W, Kilgore E. Seal finger. *J Hand Surg [Am]* 1981;6:610–612.

87. Said R, Volpin G, Grimberg B, Friedenstrom SR, Lefler E, Stahl S. Hand infections due to non-cholera Vibrio after injuries from St Peter's fish (Tilapia zillii). *J Hand Surg Br* 1998;23:808–810.

88. Letulé V, Herzinger T. Kutane Diphtherie. Dia-Klinik, 25. Fortbildungswoche praktische Dermatologie und Venerologie, Munich, Book of Abstracts 2016:79–81.

89. Raja KM, Khan AA, Hameed A, Rahman SB. Unusual clinical variants of cutaneous leishmaniasis in Pakistan. *Br J Dermatol* 1998;139:111–113.

90. Svindland HB. Subacute parathion poisoning with erysipeloid-like lesion. *Contact Dermatitis* 1981;7:177–179.

91. Maes M, Richert B, de la Brassine M. Green nail syndrome or chloronychia. *Rev Méd Liège* 2002;57:233–235.

92. Elewski BE. Bacterial infection in a patient with onychomycosis. *J Am Acad Dermatol* 1997;37:493–494.

93. Wylock P, Jaeken R, Deraemaecker R. Anthrax of the hand: Case report. *J Hand Surg Am* 1983;8: 576–578.

94. Caksen H, Arabaci F, Abuhandan M, Tuncer O, Cesur Y. Cutaneous anthrax in eastern Turkey. *Cutis* 2001;67:488–492.

95. Tekin R, Sula B, Deveci O, Tekin A, Bozkurt F, Ucmak D, Kaya S et al. Cutaneous anthrax in Southeast Anatolia of Turkey. *Cutan Ocul Toxicol* 2015;34:7–11.

96. Oncül O, Ozsoy MF, Gul HC, Koçak N, Cavuslu S, Pahsa A. Cutaneous anthrax in Turkey: A review of 32 cases. *Scand J Infect Dis* 2002;34:413–416.

97. Chakraborty PP, Thakurt SG, Satpathi PS, Hansda S, Sit S, Achar A, Banerjee D. Outbreak of cutaneous anthrax in a tribal village: A clinico-epidemiological study. *J Assoc Physicians India* 2012;60:89–93.

98. Lewis JE. Suppurative inflammatory eruption occurring in septicemia tularemia. *Cutis* 1982;30:92, 96–97, 100.

99. Young LS, Bickness DS, Archer BG, Clinton JM, Leavens LJ, Feeley JC, Brachman PS. Tularemia epidemia: Vermont, 1968. Forty-seven cases linked to contact with muskrats. *N Engl J Med* 1969;280: 1253–1260.

100. Reddy K, Lowenstein EJ. Forensics in dermatology: Part II. *J Am Acad Dermatol* 2011;64:811–824.

101. Oskouizadeh K, Zahraei-Salehi T, Aledavood S. Detection of *Bartonella henselae* in domestic cats' saliva. *Iran J Microbiol* 2010;2:80–84.

102. Arashima Y, Kumasaka K, Kawano K, Ikeda T, Munemura T, Asano R, Hokari S, Takagi A. A study on wounds caused by cats as basic materials of cat scratch disease. *Kansenshogaku Zasshi* 1994;68:734–739.

103. Pont M, Delaporte E, Patenotre P, Piette F. A cat scratch and finger swelling. *Ann Dermatol Venereol* 2000;127:1103–1104.

104. Lien SH, Lo WT, Lee CM, Cheng SN, Chu ML, Wang CC. Cat scratch disease in children at a medical center. *Acta Paediatr Taiwan* 2004;45:282–286.

105. Kordick DL, Hilyard EJ, Hadfield TL, Wilson KH, Steigerwalt AG, Brenner DJ, Breitschwerdt EB. *Bartonella clarridgeiae*, a newly recognized zoonotic pathogen causing inoculation papules, fever, and lymphadenopathy (cat scratch disease). *J Clin Microbiol* 1997;35:1813–1818.

106. Brenner DJ, O'Connor SP, Winkler HH, Steigerwalt AG. Proposals to unify the genera *Bartonella* and *Rochalimea* with descriptions of *Bartonella quintana* comb. nov., *Bartonella vinsonii* comb. nov. *Bartonella henselae* comb.nov., and *Bartonella elisabethianae* comb.nov., and to remove the family *Bartonellaceae* from the order *Rickettsiales*. *Int J Syst Bacteriol* 1993;43:777–786.

107. Jendro MC, Weber G, Brabant T, Zeidler H, Wollenhaupt J. Reactive arthritis after cat bite: A rare manifestation of cat scratch disease—Case report and overview. *Z Rheumatol* 1998;57:159–163.

108. Angelakis E, Edouard S, La Scola B, Raoult D. *Bartonella henselae* in skin biopsy specimens of patients with cat scratch disease. *Emerg Infect Dis* 2010;16:1963–1965.

109. Lin YY, Hsiao CH, Hsu YH, Lee CC, Tsai HJ, Pan MJ. Immunohistochemical study of lymph nodes in patients with cat scratch disease. *J Formos Med Ass* 2006;105:911–917.

110. Huang J, Dai L, Lei S, Liao DY, Wang XQ, Luo TY, Chen Y et al. Application of Warthin-Starry stain, immunohistochemistry and transmission electron microscopy in diagnosis of cat scratch disease. *Zhonghua Bing Li Xue Za Zhi* 2010;39:225–229.

111. Shin OR, Kim YR, Ban TH, Lim T, Han TH, Kim SY, Seo KJ. A case report of seronegative cat scratch disease, emphasizing the histopathologic point of view. *Diagn Pathol* 2014;9:62 (1–4).

112. Florin TA, Zaoutis TE, Zaoutis LB. Beyond cat scratch disease: Widening spectrum of *Bartonella henselae* infection. *Pediatrics* 2008;121:e1413–e1425.

113. Moulin C, Kanitakis J, Ranchin B, Chauvet C, Gillet Y, Morelon E, Euvrard S. Cutaneous bacillary angiomatosis in renal transplant recipients: Report of three new cases and literature review. *Transpl Infect Dis* 2012;14:403–409.

114. Beyt BE Jr, Ortbals DW, Santa Cruz DJ, Kobayashi GS, Eisen AZ, Medoff G. Cutaneous mycobacteriosis: Analysis of 34 cases with a new classification of the disease. *Medicine (Baltimore)* 1981;60:95–109.

115. Khanna D, Chakravarty P, Agarwal A, Gupta R. Tuberculous dactylitis presenting as paronychia with pseudopterygium and nail dystrophy. *Pediatr Dermatol* 2013;30:e172–176.

116. Jetton RL, Coker WL. Tuberculosis verrucosa cutis (Prosector's wart). *Arch Dermatol* 1969;100: 380–381.

117. O'Donnell TF Jr, Jurgenson PF, Weyerich NF. An occupational hazard–tuberculous paronychia. Report of a case. *Arch Surg* 1971;103:757–758.

118. Goette DK, Jacobson KW, Doty RD. Primary inoculation tuberculosis of the skin. *Prosector's paronychia. Arch Dermatol* 1978;114:567–569.

119. Hooker RP, Eberts TJ, Strickland JA. Primary inoculation tuberculosis. *J Hand Surg Am* 1979;4:270–273.

120. Hoyt EM. Primary inoculation tuberculosis. Report of a case. *JAMA* 1981;245:1556–1557.

121. Pramatarov K, Balabanova M, Miteva L, Gantcheva M. Tuberculosis verrucosa cutis associated with lupus vulgaris. *Int J Dermatol* 1993;32:815–817.

122. Hoang MP, White WA, Molberg KH. Secondary syphilis: A histologic and immunohistochemical evaluation. *J Cut Pathol* 2004;31:594–599.

123. Müller H, Eisendle K, Bräuninger W, Kutzner H, Cerroni L, Zelger B. Comparative analysis of immunohistochemistry, polymerase chain reaction and focus-floating microscopy for the detection of *Treponema pallidum* in mucocutaneous lesions of primary, secondary and tertiary syphilis. *Br J Dermatol* 2011;165:50–60.

124. Zhu K, Zhou Q, Han R, Cheng H. Acute monoarthritis in a delayed diagnosis of syphilis patient with persistent rupioid psoriasis-like lesions. *BMC Infect Dis* 2012;12:338.

125. Aparicio MA, Santos-Briz A. Unexpected immunostaining of *Mycobacterium leprae* with a polyclonal antibody against *Treponema pallidum. Am J Dermatopathol* 2012;34:559–561.

126. Belinchón Romero I, Ramos Rincón JM, Reyes Rabell F. Nail involvement in leprosy. *Actas Dermosifiliogr* 2012;103:276–284.

127. Bhushan P, Aggarwal A, Yadav R, Baliyan V. Bilateral medial fingernail dystrophy as a presenting feature in a patient with leprosy. *Lepr Rev* 2011;82:74–77.

128. Patki A, Baran R. Nail resembling cutaneous horn occurring after acral bone loss. *Cutis* 1994;54:41–42.

129. Singh PK, Nigam PK, Singh G. Terry's nails in a case of leprosy. *Indian J Lepr* 1986;58:107–109.

130. Kaur I, Chakrabarti A, Dogra S, Rai R, Kumar B. Nail involvement in leprosy: A study of 300 patients. *Int J Lepr Other Mycobact Dis* 2003;71:320–327.

131. Patki AH. Pterygium inversum unguis in a patient with leprosy. *Arch Dermatol* 1990;126:1110.

132. El Darouti MA, Hussein S, Al Tahlawy SR, Al Fangary M, Mashaly HM, El Nabarawy E, Al Tawdy A, Fawzi M, Abdel Hay RM. Clinical study of nail changes in leprosy and comparison with nail changes in diabetic patients. *J Eur Acad Dermatol Venereol* 2011;25:290–295.

133. Patki AH, Mehta JM. *Pterygium unguis* in a patient with recurrent type 2 lepra reaction. *Cutis* 1989;44:311–312.

134. Patki AH, Baran R. Significance of nail changes in leprosy: A clinical review of 357 cases. *Semin Dermatol* 1991;10:77–81.

135. Bhatia VN. Possible multiplication of *M. leprae* (?) on skin and nail bed of a laboratory worker. *Indian J Lepr* 1990;62:226–227.

136. Da Costa DA, Enokihara MM, Nonogaki S, Maeda SM, Porro AM, Tomimori J. Wade histoid leprosy: Histological and immunohistochemical analysis. *Lepr Rev* 2013;84:176–185.

137. Warren KJ, Fairley JA. Pain and swelling along the nail fold of a 51-year-old man: *Mycobacterium marinum* (fish tank granuloma). *Dermatol Online J* 1998;4(1):1.

138. Horn MS. *Mycobacterium marinum* infection. *J Ass Mil Dermatol* 1981;7(2):25.

139. Savoie JM. Infection à *Mycobacterium marinum* (forme sporotrichoïde). *Nouv Dermatol* 1989;8: 524–525.

140. Edelstein H. *Mycobacterium marinum* skin infections. *Arch Intern Med* 1994;154:1359–1364.

141. Pettit JHS. Skin tuberculosis and mycobacterial ulcers. Tropical dermatology syllabus. XVI World Cong Dermatol, Tokyo, 1985.

142. Whitaker MC, Lucas GL. Primary nontraumatic *Mycobacterium avium* complex osteomyelitis of the distal phalanx. *Am J Orthop (Belle Mead NJ)* 2004;33:248–249.

143. Winthrop KL, Abrams M, Yakrus M, Schwartz I, Ely J, Gillies D, Vugia DJ. An outbreak of mycobacterial furunculosis associated with footbaths at a nail salon. *N Engl J Med* 2002;346:1366–1371.

144. Sniezek PJ, Graham BS, Busch HB, Lederman ER, Lim ML, Poggemyer K, Kao A et al. Rapidly growing mycobacterial infections after pedicures. *Arch Dermatol* 2003;139:629–634.

145. Gira AK, Reisenauer AH, Hammock L, Nadiminti U, Macy JT, Reeves A, Burnett C et al. Furunculosis due to *Mycobacterium mageritense* associated with footbaths at a nail salon. *J Clin Microbiol* 2004;42: 1813–1817.

146. Cooksey RC, de Waard JH, Yakrus MA, Rivera I, Chopite M, Toney SR, Morlock GP, Butler WR. *Mycobacterium cosmeticum* sp. nov., a novel rapidly growing species isolated from a cosmetic infection and from a nail salon. *Int J Syst Evol Microbiol* 2004;54:2385–2391.

147. Redbord KP, Shearer DA, Gloster H, Younger B, Connelly BL, Kindel SE, Lucky AW. Atypical Mycobacterium furunculosis occurring after pedicures. *J Am Acad Dermatol* 2006;54:520–524.

148. Wertman R, Miller M, Groben P, Morrell DS, Culton DA. *Mycobacterium bolletii/Mycobacterium massiliense* furunculosis associated with pedicure footbaths: A report of 3 cases. *Arch Dermatol* 2011;147:454–458.

149. Stout JE, Gadkowski LB, Rath S, Alspaugh JA, Miller MB, Cox GM. Pedicure-associated rapidly growing mycobacterial infection: An endemic disease. *Clin Infect Dis* 2011;53:787–792.

150. Kempf W, Flaig MJ, Kutzner H. Molecular diagnostic of infectious skin diseases. *J German Soc Dermatol* 2013;11(Suppl 4):50–59.

151. Fournier A. *Traité de la Syphilis*. Paris: Masson, 1884.

152. Juvin S. Onyxis et périonyxis avec lésions osseuses chez un syphilitique non traité. *Bull Soc Fr Dermatol* 1947;54:86.

153. Fox H. Obstinate syphilitic onychia and gumma of the nose. *Arch Dermatol* 1941;44:1155.

154. Spitzer R. Kongenitale Nagelsyphilis. *Arch Dermatol Syph Berlin* 1928;154:82–83.

155. Ravaut P, Monnerot-Dumaine R. Atrophie de l'ongle d'origine hérédo-syphilitique. *Ann Dermatol Vénéréol* 1928;3:461–468.

156. Wanderer M. Nagelveränderungen bei kongenitaler Lues. *Zbl Haut-GeschlKr* 1936;52:282.

157. Srokowska R. Anonychia in individuo luetico. *Zbl Haut-GeschlKr* 1937;55:260.

158. Alkiewicz J. On the inflammation of the nail organ. *Dermatologica* 1960;121:228–239.

159. Coffin SE, Puck J. Painful discoloration of the fingernails in a 15-year-old boy. *Pediatr Infect Dis J* 1993;12:702–703; 706.

160. Murakami I, Hara H, Shigeto H, Yamada T, Isogai E, Kira J. A case of Lyme disease with the triad of neurologic manifestations (meningitis, radiculoneuritis, facial nerve palsy) and dermatitis of the nail roots. *Rinsho Shinkeigaku* 1999;39:570–572.

161. Houtman PM, Jansen TL. Nailfold capillaroscopic picture by chance. *Rheumatology (Oxford)* 2006;45:599.

162. Herzer P. 45-year-old woman with joint pain and suspected Lyme arthritis. *Dtsch Med Wochenschr* 2009;134:1741–1742.

163. Atiq N, van Meurs T. A boy with nail abnormalities. *Ned Tijdschr Geneeskd* 2013;157:A6429.

164. Moreno C, Kutzner H, Palmedo G, Goerttler E, Carrasco L, Requena L. Interstitial granulomatous dermatitis with histiocytic pseudorosettes: A new histopathologic pattern in cutaneous borreliosis. Detection of *Borrelia burgdorferi* DNA by a highly sensitive PCR-ELiSA. *J Am Acad Dermatol* 2003;48:376–384.

165. Aberer E, Klade H, Hobisch G. A clinical, histological, and immunohistochemical comparison of acrodermatitis chronica atrophicans and morphea. *Am J Dermatopathol* 1991;13:334–341.

166. López-Jodra O, Torres-Rodriguez J. Especies fúngicas poco comunes responsables de onicomicosis. *Rev Iberoam Micol.* 1999;16:S11–15.

167. Baran R, Hay RJ, Haneke E, Tosti A. *Onychomycosis —The Current Approach to Diagnosis and Therapy.* London: M Dunitz Publ, 1999.

168. Haneke E, Roseeuw D. The scope of onychomycosis: Epidemiology and clinical features. *Int J Dermatol* 1999;38(Suppl 2):7–12.

169. Burzekowski T, Molenberghs G, Abeck D, Haneke E, Hay R, Katsambas A, Roseeuw D, van de Kerkhof P, van Aelst R, Marynissen G. High prevalence of foot diseases in Europe: Results of the Achilles project. *Mycoses* 2003;46:496–505.

170. Baran R, Hay RJ, Tosti A, Haneke E. A new classification of onychomycoses. *Br J Dermatol* 1998;139: 567–571.

171. Haneke E. Fungal infections of the nail. *Sem Dermatol* 1991;10:41–53.

172. Hubka V, Dobiasova S, Lyskova P, Mallatova N, Chlebkova J, Skorepova M, Kubatova A, Dobias R, Chudickova M, Kolarik M. *Auxarthron ostraviense* sp. nov., and *A. umbrinum* associated with non-dermatophytic onychomycosis. *Med Mycol* 2013;51:614–624.

173. Haneke E. Pathogenesis of onychomycoses. *Dermatology* 1998;197:200–201.

174. Haneke E. Bedeutung der Nagelhistologie für die Diagnostik und Therapie der Onychomykosen. *Ärztl Kosmetol* 1988;18:248–254.

175. Miyajima Y, Satoh K, Uchida T, Yamada T, Abe M, Watanabe S, Makimura M, Makimura K. Rapid real-time diagnostic PCR for *Trichophyton rubrum* and *Trichophyton mentagrophytes* in patients with tinea unguium and tinea pedis using specific fluorescent probes. *J Dermatol Sci* 2013;69:229–235.

176. Winter I, Uhrlaβ S, Krüger C, Herrmann J, Bezold G, Winter A, Barth S, Simon JC, Gräser Y, Nenoff P. Molecular biological detection of dermatophytes in clinical samples when onychomycosis or tinea pedis is suspected. A prospective study comparing conventional dermatomycological diagnostics and polymerase chain reaction. *Hautarzt* 2013;64:283–289.

177. Hollemeyer K, Jager S, Altmeyer W, Heinzle E. Proteolytic peptide patterns as indicators for fungal infections and nonfungal affections of human nails measured by matrix-assisted laser desorption/ ionization time-of-flight mass spectrometry. *Anal Biochem* 2005;338:326–331.

178. Erhard M, Hipler UC, Burmester A, Brakhage AA, Wöstemeyer J. Identification of dermatophyte species causing onychomycosis and tinea pedis by MALDI-TOF mass spectrometry. *Exp Dermatol* 2008;17:356–361.

179. Nenoff P, Erhard M, Simon JC, Muylowa GK, Herrmann J, Rataj W, Gräser Y. MALDI-TOF mass spectrometry—A rapid method for identification of dermatophyte species. *Med Mycol* 2013;51:17–24.

180. Arrese JE, Piérard-Franchimont C, Greimers R, Piérard GE. Fungi in onychomycosis: A study by immunohistochemistry and dual flow cytometry. *J Eur Acad Dermatol Venereol* 1995;4:123–130.

181. Arrese JE, Quatresooz P, Piérard-Franchimont C, Piérard GE. Histomycologie unguéale. *Ann Dermatol Vénéréol* 2003;130:1254–1259.

182. Hay RJ, Baran R. Onychomycosis: A proposed revision of the clinical classification. *J Am Acad Dermatol* 2011;65:1219–1227.

183. Zaias N, Tosti A, Rebell G, Morelli R, Bardazzi F, Bieley H, Zaiac M et al. Autosomal dominant pattern of distal subungual onychomycosis caused by *Trichophyton rubrum*. *J Am Acad Dermatol* 1996;34:302–304.

184. Alkiewicz J. Candidiasis der Nägel. *Mykosen* 1957;1:52–58.

185. Hay RJ, Baran R. Deep dermatophytosis: Rare infections or common, but unrecognised, complications of lymphatic spread? *Curr Opin Infect Dis* 2004;17:77–79.

186. Baran R, McLoone N, Hay RJ. Could proximal white subungual onychomycosis be a complication of systemic spread. The lessons to be learned from Maladie Dermatophytique and other deep infections? *Br J Dermatol* 2005;153:1023–1025.

187. Baran R, Faergemann J, Hay RJ. Superficial white onychomycosis—A syndrome with different fungal causes and paths of infection. *J Am Acad Dermatol* 2007;57:879–882.

188. Weismann K, Knudsen EA, Pedersen C. White nails in AIDS/ARC due to *Trichophyton rubrum* infection. *Clin Exp Dermatol* 1988;13:24–35.

189. Badillet G. Mélanonychies superficielles. *Bull Soc Fr Med Mycol* 1988;17:335–340.

190. Meisel CW, Quadripur SA. Onychomycosis due to *Hendersonula toruloidea*. *Hautnah Myk* 1992;6:232–234.

191. Fletcher CL, Moore MK, Hay RJ. Endonyx onychomycosis due to *Trichophyton soudanense* in two Somali twins. *Br J Dermatol* 2001;145:684–648.

192. Kalter DC, Hay RJ. Onychomycosis due to *Trichophyton soudanense*. *Clin Exp Dermatol* 1988;13:221–227.

193. Tosti A, Baran R, Piraccini BM, Fanti PA. Endonyx onychomycosis: A new modality of nail invasion by dermatophyte fungi. *Acta Derm Venereol (Stockh)* 1999;79:52–53.

194. Haneke E, Djawari D: Hyperimmunglobulin E-Syndrom: Atopisches Ekzem, Eosinophilie, Chemotaxisdefekt, Infektanfälligkeit und chronische mucocutane Candidose. *Akt Dermatol* 1982;8:34–39.

195. Haneke E. Composite and heterogenous keratohyalin in the human buccal mucosa. *Arch Dermatol Res* 1982;272:127–134.

196. Roberts DT, Evans EG. Subungual dermatophytoma complicating dermatophyte onychomycosis. *Br J Dermatol* 1998 Jan;138:189–190.

197. Burkhart CN, Burkhart CG, Gupta AK. Dermatophytoma: Recalcitrance to treatment because of existence of fungal biofilm. *J Am Acad Dermatol* 2002;47:629–631.

198. Gupta AK, Baran R, Summerbell R. Onychomycosis: Strategies to improve efficacy and reduce recurrence. *J Eur Acad Dermatol Venereol* 2002;16:579–586.

199. Sommer S, Sheehan-Dare RA, Goodfield MJ, Evans EG. Prediction of outcome in the treatment of onychomycosis. *Clin Exp Dermatol.* 2003;28:425–428.

200. Lecha M, Effendy I, Feuilhade de Chauvin M, Di Chiacchio N, Baran R. Taskforce on Onychomycosis Education. Treatment options—Development of consensus guidelines. *J Eur Acad Dermatol Venereol.* 2005;19(Suppl 1):25–33.

201. Sigurgeirsson B. Prognostic factors for cure following treatment of onychomycosis. *J Eur Acad Dermatol Venereol* 2010;24:679–684.

202. Martinez-Herrera E, Moreno-Coutiño G, Fernández-Martínez RF, Finch J, Arenas R. Dermatophytoma: Description of 7 cases. *J Am Acad Dermatol* 2012;66:1014–1016.

203. Carney C, Tosti A, Daniel R, Scher R, Rich P, DeCoster J, Elewski B. A new classification system for grading the severity of onychomycosis: Onychomycosis Severity Index. *Arch Dermatol* 2011;147:1277–1282.

204. Cantrell W, Canavan T, Elewski B. Report of a case of a dermatophytoma successfully treated with topical efinaconazole 10% solution. *J Drugs Dermatol* 2015;14:524–526.

205. Bennett D, Rubin AI. Dermatophytoma: A clinicopathologic entity important for dermatologists and dermatopathologists to identify. *Int J Dermatol* 2013;52:1285–1287.

206. Martínez-Herrera EO, Arroyo-Camarena S, Tejada-García DL, Porras-López CF, Arenas R. Onychomycosis due to opportunistic molds. *An Bras Dermatol* 2015; 90:334–337.

207. Mallo-García S, Coto-Segura P, Santos-Juanes-Jiménez J. Proximal white subungual onychomycosis due to *Fusarium* species. *Actas Dermosifiliogr* 2008;99:742–743.

208. Wu CY, Chen GS, Lan CCE. Onychomycosis caused by *Fusarium solani* in a woman with diabetes. *Clin Exp Dermatol* 2009;34:e772–e774.

209. Varon AG, Nouer SA, Barreiros G, Moritz Trope B, Magalhaes F, Akiti T, Garnica M, Nucci M. Superficial skin lesions positive for *Fusarium* are associated with subsequent development of invasive fusariosis. *J Infect* 2014;68:85–89.

210. Brasch J. Dermatomykosen durch Fusarien. *Hautarzt* 2012;63:872–876.

211. Brasch J, Shimanovich I. Persistent fingernail onychomycosis caused by *Fusarium proliferatum* in a healthy woman. *Mycoses* 2012;55:86–89.

212. Ungpakorn R, Lohaprathan S, Reanghcinam S. Prevalence of foot diseases in outpatients attending the Institute of Dermatology, Bangkok, Thailand. *Clin Exp Dermatol* 2004;29:87–90.

213. Asbati M, Smythe B, Cavallera E. Onicomicosis por hongos no dematofitos. Estudio retrospectivo en 4 años. *Rev Soc Ven Microbiol* 2002;22:147–152.

214. Gupta AK, Drummond-Main C, Cooper EA, Brintnell W, Piraccini BM, Tosti A. Systematic review of nondermatophyte mold onychomycosis: Diagnosis, clinical types, epidemiology, and treatment. *J Am Acad Dermatol* 2012;66:494–502.

215. Dorko E, Jautová J, Pilipcinec E, Tkáciková L. Occurrence of *Candida* strains in cases of paronychia. *Folia Microbiol (Praha)* 2004;49:591–595.

216. Brasch J, Beck-Jendroschek V, Wohlfeil E. Recalcitrant purulent paronychia and onychomycosis caused by *Fusarium oxysporum*. *J Dtsch Dermatol Ges* 2012;10:519–520.

217. Finch J, Arenas R, Baran R. Fungal melanonychia. *J Am Acad Dermatol* 2012;66:830–841.

218. Parlak AH, Goksugur N, Karabay O. A case of melanonychia due to *Candida albicans*. *Clin Dermatol* 2006;31:398–400.

219. Lacaz CS, Pereira AD, Heins-Vaccari EM, Cuce LC, Benatti C, Nunes RS, de Melo NT, de Freitas-Leite RS, Hernández-Arriagada GL. Onychomycosis caused by *Scytalidium dimidiatum*. Report of two cases. Review of the taxonomy of the synanamorph and anmorph forms of this coelomycete. *Rev Inst Med Trop* 1999;41:318–323.

220. Boisseau-Garsaud AM, Desbois N, Guillermin ML, Ossondo M, Gueho E, Cales–Quist D. Onycohomycosis due to *Exophiala jeanselmi*. *Dermatology* 2002;204:150–152.

221. De Carvalho MLV, Mendonça I, de Oliveira JC, Val A, Hering B, Stallone C, Jimenez PA. Melanoniquia: A propósito de um caso de micotização ungueal simulando melanoma. *Dermatol Online J* 2010;16:3.

222. Amadio PC. Fungal infections of the hand. *Hand Clin* 1998;14:605–612.

223. Al-Qattan MM, Helmi AA. Chronic hand infections. *J Hand Surg Am* 2014;39:1636–1645.

224. Ramos-e-Silva M, Vasconcelos C, Carneiro S, Cestari T. Sporotrichosis. *Clin Dermatol* 2007;25:181–187.

225. Schubach A, Pacheco Schubach TM, Bastos de Lima Barros M, Wanke B. Cat-transmitted sporotrichosis, Rio de Janeiro, Brazil. *Emerg Infect Dis* 2005;11:1952–1954.

226. Hattori M, Yoshiike T, Sonoda T, Hiruma M. A case of lymphocutaneous sporotrichosis occurring at the nail bed. *Mycoses* 2011;54:e663–665.

227. Carvalho Aguinaga F, Moritz Trope B, Fernandes NC, Engel DC, Ramos-e-Silva M. Sporotrichosis with bone involvement: An alert to an occupational disease. *Case Rep Dermatol* 2014;6:114–118.

228. Conti-Díaz I. Estudio micológico de 85 casos de onicopatías. *An Fac Med Univ Montevideo* 1964;49:535–540.

229. Cruz R, Vieille P, Opazo D, Soto I. A islamiento de *Sporothrix pallida* y Trichophyton rubrum en onicomicosis de mano. *Bol Micol* 2013;28:26–30.

230. Cruz Choappa RM, Vieille Oyarzoa PI, Carvajal Silva LC. Aislamiento de *Sporothrix pallida* complex en muestras clínicas y ambientales de Chile. *Rev Argent Microbiol.* 2014;46:311–314.

231. Larone DH. *Medically Important fungi: A Guide to Identification*, 4th edn. Washington, DC: ASM Press, 2002.

232. Morris-Jones R. Sporotrichosis. *Clin Exp Dermatol* 2002;27:427–431.

233. Male O. Diagnostische und therapeutsiche Probleme bei der kutanen Sporotrichose. *Z Hautkr* 1974;49:505–515.

234. Marques MEA, Coelho KIR, Sotto MN, Bacchi CE. Comparison between histochemical and immunohistochemical methods for diagnosis of sporotrichosis. *J Clin Pathol* 1992;45:1089–1093.

235. Quintella LP, Passos SRL, de Miranda LHM, Cuzzi T, Barros MB de L, Francesconi-do-Vale AC et al. Proposal of a histopathological predictive rule for the differential diagnosis between American tegumentary leishmaniasis and sporotrichosis skin lesions. *Br J Dermatol* 212;167:837–846.

236. Lobo JO. Nova especie de blastomicose. *Brasil Med* 1930;44:1227.

237. Paniz-Mondolfi A, Talhari C, Sander Hoffmann L, Connor DL, Talhari S, Bermudez-Villapol L, Hernandez-Perez M, Van Bressem M F. Lobomycosis: An emerging disease in humans and delphinidae. *Mycoses* 2012;55:298–309.

238. Cardoso de Brito A, Simões Quaresma JA. Lacaziosis (Jorge Lobo's disease): Review and update. *An Bras Dermatol* 2007;82:461–474.

239. Borelli D. Lobomicose: Nomenclatura de su agente (revisión critica). *Med Cutanea* 1968;3:151–156.

240. Taborda PR, Taborda VA, McGinnis MR. *Lacazia loboi* General Nov, comb. Nov, the etiologic agent of lobomycosis. *J Clin Microbiol* 1999;37: 2031–2033.

241. Migaki G, Valerio MG, Irvine B, Garner FM. Lobo's disease in an Atlantic bottle-nosed dolphin. *J Am Vet Med Assoc* 1971;159:582.

242. Caldwell DK, Caldwell MC, Woodard JC, Ajello L, Kaplan W, McLure HM. Lobomycosis as a disease of the Atlantic bottle-nosed dolphin (*Tursiops truncatus* Montagu, 1821). *Am J Trop Med Hyg* 1975;24:105–114.

243. Paniz Mondolfi AE, Sander-Hoffmann L. Lobomycosis in inshore and estuarine dolphins. *Emerg Infect Dis* 2009;15:672–673.

244. Symmers WStC. A possible case of Lobo's disease acquired in Europe from a bottle-nosed dolphin (*Tursiops truncatus*). *Bull Soc Pathol Exot* 1983;76:777–784.

245. Rotstein DS, Burdett LG, McLellan W, Schwacke L, Rowles T, Terio KA, Schultz S, Pabst A. Lobomycosis in offshore bottlenose dolphins (*Tursiops truncatus*). North Carolina. *Emerg Infect Dis* 2009;15:588–590.

246. Talhari S, Talhari C. Lobomycosis. *Clin Dermatol* 2012;30:420–424.

247. Baruzzi RG, Lacaz de S, Souza PA. Historia natural de doença de Jorge Lobo; ocurrência entre os indios Caiabi (Brasil Central). *Rev Med Trop São Paulo* 1979;21:302–338.

248. Brito A. Lobomicose. 67th Cong Soc Bras Dermatol, Rio de Janeiro, Sept 1–5, 2012.

249. Esterre P, Pradineau R, Ravisse P. Etude immuno-histochimique de la lésion cutanée de lobomycose. *J Mycol Méd* 1991;1:276–283.

250. Talhari C, Chrusciak-Talhari A, de Souza JV, Araújo JR, Talhari S. Exfoliative cytology as a rapid diagnostic tool for lobomycosis. *Mycoses* 2009;52: 187–189.

251. Rosa PS, Belone AF, Lauris JR, Soares CT. Fine-needle aspiration may replace skin biopsy for the collection of material for experimental infection of mice with *Mycobacterium leprae* and *Lacazia loboi*. *Int J Infect Dis* 2010;14(Suppl 3):e49–e53.

252. Rubin HA, Bruce S, Rosen T, McBride ME. Evidence for percutaneous inoculation as the mode of transmission of chromoblastomycosis. *J Am Acad Dermatol* 1991;25:951–954.

253. Silva JP, de Souza W, Rozental S. Chromoblastomycosis: A retrospective study of 325 cases on Amazonic Region (Brazil). *Mycopathologia* 1998–99;143:171–175.

254. Gall FL, Lulin J, Couatarmanac'h A, Cotton F, Chevrant-Breton J, Ramee MP. A cutaneous parasitosis rarely observed in France: Chromomycosis. *Ann Pathol* 1993;13:123–127.

255. Putkonen T. Chromomycosis in Finland. The possible role of the Finnish sauna in its spreading. *Hautarzt* 1966;17:507–509.

256. Pindycka-Piaszczyńska M, Krzyściak P, Piaszczyński M, Cieślik S, Januszewski K, Izdebska-Straszak G, Jarząb J, de Hoog S, Jagielski T. Chromoblastomycosis as an endemic disease in temperate Europe: First confirmed case and review of the literature. *Eur J Clin Microbiol Infect Dis* 2014;33:391–398.

257. Sarti HM, Vega-Memije ME, Domínguez-Cherit J, Arenas R. Longitudinal melanonychia secondary to chromoblastomycosis due to *Fonsecaea pedrosoi*. *Int J Dermatol* 2008;47:764–765.

258. Ko CJ, Sarantopoulos GP, Pai G, Binder SW. Longitudinal melanonychia of the toenails with presence of Medlar bodies on biopsy. *J Cutan Pathol* 2005;32:63–65.

259. de Bièvre C. Comparative study of Cladosporium isolated from various human lesions. *Bull Soc Pathol Exot Filiales* 1982;75:390–399.

260. Alcland KM, Hay RJ, Groves R. Cutaneous infection with *Alternaria alternata* complicating immunosuppression: Successful treatment with itraconazole. *Br J Dermatol* 1998;138:354–356.

261. Gilmour TK, Rytina E, O'Connell PB, Sterling JC. Cutaneous alternariosis in a cardiac transplant recipient. *Aust J Dermatol* 2001;42:46–49.

262. Lyke KE, Miller NS, Topwne L, Merz WG. A case of cutaneous ulcerative alternariosis: Rare association with diabetes mellitus and unusual failure of itraconazole treatment. *Clin Infect Dis* 2001;32:1178–1187.

263. Uenotsuchi T, Moroi Y, Urabe K, Fukagawa S, Tsuji G, Matsuda T, Furue M. Cutaneous alternariosis with chronic granulomatous disease. *Eur J Dermatol* 2005;15:406–408.

264. Mayser P, Nilles M, de Hoog GS. Case report. Cutaneous phaeohyphomycosis due to *Alternaria alternata*. *Mycoses* 2002;45:338–340.

265. Vezon G, Desbois N, Boisseau-Garsaud AM, Helenon R, Jouannelle A, Saint-Cyr I, Cales-Quist D. Microsporum canis mycetoma of the scalp. *Ann Dermatol Venereol* 2000;127:729–731.

266. Tirado-González M, Ball E, Ruiz A, Rodriguez Y, Goudet CE, Finkel O, Golan H et al. Disseminated dermatophytic pseudomycetoma caused by *Microsporum* species. *Int J Dermatol* 2012;51:1478–1482.

267. Zaias N, Taplin D, Rebell G. Mycetoma. *Arch Dermatol* 1969;99:215–225.

268. Graupmann-Kuzma A, Valentine BA, Shubith LF, Dial SM, Watrous B, Tornquist SJ. Coccidioidomycosis in dogs and cats: A review. *J Am Anim Hosp Ass* 2008;44:226–235.

269. Schwartz RA, Lamberts RJ. Isolated nodular cutaneous coccidioidomycosis: The initial manifestion of disseminated disease. *J Am Acad Dermatol* 1981;4:38.

270. Timble JR, Doucette J. Primary cutaneous coccidioidomycosis: Report of a case of a laboratory infection. *Arch Dermatol* 1956;74:405.

271. Carroll GF, Haley LD, Brown JM. Primary cutaneous coccidioidomycosis. *Arch Dermatol* 1977;113:933.

272. Levan NE, Huntington RW Jr. Primary cutaneous coccidioidomycosis in an agricultural worker. *Arch Dermatol* 1965;92:215.

273. Winn WA. Primary cutaneous coccidioidomycosis: Reevaluation of its potentiality based on study of three new cases. *Arch Dermatol* 1965;91:221.

274. Carpenter JB, Feldman JS, Leyva W, DiCaudo D. Clinical and pathologic characteristics of disseminated cutaneous coccidioidomycosis. *J Am Acad Dermatol* 2010;62:831–837.

275. Lutz A. Uma mycose pseudococcidica localisada na bocca e observada no Brazil. Contribuição ao conhecimento das hyphoblastomycose americanas. *Bras Méd* 1908;22:121–124.

276. Theodoro RC, Teixeira MdM, Felipe MSS, Paduan KdS, Ribolla PM, San-Blas G, Bagagli E. Genus *Paracoccidioidis*: Species recognition and biogeographic aspects. *PLoS ONE* 2012;7(5):e37694. doi:10.1371/journal.pone.0037694

277. Hernández O, Tamayo D, Torres I, Restrepo Á, McEwen JG, García AM. Kinetic analysis of gene expression during mycelium to yeast transition and yeast to mycelium germination in *Paracoccidioidis brasiliensis*. *Biomédica* 2011;31:570–579.

278. Santos WA, da Silva BM, Passos ED, Zandonade E, Falqueto A. Association between smoking and paracoccidioidomycosis: A case-control study in the State of Espírito Santo, Brazil. *Cad Saude Publ* 2003;19:245–253.

279. Londero AT, Ramos CD. Paracoccidioidomycosis: A clinical and mycologic study of forty-one cases observed in Santa Maria, RS, Brazil. *Am J Med* 1972;52:771–775.

280. Nascimento CR, Delanina WFB, Soares CT. Paracoccidioidomycosis: Sarcoid-like form in childhood. *An Bras Dermatol* 2012;87:486–487.

281. Bernard G. An overview of the immunopathology of human paracoccidioidomycosis. *Mycopathologia* 2008;165:209–221.

282. Salfelder K, Doehnert G, Doedhnert H-R. Paracoccidioidomycosis: Anatomic study with complete autopsies. *Virchows Arch Pathol* 1969;348:51–76.

283. Murray HW, Littman MI. Disseminated paracoccidioidomycosis (South American blastomycosis) in the United States. *Am J Med* 1974;56:209–220.

284. Marques AS, Camargo RMP, Marques MEA, Tangoda LK, Stolf HO. Paraccidioidomycosis of external genitalia: Report of six new cases and review of the literature. *An Bras Dermatol* 2012;87:235–240.

285. Castro RM, Cucé LC, Fava-Netto C. Paracoccidioidomicose: Inoculação acidental "in animanobile". *Relato de um caso. Med Cut Ibero Lat Am* 1975;4:282–289.

286. Albornoz MB, Fuenmayor F. Paracoccidioidomicose cutánea. *Rev Inst Med Trop Sao Paulo* 1983;25:82–86.

287. Nakamura R, Valgas N, Bichara RM, Brazuna D, Leverone A. Paracoccidioidomycosis: Chronic adult unifocal form. *Int J Dermatol* 2012;51:195–196.

288. Tosh FE, Balhuizen J, Yates JL, Brasher CA. Primary cutaneous histoplasmosis. *Arch Intern Med* 1964;114:118–119.

289. Tesh RB, Schneidau JD Jr. Primary cutaneous histoplasmosis. *New Engl J Med* 1966;275:597–599.

290. Tesh RB, Schneidau JD Jr. Histoplasmosis: A review of the cutaneous and adjacent mucous membrane manifestations with a report of three cases. *J Am Ass Med* 1947;134:1217.

291. Chanda JJ, Callen JP. Isolated nodular cutaneous histoplasmosis: The initial manifestation of recurrent disseminated disease. *Arch Dermatol* 1978;114:1197–1198.

292. Merin MR, Fung MA, Eisen DB, Lin LK. Histoplasmosis presenting as a cutaneous malignancy of the eyelid. *Ophthal Plast reconstr Surg* 2011;27:e41–e42.

293. Bonifaz A, Chang P, Moreno K, Fernández-Fernández V, Montes de Oca G, Araiza J, Ponce RM. Disseminated cutaneous histoplasmosis in acquired immunodeficiency syndrome: Report of 23 cases. *Clin Exp Dermatol* 2009;34:481–486.

294. Dumont A, Piché C. Electron microscopic study of human histoplasmosis. *Arch Pathol* 1969;87:168–178.

295. Bradsher RW, Chapman SW, Pappas PG. l Blastomycosis. *Infect Clin Dis North Am* 2003;17:21–40.

296. López-Martínez R, Méndez-Tovar LJ. Blastomycosis. *Clin Dermatol* 2012;30:360–372.

297. Wiener E. Blastomykose der Nägel mit Paronychien und Polypen der Nagelbetten. *Zbl Haut- GeschlKr* 1928;27:243.

298. Kaplan W, Kraft DE. Demonstration of pathogenic fungi in formalin-fixed tissues by immunofluorescence. *Am J Clin Pathol* 1969;52:420–432.

299. Russell B, Beckett JH, Jacobs PH. Immunoperoxidase localization of *Sporothrix schenckii* and *Cryptococcus neoformans*. *Arch Dermatol* 1979;115:443–435.

300. Ferreyra Dillon R, Lascano CD, Riera F, Albiero E. Cutaneous cryptococosis in a patient with Behçet's disease and colon cancer. *Reumatol Clin* 2011;7:147–148.

301. Chayakulkeeree M. Cryptococcosis. *Infect Dis Clin North Am* 2006;20:507–544.

302. Pappas P. Invasive fungal infections among organ transplant recipients: Results of the Transplant-Associated Intection Surveillance Network (TRANSNET). *Clin Infect Dis* 2010;50:1101–1111.

303. Santos T, Aguiar B, Santos L, Romaozinho C, Tome R, Macario F, Alves R, Campos M, Mota A. Invasive fungal infections after kidney transplantation: A single center experience. *Transplantation Proc* 2015;47:971–975.

304. Singh N. Cryptococcosis in solid organ transplant recipients: Current state of the science. *Clin Infect Dis* 2008;47:1321–1327.

305. Revenga F, Paricio JF, Merino FJ, Nebreda T, Ramírez T, Martínez AM. Primary cutaneous cryptococcosis in an immunocompetent host: Case report and review of the literature. *Dermatology* 2002; 204:145–149.

306. Virgili A, Zampino MR, Mantovani L. Fungal skin infections in organ transplant recipient. *Am J Clin Dermatol* 2002;3:19–35.

307. Sentamil Selvi G, Kamalam A, Ajithados K, Janaki C, Tambiah AS. Clinical and dermatological features of dermatophytosis in renal transplant recipients. *Mycoses* 1999;42:75–80.

308. Tilak R, Prakash P, Nigam C, Gambhir IS, Gulati AK. Cryptococcal meningitis with an antecedent cutaneous cryptococcal lesion. *Dermatol Online J* 2009;15:12.

309. Jain K, Mruthyunjaya, Ravishankar R. Cryptococcal abscess and osteomyelitis of the proximal phalanx of the hand. *Indian J Pathol Microbiol.* 2011;54:216–218.

310. Manrique P, Mayo J, Alvarez JA, Ganchegui X, Zabalza I, Flores M. Polymorphous cutaneous cryptococcosis: Nodular, herpes-like, and molluscum-like lesions in a patient with the acquired immunodeficiency syndrome. *J Am Acad Dermatol* 1992;26:122–124.

311. Tabassum S, Rahman A, Herekar F, Masood S. Cryptococcal meningitis with secondary cutaneous involvement in an immunocompetent host. *J Infect Dev Ctries* 2013;7:680–685.

312. Verneuil L, Dompmartin A, Duhamel C, Cren P, Six M, Le Maitre M, Le Maitre M, Galateau F, Moreau A, Leroy D. Panaris cryptococcique chez un malade VIH positif. *Ann Dermatol Venereol* 1995;122:688–691.

313. Neuville S, Dromer F, Morin O, Dupont B, Ronin O, Lortholary O. Primary cutaneous crytococcosis: A distinct clinical entity. *Clin Infect Dis* 2003;36:337–347.

314. Allegue F, Pérez de Lis M, Pérez-Álvarez R. Primary cutaneous cryptococcosis presenting as a whitlow. *Acta Derm Venereol* 2007;87:443–444.

315. Casadevall A, Perfect JR. *Cryptococcus neoformans.* Washington: The American Society for Microbiology, ASM Press, 1998.

316. Schwartz DA. Characterization of the biological activity of Cryptococcus infections in surgical pathology. The budding index and carminophilic index. *Ann Clin Lab Sci* 1988;18:388–397.

317. Perfect JR, Casadevall A. Cryptococcosis. *Infect Dis Clin N Amer* 2002;16:837–874.

318. Harding SA, Scheld WM, Feldmn PS, Sande MA. Pulmonary infection with capsule-deficient *Cryptococcus neoformans. Virchows Arch A Path Anat Histol* 1979;382:113–118.

319. Töröcsik D, Gergely L, Veres I, Remenyik É, Bégány Á. Cutaneous cryptococcosis mimicking basal cell carcinoma in a patient with Sézary syndrome. *Acta Derm Venereol* 2012;92:286–287.

320. Latino GA, Gago E, Vidau P, Vivanco B. Cutaneous cryptococcosis in a patient on chronic haemodialysis. *Nefrologia* 2012;32:697–698.

321. Lingegowda BP, Koh TH, Ong HS, Tan TT. Primary cutaneous cryptococcosis due to *Cryptococcus gattii* in Singapore. *Singapore Med J* 2011;52(7):e160–e162.

322. Kwon-Chung KJ, Hill WB, Bennett JE. New, special for histopathological diagnosis of cryptococcosis. *J clin Microbiol* 1981;13:383–387.

323. Lazcano O, Speights VO Jr, Bilbao J, Becker J, Diaz J. Combined Fontana-Masson-Mucin staining of *Cryptococcus neoformans. Arch Path Lab Med* 1991;115:1145–1149.

324. Gazzoni AF, Severo CB, Barra MB, Severo LC. Atypical micromorphology and uncommon location of cryptococcosis: A histopathologic study using special histochemical techniques (one case report). *Mycopathologia* 2009;167:197–202.

325. Gazzoni AF, Pegas KL, Severo LC. Histopathological techniques for diagnosing cryptococcosis due to capsule-deficient Cryptococcus: Case report. *Rev Soc Bras Med Trop* 2008;41:76–78.

326. Gazzoni AF, Severo CB, Salles EF, Severo LC. Histopathology, serology and cultures in the diagnosis of cryptococcosis. *Rev Inst Med Trop S Paulo* 2009;51:255–259.

327. Van Burik JA, Colven R, Spach DH. Cutaneous aspergillosis. *J Clin Microbiol* 1998;36:3115–3121.

328. Yuanjie Z, Jingxia D, Hai W, Jianghan C, Julin G. Primary cutaneous aspergillosis in a patient with cutaneous T-cell lymphoma. *Mycoses* 2008;52:462–464.

329. Ramos A, Ussetti P, Laporta R, Lazaro MT, Sanchez-Romero I. Cutaneous aspergillosis in a lung transplant recipient. *Transplant Infect Dis* 2009;11:471–473.

330. Cahill KM, Mofty AM, Kawaguchi TP. Primary cutaneous aspergillosis. *Arch Dermatol* 1967;96:545–547.

331. Romano C, Miracco C. Primary cutaneous aspergillosis in an immunocompetent patient. *Mycoses* 2003;46:56–59.

332. Craiglow B, Hinds G, Antaya R, Girardi M. Primary cutaneous aspergillosis in an immunocompetent patient: Successful treatment with oral voriconazole. *Pediatr Dermatol* 2009;26:493–495.

333. Chen Z, Li HM, Han W, Sang JH, Du J, Zhang WJ Zhang JZ. Genital cutaneous lesions in an allogeneic haematopoietic stem cell transplant recipient with aspergillosis. *Clin Exper Dermatol* 2009;34:552–558.

334. Tunçcan ÖG, Akı ŞZ, Akyürek N, Sucak G, Şenol E. Isolated cutaneous aspergillosis in an acute lymphoblastic leukemia patient after allogeneic stem cell transplantation. *J Infect Dev Ctries* 2011;5:406–409.

335. Chakrabarti A, Gupta V, Biswas G, Kumar B, Sakhuja VK. Primary cutaneous aspergillosis: Our experience in 10 years. *J Infect* 1998;37:24–27.

336. Nakashima K, Yamada N, Yoshida Y, Yamamoto O. Primary cutaneous aspergillosis. *Acta Derm Venereol* 2010;90:519–520.

337. Zhang QQ, Li L, Zhu M, Zhang CY, Wang JJ. Primary cutaneous aspergillosis due to *Aspergillus flavus*: A case report. *Chin Med J* 2005;118:255–257.

338. Mammatas LH, Regelink JC, Klein IE, Barbé E, Huijgens PC. Palmar necrosis during the treatment of acute myeloid leukaemia. *Netherl J Med* 2010;468:472.

339. Bernadeschi C, Foulet F, Ingen-Housz-Oro S, Ortonne O, Sitbon K, Quereux G, Lorthorary O, Chosidow O, Bretagne S, French Mycosis Study Group. Cutaneous

invasive aspergillosis: Retrospective multicenter study of the French Invasive-Aspergillosis Registry and literature review. *Medicine* 2015;94:1–9.

340. Lopes Bezerra LM, Filler SG. Interactions of *Aspergillus fumigatus* with endothelial cells: Internalization, injury, and stimulation of tissue factor activity. *Blood.* 2004;103:2143–2149.

341. Konishi M, Yonekawa S, Nakagawa C, Uno K, Kasahara K, Yoshimoto E, Maeda K, Mikasa K. Case of *Scedosporium apiospermum* cutaneous soft tissue infection treated with voriconazole. *Kansenshogaku Zasshi* 2008;82:82–85.

342. Maschmeyer G, Haas A, Cornely OA. Invasive aspergillosis: Epidemiology, diagnosis and management in immunocompromised patients. *Drugs* 2007;67:1567–1601.

343. Chacon AH, Farooq U, Shiman MI, Nolan B, Elgart GW. Cutaneous aspergillosis masquerading as Sweet's syndrome in a patient with acute myelogenous leukemia. *J Cut Pathol* 2013;40:66–68.

344. Bodey GP, Boktour M, Mays S, Duvic M, Kontoyiannis D, Hachem R, Raad I. Skin lesions associated with *Fusarium* infection. *J Am Acad Dermatol* 2002;47:659–666.

345. Halpern M, Balbi E, Carius L, Roma J, Gonzalez AC, Agoglia L, Covelo M et al. Cellulitis and nodular skin lesions due to *Fusarium* spp. in liver transplant: Case report. *Transplantation Proc* 2010;42:599–600.

346. Yang Y-S, Ahn J-J, Shin M-K, Lee M-H. *Fusarium solani* onychomycosis of the thumbnail coinfected with *Pseudomonas aeruginosa*: Report of two cases. *Mycoses* 2011;54:168–171.

347. Baran R, Tosti A, Piraccini BM. Uncommon clinical patterns of *Fusarium* nail infection: Report of three cases. *Br J Dermatol* 1997;136:424–427.

348. Nucci M Anaissie E. Cutaneous infection by *Fusarium* species in healthy and immunocompromised hosts: Implications for diagnosis and management. *Clin Infect Dis* 2002;35:909–920.

349. Brasch J, Köppl G. Persisting onychomycosis caused by *Fusarium solani* in an immunocompetent patient. *Mycoses* 2009;52:285–286.

350. Girmenia C, Arcese W, Micozzi A, Martino P, Bianco P, Morace G. Onychomycosis as a possible origin of disseminated *Fusarium solani* infection in a patient with severe aplastic anemia. *Clin Infect Dis* 1992;14:1167.

351. Arrese JE, Piérard-Franchimont C, Piérard GE. Fatal hyalohyphomycosis following Fusarium onychomycosis in an immunocompromised patient. *Am J Dermatopathol* 1996;18:196–198.

352. Schollenberger M, Müller HM, Rüfle M, Suchy S, Plank S, Drochner W. Natural occurence of 16 Fusarium toxins in grains and feedstuffs of plant origin from Germany. *Mycopathologia* 2006;161:43–52.

353. Nucci M, Anaissie E. *Fusarium* infections in immunocompromised patients. *Clin Microbiol Rev* 2007;20:695.

354. Melcher GP, McGough DA, Fothergill AW, Norris C, Rinaldi M. Disseminated hyalophyphomycosis caused by a novel human pathogen, *Fusarium napiforme. J Clin Microbiol* 1993;31:1461–1467.

355. Dignani MC, Anaissie E. Human fusariosis. *Clin Microbiol* 2004;10(Suppl 1):67–75.

356. Hsu C-K, Hsu MM-L, Lee JYY. Fusariosis orccurring in an ulcerated cutaneouss CD8+ T cell lymphoma tumor. *Eur J Dermatol* 2006;16:297–301.

357. Gardner JM, Nelson MM, Heffernan MP. Chronic cutaneous fusariosis. *Arch Dermatol* 2005;141:794.

358. King BA, Seropian S, Fox LP. Disseminated Fusarium infection with muscle involvement. *J Am Acad Dermatol* 2011;65:237–239.

359. Fierro-Arias L, Ramírez-Dovala SM, Araiza-Santibáñez J, Amelia Peniche-Castellanos A, Bonifaz A. Frecuencia de infecciones micóticas oportunistas tras intervención quirúrgica del aparato ungueal en la Unidad de Dermato-Oncología y Cirugía Dermatológica del Hospital General de México Dr. Eduardo Liceaga. *Dermatol Rev Mex* 2015;59:19–25.

360. Martino P, Gastaldi R, Raccah R, Girmenia C. Clinical patterns of *Fusarium* infections in immunocompromised patients. *J Infect* 1994;28(Supp 1):7–15.

361. Boucher HW, Groll AH, Chiou CC, Walsh TJ. Newer systemic antifungal agents: Pharmacokinetics, safety and efficacy. *Drugs* 2004;64:1997–2020.

362. Haneke E. Mucor mycosis and neonatal fat necrosis in a premature neonate. Clear-cell syringomatous carcinoma. Fusariosis. Coll Dermato-Pathol Unna-Darier, Zürich, Sept 1–3, 2000.

363. Esnakula AK, Summers I, Naab TJ. Fatal disseminated Fusarium infection in a human immunodeficiency virus positive patient. *Case Reports in Infectious Diseases* 2013;Article ID 379320:1–5.

364. Nelson PE, Dignani MC, Anaissie EJ. Taxonomy, biology and clinical aspects of *Fusarium* species. *Clin Microbiol Rev* 1994;7:479–504.

365. Pérez-Pérez L, Pereiro M Jr, Sánchez-Aguzilar D, Toribio J. Ulcerous lesions disclosing cutaneous infection with *Fusarium solani. Acta Derm Venereol* 2007;87:422–424.

366. Gonzalez CE, Rinaldi MG, Sugar AM. Zygomycosis. *Infect Dis Clin North Am* 2002;16:895–914.

367. Rees JR, Pinner RW, Hajjeh RA, Brandt ME, Reingold AL. The epidemiological features of invasive mycotic infections in the San Francisco Bay area, 1992–1993: Results of population-based laboratory active surveillance. *Clin Infect Dis* 1998;27:1138–1147.

368. Bonifaz A, Vázquez-González D, Tirado-Sánchez A, Rosa Ponce-Olivera RM. Cutaneous zygomycosis. *Clin Dermatol* 2012;30:413–419.

369. Eucker J, Sezer O, Graf B, Possinger K. Mucormycosis. *Mycoses* 2001;44:253–260.

370. Spellberg B, Edwards J Jr, Ibrahim A. Novel perspectives on mucormycosis: Pathophysiology, presentation, and management. *Clin Microbiol Rev* 2005;18:556–559.

371. Brown J. Zygomycosis: An emerging fungal infection. *Am J Health Syst Pharm* 2005;62:2593–2596.

372. Desai RP, Joseph NM, Ananthakrishnan N, Ambujam S. Subcutaneous zygomycosis caused by *Mucor hiemalis* in an immunocompetent patient. *Australasian Med J* 2013;6:374–377.

373. Roden MM, Zaoutis TE, Buchanan WL, Knudsen TA, Sarkisova TA. Schaufele RL, Chiou CC, Chu JH, Kontoyiannis DP, Walsh TJ. Epidemiology and outcome of zygomycosis: A review of 929 reported cases. *Clin InfectDis* 2005;41:634–53.

374. Mantadakis E, Samonis G. Clinical presentation of zygomycosis. *Clin Microbiol Infect* 2009;15(Suppl 5):15–20.

375. Ellis DH. Systemic zygomycosis. In: Merz WG, Hay RJ, eds. *Topley and Wilson' Microbiology and Microbial Infections. Medical Mycology*, 10th edn. London: Edward Arnold, 2005; 659–686.

376. Hata DJ, Buckwalter SP, Pritt BS, Roberts DG, Wengenack NL. Real-time PCR method for detection of zygomycetes. *J Clin Microbiol* 2008;46: 2353–2358.

377. Alvarez E, Sutton DA, Cano J, Fothergill AW, Stchigel A, Rinaldi MG, Guarro J. Spectrum of zygomycetes species identified in clinically significant specimens in the United States. *J Clin Microbiol* 2009;47:1650–1656.

378. Rogers TR. Treatment of zygomycosis: Current and new options. *J Antimicrob Chemother* 2008;61(Suppl 1):i35–40.

379. Ribes JA, Vanover-Sams CL, Baker DJ. Zygomycetes in human disease. *Clin Microbiol Rev* 2000;13: 236–301.

380. Wirth FA, Passalacqua JA, Kao G. Disseminated cutaneous protothecosis in an immunocompromised host: A case report and a literature review. *Cutis* 1999;63:185–188.

381. Hernandez M, Gonzalez-Serva A, Downey K. O'Brien KJ. Protothecosis of the nail: A rare subungual presentation of algal disease. *J Cut Pathol* 2010;37:119.

382. Rodríguez-Salinas E, González Halphen D. Los genomas mitocondriales: Qué nos dicen sobre la evolución de las algas verdes? *Rev Latinoam Microbiol* 2009;51:44–57.

383. Lass-Flord MA. Human protothecosis. *Clin Microbiol Rev* 2007;20:230–242.

384. Pfaller MA, Diekema DJ. Unusual fungal and pseudofungal infections of humans. *J Clin Microbiol* 2005;43:1495–1504.

385. Ramsay E, Chandler FW, Connor DH, Lack EE. Protothecosis. In: Connor DH, Chandler FW, eds. *Pathology of Infectious Diseases*, 1st edn. New York: McGraw-Hill Professional, 1997; 1067–1072.

386. Mayorga J, Fernando Barba-Gómez J, Verduzco-Martínez AP, Muñoz-Estrada VF, Welsh O. Protothecosis. *Clin Dermatol* 2012;30:432–436.

387. Sudman MS, Kaplan W. Identification of the Prototheca species by immunofluorescence. *Appl Microbiol* 1973;25:981–990.

388. Ghorpade A. Polymorphic cutaneous rhinosporidiosis. *Eur J Dermatol* 2006;16:190–192.

389. Choi CM, Lerner EA. Leishmaniasis as an emerging infection. *J Invest Dermatol Symp Proc* 2001;6:175–182.

390. Haneke E, Schell H. Ultrastructure of Leishmania tropica. 14th Ann Meeting Soc Cut Ultrastructure Res, Edinburgh, 9–10 July 1987.

391. Ogawa MM, Macedo FS, Alchorne MM, Tomimori-Yamashita J. Unusual location of cutaneous leishmaniasis on the hallux in a Brazilian patient. *Int J Dermatol.* 2002;41:439–440.

392. Jha AK, Anand V, Mallik SK, Kumar A. Post kala azar dermal leishmaniasis (PKDL) presenting with ulcerated chronic paronychia like lesion. Kathmandu Univ Med J (KUMJ) 2012;10(40):87–90.

393. Kenner Jr, Aronson NF, Brathauer GL, Turnicky RP, Jackson JE, Tang DB, Sau P. Immunohistochemistry to identify *Leishmania* in fixed tissues. *J Cutan Pathol* 1999;26:130–136.

394. Safaei A, Motazedian MH, Vasei M. Polymerase chain reaction for diagnosis of cutaneous leishmaniasis in histologically positive, suspicious and negative skin biopsies. *Dermatology* 2002;205:18.

395. Libow LF, Beltrani VP, Silvers DN, Grossman ME. Post-cardiac transplant reactivation of Chagas' disease diagnosed by skin biopsy. *Cutis* 1991;48: 37–40.

396. Hall CS, Fields K. Cutaneous presentation of Chagas' disease reactivation in a heart-transplant patient in Utah. *J Am Acad Dermatol* 2008;58:529–530.

397. Sellheyer K, Haneke E. Protozoan diseases and parasitic manifestations. In: Elder DE, Elenitsas R, Johnson BL Jr, Murphy GF, Xu X, eds. *Lever's Histopathology of the Skin*, 10th edn. Philadelphia: Lippincott Williams & Wilkins, 2009; 621–636.

398. Van Neste D, Minne G, Thomas P, Gosselin X. Hyperkeratotic (Norwegian) scabies and onychomycosis in an immunosuppressed patient. *Dermatologica* 1985;170:142–144.

399. Saruta T, Nakamizo Y. Usual scabies with nail infestation. *Arch Dermatol* 1978;114:956–957.

400. Judge MR, Kobza-Black A. Crusted scabies in pregnancy. *Br J Dermatol* 1995;132:116–119.

401. Isogai R, Kawada A, Aragane Y, Tezuka T. Nail scabies as an initial lesion of ordinary scabies. *Br J Dermatol* 2002;147:603.

402. Markelov VP. Lesions of the nail plate in an infant with scabies. *Vestn Dermatol Venerol* 1969;43(9): 83–84.

403. Kocsard E. The dystrophic nail of keratotic scabies. *Am J Dermatopathol* 1984;6:308–309.

404. Scher RK. Subungual scabies. *J Am Acad Dermatol* 1985;12:577–578.

405. Bezerra SM, Cantarelli DL. Crusted scabies: An unusual clinical manifestation. *Int J Dermatol* 1993;32:734–736.

406. Weatherhead SC, Speight EL. Crusted scabies as a cause of longitudinal nail splitting. *Clin Exp Dermatol* 2004;29:315.

407. Witkowski JA, Parish LC. Scabies. Subungual areas harbor mites. *J Ass Med Assoc* 1984;252:1318–1319.

408. Bonaduce F. Scabbia delle lamine ungueali. *Il Dermosif A* 1929;IV:503.

409. De Paoli RT, Marks VJ. Crusted (Norwegian) scabies: Treatment of nail involvement. *J Am Acad Dermatol* 1987;17:136–139.

410. Sokolova TV, Sizov IE. Involvement of fingernails in scabies in an infant. *Vestn Dermatol Venerol* 1989;2:68–69.

411. Paasch U, Haustein UF. Treatment of endemic scabies with allethrin, permethrin and ivermectin. Evaluation of a treatment strategy. *Hautarzt* 2001;52:31–37.

412. Ohtaki N, Taniguchi H, Ohtomo H. Oral ivermectin treatment in two cases of scabies: Effective in crusted scabies induced by corticosteroid but ineffective in nail scabies. *J Dermatol* 2003;30:411–416.

413. Scher RK. Biopsies of nails. Subungual scabies. *Am J Dermatopathol* 1983;5:187–189.

414. Martin WE, Wheeler CE Jr. Diagnosis of human scabies by epidermal shave biopsy. *J Am Acad Dermatol* 1979;1:335–337.

415. Kristjansson AK, Smith MK, Gould JW, Gilliam AC: Pink pigtails are a clue to the diagnosis of scabies. *J Am Acad Dermatol* 2007;57:174–175.

416. Feldmeier H, Sentongo E, Krantz I. Tungiasis (sand flea disease): A parasitic disease with particular challenges for public health. *Eur J Clin Microbiol Infect Dis* 2013;32:19–26.

417. Karunamoorthi K. Tungiasis: A neglected epidermal parasitic disease of marginalized populations—A call for global science and policy. *Parasitol Res* 2013;112:3635–3643.

418. Borovaya A, Varga R, Flaig MJ, Maier T. Tungiasis. Dia-Klinik, 24. Fortbildungswoche für praktische Dermatologie und Venerologie, Munich, 19–25 July 2014:65–67.

419. Lapczynski N, Kapser C, Hartmann C. Subunguale Myiasis. Dia-Klinik, 25. Fortbildungswoche praktische Dermatologie und Venerologie, Munich, Book of Abstracts 2016; 46–47.

420. Guse ST, Tieszen ME. Cutaneous myiasis from *Dermatobia hominis*. *Wilderness Environment Med* 1997;8:156–160.

421. Hausdörfer-Scheiff S, Bourlond A, Pirard C. Histopathological aspects of myiasis. *Dermatology* 1993;186:298–300.

422. Noutsis C, Millikan LE. Myiasis. *Dermatol Clin* 1994;12:729–736.

423. Jelinek T, Maiwald H, Nothdurft HD, Löscher T. Cutaneous larva migrans in travelers: Synopsis of histories, symptoms and treatment of 98 patients. *Clin Inf Dis* 1994;19:1062–1066.

424. Caumes E, Danis M. From creeping eruption to hookworm-related cutaneous larva migrans. *Lancet Infect Dis* 2004;4:659.

425. Balfour E, Zalka A, Lazova R. Cutaneous larva migrans with parts of the larva in the epidermis. *Cutis* 2002;69:368–370.

426. Diemer JT. Isolated pediculosis. *J Am Podiat Med Ass* 1985;75:99–101.

427. Lin YC, Chan ML, Ko CW, Hsieh MY. Nail infestation by *Liposcelis bostrychophila* Badonnei. *Clin Exp Dermatol* 2004;29:620–621.

Nail changes in systemic diseases and drug reactions

5

There are a vast number of systemic disorders potentially causing or being associated with nail changes.[1] Some of them are dealt with in other chapters when the systemic cause is not certain or the condition is better known as a nail disease of its own (see Chapters 3, 11, and 14).

5.1 NAIL CHANGES IN CARDIOVASCULAR DISORDERS

5.1.1 Clubbing

Clubbing is a phenomenon involving the entire distal phalanx of the digits.[2] Described as early as 400 BC by Hippocrates, its exact etiology and pathogenesis are still not completely elucidated. Hippocratic fingers, drumstick fingers, or watch-glass nails may be observed as a sign of chronic hypoxia due to cor pulmonale or other heart and lung diseases, rarely in chronic intestinal, hepatic, and kidney disorders, but also as a part of hypertrophic osteoarthropathy[3] or pachydermoperiostosis.[4] The latter syndromes have different etiologies and clubbing may be primary or secondary. Incomplete hypertrophic osteoarthropathy may cause clubbing only.[5] Unilateral clubbing may be a sign of hemiplegia,[6] an arterio-venous shunt,[7] thromboembolism, or obliteration of a large artery of an extremity[8,9] whereas single digit clubbing may be due to a vascular phenomenon or be observed after surgery of the digit. Most of these conditions have digital hypoxia in common.[2]

The pathogenesis of clubbing is still not clear. Of the many hypotheses, that of insufficient fragmentation of megakaryocytes in the lungs is the most widely accepted one.[10] Disturbance in the normal pulmonary circulation would allow megakaryocytes to enter the general circulation and be trapped in the capillaries of the nail where they fragment to thrombocytes that release their cocktail of growth factors, in particular platelet derived growth factor. This promotes growth, vascular permeability, and monocyte and neutrophil chemotaxis. It also leads to an increase in vascular smooth muscle cells and fibroblasts. Most of these events are seen in the pathology of clubbing. Inflammatory bowel disease may also be associated with an increase in the number of platelets. Liver disease can be associated with pulmonary arteriovenous malformations.[10] Autopsy showed more thrombocyte microthrombi in clubbed fingers than in control persons.[11] However, cyanosis appears to be another necessary factor in the development of digital clubbing.[12]

Clubbing usually occurs in stages, beginning with a periungual erythema and a softening of the nail bed.[13] This gives the impression of the nail bed being spongy on palpation. Then the normal angle of 160° formed by the proximal nail fold's free margin and the nail plate increases to over 180°; this is called Lovibond's angle.[14] The increased angle causes the nail to develop a longitudinal convexity. This in turn is associated with a decrease of the angle between the dorsal aspect of the middle and distal phalanges.[15] Placing the back surfaces of opposite terminal phalanges together normally gives a diamond-shaped window, which is obliterated in clubbing.[16] The depth of the finger pulp is greater than the interphalangeal depth.[17] With time, the nail and periungual skin appear shiny and the lunula becomes excessively large. Sometimes, the nail will be longitudinally ridged. The entire distal phalanx gets thicker giving it the aspect of a drumstick. The distal interphalangeal joint may become hyperextensible.[6] Most commonly, clubbing insidiously develops over many years. Subacute development may be a hint at a malignancy.

In most cases, imaging does not help to make the diagnosis. Plain radiographs do not show any alterations in clubbing except for hypertrophic osteoarthropathy. Capillary microscopy shows more splayed and arborized capillary loops and greater capillary plexus formation.[17] Angiography was claimed to show hypervascularization,[18,19] but this was not confirmed by other groups.[20] Positron emission tomography shows a higher metabolic rate in clubbed digits as compared to normal ones.[21] Magnetic resonance imaging also suggests an increased vascularization.[22,23]

The clinical differential diagnosis includes all lesions potentially increasing the space under the nail. When all nails are involved, clubbing may be due to circulatory, gastrointestinal, infectious, and other causes or be part of hypertrophic osteoarthropathy. Clubbing of one extremity is associated with a disturbance in the circulation of that limb. Single-digit clubbing raises the question of a subungual tumor. Familial clubbing was associated with a mutation of the gene for a major prostaglandin catabolizing enzyme.[24]

5.1.1.1 Histopathology

There are amazingly few reports on the histopathology of digital clubbing and almost all deal with the skin in hypertrophic osteoarthropathy.[25] The endothelial cells are diffusely hyperplastic with partial occlusion of the capillary lumen. There is a pericapillary lymphohistiocytic infiltrate, and hyalinosis and even sclerosis with thickening and packing of collagen fibers may be found. Sebaceous and eccrine hypertrophy are features of hypertrophic osteoarthropathy.[26] Electron microscopy of the fingertip skin showed both ectatic and hypertrophic capillaries, activated endothelia, thickened, reduplicated capillary basal membranes, and a perivascular infiltrate.

(a)

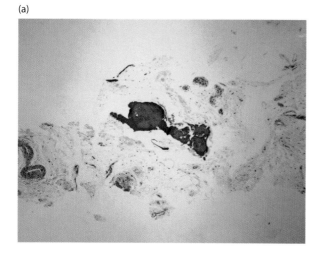

(b)

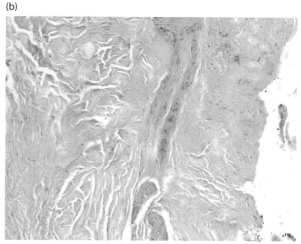

Figure 5.1 Subungual tissue from a patient with idiopathic digital clubbing. (a) H&E stain shows very loose tissue without inflammation and a tiny piece of bone (due to the biopsy technique). (b) Alcian blue exhibits diffuse positivity and an apparently acellular connective tissue. (Courtesy of Dr. N. G. Di Chiacchio, São Paulo, Brazil.)

The nail is said to be hypertrophic and more intensely stained occasionally showing some pits.[27–29] In the beginning, the connective tissue is increased with hyaline degeneration of the ground substance later. Marked clubbing is said to exhibit an increase in vascularization, edematization, and an infiltrate made up of fibroblasts, lymphocytes, and plasma cells. The largest study on the pathology of finger clubbing did not show differences between the microscopic appearance of sections of clubbed phalangeal tissue compared with normal phalangeal tissue.[20] A decrease in mast cells in the tissues just superficial under the nail may be seen.[30] The removal of the nail bed and matrix dermis in an attempt to increase the aesthetic aspect in a case of idiopathic clubbing of all fingers of a healthy 38-year-old man showed a very loose tissue with much mucin and no inflammatory infiltrates (unpublished observation) (Figure 5.1).

5.1.1.2 Differential diagnosis

Clubbed digits are rarely biopsied. Judging from the few reports of histopathology of clubbing, any "invisible" nail disease may be considered.

5.1.2 Splinter hemorrhages

Splinter hemorrhages are narrow dark lines in the nail bed due to thrombotization of the longitudinally arranged nail bed capillaries. They are said to be a hallmark of bacterial endocarditis, but in fact they may occur in a large number of very different systemic conditions and dermatological diseases or be due to medications and are rarely a sign of a specific disorder. It appears that most splinter hemorrhages are idiopathic.[31] They are mostly seen in the distal nail bed.

5.1.2.1 Histopathology

Splinter hemorrhages are clinically very typical and therefore rarely biopsied; however, they are not rare as a chance observation. They are seen in the immediate subungual keratosis that has a papillomatous aspect, as round to oval globules of condensed erythrocytes. They are positive with the benzidine stain; Prussian blue stain is negative. Rarely, intraungual small blood globules are observed (Figure 5.2).

5.1.2.2 Differential diagnosis

Common subungual hematomas are seen as large lakes of blood that are truly under the nail in very acute cases and become included in the nail in older cases.

5.1.3 Thrombangitis obliterans

This condition is also known as Bürger's disease and is characterized by obstruction of intermediate and small arteries that result in digit ischemia and finally gangrene. In the beginning, painful vesicles may develop in the digital tip with hypersensitivity and hyperemia.[32] Nail growth abnormalities, splinter hemorrhages, and finally

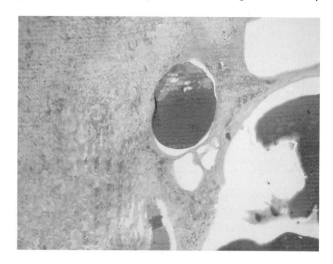

Figure 5.2 Intraungual blood globules in a patient taking an anticoagulant.

ulceration and gangrene may develop. This explains why a biopsy from the tip of the digit is rarely performed.

5.1.3.1 Histopathology

Typically, active lesions show a thrombotic occlusion of the arterial lumen and a mixed infiltrate of inflammatory cells in the vessel wall, often with microabscesses. In the late stage, the thrombus is organized and finally the lumen may be recanalized.

5.1.3.2 Differential diagnosis

Once believed to be specific, the histologic findings are now thought to be nonspecific and occur in a variety of other conditions.

5.1.4 Osler's nodes

Osler's nodes are thought to be a manifestation of septic microthrombi. They are small tender red nodules around the nail developing within hours or days.

5.1.4.1 Histopathology

The characteristic histopathological alterations consist of dermal neutrophilic abscesses and masses of gram-positive bacteria in the vessels.[33]

5.1.4.2 Differential diagnosis

Septic vasculitis and intravascular coagulation have to be ruled out.

5.1.5 Ischemia and gangrene

A great number of conditions obstructing arteries can lead to symmetrical or asymmetrical digit gangrene.[34] Once this has developed, it is rarely possible to define the underlying disorder. In the early phase of obstructive arterial disease, the nail becomes dystrophic, thin, brittle, and fragile. Onycholysis and onychorrhexis may follow. Intermittent vascular compromise to the nails may cause Beau's lines.

5.1.5.1 Histopathology

There is a diffuse imbibition of the tissue with blood and a loss of cytological details. The epithelium may be detached from the dermis. The nail plate is not altered.

5.1.5.2 Differential diagnosis

All hemorrhagic necroses have to be considered.

5.2 RESPIRATORY DISEASES

A variety of nail changes may develop in lung diseases that are also seen in cardiovascular disorders such as clubbing and splinter hemorrhages. Histopathology does not allow their etiology to be determined.

5.2.1 Sarcoidosis

Sarcoidosis is a granulomatous multisystem disorder with predominant lung involvement. It may rarely be acute or much more frequently chronic. Blau syndrome is a hereditary early onset sarcoidosis due to an NOD2 mutation.[35,36] Roughly one-quarter of sarcoidosis patients develop cutaneous lesions, but one-quarter of patients with sarcoidosis presenting in dermatology have only skin involvement.[37,38] Between 0.25% and 1.5% of sarcoidosis patients develop nail involvement.[39,40] In many cases, there is also radiological evidence of bone alterations of the distal phalanx known as ostitis multiplex cystoides of Jüngling,[41,42] but cases without bone involvement have been described.[43–45] The nail lesions are very variable with nail dystrophy to painful clubbing, massive painful swelling of the distal phalanx, or lupus pernio. A necrotizing sarcoidal distal dactylitis was observed in black South Africans.[46] Splinter hemorrhages, onycholysis, subungual hyperkeratosis, and brown discoloration of the nail bed may occur. Pterygium formation and cicatricial nail atrophy were seen.[47,48] Treatment with prednisone and chloroquine or intralesional steroid injections may improve the nail lesions.[38,49] The cystic ostitis has to be differentiated from phalangeal microgeodic syndrome.[50]

5.2.1.1 Histopathology

The classical sarcoidal lesions are seen in the nail bed and matrix as circumscribed noncaseating epithelioid granulomas (Figure 5.3). Giant cells are rare and may contain asteroid bodies that are star-shaped eosinophilic structures, and Schaumann bodies, which are round to oval calcified and therefore basophilic structures. There may be a perigranulomatous lymphocytic infiltrate. When the granulomas involute, a fibrosis develops from the margins to the center.

The visible nail plate changes are thought to be the consequence of matrix granulomas interfering with onychotization.[51,52] Longitudinal ridging and onychorrhexis are believed to result from compression of sarcoidal granulomas between the phalangeal bone and nail plate. They may cause destruction of the matrix, nail bed, and hyponychium.[53]

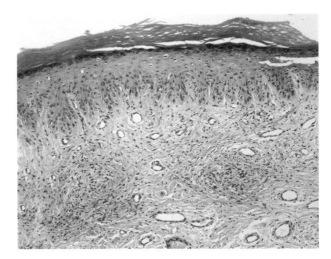

Figure 5.3 Subungual sarcoidosis of the distal nail bed with subungual orthokeratosis causing mild onycholysis. (Courtesy of Dr. A. Michalany, São Paulo, Brazil.)

5.2.1.2 Differential diagnosis

Sarcoidal foreign body granulomas can be identical to single sarcoid granulomas, and multisystem sarcoidosis has been observed to develop from scar and tattoo sarcoidal granulomas. Polarization microscopy is able to identify birefringent structures such as silica and starch; however, this does not safely exclude sarcoidosis.[54] Mycobacterial infections such as lupus vulgaris and leprosy are difficult to distinguish particularly when they are paucibacillary.

5.2.2 Yellow nail syndrome

Yellow nail syndrome is a relatively rare disorder consisting of the triad of yellow nails, edema of the distal extremities, and chronic sinu-broncho-pulmonary disease, but only approximately one-quarter of the cases display all three signs. On the other hand, several other associations, particularly with cancers, were recently described.[55–60] The nails are slow growing, very hard, markedly overcurved both longitudinally as well as transversely, intransparent, onycholytic, and may develop onychomadesis before they fall off. They often take on another color, particularly a greenish hue due to secondary bacterial colonization or infection. The cuticle is lost and the lunula is no longer visible. The proximal nail fold may be swollen.

The etiopathogenesis is not yet clear. Lymphedema appears to play a role and lymphangiograms have shown abnormal results with peripheral lymphatic atresia, hypoplasia, and focal dilatations.[61] This defective lymphatic drainage was thought to be the cause for slow growth and thickening of the nail.

Treatment of yellow nail syndrome consists of long-term antibiotherapy for the chronic respiratory infection.[62] Systemic and topical vitamin E has also been given with variable results.[63]

5.2.2.1 Histopathology

The nail plate does not show obvious changes except for a bacterial biofilm seen at the undersurface of greenish nails, which most probably represents *Pseudomonas aeruginosa*.

In some patients, the nail bed was normal without alterations of the dermal vessels. In other cases, the dermis consisted of dense fibrous tissue with numerous ectatic endothelium-lined vessels very similar to the histopathology of pleural lesions of the yellow nail syndrome; this gave rise to the hypothesis that the primary stromal sclerosis may lead to lymphatic obstruction explaining the clinical manifestations.[64] Keratohyalin granules were found in the matrix and thought to be the cause for slow nail growth; however, almost any condition with extremely slow nail growth develops a granular layer in the matrix.[65]

5.2.2.2 Differential diagnosis

Yellow nail syndrome can be diagnosed clinically with certainty. Nail plate histopathology has to rule out leukonychia. Any fibrosing and sclerosing condition of the nail bed and matrix has to be considered. Diffuse lymphectasias were seen in a case of congenital nail hypoplasia of the hand with lymphangiectasias.[66]

5.2.3 Hypertrophic osteoarthropathy

Hypertrophic osteoarthropathy (HOP) is subdivided into the primary familial type of Touraine-Solente-Golé, of which an autosomal dominant and a recessive and possibly also an X-linked type exist, and the secondary pulmonary HOP of Bamberger-Pierre-Marie. It is characterized by clubbing of fingers and toes, very coarse skin with thick folds and glandular hypertrophy, thickening of the palmar and plantar skin with hyperhidrosis, acromegalic hypertrophy of the extremities with bone pain and pathology due to osteoblast proliferation, acroosteolysis due to osteoclast stimulation, joint swelling and pain, peripheral neurovascular disease, and muscle weakness. The bone changes are seen radiologically as a proliferative periostitis with a thin translucent line between the periosteal apposition and the thick cortex. The peripheral neurovascular disease presents a cyanosis and paresthesia. Primary HOP with clubbing is due to a mutation of the 15-hydroxyprostaglandin dehydrogenase gene encoding the major prostaglandin PGE_2 catabolizing enzyme.[67,68] In autosomal recessive HOP, the transporter gene SCLO2A1 is mutated.[69,70] Secondary HOP is mainly seen in patients with lung carcinoma, lung metastases, pleural tumors, and other intrathoracic neoplasms.[71]

5.2.3.1 Histopathology

Whereas the skin shows thickening of the dermis with thick fibrous bands and an increase in fibroblasts and hyaluronic acid-rich ground substance as well as sebaceous hyperplasia, the nail lesions are identical to common clubbing (see Section 5.1.1). The histopathology of osteoblast and osteoclast proliferation has not been studied.[72]

5.2.3.2 Differential diagnosis

The main conditions to be considered are common clubbing and acromegaly.

5.2.4 Acrokeratosis paraneoplastica of Bazex

This characteristic paraneoplastic dermatosis is almost exclusively seen in patients with cancers of, or metastases to, the upper respiratory and digestive tract.[73] Most patients were French males although this condition has also been described in many other countries. The disease is characterized by symmetrical erythematous to violaceous keratotic areas on the nose, the pinna, hands, and feet with marked psoriasiform involvement of the distal phalanges. The nails are the first to be affected with thin brittle nail plates and then onycholysis and dystrophy. Nail shedding may be seen and the nail bed replaced by smooth epidermis with hyperkeratotic debris. The proximal nail folds are often erythemato-squamous with papules and/or a paronychia-like aspect. The toes are more severely affected than the fingers. Acrokeratosis paraneoplastica may precede the cancer by some months and disappear with successful surgery.

5.2.4.1 Histopathology

The histopathologic alterations are nonspecific with mostly psoriasiform acanthosis and focal parakeratosis, a mild perivascular lymphocytic infiltrate in the superficial dermis with some pycnotic neutrophils. Hyalinization of single keratinocytes and focal vacuolar degeneration of the basal cells may occur.[74]

5.2.4.2 Differential diagnosis

Psoriasis, pityriasis rubra pilaris, other diseases leading to nail dystrophy such as amyloidosis, and scabies crustosa have to be differentiated. The condition published as paraneoplastic syndrome with papulo-keratotic lesions of the extremities and diffuse keratosis pilaris spinulosa[75] is probably a variant of Bazex syndrome.

5.3 GASTROINTESTINAL DISEASES

Several gastrointestinal disorders may cause nail alterations, which are often not specific and may also be seen in other system diseases. Clubbing and hypertrophic osteo-arthropathy were observed in Crohn's disease and colitis ulcerosa.[76,77] Nail dystrophy occurs in several deficiency states. Beau's lines were typically observed in typhoid.[78]

5.3.1 Cronkhite–Canada syndrome

Cronkhite–Canada syndrome is a very rare condition characterized by nonhereditary gastrointestinal polyposis with diarrhea, dysgeusia, fatigue, weight loss, skin hyperpigmentation, alopecia, and nail dystrophy. Fecal occult blood is often positive. Hemoglobin, serum potassium, calcium, and protein may be below the normal range. Colonoscopy reveals multiple polyps of different types.[79] Nail alterations are almost always present with a peculiar soft spongy area of the proximal nail and thickened irregular hard distal nail.[80] Nail shedding often occurs.[81] The disease is usually progressive and may eventually be fatal. Recently, an autoimmune pathogenesis was assumed as there is a strong IgG4 staining in the polyps.[82] The risk of colorectal cancer is estimated to be 25%. Nutritional support and systemic corticosteroids are the treatment of choice.[83]

5.3.1.1 Histopathology

Systematic nail examinations are lacking. Nail clippings from the distal part reveal irregular nail substance without any diagnostic features.

5.3.1.2 Differential diagnosis

The histopathological examination of nail clippings does not give any hint at the primary diagnosis. The polyposis has to be differentiated from familial adenomatous polyposis, Peutz–Jeghers syndrome, Cowden disease, and juvenile polyposis.[84]

5.3.2 Peutz–Jeghers syndrome

Intestinal polyps and pigmented macules of the lips, peri-orificially, on fingers, toes, and nails are the diagnostic criteria for this syndrome. Longitudinal melanonychia has been seen.[85] Pigment spots on the distal phalanx may occur.[86] Malignant degeneration of polyps is the most serious complication.[87]

5.3.2.1 Histopathology

Using special stains such as Fontana-Masson's argentaffin reaction shows melanin in the nail plate. It may be assumed that there is also a numerical increase in the number of melanocytes (see Chapter 15).

5.3.2.2 Differential diagnosis

Laugier–Hunziker–Baran syndrome shows lenticular brown spots of the oral mucosa and brown streaks in one or more nails that are usually lighter than those of Peutz–Jeghers syndrome. Histopathology shows little pigment in the nail plate and melanocyte activation in the matrix or a slight increase in the number of melanocytes (see Chapter 15).

5.3.3 Pyodermatitis pyostomatitis vegetans

This disease that is clinically similar to pemphigus vegetans is said to be a marker of inflammatory bowel disease, most commonly colitis ulcerosa and Crohn's disease.[88–90] Annular pustular lesions of the skin are associated with extensive vegetating oral lesions and "snail-track" mucosal pustules.[91] The skin of the digital tips is raw, red, oozing, and covered with pustules.

5.3.3.1 Histopathology

The epidermis is hyperplastic with intra- and subepithelial neutrophils and eosinophils that may form microabscesses. Immunofluorescence for pemphigus antibodies is negative.

5.3.3.2 Differential diagnosis

The most important disease to be ruled out is pemphigus vegetans, which is positive for direct and indirect immunofluorescence. Acrodermatitis continua suppurativa is another important differential diagnosis. Vegetating candidiasis may be very similar and requires a PAS stain.

5.3.4 Glucagonoma syndrome

Glucagonoma may cause a characteristic paraneoplastic disease with weight loss, diabetes mellitus, necrolytic migratory erythema, erosive stomatitis, angular cheilitis, paronychia, and very thin and brittle nails.[92,93] Granulation tissue may appear.[94]

5.3.4.1 Histopathology

The histopathology of glucagonoma dermatitis is very characteristic though almost identical with that of acute pellagra, acrodermatitis enteropathica, acrodermatitis acidemica, and acquired zinc deficiency dermatitis. The epidermis exhibits a thick parakeratotic layer due to necrosis of the upper stratum spinosum and a typical epidermal pallor of the upper half of the epidermis due to massive keratinocyte swelling with small pycnotic basophilic nuclei. The lower half of the epidermis is unaltered

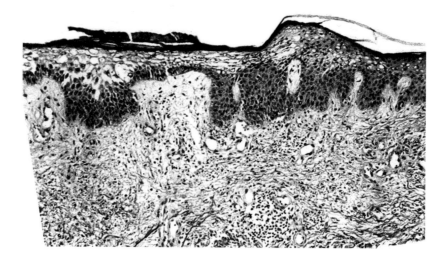

Figure 5.4 Acute zinc deficiency dermatitis. The upper half of the epidermis is very pale due to large empty-appearing keratinocytes.

except for a mild spongiosis. Neutrophils may be found in the uppermost layers giving a psoriasiform aspect. With increasing age of the lesions, the psoriasiform character increases. The dermis is surprisingly devoid of inflammatory changes. Both bacteria as well as yeasts may be found on erosive surfaces.

5.3.4.2 Differential diagnosis

Pellagra, zinc deficiency (Figure 5.4), biotin-responsive multiple carboxylase deficiency,[95] but also kwashiorkor and subacute psoriasis may mimic glucagonoma dermatitis. Other dermatoses with a disturbance of epidermal maturation such as subacute cutaneous lupus erythematosus, dermatomyositis, drug eruptions, pityriasis rubra pilaris, and graft-versus-host disease may be similar.

5.4 HEPATIC DISEASES

Although a variety of hepatic disorders are associated with nail changes, they are usually not specific enough to allow a clinical or histopathological diagnosis to be made from them. Clubbing, periungual erythema, splinter hemorrhages, diffuse leukonychia and Terry's nails, flat fingernails, red lunulae, and melanonychia may be seen.[1]

5.4.1 Terry's nails

White nails were found in 82 of 100 patients with liver cirrhosis.[96] The nails appear ground-glass-like over almost the entire length leaving a distal pink to brownish band of 1–2 mm width. The lunula can no longer be discerned. Terry's nails were later redefined as having a distal pink band of 0.5–3 mm in width, the distal band is not obscured by decreased venous return, a white or pink proximal nail, the lunula is visible or not, and at least 10 nails are affected.[97]

5.4.1.1 Histopathology

Three patients underwent lateral longitudinal nail biopsies. Histopathology revealed telangiectasiae in the upper

dermis of the distal band whereas the proximal nail bed was poor in vessels.

5.4.1.2 Differential diagnosis

Clinically, half-and-half nails (see Section 5.5) and Neapolitan nails have to be differentiated.

5.4.2 Necrolytic acral erythema (NAE)

NAE has only been observed in patients with hepatitis C and is considered to be pathognomic for this viral infection[98,99] although its prevalence is low.[100] More than three-quarters of the patients were diagnosed as having hepatitis C on the basis of the skin lesions.[101] The skin lesions vary according to the stage of the skin alterations: acute lesions are red scaly plaques often with flaccid bullae at their periphery. With time, thick scaly plaques with erosions and crusting develop mostly in acral locations with more intense lesions on the lower extremities, particularly the dorsal feet, but involvement of the palms, soles, periungual skin, and nails is possible.[102] Laboratory examinations should rule out glucagonoma dermatitis, and zinc and amino acid deficiencies.[103] Despite normal serum zinc levels, the initial treatment of choice is oral zinc often leading to dramatic improvement.[104] However, effective therapy of hepatitis C usually gives long-lasting effects.[105,106] The pathogenesis of this condition is not yet clear.

5.4.2.1 Histopathology

Early stage NAE exhibits acanthosis, spongiosis, and a superficial perivascular infiltrate similar to nummular eczema. These lesions develop to marked psoriasiform hyperplasia, prominent papillomatosis, parakeratosis, subcorneal pustules, epidermal pallor, and widespread, often confluent necrosis of superficial keratinocytes leading to cleft formation. Dermal papillary vessels are dilated.[107]

Electron microscopy and polymerase chain reaction (PCR) failed to demonstrate virus particles or hepatitis C virus-ribonucleic acid (HCV-RNA) in the skin lesions.

5.4.2.2 Differential diagnosis

In the early stage, nummular eczema (dermatitis) has to be considered. The epidermal hyperplasia may lead to the misdiagnosis of psoriasis. Epidermal pallor, keratinocyte necrosis, and cleft formation are also characteristic for other types of necrolytic erythemas, such as seen in the glucagonoma syndrome, pellagra, or zinc deficiency.[108] A high degree of suspicion is necessary to make the correct diagnosis.[109] Acral peeling skin syndrome shows a lamellar exfoliation of the horny layer of the normal epidermis without an inflammatory infiltrate.[110]

5.5 RENAL AND GENITOURINARY DISEASES

Several renal disorders may be associated with nail changes. Nail alterations are even seen in 98% of patients under chronic hemodialyis; the nail changes included absence of the lunula (55%), half-and-half (51%), splinter hemorrhages (36%), subungual hyperkeratosis (34%), onychomycosis (31%), koilonychia (19%), and onycholysis (9%).[111] Muehrke's lines are two pale bands in the nail beds of patients with hypalbuminemia under 2.2 g/100 mL. Pressure makes the bands that run parallel to the lunula disappear. No specific pathology can be attributed to them. Calciphylaxis may cause acral necrosis,[112] but is rare in the tip of the digit. Half-and-half nails are said to be characteristic for chronic renal failure and azotemia. The proximal nail half is opaque and ground-glass-like whereas the distal half is red, pink, or brown.

5.5.1 Histopathology

The red color of the distal band in half-and-half nails is thought to be due to an increase of capillaries with thickening of their walls.[113]

5.5.2 Differential diagnosis

Terry's nails have to be differentiated.

5.6 DISEASES OF THE REPRODUCTIVE SYSTEM

Menstruation and pregnancy can have a profound impact on the nails. Transverse leukonychia, sometimes as a repeated phenomenon, may be seen due to menstruation.[114] The nails grow faster during pregnancy, but may become softer and brittle.[115] Leukonychia may disappear during pregnancy.[116] Hyperpigmentation and longitudinal melanonychia are particularly common in darkly pigmented women.[117,118]

5.6.1 Histopathology

The histopathology of leukonychia (see Chapter 7) and longitudinal melanonychia (see Chapter 15) is not different from that of other causes.

5.6.2 Differential diagnosis

They are identical with those of other etiologies.

5.7 ENDOCRINE DISEASES

Although there are a plethora of nail changes associated with diabetes mellitus, pituitary, adrenal, and thyroid diseases, they are not specific for any of these conditions and do not allow a specific diagnosis to be made with certainty.

5.7.1 Histopathology

There are no characteristic pathognomonic histopathologic changes for most endocrine-induced nail changes. Anorexia nervosa and bulimia cause brittle nails.

5.7.2 Differential diagnosis

Nail alterations of other etiologies have to be considered.

5.7.3 Sertoli–Leydig cell (androgen-) producing tumor

Recently, peculiar fingernail changes mimicking spoon nails were observed in a case of Sertoli–Leydig cell tumor in a postmenopausal woman.

5.7.3.1 Histopathology

In the Sertoli–Leydig cell tumor, increased androgen receptors were found in the distal nail bed. As the nail changes receded after successful surgery, it was assumed that the upward curving of the distal nail plates was due to the high androgen levels in this rare sex cord stromal tumor.[119]

5.7.3.2 Differential diagnosis

Nail alterations of other etiologies have to be considered.

5.7.4 Acromegaly

Acromegaly is due to human growth hormone overproduction, in most cases by a pituitary eosinophil adenoma, and characterized by hypertrophy of the soft tissues as well as growth of the hands, feet, and tongue as well as joint pain. The skin is enlarged and doughy.

Nail changes are not often observed, but they may be large, hard, or brittle, occasionally pigmented and koilonychotic.[120] The nail folds may be hypertrophic.[121]

5.7.4.1 Histopathology

There are few histological skin examinations in acromegaly and apparently none specifically of the nails. However, the available data can most probably also be applied to the periungual skin. Collagen-bundles are coarse and there are acidic glycosaminoglycan deposits. Dermal dendrocytes may be markedly reduced in numbers, but those present are plump with few dendrites. A negative correlation is found between dermal dendrocyte numbers and the maximum insulin-like growth factor (IGF)-1 dosages given to the patients. The dendrocyte changes are persistent even after treatment.[122]

5.7.4.2 Differential diagnosis

Myxedema in hypothyroidosis may also cause swollen hands and feet with a tendency to hyperplastic nail folds.

5.8 MUSCULOSKELETAL DISEASES

They rarely cause characteristic signs in the nails.

5.8.1 Trichinosis

Trichinosis, an infestation mainly of the muscles by *Trichinella spiralis*, causes symptomatic diarrhea, continuous fever, headache, muscle pain that has similarity to dermatomyositis, and allergic lid and facial edema. Blood eosinophilia is high. It was reported to cause splinter-like hemorrhages in 10%–30% of the larval migrating phase. In contrast to virtually all other causes, some of these splinters are not arranged longitudinally and may be painful.[123–125] These splinters may be much larger, up to 2 mm wide and 4–5 mm long, first red, then plum-colored and later black.[126] The source of infestation is mainly undercooked or raw meat of domestic pigs and wild boar.[127] Treatment in the acute stage is with albendazole or mebendazole.[128]

5.8.1.1 Histopathology

Nail bed biopsy in the acute phase of larval migration revealed *Trichinella spiralis* organisms.[129] Usually, there are *Trichinella* cysts that may die and calcify over the course of years. However, in experimental trichinosis in cats, larvae were exclusively found in muscles.[130]

5.8.1.2 Differential diagnosis

The diagnosis depends on the demonstration of the larvae. Chronic meningococcemia and rheumatic fever may cause similar splinter hemorrhages.[131] Clinically and histologically, anatrichosomiasis, an infection of the trichuroid nematode *Anatrichosoma* and mainly of skin and mucosa of non-human primates, has to be considered; *Anatrichosoma* does not encyst and may also be located in the epithelium.[132]

5.9 CONNECTIVE TISSUE DISEASES

Nail changes seen in lupus erythematosus, dermatomyoisitis, mixed connective tissue disease, and scleroderma are dealt with in Chapter 3.

5.9.1 Rheumatoid arthritis

Approximately half of the patients with rheumatic arthritis display nail changes of variable types. Particularly, dilated nail fold capillaries have attracted much attention among rheumatologists. Brittle nails, onychorrhexis, and onycholysis with subungual hyperkeratosis and splinter hemorrhages are frequent.[133] Immobility due to joint pain may favor onychogryposis.

5.9.1.1 Rheumatoid nodules

Rheumatoid nodules occur in one-fifth of patients with rheumatoid arthritis although mainly over extensor surfaces at the elbows, metacarpophalangeal and interphalangeal joints. Rarely, they are seen on the distal pads, the free margin of the nails, and the dorsal aspect of the fingers. They may even occur without typical rheumatoid arthritis, particularly in accelerated rheumatoid nodulosis.[134,135]

5.9.1.1.1 Histopathology

In the dermis and subcutis, nodules with one or more areas of central fibrinoid collagen degeneration being homogenously eosinophilic are found. Both nuclear fragments and basophilic material may be present. Around the degenerative foci, palisading histiocytes are seen. Foreign body giant cells are often present. Proliferating blood vessels are found in the surrounding fibrosis. The inflammatory infiltrate is sparse to moderate with lymphocytes and neutrophils predominating. Perforation with transepidermal elimination of the degenerated fibrinoid material may occur.[136]

5.9.1.1.2 Differential diagnosis

The most important differential diagnosis is subcutaneous granuloma annulare. In contrast to deep-seated granuloma annulare, rheumatoid nodules are usually devoid of mucin. Epithelioid sarcoma may mimic rheumatoid nodules. Suture granulomas, particularly when the suture material is not included in the section, may be difficult to rule out on histological grounds alone.[137] Rheumatic nodules occurring in rheumatic fever do not exhibit the central fibrinoid necrosis.[138,139] Multicentric reticulohistiocytosis presents in about one-half of the patients with warty to flesh-colored nodules in a coral bead distribution along the free margin of proximal nail folds; this may be isolated or in association with an erosive arthritis, and malignant neoplasms are found in approximately 25%. Histologically, oncocytic macrophages and numerous multinucleate giant cells with eosinophilic finely granular cytoplasm giving the aspect of ground glass are characteristic.[140] Pernio is a distinct injury induced by humid cold characterized by painful, burning, or pruritic violaceous or erythematous papules and infiltrates on fingers, toes, and distal extremities; histologically they are characterized by a marked T-lymphocytic perivascular infiltrate around superficial and deep vessels and endothelial swelling, with edema in the papillary dermis but without fibrinoid necrosis. Epidermal pallor may be present. An interface dermatitis with vacuolar basal cell degeneration is typical for chilblain lupus erythematosus. Cold-induced blister, for example, after cryotherapy of warts, shows a loss of cellular outline of the keratinocytes and ghost-like alterations of the epidermis.[141] Dermal and deep-seated infections to mycobacteria and some fungi may require special stains to be ruled out.

5.9.1.2 Ischemic-hemorrhagic distal finger lesions of Bywaters

Small painless hemorrhagic necroses of elbows, hands, finger pulps, nail folds, and edges due to obstruction of digital arteries at different levels are said to be characteristic for rheumatoid arthritis.[142] They start as periungual swelling, which develops into a skin infarction turning into an eschar that heals with or without leaving a pigmented scar. Larger necroses do occur, but are rare. Sometimes, they look like paronychia. Grooving and ridging may develop.[143]

5.9.1.2.1 Histopathology

Histopathologically, a concentric intimal proliferation and thrombosis without an adventitial reaction may be seen.

Depending on the level of sectioning, some neutrophils may be present around the fibrin thrombi. In severe cases, full-blown necrosis develops.[144]

5.9.1.2.2 Differential diagnosis

Vascular changes in scleroderma, lupus erythematosus, polyarteritis nodosa,[145] and Bürger's disease have to be ruled out. Cholesterol crystal embolization may cause blisters and gangrene of the distal extremities.[146,147] Isolated necrotizing vasculitis with neutrophils in the necrotic walls of small superficial vessels may occur.[148,149] Small vessel necrotizing vasculitis is seen in Wegener granulomatosis.[150,151] The antisynthetase syndrome with anti-Jo1 antibodies may also cause periungual ischemia and fingertip necroses due to severe arteritis.[152] Septic vasculitis in gonorrhea and meningitis may involve the nail folds.

5.10 IMMUNOLOGICAL DISEASES

A great many immunologic disorders may be associated with nail changes. Virtually none of them is specific for a certain type of immune disease. Clubbing, brittle nails, Beau's lines, periungual erythema, melanonychia, digital tip necroses, onychomycoses, psoriasiform dermatitis, and yellow nails may be due to the immune disease itself or, more frequently, to another disease subsequent to immunodeficiency.

5.10.1 Graft-versus-host disease

Approximately one-half to two-thirds of patients with graft-versus-host disease (GvHD) develop nail changes of various kinds. Most of them are nonspecific. Their severity depends on the duration of the GvHD. On the digits, periungual erythema is the first sign, often followed by telangiectasiae, onychomadesis, and shedding.[153] In chronic GvDH, the nails may look like in ungual lichen planus or amyloidosis with longitudinal ridging, fragility, roughness, and pterygium formation.[154–156]

5.10.1.1 Histopathology

Nail changes in chronic cutaneous GvHD are microscopically similar to those of ungual lichen planus. There is hydropic basal cell degeneration and an epitheliotropic infiltrate of variable density and acanthosis, hypergranulosis, hyperkeratosis, and apoptosis in the epithelium of the matrix, undersurface of the proximal nail fold, and in the nail bed. Pigmentary incontinence may be seen in deeply pigmented individuals. In the late sclerodermiform stage, the epithelium is flattened and the inflammatory infiltrate is minimal. The nail dermis is fibrotic. Immunophenotyping exhibited a predominance of T lymphocytes and epidermal HLA-DR expression.[157]

5.10.1.2 Differential diagnosis

Lichen planus is the major differential diagnosis. Dyskeratosis congenita, amyloidosis, and erythema multiforme have to be ruled out.

5.10.2 Atypical rejection of hand allograft

The skin of the first hand allograft was sequentially followed histologically and immunohistochemically.[158] Nail growth was not impaired; to the contrary, there was an impression that the nails of the allograft grew faster than those of the recipient's own hand. Due to noncompliance to the immunosuppressive treatment, the skin developed lichenoid papules from month 15 onward that progressively spread coalescing to diffuse erythematous-scaly areas over the allografted hand. Histopathology showed the aspect of a chronic lichenoid cutaneous graft-versus-host disease. At month 29, the allograft hand had to be amputated presenting erosive and necrotic changes. Histopathologic examination of the allograft showed the most severe changes in the skin whereas only mild inflammation was present in muscles and tendons. The bones, bone marrow, and joints were uninvolved. The nails were not specifically examined.[159] A 30-year-old patient with two allotransplanted hands was observed over 60 months; he developed three rejection episodes during this period.[160] During the first month after transplantation, he developed a rejection with transverse leukonychia and ridging that improved rapidly within 2 weeks. The third rejection episode occurred at month 60 post-transplantation and showed lesions of the palmar skin and nails. The skin lesions were psoriasiform whereas the nails presented with severe onycholysis leading to nail loss due to a rejection Banff grade III. Despite intensification of the immunosuppressive treatment, the lesions got worse in the following month to finally normalize after another 74 days.[161] The appearance of skin lesions associated with nail changes, volar skin involvement, and the response to immunosuppressant is called atypical rejection and appears to be characteristic for hand allograft.[162]

5.10.2.1 Histopathology

The nail biopsy of Banff rejection grade III showed a very dense lymphocytic infiltrate in the dermis invading the overlying epithelium.[147] Vacuolar basal cell degeneration is not very prominent. Apoptoses are also not frequent. Immunophenotyping exhibits mainly CD3+ with predominantly CD4+ and fewer CD8+ cells and CD68+ macrophages. B cells (CD20+, CD79a+) are few in number. FOXP3 cells may increase over time. Cytoid bodies may occur.

5.10.2.2 Differential diagnosis

The patient history is obvious and should allow the diagnosis to be made. In classical graft-versus-host reaction, the nail changes are more lichenoid. Nail changes were also seen in renal transplant patients under immunosuppression,[163] during mycophenolate[164] and rapamycin treatment.[165]

5.11 NERVOUS SYSTEM DISEASES

Nail involvement in neurofibromatosis and tuberous sclerosis are described in the respective chapters on tumors (see Chapters 9 and 12).

5.12 PSYCHOLOGICAL DISTURBANCES AND PSYCHIATRIC DISEASES

A variety of habit tics, onychophagia, onychotillomania, onychoteiromania, and onychodaknomania cause clinically characteristic nail changes, which have not yet been studied histopathologically.[166]

5.13 HEMATOLOGICAL DISEASES

As in many other systemic disorders, hematological conditions may cause many different mostly unspecific nail changes.[1] Pallor of the nail bed is seen in anemia, koilonychia is said to be characteristic for iron deficiency anemia, red nail beds are observed in polycythemia, splinter hemorrhages and ulcero-necrotic lesions may be a sign of thrombocytopenia. Sickle cell anemia may cause symmetrical peripheral gangrene and phalangeal osteomyelitis. Digital necroses were also seen in gamma-heavy chain disease. Nail fold telangiectasiae, purple fingertips, subungual hemorrhage, and painful digital necrosis were observed in cryoglobulinemia. Hereditary hemorrhagic telangiectasia of Weber-Osler-Rendu is characterized by giant nail fold and subungual capillaries. Pale gray nail beds may be a sign of parasitemia in children with malaria.[167] Plasmocytoma caused a subungual nodule. Osteolytic areas in the distal phalanges were seen in multiple myeloma. Clubbing was seen in a case of POEMS syndrome. Castleman tumor often causes severe erosive nail changes due to paraneoplastic pemphigus.[168] This has recently also been observed in a follicular lymphoma.[169]

5.13.1 Hematological neoplasms

See Chapter 14.

5.14 METABOLIC DISEASES

Many metabolic diseases cause nail changes similar to those seen in various malnutrition conditions. Most are nonspecific. Clubbing and half-and-half nails were seen in a case of citrullinemia but thought to be nonspecific.[170]

5.14.1 Hyperhomocysteinemia

Hyperhomocysteinemia is associated with atherosclerotic disease and venous thrombosis. It is due to a mutation in the methylene-tetra-hydrofolate-reductase gene. Treatment is with folic acid. A case with acral purpura of the nail beds and onycholysis was observed.[171]

5.14.1.1 Histopathology

Histologic sections show thromboses of the cutaneous vessels without vasculitis.

5.14.1.2 Differential diagnosis

Many other conditions with intravascular thrombosis have to be considered.

5.14.2 Gout

Gout is due to hyperuricemia. It usually becomes manifest by recurring attacks of painful arthritis, often of the

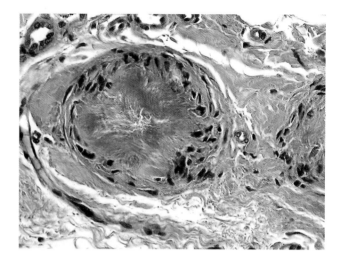

Figure 5.5 Small gout tophus under the distal nail bed.

metatarsophalangeal hallux joint; therefore it was called podagra in earlier times. Approximately 3% of gout patients develop tophi, which represent deposits of uric acid crystals.[172] They are typically found on the helix, over the elbows, and on fingers and toes and rarely the fingertips.[173] Their size may reach from a few millimeters to over 5 centimeters. Large tophi may discharge a milky-white chalky material.

5.14.2.1 Histopathology

Usually there are deposits of amorphous material with a feathery aspect surrounded by foreign body giant cells and macrophages (Figure 5.5). Secondary calcification is possible. When fresh material is available it should be fixed in absolute alcohol or Carnoy's solution as they do not dissolve the urate crystals like aqueous fixatives.[174] The urate crystals can be recognized under polarized light due to their strong birefringence. Thick unstained sections of formalin-fixed biopsies also show birefringent urate crystals in about half of the cases.[175]

Clippings of the nail with subungual hyperkeratosis may reveal urate crystals in unstained thick sections.[176]

5.14.2.2 Differential diagnosis

The urate crystal tophi are highly characteristic for gout.

5.14.3 Oxalosis

The deposition of calcium oxalate crystals in renal and extrarenal tissues is called oxalosis. Three genetic disorders of glyoxalate metabolism are known all associated with hyperoxaluria.[177] A secondary form results from ingestion of oxalates, oxalic acid precursors, or renal failure. Oxalate crystals may be deposited under the nail.[178,179] Other signs of oxalosis are acrocyanosis, Raynaud phenomenon, loss of distal pulses, peripheral gangrene, and cutaneous calcifications of the fingers.

5.14.3.1 Histopathology

The biopsy demonstrates needle-like crystals that are arranged in rosette-like arrays typical for oxalate crystals.

There is a lymphocytic and neutrophilic infiltrate surrounding these deposits. Polarization microscopy shows the crystals to be birefringent.

5.14.3.2 Differential diagnosis

The diagnosis is obvious when the hyperoxaluria is diagnosed in the laboratory. Needle-like crystals may look similar to gout.

5.14.4 Ochronosis

Ochronosis is a rare autosomal recessive disorder caused by a deficiency of the enzyme homogentisic acid oxidase. This leads to alkaptonuria, staining the urine dark. Homogentisic acid accumulates in ear, nose, and joint cartilage, ligaments and tendons, sclerae, and after a long time in the dermis it causes a dirty brown pigmentation, similar to that seen in localized exogenous ochronosis due to long-term topical application of hydroquinone cream. A bluish-brown subungual pigmentation may develop.[180,181] A bluish nail bed may occur.

Particularly in darkly pigmented individuals, the proximal nail folds often are very dark and may be treated with hydroquinone-containing creams that over the long run may cause exogenous ochronosis. This is histologically identical.

5.14.4.1 Histopathology

The hallmark of ochronosis is thick yellow-brown to ochre collagen bundles in the dermis without an inflammatory reaction. These fibers often have a bizarre shape, appear rigid, and tend to break with jagged ends. Short collagen segments appear as brown clumps. Staining with methylene blue and cresyl violet turns them black.[182] Fine free pigment granules may be seen in the tissue, basement membrane, endothelial cells, secretory sweat gland cells, and some macrophages. These granules are negative with silver stain.

5.14.4.2 Differential diagnosis

Nail bed pigmentation due to minocycline[183–185] and hydroxychloroquine[186–189] may look similar. In amalgam tattoos, the elastic fibers are imbibed with the silver-mercury alloy and look yellowish-brown in H&E stains. In mucocutaneous and nail bed pigmentation due to ezogabine, perivascular and periadnexal cells were heavily laden with coarse melanin granules that were electron micoscopically proven to be intracellular.[190]

5.14.5 Porphyria cutanea tarda

Of the seven types of porphyrias, porphyria cutanea tarda (PCT) is the most common one. Almost all porphyrias, except acute intermittent porphyria, are characterized by sensitivity to near ultraviolet A and visible light. PCT is either sporadic due to toxic liver disease, familial, or hepatoerythropoietic.[191] This is due to a reduced activity of uroporphyrinogen decarboxylase in the liver. Alcohol, estrogens, iron supplementation, and hepatitis are the most common precipitating factors.[192] Clinically, sun-exposed skin becomes extremely vulnerable and blisters and erosions develop mainly in the face, bald scalp, and dorsa of the hands and fingers, also around the nails. They may heal with milia. Hypertrichosis malaris is typical in men. A simple qualitative laboratory test is urine fluorescence with Wood light excitation: a test tube with fresh urine is irradiated from the side and looked at from the top. Uropoporphyrin III shows bright red fluorescence.[193] Exact determination of porphyrins in blood, urine, and feces as well as molecular genetic studies are now the standard to diagnose porphyrias.[194]

5.14.5.1 Histopathology

Typical blisters of PCT are subepidermal with the basal lamina remaining at the bottom in most cases. Characteristic for PCT is that the dermal papillae remain and extend into the blister lumen (Figure 5.6). This is called festooning. PAS stain shows positive material around capillaries in the upper dermis, and it is believed that this material makes the dermal papillae rigid so that they do not flatten in the blisters. The epidermal roof of the blisters may contain elongate eosinophilic PAS-positive bodies referred to as caterpillar bodies.

5.14.5.2 Differential diagnosis

PAS-positive hyaline substances are also found in erythropoietic protoporphyria and in the other porphyrias with skin lesions. Autoimmune blistering diseases are associated with inflammatory infiltrates. Pseudoporphyria cutanea in patients under long-term hemodialysis is histologically virtually identical with mild PCT.

5.14.6 Amyloidosis

Several forms of amyloidosis are known. Systemic amyloidosis involving the skin is also called primary amyloidosis. It is usually due to a plasma cell dyscrasia and the production of monoclonal light chain immunoglobulins. These can involve the heart, muscle, kidney, liver, spleen, lung, and skin.[195] The latter involvement may cause petechiae and ecchymoses as well as pseudoxanthelasma. Amyloid

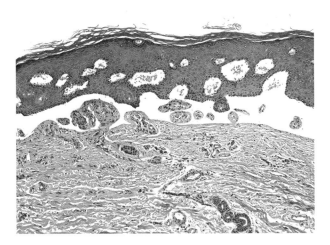

Figure 5.6 Biopsy of a blister on the proximal nail fold of a patient with porphyria cutanea tarda demonstrating the festooning of the dermal papillae into the lumen.

deposition around hair follicles causes alopecia, around and in salivary and sweat glands results in dry mouth and skin, in the nail unit a lichen-planus-like nail dystrophy, splinter hemorrhages, distal onycholysis, and subungual hyperkeratosis may develop.[196,197] One case presented subungual verrucous masses.[198]

5.14.6.1 Histopathology

Skin biopsies show a pale eosinophilic fissured material in the papillary dermis and also around blood vessels of the subcutis. Scalp biopsies reveal perifollicular amyloid deposits suffocating the follicles. Salivary gland acini are substituted by amyloid masses and become atrophic. In nail biopsies, the most striking feature is a very thin nail that exhibits staining characteristics more like stratum corneum than nail plate. The matrix shows a broad granular layer, but its rete relief is preserved. Faintly eosinophilic material may be seen subepithelially that stains more intensely with Congo red and then exhibits an apple-green birefringence under polarized light (Figure 5.7).[199] Thioflavin T causes an intense fluorescence,[200] and when excited with UV this is a bright whitish-blue relatively specific for amyloid. Specialized immunohistochemistry allows the type of amyloidosis to be defined.[201]

5.14.6.2 Differential diagnosis

Chronic lichen planus and postlichen condition may look very similar.

5.14.7 Scleromyxedema and lichen myxoedematosus

Scleromyxedema is a rare disease characterized by generalized papular and sclerodermoid changes and mucin deposition in the skin often associated by IgGκ[202] or IgGλ paraproteinemia.[203] The risk to develop multiple myeloma is >10%. No paraproteins are found in lichen myxoedematosus. There is no hypothyroidosis in any of these conditions.[204] The skin is thickened and slightly harder. Waxy

lichenoid papules are mainly seen on the head and neck, upper trunk, and hands that may also involve the dorsa of the fingers and nail folds.[205,206]

5.14.7.1 Histopathology

The histopathologic changes in scleromyxedema and lichen myxoedematosus are identical. The epidermis is usually normal or may become slightly flattened. There is a diffuse mucin deposition in the papillary and less pronounced in the reticular dermis with an increase in the number of fibroblasts and fibrosis. Inflammatory infiltrates are not common.[207]

5.14.7.2 Differential diagnosis

In myxedema, there is only mucin deposition without fibroblast proliferation. Nephrogenic fibrosing dermopathy is characterized by an enormous increase in fibroblasts and collagen without mucin. Scleredema is mainly seen in the shoulder girdle and has no lichenoid papules. Scleroderma is characterized by increased hardness of the skin and sclerosis of the dermis without mucinosis.

5.15 NUTRITIONAL DISEASES

Malnutrition, kwashiorkor, marasmus, anorexia nervosa, bulimia, and many deficiencies of vitamins and essential elements cause nail growth disturbance, brittle, and dystrophic nails. Vitamin A deficiency causes thin white curved nails called eggshell nails.[208]

5.15.1 Pellagra

Vitamin B$_3$ (niacinamide) plus protein deficiency causes pellagra. Clinically, transverse leukonychia, Beau's lines, loss of nail transparency, onycholysis, koilonychia, and half-and-half nails were observed. However, it is characterized by the 4 Ds: dermatitis, diarrhea, dementia, and death. The skin lesions are a photoinduced, intensely erythematous psoriasiform dermatitis, painful erosions in the genital and perineal area, and a rash similar to seborrheic

(a)

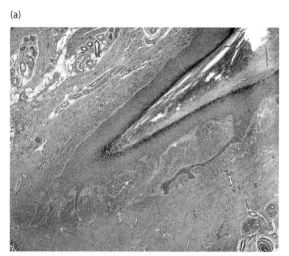

(b)

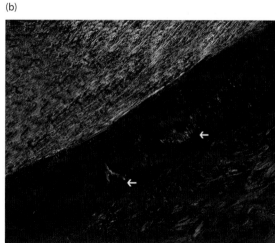

Figure 5.7 (a) Amyloidosis of the nail with submatrical amyloid deposit stained more intensely with Congo red. (b) Polarization microscopy reveals apple-green birefringence.

dermatitis in the face, scalp, and neck. Oral lesions are beefy red fissured lips and tongue with loss of papillae. Periungual psoriasiform lesions may be present.

5.15.1.1 Histopathology

The periungual lesions are psoriasiform with marked parakeratosis and loss of the granular layer, pallor of the upper half of the epidermis, some necrotic keratinocytes, and altered epidermal maturation.

5.15.1.2 Differential diagnosis

As outlined above, glucagonoma dermatitis, acquired zinc deficiency, and acrodermatitis enteropathica are histologically very similar. Hartnup disease, an autosomal recessive congenital vitamin B_3 deficiency with niacin-unresponsive skin lesions, neurological signs, and aminoaciduria, is very similar to pellagra but specific nail lesions have not yet been described.

5.15.2 Acquired zinc deficiency

The histopathological alterations (Figure 5.4) are identical to acrodermatitis enteropathica and very similar to those of glucagonoma dermatitis, pellagra, and acrodermatitis acidemica[209-211] (see Section 5.3.4 and Figure 5.4).

5.16 INTOXICATIONS

Deleterious toxic effects can already develop *in utero* as is evidenced by dysplasia or absence of nails in approximately 20% of patients with the fetal alcohol syndrome.[212]

Arsenic intoxication may cause transverse leukonychia, Beau's lines, onychomadesis, and brown bands or diffuse blackish nail discoloration and clubbing. The nails are a valuable source of examination for arsenic intoxication by drinking water and in forensic medicine (see Chapter 1). Mee's lines are transverse white bands arranged parallel to the lunula border and growing out with the nail. They are due to parakeratosis in the nail plate.[213] Similar nail alterations are seen in cadmium poisoning.

Mercury poisoning causes acrodynia, swollen hands, and red soles and fingers in addition to a variety of internal and neuropsychiatric symptoms. The clinical differential diagnosis may be atypical Kawasaki disease.[214]

5.17 DRUG REACTIONS

Drug-induced nail alterations are very varied and may be classified according to the drug classes, their indications, or the particular nail lesions they cause. Some drugs accumulate in the nail, which may be intended for antifungals used in the treatment of onychomycoses. Nails are also used to monitor drug intake and intoxications (see Section 5.16). Many drug nail reactions are described as single or few-case reports and most of them do not allow the specific drug to be defined with certainty. Brittle nails, Beau's lines, onychomadesis, subungual hyperkeratosis, onycholysis, and splinter hemorrhages are frequent and nonspecific. Sometimes it is not clear whether the nail changes seen are due to the drug or to the original disease. Some reactions often attributed to drugs such as ingrown nails after

successful onychomycosis treatment with terbinafine[215,216] or ingrowing nails with granulation tissue, often wrongly called pyogenic granulomas (see Chapter 10), during treatment with retinoids,[217,218] reverse transcriptase inhibitors for HIV infection,[219,220] anti-CD20,[221] tumor necrosis factor-a inhibitor,[222] or epidermal growth factor receptor (EGFR) inhibitors[223] are indirect effects.[224-226] Taxans were observed to cause subungual hemorrhagic abscesses and pyogenic granulomas (probably granulation tissue).[227,228]

A number of cytostatic drugs cause periungual and palmar erythema that often turns into a scaling lesion. This starts with masses of single keratinocyte necroses (Figure 5.8). Nail pigmentation,[229] probably via stimulation of matrix melanocytes, is also quite common. Melanonychia may be longitudinal, diffuse, or even transverse[230,231] and some drugs like hydroxyurea are particularly frequently the cause[232,233] (see Chapter 15). Transverse grayish melanonychia developed under topical 5-fluorouracil treatment for periungual warts.[234] Nail pigmentation and darkening of already pigmented nails in dark-skinned individuals is seen in about 5% of patients with HIV infection; it is often not clear whether this is idiopathic, due to the infection itself, the drug, or a combination of them.[235] Melanonychia developed in 9% of patients treated with interferon-α for hepatitis C.[236]

Lichenoid nail changes are seen to develop under therapy with β-blockers, angiotensin-converting enzyme inhibitors,[237] thyrostatic drugs,[238] mitoxantrone,[239] etanercept,[240] and EGFR inhibitors.[241,242] Histologically, these changes are similar to ungual lichen planus.

Photoonycholysis is a peculiar reaction said to occur in four different morphological types.[243] It may be due to drugs, porphyria cutanea tarda, other porphyrias such as erythropoietic protoporphyria, erythropoietic porphyria, porphyria variegata, and pseudoporphyria.[244] Spontaneous photoonycholysis is very rare.[245] It may occur

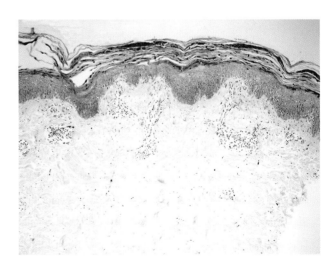

Figure 5.8 Periungual erythema due to cytostatic treatment. There are mitoses and many necrotic keratinocytes in the epidermis and the horny layer; the latter stain dark blue with Giemsa in the horny layer.

together with cutaneous photosensitization or without. The drugs most commonly encountered are tetracyclines, psoralens, and fluoroquinolones. It usually does not develop before 2 weeks of drug intake. The sequence of cutaneous photosensitivity, nail discoloration, and photoonycholysis is called Segal's triad.[246] Photoonycholysis cannot be reproduced by skin testing or UV light provocation. As it is now known that almost no UV light can penetrate the nail, the concept of photoonycholysis may have to be revised.

The histopathologic changes of most drug reactions have not systematically been examined. It may be assumed that they are identical to those with the same morphology but seen in other conditions.

5.17.1 Argyrosis (Argyria)

Ingestion of silver preparations was once commonplace against a variety of gastrointestinal problems, but silver-containing lozenges were also taken by patients with sore throat. Although these drugs usually carried a warning against long-term use, these were often not followed by the patients. Generalized silver deposits would develop in the light-exposed areas due to the photochemical reaction of silver ions to metallic silver. A grayish appearance particularly of the face and hands was the most obvious sign. Long-term use of silver-containing eye drops or large area application of silver-protein for burn patients provoked localized argyria. This is called imbibition argyria.[247] Causes of generalized argyrosis about 80 years ago were injections of Kollargol and silver-salvarsan in syphilis. About 20–30 g of silver were said to be needed for systemic argyrosis although much lower amounts were also proven to cause argyrosis.[248] Nail involvement was repeatedly described, mainly as azure lunulae.[249–256] In recent years, more cases were described due to ingestion of food additives and other over-the-counter health products or to medical applications containing silver.[257–263] Recently, silver preparations became a fashion for health addicts and people with orthorexia.[264]

5.17.1.1 Histopathology

In severe generalized argyrosis, skin, mucosal membranes, and internal organs are impregnated with minute silver grains. In the skin, the epidermis is free from silver. Under the epidermis, there may be a band of fine silver granules that can also be seen in the perifollicular connective tissue, the arrector pili muscles, and particularly around the sweat glands. Often, silver granules impregnate elastic fibers, similar to what is usually seen in amalgam tattoos of the oral mucosa. The silver granules are extracellular and do not provoke any inflammatory reaction. This is also proven by electron microscopy.[265] Dark-field microscopy makes the detection of the silver granules very easy.[1] In the nail bed, fine granules are seen in the dermis. Electron microscopy revealed electron dense granules in the nailbed dermis in the extracellular space, but as phagolysosomes also in some macrophages. The nail plate is free from silver particles.[266]

5.17.1.2 Differential diagnosis

All causes of slate gray to azure diffuse nail or lunula discoloration have to be ruled out. Melanin is not a cause of such a pigmentation although when located deep subcutaneously it may provoke a more gray to bluish gray color as is seen in blue nevi; however, this is never as diffuse as in systemic argyrosis. In Wilson's disease, the copper may cause a similar azure color of the lunulae.[249,267–269] Gold therapy may lead to yellow to dark brown nail pigmentation, called chrysiasis.[270–272] Mercury can also cause nail pigmentation.[273,274] In ochronosis, the homogentisinic acid causes a diffuse yellow-brown to ochre imbibition of the collagen bundles that are homogenized and appear swollen and broken. The granular nature of the ochronotic pigment is not evident at first glance. These granules are free in the dermal connective tissue and in endothelial cells of blood vessels.[275] Diffuse nail staining may also be seen due to antimalarials such as atabrine,[276] mepacrine,[277] amodiaquine,[278] quinacrine,[279] or chloroquine.[280] It is worth noting that silver nitrate application on the nail, for example, in the treatment of granulation tissue due to ingrown nails, is completely different from systemic argyrosis (see Chapter 7).

REFERENCES

1. Holzberg M. The nail in systemic disease. In: Baran R, de Berker DAR, Holzberg M, Thomas L, eds. *Baran & Dawber's Diseases of the Nails and Their Management*, 4th edn. Oxford: John Wiley & Sons, 2012; 315–412.
2. Spicknall KE, Zirwas MJ, English JC III. Clubbing: An update on diagnosis, differential diagnosis, pathophysiology, and clinical relevance. *J Am Acad Dermatol* 2005;52:1020–1028.
3. Martinez-Lavin M, Matucci-Cerinic M, Jajic I, Pineda C. Hypertrophic osteoarthropathy: Consensus on its definition, classification, assessment, and diagnostic criteria. *J Rheumatol* 1993;20:1386–1387.
4. Matucci-Cerinic M, Lotti T, Jajic I, Pignone A, Bussani C, Cagnoni M. The clinical spectrum of pachydermoperiostosis (primary hypertrophic osteoarthropathy). *Medicine (Baltimore)* 1991;70:208–214.
5. Seaton DR. Familial clubbing of the fingers and toes. *Br Med J* 1938;1:614–615.
6. Alvarez S, McNair D, Wildman J, Hewson JW. Unilateral clubbing of the fingernails in patients with hemiplegia. *Gerontol Clin* 1975;17:1–6.
7. Leb DE, Sharma JK. Clubbing secondary to an arteriovenous fistula used for hemodialysis. *J Am Med Ass* 1978;240:142–143.
8. Kaditis AG, Nelson AM, Driscoll DJ. Takayasu's arteritis presenting with unilateral digital clubbing. *J Rheumatol* 1995;22:2346–2348.
9. De Waele M, Lauwers P, Hendriks J, Van Schil P. Fibromuscular dysplasia of the brachial artery associated with unilateral clubbing. *Interact Cardiovasc Thorac Surg* 2012;15:1080–1081.

10. Dickinson CJ, Martin JF. Megakaryocytes and platelet clumps as the cause of finger clubbing. *Lancet* 1987;2:1434–1435.

11. Fox SV, Day CA, Gatter KC. Association between platelet microthrombi and finger clubbing. *Lancet* 1991;338:313–314.

12. Silveira LH, Martinez-Levin M, Pineda C, Fonseca M-C, Navarro C, Nava A. Vascular endothelial growth factor and hypertrophic osteoarthropathy. *Clin Exp Rheumatol* 2000;18:57–62.

13. Altman RD, Tenenbaum J. Hypertrophic osteoarthropathy. In: Ruddy S, Harris EPJ, Sledge CB, eds. *Kelly's Textbook of Rheumatology*, 6th edn. Philadelphia: WB Saunders, 2001; 1589.

14. Lovibond JL. Diagnosis of clubbed fingers. *Lancet* 1938;1:363–364.

15. Curth HO, Firschein IL, Alpert M. Familial clubbed fingers. *Arch Dermatol* 1961;83:828–836.

16. Schamroth L. Personal experience. *S Afr Med J* 1976;50:297–300.

17. Myers KA, Farquhar DR. Does this patient have clubbing? *J Am Med Ass* 2001;286:341–347.

18. Takaro T, Hines EA. Digital arteriography in occlusive arterial disease and clubbing of the fingers. *Circulation* 1967;35:682–689.

19. Jajic I, Pecina M, Krstulovic B, Kovacevic D, Pavicic F, Spaventi S. Primary hypertrophic osteoarthropathy (PHO) and changes in the joints. *Scand J Rheumatol* 1980;9:89–96.

20. Currie AE, Gallagher PJ. The pathology of clubbing: Vascular changes in the nail bed. *Br J Dis Chest* 1988;82:382–385.

21. Ward RW, Chin R, Keyes JW, Haponik EF. Digital clubbing: Demonstration with positron emission tomography. *Chest* 1995;107:1172–1773.

22. Wiesmann F, Beer M, Krause U, Pabst T, Kenn W, Hahn D, Ertl G. Clubbing due to peripheral hypervascularization. *Circulation* 2001;104:2503.

23. Nakamura J, Halliday NA, Fukuba E, Radjenovic A, Tanner SF, Emery P, McGonagle D, Tan AL. The microanatomic basis of finger clubbing—A high-resolution magnetic resonance imaging study. *J Rheumatol* 2014;41:523–537.

24. Tariq M, Azeem Z, Ali G, Chishti MS, Ahmad W. Mutation in the HPGD gene encoding NAD+ dependent 15-hydroxyprostaglandin dehydrogenase underlies isolated congenital nail clubbing (ICNC). *J Med Genet* 2009;46:14–20.

25. Matucci-Cerinic M, Cinti S, Morroni M, Lotti T, Nuzzaci G, Lucente E, di Lollo S, Ceruso M, Cagnoni M. Pachydermoperiostosis (primary hypertrophic osteoarthropathy): Report of a case with endothelial and connective tissue involvement. *Ann Rheum Dis* 1989;48:240–246.

26. Fara EF, Baughman RP. A study of capillary morphology in the digits of patients with acquired clubbing. *Am Rev Resp Dis* 1989;140:1063–1066.

27. Lovell RH. Observations on the structure of clubbed fingers. *Clin Sci* 1950;9:299.

28. Lewin BL. The finger nail in general disease. *Br J Dermatol* 1955;77:431.

29. Stone OJ, Maberry JD. Spoon nails and clubbing. Review and possible structure mechanisms. *Tex J Med* 1965;61:620–627.

30. Marshall R. Observations of the pathology of clubbed fingers with special reference to mast cells. *Am Rev Respir Dis* 1976;113:395–397.

31. Saladi RN, Persaud AN, Rudikoff D, Cohen SR. Idiopathic splinter hemorrhages. *J Am Acad Dermatol* 2004;50:289–292.

32. Quenneville JG, Gossard D. Subungueal splinter hemorrhage an early sign of thromboangitis obliterans. *Angiology* 1981;32:424–432.

33. Cardullo AC, Silvers DN, Grossman ME. Janeway lesions and Osler's nodes: A review of histopathologic findings. *J Am Acad Dermatol* 1990;22:1088–1090.

34. Kerdel FA. Subclavian occlusive disease presenting as a painful nail. *J Am Acad Dermatol* 1984;10:523–525.

35. Blank N, Max R, Autschbach F, Libicher M, Lorenz HM. Familial early onset sarcoidosis with bone cysts and erosions. *Skeletal Radiol* 2007;36:891–893.

36. Wouters CH, Maes A, Foley KP, Bertin J, Rose CD. Blau syndrome, the prototypic auto-inflammatory granulomatous disease. *Pediatr Rheumatol Online J* 2014;12(33):1–9.

37. Olive KE, Kataria YP. Cutaneous manifestations of sarcoidosis. *Arch Int Med* 1985;145:1811–1814.

38. Hanno R, Needelman A, Eiferman RA, Callen JP. Cutaneous sarcoidal granulomas and the development of systemic sarcoidosis. *Arch Dermatol* 1981;117:203–207.

39. Patel KB, Sharma OP. Nails in sarcoidosis: Response to treatment. *Arch Dermatol* 1983;119:277–278.

40. Veien NK, Stahl D, Brodthagen H. Cutaneous sarcoidosis in Caucasians. *J Am Acad Dermatol* 1987;16:534–540.

41. Baltzer G, Behrend H, Behrend T, Dombrowski H. Incidence of cystic bone alterations (ostitis cystoides multiplex Jüngling) in sarcoidosis. *Dtsch Med Wochenschr* 1970;95:1926–1929.

42. Studler U, Wiesner W, Bongartz G. Bone manifestations of sarcoidosis Jüngling ostitis multiplex cystoides. *Praxis (Bern 1994)* 2000;89:1925–1928.

43. Momen SE, Al-Niaimi F. Sarcoid and the nail: Review of the literature. *Clin Exp Dermatol* 2013;38:119–124; quiz 125.

44. Kawaguchi M, Suzuki T. Nail dystrophy without bony involvement in a patient with chronic sarcoidosis. *J Dermatol* 2014;41:194–195.

45. Noriega L, Criado P, Gabbi T, Avancini J, Di Chiacchio N. Nail sarcoidosis with and without systemic involvement: Report of two cases. *Skin Appendage Disorders* 2015;1:87–90.

46. Leibowitz MR, Essop AR, Schamroth CL, Blumsohn D, Smith EH. Sarcoid dactylitis in black South African patients. *Semin Arthritis Rheum* 1985;14:232–237.

47. Kalb RE, Grossmann ME. Pterygium formation due to sarcoidosis. *Arch Dermatol* 1985;121:276–277.

48. Santoro F, Sloan SB. Nail dystrophy and bony involvement in chronic sarcoidosis. *J Am Acad Dermatol* 2009;60:1050–1052.

49. Rajan S, Melegh Z, de Berker D. Subungual sarcoidosis: A rare entity. *Clin Exp Dermatol* 2014;39:720–722.

50. MacCarthy J, O'Brien N. Phalangeal microgeodic syndrome of infancy. *Arch Dis Child* 1976;51:472–474.

51. Wakelin SH, James P. Sarcoidosis: Nail dystrophy without underlying bone changes. *Cutis* 1995;55:344–346.

52. Tosti A, Peluso AM, Misciali C. Systemic sarcoidosis presenting with nail dystrophy. *Eur J Dermatol* 1997;7:69–70.

53. Losada-Campa A, De la Torre-Fraga C, Gomez de Liaño A, Cruces-Prado MJ. Histopathology of nail sarcoidosis. *Acta Derm Venereol* 1995;75:404–405.

54. Mangas C, Fernández-Figueras MT, Fité E, Fernández-Chico N, Sàbat M, Ferrándiz C. Clinical spectrum and histological analysis of 32 cases of specific cutaneous sarcoidosis. *J Cutan Pathol* 2006;33:772–777.

55. Dhillon SS. Yellow nail syndrome. *Am J Respir Crit Care Med* 2012;186:e10.

56. Tidder J, Pang CL. A staged management of prolonged chylothorax in a patient with yellow nail syndrome. *BMJ Case Rep* 2012. pii: bcr2012006469. doi: 10.1136/bcr-2012-006469

57. Modrzewska K, Fijołek J, Ptak J, Wiatr E. Yellow nail syndrome in a patient with membranous glomerulonephritis. *Pneumonol Alergol Pol* 2012;80:158–162.

58. Letheulle J, Deslée G, Guy T, Lebargy F, Jego P, Delaval P, Desrues B, Jouneau S. Le syndrome des ongles jaunes: Presentation de cinq cas. *Rev Mal Respir* 2012;29:419–425.

59. Noël-Savina E, Paleiron N, Leroyer C, Descourt R. Découverte d'un syndrome des ongles jaunes lors d'une insuffisance thyroidienne majeure. *Rev Pneumol Clin* 2012;68:315–317.

60. Taki H, Tobe K. Yellow nail syndrome associated with rheumatoid arthritis, thiol-compound therapy and early gastric cancer. *BMJ Case Rep* 2012. pii: bcr1120115183. doi: 10.1136/bcr.11.2011.5183

61. Bull RH, Fenton DA, Mortimer PS. Lymphatic function in the yellow nail syndrome. *Br J Dermatol* 1996;134:307–312.

62. Suzuki ML, Yoshizawa A, Sugiyama H, Ichimura Y, Morita A, Takasaki J, Naka G et al. A case of yellow nail syndrome with dramatically improved nail discoloration by oral clarithromycin. *Case Rep Dermatol* 2011;3:251–258.

63. Piraccini BM, Urciuoli B, Starace M, Tosti A, Balestri R. Yellow nail syndrome: Clinical experience in a series of 21 patients. *J Dtsch Dermatol Ges* 2014;12:131–137.

64. DeCoste SD, Imber MJ, Baden HP. Yellow nail syndrome. *J Am Acad Dermatol* 1990;22:608–611.

65. Pavlidakey GP, Hashimoto K, Blum D. Yellow nail syndrome. *J Am Acad Dermatol* 1984;11:509–512.

66. Fernandes-Flores A, Manjon JA. Congenital hyponychia of the hand with lymphangiectases: A new entity? *J Clin Diagn Res* 2015;9(3):WD01–WD02.

67. Uppal S, Diggle CP, Carr IM, Fishwick CW, Ahmed M, Ibrahim GH, Helliwell PS et al. Mutations in 15-hydroxyprostaglandin dehydrogenase cause primary hypertrophic osteoarthropathy. *Nat Genet* 2008;40:789–793.

68. Bergmann C, Wobser M, Morbach H, Falkenbach A, Wittenhagen D, Lassay L, Ott H, Zerres K, Girschick HJ, Hamm H. Primary hypertrophic osteoarthropathy with digital clubbing and palmoplantar hyperhidrosis caused by 15-PGHD/HPGD loss-of-function mutations. *Exp Dermatol* 2011;20:531–533.

69. Zhang Z, Xia W, He J, Zhang Z, Ke Y, Yue H, Wang C et al. Exome sequencing identifies SLCO2A1 mutations as a cause of primary hypertrophic osteoarthropathy. *Am J Hum Genet* 2012;90:125–132.

70. Busch J, Frank V, Bachmann N, Otsuka A, Oji V, Metze D, Shah K et al. Mutations in the prostaglandin transporter SLCO2A1 cause primary hypertrophic osteoarthropathy with digital clubbing. *J Invest Dermatol* 2012;132:2473–2476.

71. Coury C. Hippocratic fingers and hypertrophic osteoarthropathy: Study of 350 cases. *Br J Dis Chest* 1960;54:202–209.

72. Castori M, Sinibaldi L, Mingarelli R, Lachman RS, Rimoin DL, Dallapiccola B. Pachydermoperiostosis: An update. *Clin Genet* 2005;68:477–486.

73. Bazex A, Salvador R, Dupré A. Syndrome paranéoplasique à type d'hyperkératose des extrémités: Guérison après traitement de l'épithélioma laryngé. *Bull soc Fr Dermatol Syphil* 1965;72:182.

74. Bazex A, Griffiths A. Acrokeratosis paraneoplastica: A new cutaneous marker of malignancy. *Br J Dermatol* 1980;102:301–306.

75. Nazzaro P, Argentieri R, Balus L, Bassetti F, Fazio M, Giacalone B, Ponno R. Syndrome paranéoplasique avec lésions papulokératosiques des extrémités et kératose pilaire spinulosique diffuse. *Ann Dermatol Vénéréol* 1974;101:411–413.

76. Kitis G, Thompson H, Allan RH. Finger clubbing in inflammatory bowel disease, its prevalence and pathogenesis. *Br Med J* 1979;2:825–828.

77. Young JR. Ulcerative colitis and finger clubbing. *Br Med J* 1966;1:278–279.

78. Beau JH. Note sur certains caractères de séméiologie rétrospective présentés par les ongles. *Arch Gén Méd* 1846;11:447.

79. Goto A. Cronkhite–Canada syndrome: Epidemiological study of 110 cases reported in Japan. *Nippon Geka Hokan* 1995;64:3–14.

80. Herzberg AJ, Kaplan DJ. Cronkhite–Canada syndrome: Light and electron microscopy of the cutaneous pigmentary abnormalities. *Int J Dermatol* 1990;29:121–125.

81. Cunliffe WJ, Anderson J. Cronkhite–Canada syndrome with associated jejunal diverticulosis. *Br Med J* 1967;4:601–602.

82. Sweetser S, Ahlquist DA, Osborn NK, Sanderson SO, Smyrk TC, Chari ST, Boardman LA. Clinicopathologic features and treatment outcomes in Cronkhite–Canada syndrome: Support for autoimmunity. *Dig Dis Sci* 2012;57:496–502.

83. Wen XH, Wang L, Wang YX, Qian JM. Cronkhite–Canada syndrome: Report of six cases and review of literature. *World J Gastroenterol* 2014;20:7518–7522.

84. Sweetser S, Boardman LA. Cronkhite–Canada syndrome: An acquired condition of gastrointestinal polyposis and dermatologic abnormalities. *Gastroenterol Hepatol* 2012;8:201–203.

85. Valero A, Sherf K. Pigmented nails in Peutz–Jeghers syndrome. *Am J Gastroenterol* 1965;43:56–58.

86. Daniel CR. Nail pigmentation abnormalities. *Dermatol Clin* 1985;3:431–443.

87. Archord JL, Proctor HD. Malignant degeneration and mestatasis in Peutz–Jeghers syndrome. *Arch Int Med* 1963;111:498–502.

88. Storwick GS, Prihoda MB, Fulton RJ, Wood WS. Pyodermatitis-pyostomatitis vegetans: A specific marker for inflammatory bowel disease. *J Am Acad Dermatol* 1994;31:336–341.

89. Shah S, Cotliar J. Images in clinical medicine. Pyostomatitis vegetans. *N Engl J Med* 2013;368:1918.

90. Lankarani KB, Sivandzadeh GR, Hassanpour S. Oral manifestation in inflammatory bowel disease: A review. *World J Gastroenterol* 2013;19:8571–8579.

91. Merkourea SS, Tosios KI, Merkoureas S, Sklavounou-Andrikopoulou A. Pyostomatitis vegetans leading to Crohn's disease diagnosis. *Ann Gastroenterol* 2013;26:187.

92. Guillausseau PJ, Guillausseau C, Villet R, Kaloustian E, Valleur P, Hautefeuille P, Lubetzki J. Les glucagonomes. Aspects cliniques, biologiques, anatomopathologiques et thérapeutiques (revue générale de 130 cas). *Gastroenterol Clin Biol* 1982;6: 1029–1041.

93. Chao SC, Lee JY. Brittle nails and dyspareunia as first clues to recurrences of malignant glucagonoma. *Br J Dermatol* 2002;146:1071–1074.

94. Picard C, Mazer JM, Bilet S, Villette B, Penchet A, Toublanc M, Grossin M, Debussche X, Assan R, Belaïch S. Syndrome du glucagonome. *Ann Dermatol Venereol* 1988;115:1142–1145.

95. Seymons K, De Moor A, De Raeve H, Lambert J. Dermatologic signs of biotin deficiency leading to the diagnosis of multiple carboxylase deficiency. *Ped Dermatol* 2004;21:231–235.

96. Terry RB. White nails in hepatic cirrhosis. *Lancet* 1954;1:757–759.

97. Holzberg M, Walker HK. Terry's nails: Revised definition and new correlations. *Lancet* 1984;1:896–899.

98. Darouti M, Abu el Ela M. Necrolytic acral erythema: A cutaneous marker of viral hepatitis C. *Int J Dermatol* 1996;35:252–256.

99. Abdallah MA, Ghozzi MY, Monib HA, Hafez AM, Hiatt KM, Smoller BR, Horn TD. Necrolytic acral erythema: A cutaneous sign of hepatitis C virus infection. *J Am Acad Dermatol* 2005;53:247–251.

100. Raphael BA, Dorey-Stein ZL, Lott J, Amorosa V, Lo Re VIII, Carrie Kovarik C. Low prevalence of necrolytic acral erythema in patients with chronic hepatitis C virus infection. *J Am Acad Dermatol* 2012;67:962–968.

101. El-Ghandour TM, Sakr MA, El-Sebai H, El-Gammal TF, El-Sayed MH. Necrolytic acral erythema in Egyptian patients with hepatitis C virus infection. *J Gastroenterol Hepatol* 2006;21:1200–1206.

102. Bentley D, Andor A, Holzer A, Elewski B. Lack of classic histology should not prevent diagnosis of acral necrolytic erythema. *J Am Acad Dermatol* 2009;60:504–507.

103. Najarian DJ, Lefkowitz I, Balfour E, Pappert AS, Rao BK. Zinc deficiency associated with necrolytic acral erythema. *J Am Acad Dermatol* 2006;55(Suppl 5):S108–S110.

104. Abdallah MA, Hull C, Horn TD. Necrolytic acral erythema: A patient from the United States successfully treated with oral zinc. *Arch Dermatol* 2005;141:85–87.

105. Khanna VJ, Shieh S, Benjamin J, Somach S, Zaim MT, Dorner WJr, Shill M, Wood GS. Necrolytic acral erythema associated with hepatitis C: Effective treatment with interferon alfa and zinc. *Arch Dermatol* 2000;136:755–757.

106. Hivnor CM, Yan AC, Junkins-Hopkins JM, Honig PJ. Necrolytic acral erythema: Response to combination therapy with interferon and ribavirin. *J Am Acad Dermatol* 2004;50(Suppl 5):S121–S124.

107. Abdallah MA, Ghozzi MY, Monib HA, Hafez AM, Hiatt KM, Smoller BR, Horn TD. Histological study of necrolytic acral erythema. *J Ark Med Soc* 2004;100:354–355.

108. Nofal AA, Nofal E, Attwa E, El-Assar O, Assaf M. Necrolytic acral erythema: A variant of necrolytic migratory erythema or a distinct entity? *Int J Dermatol* 2005;44:916–921.

109. Fielder LM, Harvey VM, Kishor SI. Necrolytic acral erythema: Case report and review of the literature. *Int J Dermatol* 2005;44:916–921.

110. Cañueto J, Bueno E, Rodríguez-Diaz E, Vicente-Díaz MA, Álvarez-Cuesta CC, Gonzalvo-Rodríguez P, González-Sarmiento R. Acral peeling syndrome resulting from mutations in *TGM5*. *J Eur Acad Dermatol Venereol* 2016;30:477–480.

111. Onelmis H, Sener S, Sasmaz S, Ozer A. Cutaneous changes in patients with chronic renal failure on hemodialysis. *Cutan Ocul Toxicol* 2012;31:286–291.

112. Scheinman IL, Helm KF, Fairley JA. Acral necrosis in a patient with chronic renal failure. *Arch Dermatol* 1991;127:247–252.

113. Kint A, Bussels L, Fernandes M, Ringoir S. Skin and nail disorders in relation to chronic renal failure. *Acta Derm Venereol* 1974;54:137–140.

114. Colver GB, Dawber RP. Multiple Beau's lines due to dysmenorrhoea? *Br J Dermatol* 1984;111:111–113.

115. Wong RC, Ellis CN. Physiologic skin changes in pregnancy. *J Am Acad Dermatol* 1984;10:929–940.

116. Chaudhry SI, Black MM. True transverse leuconychia with spontaneous resolution during pregnancy. *Br J Dermatol* 2006;154:1212–1213.

117. Fryer JM, Werth VP. Pregnancy associated hyperpigmentation: Longitudinal melanonychia. *J Am Acad Dermatol* 1992;26:493–494.

118. Monteagudo B, Suárez O, Rodríguez I, Ginarte M, León A, Pereiro M, Pereiro M Jr. Melanoniquia longitudinal en el embarazo. *Actas Dermosifiliogr* 2005;96:550.

119. Moghazy D, Sharan C, Malika Nair M, Rackauskas C, Burnette R, Diamond M, Al-Hendy O, Al-Hendy A. Sertoli–Leydig cell tumor with unique nail findings in a post-menopausal woman: A case report and literature review. *J Ovar Res* 2014;7:83(1–8).

120. Haneke E. Nagelveränderungen bei Erkrankungen des Endokriniums. *Therapiewoche* 1987;37:4379–4382.

121. Keefe M, Chapman RS, Peden NR. Ingrowing fingernails: An unusual complication of acromegaly successfully treated by conservative means. *Clin Exp Dermatol* 1987;12:343–344.

122. Quatresooz P, Hermanns-Lê T, Ciccarelli A, Beckers A, Piérard GE. Tensegrity and type 1 dermal dendrocytes in acromegaly. *Eur J Clin Invest* 2005;35:133–139.

123. Pfister R. Pathological changes of the nails and their relationships to systemic diseases. Part II. *Hautarzt* 1969;20:341–347.

124. Samman PD. *The Nails in Disease*, 3rd edn. Chicago: Yearbook Med Publ, 1978.

125. Young JB, Will EJ, Mulley GP. Splinter haemorrhages: Facts and fiction. *J R Coll Phys Lond* 1988;22:240–243.

126. Fisher AA. Subungual splinter hemorrhages associated with trichinosis. *Arch Dermatol* 1957;75:752–754.

127. Murrell KD, Pozio E. Worldwide occurrence and impact of human trichinellosis, 1986–2009. *Emerg Infect Dis* 2011;17:2194–2202.

128. Watt G, Saisorn S, Jongsakul K, Sakolvaree Y, Chaicumpa W. Blinded, placebo-controlled trial of antiparasitic drugs for trichinosis myositis. *J Infect Dis* 2000;182:371–374.

129. Farah FS. Protozoan and helminth infections. In: Fitzpatrick TB, Eisen AZ, Wolff K, eds. *Dermatology in General Medicine*, 2nd edn. New York: McGraw-Hill, 1987;2483–2486.

130. Ribicich M, Krivokapich S, Pasqualetti M, Gonzalez Prous CL, Gatti GM, Falzoni E, Aronowicz T, Arbusti P, Fariña F, Rosa A. Experimental infection with Trichinella T12 in domestic cats. *Vet Parasitol* 2013;194:168–170.

131. Angoff GH, Czarnecki B, Wolinsky E. A case of chronic meningococcemia with unusual features. *Am J Med* 1975;269:243–246.

132. Eberhard ML, Mathison B, Bishop H, Handoo NQ, Hellstein JW. Zoonotic anatrichosomiasis in an Illinois resident. *Am J Trop Med Hyg* 2010;83:342–344.

133. Tunc SE, Ertam I, Pirildar T, Turk T, Ozturk M, Doganavsargil E. Nail changes in connective tissue diseases: Do nail changes provide clues for the diagnosis? *J Eur Acad Dermatol Venereol* 2007;21:497–503.

134. Rongioletti F, Cestari R, Cozzani E. Nodules rhumatoides bénins chez un adulte (évaluant depuis 16 années). *Nouv Dermatol* 1990;9:655–656.

135. Williams FM, Cohen PR, Arnett FC. Accelerated cutaneous nodulosis during methotrexate therapy in a patient with rheumatoid arthritis. *J Am Acad Dermatol* 1998;39:359–362.

136. Horn RT Jr, Goette DK. Perforating rheumatoid nodule. *Arch Dermatol.* 1982;118:696–697.

137. Alguacil-Garcia A. Necrobiotic palisading suture granulomas simulating rheumatoid nodule. *Am J Surg Pathol* 1993;17:920–923.

138. Keil H. The rheumatic subcutaneous nodules and simulating lesions. *Medicine (Baltimore)* 1938;17:261–380.

139. Moore CP, Wilkens RF. The subcutaneous nodule: Its significance in the diagnosis of rheumatic disease. *Sem Arthritis Rheum* 1977;7:63–79.

140. Zelger B, Cerio R, Soyer HP, Misch K, Orchard G, Wilson-Jones E. Reticulohistiocytoma and multicentric reticulohistiocytosis. Histopathologic and immunophenotypic distinct entities. *Am J Dermatopathol* 1994;16:577–584.

141. Page EH, Shear NH. Temperature-dependent skin disorders. *J Am Acad Dermatol* 1988;18:1003–1019.

142. Bywaters EGL. Peripheral vascular obstruction in rheumatoid arthritis and its relationship to other vascular lesions. *Ann Rheum Dis* 1957;16:84–103.

143. Bywaters EGL, Scott JT. The natural history of vascular lesions in rheumatoid arthritis. *J Chron Dis* 1963;16:905–914.

144. Scott JT, Hourihane DO, Doyle FH, Seiner RE, Laws JW, Dixon ASJ, Bywaters EGL. Digital arteritis in rheumatoid disease. *Ann Rheuma Dis* 1961;20:224–234.

145. Broussard RK, Baethge BA. Peripheral gangrene in polyarteritis nodosa. *Cutis* 1990;46:53–55.

146. Colt HG, Begg RJ, Saporito JJ, Cooper WM, Shapiro AP. Cholesterol embolization after cardiac catheterization: Eight cases and review of the literature. *Medicine (Baltimore)* 1988;67:389–400.

147. Khan AM, Jacobs S. Trash feet after coronary angiography. *Heart* 2003;89:e17.

148. O'Quinn SE, Kennedy BC, Baker DT. Peripheral vascular lesions in rheumatoid arthritis. *Arch Dermatol* 1965;92:489–494.

149. Watts RA, Carruthers DM, Scott DG. Isolated nail fold vasculitis in rheumatoid arthritis. *Ann Rheuma Dis* 1995;54:927–929.

150. Spigel GT, Krall RA, Hilal A. Limited Wegener's granulomatosis. Unusual cutaneous, radiographic, and pathologic manifestations. *Cutis* 1983;32:41–44, 46, 49–51.

151. Schattner A, Kozak N, Friedman J. Pulmonary nodules and splinter haemorrhages. *Postgrad Med J* 2001;77:785, 792–794.

152. Disdier P, Bolla G, Harle JR, Pache X, Weiller-Merli C, Marco MS, Figarella-Branger D, Weiller PJ. Nécroses digitales révélatrices d'un syndrome des antisynthétases. *Ann Dermatol Venereol* 1994;121:493–495.

153. Horwitz LJ, Dreizen S. Acral erythemas induced by chemotherapy and graft-versus-host disease in adults with hematogenous malignancies. *Cutis* 1990;46:397–404.

154. Sanli H, Ekmekçi P, Arat M, Gürman G. Clinical manifestations of cutaneous graft-versus-host disease after allogeneic haematopoietic cell transplantation: Long-term follow-up results in a single Turkish centre. *Acta Derm Venereol* 2004;84:296–301.

155. Liddle BJ, Cowan MA. Lichen planus-like eruption and nail changes in a patient with graft-versus-host disease. *Br J Dermatol* 1990;122:841–843.

156. Müller-Serten B, Vakilzadeh F. Chronische sklerodermiforme Graft-versus-Host Disease. *Hautarzt* 1994;45:772–775.

157. Brun P, Baran R, Desbas C, Czernielewski J. Dystrophie lichénienne isolée des 20 onlges. Etude en immunofluorescence par les anticorps monoclonaux. Conséquence pathologiques. *Ann Dermatol Vénéréol* 1985;112:215.

158. Kanitakis J, Jullien D, Nicolas JF, Frances C, Claud A, Revillard J-P, Owen E, Dubernard J-M. Sequential histological and immunohistochemical study of the skin of the first human hand allograft. *Transplantation* 2000;69:1380–1385.

159. Kanitakis J, Jullien D, Petruzzo P, Hakim N, Claudy A, Revillard JP, Owen E, Dubernard JM. Clinicopathologic features of graft rejection of the first human hand allograft. *Transplantation* 2003;76:688–693.

160. Landin L, Cavadas PC, Garcia-Cosmes P, Thione A, Vera-Sempere F. Perioperative ischemic injury and fibrotic degeneration of muscle in a forearm allograft: Functional follow-up at 32 months post transplantation. *Ann Plast Surg* 2011;66:202–209.

161. Thione A, Cavadas PC, Lorca-García C, Pérez-García A, Alfaro L. Late nail lesions rejection in a stable bilateral forearm allograft at 60 months post-transplantation. *Ann Plast Surg* 2014;73:612–614.

162. Schneeberger S, Gorantla VS, van Riet RP, Lanzetta M, Vereecken P, van Holder C, Rorive S et al. Atypical acute rejection after hand transplantation. *Am J Transplant* 2008;8:688–696.

163. Saray Y, Seckin D, Gulec AT, Akgun S, Haberal M. Nail disorders in hemodialysis patients and renal transplant recipient: A case-control study. *J Am Acad Dermatol* 2004;50:197–202.

164. Rault R. Mycophenolate-associated onycholysis. *Ann Intern Med* 2000;133:921–922.

165. Mahe E, Morelon E, Lechaton S, Kreis H, De Prost Y, Bodemer C. Sirolimus-induced onychopathy in renal transplant recipients. *Ann Dermatol Venereol* 2006;133:531–535.

166. Haneke E. Autoaggressive nail disorders. Trastornos de autoagresión hacia las uñas (Engl & Span). *Dermatol Rev Mex* 2013;57:225–234.

167. Redd SC, Kazembe PN, Luby SP, Nwanyanwu O, Hightower AW, Ziba C, Wirima JJ, Chitsulo L, Franco C, Olivar M. Clinical algorithm for treatment of Plasmodium falciparum malaria in children. *Lancet* 1996;347(8996):223–227.

168. Jansen T, Plewig G, Anhalt GJ. Paraneoplastic pemphigus with clinical features of erosive lichen planus associated with Castleman's tumor. *Dermatology* 1995;190:245–250.

169. Liang JJ, Cordes SF, Witzig TE. More than skin deep. *Cleve Clin J Med* 2015;80:632–633.

170. Bonafé JL, Pieraggi MT, Abravanel M, Benque A, Abravanel G. Skin, hair and nail changes in a case of citrullinemia with late manifestation. *Dermatologica* 1984;168:213–218.

171. Boeckler P, Grange F, Krzisch S, Grosshans E, Guillaume JC. Acral purpura and hyperhomocysteinemia. *Ann Dermatol Venereol* 2003;130:542–545.

172. O'Duffy JD, Hunder GG, Kelly PJ. Decreasing prevalence of tophaceous gout. *DMayo Clin Proc* 1975;20:227–228.

173. López Redondo MJ, Requena L, Macía M, Schoendorff C, Sánchez Yus E, Robledo A. Fingertip tophi without gouty arthritis. *Dermatology* 1993;187:140–143.

174. King DE, King LA. The appropriate processing of tophi for microscopy. *Am J Dermatopathol* 1982;4:239.

175. Weaver J, Somani N, Bauer TW, Piliang M. Simple non-staining method to demonstrate urate crystals in formalin-fixed, paraffin-embedded skin biopsies. *J Cutan Pathol* 2009;36:560–564.

176. Tirado-González M, González-Serva A. The nail plate biopsy may pick up gout crystals and other crystals. *Am J Dermatopathol* 2011;33:351–353.

177. Spiers EM, Sanders DY, Omura EF. Clinical and histologic features of primary oxalosis. *J Am Acad Dermatol* 1990;22:952–956.

178. Sina B, Lutz LL. Cutaneous oxalate granuloma. *J Am Acad Dermatol* 1990;22:316–317.

179. Gregoriou S, Kalapothakou K, Kontochristopoulos G, Belyayeva H, Chatziolou E, Rigopoulos D. Subungual oxalate deposits in a patient with secondary hyperoxaluria. *Acta Derm Venereol* 2011;91:195–196.

180. ter Borg EJ. Clinical image: Bluish discoloration of the nails in ochronosis. *Arthritis Rheum* 1998;41:1895.

181. Murgić L, Grubišić F, Jajić Z. Unrecognized ochronosis—A case report. *Acta Clin Croat* 2008;47: 105–109.

182. Laymon CW. Ochronosis. *Arch Dermatol* 1953;67: 553–560.

183. Gordon G, Sparano BM, Iatropoulos MJ. Hyperpigmentation of the skin associated with minocycline therapy. *Arch Dermatol* 1985;121:618–623.

184. Ban M, Kitajima Y. Nail discoloration occurring after 8 weeks of minocycline therapy. *J Dermatol* 2007;34:699–701.

185. Tavares J, Leung WW. Discoloration of nail beds and skin from minocycline. *Can Med Ass J* 2011;183:224.

186. Dereure O. Drug-induced skin pigmentation epidemiology, diagnosis and treatment. *Am J Clin Dermatol* 2001;2:253–262.

187. Melikoglu MA, Melikoglu M, Gurbuz U, Budak BS, Kacar C. Hydroxychloroquine-induced hyperpigmentation: A case report. *J Clin Pharm Ther* 2008;33:699–701.

188. Kalabalikis D, Patsatsi A, Trakatelli MG, Pitsari P, Efstratiou I, Sotiriadis D. Hyperpigmented forearms and nail: Hydroxychloroquine-induced skin and nail pigmentation. *Acta Derm Venereol* 2010;90:657–659.

189. Sifuentes Giraldo WA, Grandal Platero M, de la Puente Bujidos C, Gámir Gámir ML. Generalized skin hyperpigmentation and longitudinal melanonychia secondary to treatment with hydroxychloroquine in systemic lupus erythematosus. *Reumatol Clin* 2013;9:381–382.

190. Garin Shkolnik T, Feuerman H, Didkovsky E, Kaplan I, Bergman R, Pavlovsky L, Hodak E. Blue-gray mucocutaneous discoloration: A new adverse effect of ezogabine. *JAMA Dermatol* 2014;150:984–989.

191. Elder GH. Recent advances in the identification of enzyme deficiencies in the porphyrias. *Br J Dermatol* 1983;108:729.

192. Haneke E, Schwartze G. Gleichzeitiges Vorkommen von Porphyria cutanea tarda und Erythematodes chronicus. *Dermatol Mschr* 1971;157:168–174.

193. Schwartze G, Haneke E. Über Beziehungen zwischen Porphyrinausscheidung und Harnvolumen. *Z ges Inn Med* 1972;27:518–523.

194. Aarsand AK, Villanger JH, Støle E, Deybach JC, Marsden J, To-Figueras J, Badminton M, Elder GH, Sandberg S. European specialist porphyria laboratories: Diagnostic strategies, analytical quality, clinical interpretation, and reporting as assessed by an external quality assurance program. *Clin Chem* 2011;57:1514–1523.

195. Röcken C, Shakespeare A. Pathology diagnosis and pathogenesis of AA amyloidosis. *Virchows Arch* 2002;440:111–122.

196. Fernandez-Flores A, Castañón-González JA, Guerrero-Ramos B, Castro-Gaytan A, Saeb-Lima M. Systemic amyloidosis presenting with glans penis involvement. *J Cutan Pathol* 2014;41:791–796.

197. Étienne M, Denizon N, Maillard H. Anomalies unguéales revélant une amylose systémique AL. *Rév Méd Interne* 2015;36:356–358.

198. Tausend W, Neill M, Kelly B. Primary amyloidosis-induced nail dystrophy. *Dermatol Online J* 2014;20(1):21247.

199. Renker T, Borradori L, Röcken C, Haneke E. Systemic AL amyloidosis revealed by progressive nail involvement, diffuse alopecia and sicca syndrome. Report of an unusual case with review of the literature. *Dermatology* 2014;228:97–102.

200. Pink AE, Stefanato CM, Breathnach SM. An unusual presentation of systemic AL amyloidosis: Bullae, milia and nail dystrophy. *Clin Exp Dermatol* 2012;37:788–790.

201. Schönland SO, Hegenbart U, Bochtler T, Mangatter A, Hansberg M, Ho AD, Lohse P, Röcken C. Immunohistochemistry in the classification of systemic forms of amyloidosis: A systematic investigation of 117 patients. *Blood* 2012;119:488–493.

202. Salas-Alanis JC, Martinez-Jaramillo B, Gomez-Flores M, Ocampo-Candiani J. Scleromyxedema, a therapeutic dilemma. *Indian J Dermatol* 2015;60:215.

203. Bogner RR, Wetter DA, Dingli D. Scleromyxedema. *Intern Med* 2014;53:2561–2562.

204. Rongioletti F, Rebora A. Updated classification of papular mucinosis, lichen myxedematosus, and scleromyxedema. *J Am Acad Dermatol* 2001;44:273–281.

205. Rongioletti F, Merlo G, Cinotti E, Fausti V, Cozzani E, Cribier B, Metze D et al. Scleromyxedema: A multicenter study of characteristics, comorbidities, course, and therapy in 30 patients. *J Am Acad Dermatol* 2013;69:66–72.

206. Krause W. Hauterscheinungen bei Erkrankungen endokriner Organe. Der weitreichende Einfluss der Hormone. *Hautnah* 2015;31(3):40–45.

207. Allam M, Ghozzi M. Scleromyxedema: A case report and review of the literature. *Case Rep Dermatol* 2013;5:168–175.

208. Bereston ES. Diseases of the nails. *Clin Med* 1950;238–240.

209. Koopman RJJ, Happle R. Cutaneous manifestations of methylmalonic acidemia. *Arch Dermatol Res* 1990;282:272–273.

210. Niiyama S, Koelker S, Degen I, Hoffmann GF, Happle R, Hoffmann R. Acrodermatitis acidemica secondary to malnutrition in glutaric aciduria type I. *Eur J Dermatol* 2001;11:244–246.

211. Niiyama S, Okiyama R, Nagahashi K, Kaneko S, Aiba S, Mukai H. Acrodermatitis acidemica with an eating disorder. *Eur J Dermatol* 2006;16:318–319.

212. Crain LS, Fitzmaurice NE, Mondry C. Nail dysplasia and fetal alcohol syndrome. Case report of a heteropaternal sibship. *Am J Dis Child* 1983;137: 1069–1072.

213. Grossman M, Scher RK. Leuconychia: Review and classification. *Int J Dermatol* 1990;29:535–541.

214. Beck C, Krafchik B, Traubici J, Jacobson S. Mercury intoxication: It still exists. *Ped Dermatol* 2004;21:254–259.

215. Weaver TD, Jespersen DL. Multiple onychocryptosis following treatment of onychomycosis with oral terbinafine. *Cutis* 2000;66:211–212.

216. Bonifaz A, Paredes V, Fierro L. Onychocryptosis as consequence of effective treatment of dermatophytic onychomycosis. *J Eur Acad Dermatol Venereol* 2007;21:699–700.

217. Armstrong K, Weinstein M. Pyogenic granulomas during isotretinoin therapy. *J Dermatol Case Rep* 2011;5:5–7.

218. Piraccini BM, Venturi M, Patrizi A. Periungual pyogenic granulomas due to topical tazarotene for nail psoriasis. *G Ital Dermatol Venereol* 2014;149:363–366.

219. Bouscarat F, Bouchard C, Bouhour D. Paronychia and pyogenic granuloma of the great toes in patients treated with indinavir. *N Engl J Med* 1998;338:1776–1777.

220. Williams LH, Fleckman P. Painless periungual pyogenic granulomata associated with reverse transcriptase inhibitor therapy in a patient with human immunodeficiency virus infection. *Br J Dermatol* 2007;156:163–164.

221. Wollina U. Multiple eruptive periungual pyogenic granulomas during anti-CD20 monoclonal antibody therapy for rheumatoid arthritis. *J Dermatol Case Rep* 2010;4:44–46.

222. Patruno C1, Balato N, Cirillo T, Napolitano M, Ayala F. Periungual and subungual pyogenic granuloma following anti-TNF-α therapy: Is it the first case? *Dermatol Ther* 2013;26:493–495.

223. Nam Choi J. Chemotherapy-induced iatrogenic injury of skin: New drugs and new concepts. *Clin Dermatol* 2011;29:587–601.

224. High WA. Gefitinib: A cause of pyogenic granulomalike lesions of the nail. *Arch Dermatol* 2006;142:939.

225. Dika E, Barisani A, Vaccari S, Fanti PA, Ismaili A, Patrizi A. Periungual pyogenic granuloma following imatinib therapy in a patient with chronic myelogenous leukemia. *J Drugs Dermatol* 2013;12:512–513.

226. Robert C, Sibaud V, Mateus C, Verschoore M, Charles C, Lanoy E, Baran R. Nail toxicities induced by systemic anticancer treatments. *Lancet Oncol* 2015;16:e181–e189.

227. Devillers C, Vanhooteghem O, Henrijean A, Ramaut M, de la Brassinne M. Subungueal pyogenic granuloma secondary to docetaxel therapy. *Clin Exp Dermatol* 2009;34:251–252.

228. Paul LJ, Cohen PR. Paclitaxel-associated subungual pyogenic granuloma: Report in a patient with breast cancer receiving paclitaxel and review of drug-induced pyogenic granulomas adjacent to and beneath the nail. *J Drugs Dermatol* 2012;11:262–268.

229. Ranawaka RR. Patterns of chromonychia during chemotherapy in patients with skin type V and outcome after 1 year of follow-up. *Clin Exp Dermatol* 2009;34:e920–e926.

230. Dasanu CA, Wiernik PH, Vaillant J, Alexandrescu DT. A complex pattern of melanonychia and onycholysis after treatment with pemetrexed for lung cancer. *Skinmed* 2007;6:95–96.

231. Borecky DJ, Stephenson JJ, Keeling JH, Vukelja SJ. Idarubicin-induced pigmentary changes of the nails. *Cutis* 1997;59:203–204.

232. Pirard C, Michaux JL, Bourlond A. Longitudinal melanonychia and hydroxyurea. *Ann Dermatol Venereol* 1994;121:106–109.

233. Issaivanan M, Mitu PS, Manisha C, Praveen K. Cutaneous manifestations of hydroxyurea therapy in childhood: Case report and review. *Pediatr Dermatol* 2004;21:124–127.

234. De Anda MC, Dominguez JG. Melanonychia induced by topical tretment of periungual warts with 5-fluorouracil. *Dermatol Online J* 2013;19(3):10.

235. Kore SD, Kanwar AJ, Vinay K, Wanchu A. Pattern of mucocutaneous manifestations in human immunodeficiency virus-positive patients in North India. *Indian J Sex Transm Dis* 2013;34:19–24.

236. Tsilika K, Tran A, Trucchi R, Pop S, Anty R, Cardot-Leccia N, Lacour JP, Ortonne JP, Passeron T. Secondary hyperpigmentation during interferon alfa treatment for chronic hepatitis C virus infection. *JAMA Dermatol* 2013;149:675–677.

237. Bories A, Denis P. Lichenoid nail dystrophy induced by angiotensin 2 receptor antagonists. *Ann Dermatol Venereol* 2005;132:265–267.

238. Saito M, Nakamura K, Kaneko F. Lichenoid drug eruption of nails induced by propylthiouracil. *J Dermatol* 2007;34:696–698.

239. Reinsberger C, Meuth SG, Wiendl H. Dose-dependent melanonychia by mitoxantrone. *Mult Scler* 2009;15:1131–1132.

240. Musumeci ML, Lacarrubba F, Micali G. Onset of lichen planus during treatment with etanercept. *Am J Clin Dermatol* 2010;11(Suppl 1):55–56.

241. Wahiduzzaman M, Pubalan M. Oral and cutaneous lichenoid reaction with nail changes secondary to imatinib: Report of a case and literature review. *Dermatol Online J* 2008;14(12):14.

242. Zhang JA, Yu JB, Li XH, Zhao L. Oral and cutaneous lichenoid eruption with nail changes due to imatinib treatment in a Chinese patient with chronic myeloid leukemia. *Ann Dermatol* 2015;27:228–229.

243. Baran R, Juhlin L. Photoonycholysis. *Photodermatol Photoimmunol Photomed* 2002;18:202–207.

244. Green JJ, Manders SM. Pseudoporphyria. *J Am Acad Dermatol* 2001;44:100–104.

245. Baran R, Jeanmougin M, Cesarini JP. Spontaneous photoonycholysis in a West Indian with type V skin. *Acta Derma Venereol* 1997;77:169–170.

246. Segal BM. Photosensitivity, nail discoloration and onycholysis. Side effects of tetracycline therapy. *Arch Int Med* 1963;112:165–167.

247. Arzt L, Zieler K, eds. *Die Haut- und Geschlechtskrankheiten. Eine zusammenfassende Darstellung für die Praxis.* Berlin Wien: Urban & Schwarzenberg, 1935; Vol II:110–114.

248. Siemund J, Stolp A. Argyrose. *Z Hautkr* 1968;43:71.

249. Harker JM, Hunter D. Occupational argyria. *Br J Dermatol Syph* 1935;47:441.

250. Bearn AG, McKusick VA. Azure lunulae; an unusual change in the fingernails in two patients with hepatolenticular degeneration (Wilson's disease). *J Am Med Ass* 1958;166:904–906.

251. Weyhbrecht H. Allgemeine Argyrose bei gleichzeitiger Hepatopathie (Trichloräthylen-Intoxikation?) und die Beziehung der beiden Krankheitszustände zueinander. *Dermatol Wschr* 1953;127:494.

252. Koplon BS. Azure lunulae due to argyria. *Arch Dermatol* 1966;94:333–334.

253. Whelton MJ, Pope FM. Azure lunulae in argyria. Corneal changes resembling Kayser-Fleischer Rings. *Arch Intern Med* 1968;121:267–269.

254. Zaias N, Baden HP. Disorders of nails. In: Fitzpatrick TB, ed. *Dermatology in General Mediciney.* New York: McGrw-Hill, 1971; 331–353.

255. Samman PD. *The Nails in Disease*, 2nd edn. London: Heinemann Med Books, 1972; 91–92.

256. Korting GW, Denk R. *Dermatologische Differentialdiagnose.* Stuttgart New York: FK Schattauer, 1974; 375–376.

257. Pardo-Peret P, Sans-Sabrafen J, Boleda Relats M. Argyriasis. Report of a case. *Med Clin (Barc)* 1979;73:386–388.

258. Gulbranson SH, Hud JA, Hansen RC. Argyria following the use of dietary supplements containing colloidal silver protein. *Cutis* 2000;66:373–374.

259. Sue YM, Lee JY, Wang MC, Lin TK, Sung JM, Huang JJ. Generalized argyria in two chronic hemodialysis patients. *Am J Kidney Dis* 2001;37:1048–1051.

260. McKenna JK, Hull CM, Zone JJ. Argyria associated with colloidal silver supplementation. *Int J Dermatol* 2003;42:549.

261. Tran HA, Song S. Silver toxicity masquerading as hypocaeruloplasminaemia. *Pathology* 2007;39:456–458.

262. Kalouche H, Watson A, Routley D. Blue lunulae: Argyria and hypercopprecaemia. *Australas J Dermatol* 2007;48:182–184.

263. Kim Y, Suh HS, Cha HJ, Kim SH, Jeong KS, Kim DH. A case of generalized argyria after ingestion of colloidal silver solution. *Am J Ind Med* 2009;52:246–250.

264. Butzmann CM, Technau-Hafsi K, Bross F. "Silver man" argyria of the skin after ingestion of a colloidal silver solution. *J Dtsch Dermatol Ges* 2015;13:1030–1032.

265. Sakai N, Aoki M, Miyazawa S, Akita M, Takezaki S, Kawana S. A case of generalized argyria caused by the use of silver protein as a disinfection medicine. *Acta Derm Venereol* 2007;8:186–187.

266. Plewig G, Lincke H, Wolff HH. Silver-blue nails. *Acta Derm Venereol* 1977;57:413–419.

267. Rice EW, Goldstein NP. Copper content of hair and nails in Wilson's disease (hepatolenticular degeneration). *Metabolism* 1961;10:1085–1087.

268. Martin GM. Copper content of hair and nails of normal invididuals and of patients with hepatolenticular degeneration. *Nature* 1964 30;202:903–904.

269. Seyhan M, Erdem T, Selimoğlu MA, Ertekin V. Dermatological signs in Wilson's disease. *Pediatr Int* 2009;51:395–398.

270. Altmeyer P, Hufnagl D. Chrysiasis. Nebenwirkungen einer intramusckulären Goldtherapie. *Hautarzt* 1975;26:330–333.

271. Fam AG, Paton TW. Nail pigmentation after parenteral gold therapy for rheumatoid arthritis: "gold nails." *Arthritis Rheum* 1984;27:119–120.

272. Roest MA, Ratnavel R. Yellow nails associated with gold therapy for rheumatoid arthritis. *Br J Dermatol* 2001;145:855–856.

273. Butterworth T, Strean LP. Mercurial pigmentation of nails. *Arch Dermatol* 1963;88:55–57.

274. Böckers M, Wagner R, Oster O. Nageldyschromie als Leitsymptom einer chronischen Quecksilberintoxikation durch ein kosmetisches Bleichmittel. *Z Hautkr* 1985;60:821–829.

275. Friederich H-C, Nikolowski W. Endogene Ochronose. *Arch Derm Syph (Berlin)* 1951;192:273.

276. Barr JF. Subungual pigmentation following prolonged atabrine therapy. *US Nav Med Bull* 1944;43:929.

277. Dodd J, Sarkany I. Chronic discoid lupus erythematosus with mepacrine pigmentation bands in the nails. *Br J Dermatol* 1980;119(Suppl 33):74–75.

278. Young E. Melanosis caused by Camoquin. *Dermatologica* 1958;116:389–395.

279. Kleinegger CL, Hammond HL, Finkelstein MW. Oral mucosal hyperpigmentation secondary to antimalarial drug therapy. *Oral Surg Oral Med Oral Pathol Oral Radiol Endod* 2000;90:189–194.

280. Daniel CR 3rd, Scher RK. Nail changes caused by systemic drugs or ingestants. *Dermatol Clin* 1985;3:491–500.

Genodermatoses affecting the nail 6

The number of skin diseases with a genetic background and exhibiting nail alterations is vast. They comprise chromosomal abnormalities and conditions defined by mutations of a single gene that may lead to structural or metabolic alterations, but many genetic nail conditions are not yet defined on a molecular basis. Nail aplasia, hypoplasia, hyperplasia, or even dystrophies developing later in life are quite common. With the exception of very few genodermatoses, there are no reports on the specific histopathology of their nail alterations. One may assume that the more than 200 genetically defined nail dystrophies may show a hypoplastic nail matrix and/or nail bed, but this has yet to be proven. Even in autopsy cases, no nail histopathology was done.[1]

Some recently described genodermatoses exhibit considerable hyperkeratoses of the periungual skin and although this region has not been specifically biopsied it is expected that they show the same histopathologic changes like the body skin.

A workable (rational) classification of the many genodermatoses potentially affecting the nail unit is difficult and always arbitrary.

1. Ichthyoses (Mendelian disorders of cornification)
2. Palmar and plantar keratoses
3. Pachyonychia congenita
4. Porokeratoses
5. Acantholytic disorders
6. Acrokeratosis verruciformis of Hopf
7. Dyskeratosis congenita
8. Rothmund–Thomson syndrome
9. Ectodermal dysplasias
10. The group of epidermolysis bullosa (skin fragility disorders)
11. Incontinentia pigmenti
12. Pachydermoperiostosis
13. Focal dermal hypoplasia
14. The group of aplasia cutis congenita
15. Ehlers–Danlos syndrome
16. Tuberous sclerosis complex (see Chapter 9)
17. Bloom's syndrome
18. Ataxia-telangiectasia (Louis–Bar syndrome)
19. Xeroderma pigmentosum
20. Werner syndrome
21. FOXN1 deficiency

6.1 ICHTHYOSES

Ichthyoses, now also called Mendelian disorders of cornification (MeDOC), are defined by visible scaling and/or hyperkeratosis of the skin.[2,3] Most are hereditary, either autosomal dominant, X-linked, or autosomal recessive. Many mutations in various different genes important for keratinocyte differentiation and epidermal barrier function are known. The current classification of this large heterogeneous group of skin disorders is still clinically based and poses a particular diagnostic challenge to all physicians facing a patient with scaling skin. Nail changes are not often described. Loss-of-function mutations in the filaggrin gene are the basis for autosomal dominant ichthyosis vulgaris (ADIV, OMIM 146700), which is histologically and electron microscopically seen as an almost absent granular layer with hypoplastic keratohyalin granules.[4] Trachyonychia was reported in one case of ADIV.[5] Thick striated nails were observed in lamellar ichthyosis (OMIM 146750).[6,7] Epidermolytic ichthyosis of Brocq (OMIM 113800) is due to mutations in the keratin genes 1 or 10.[8] Subungual hyperkeratosis is observed in keratitis-ichthyosis-deafness (KID, OMIM 148210) syndrome (missense mutations in the GJB2 (gap junction β-2) gene encoding for connexin26 protein, which clusters at chromosome 13q12).[9] Thick overcurved nails were seen in ichthyosis hystrix, which is characterized by a heterozygous mutation in exon 9 of keratin 1 (OMIM 146590)[10] and in another hystrix-like ichthyosis with nail and joint involvement.[11] Pachyonychia occurred in the follicular ichthyosis–atrichia–photophobia syndrome (IFAP) (OMIM 308205).[12] However, in most forms of ichthyoses, the nails appear normal although nail clippings permit steroid sulfatase activity to be determined for the diagnosis of X-linked recessive ichthyosis (OMIM 308100).[13]

CHILD syndrome is characterized by congenital hemidysplasia with ichthyosiform nevus and limb defects (OMIM 308050).[14,15] It is a rare but striking dermatosis. This X-linked dominant, male-lethal multisystem MeDOC is due to a mutation of NSDHL (NAD(P)H steroid dehydrogenase-like protein) at chromosome Xq28, which is involved in the distal cholesterol biosynthesis pathway.[16] The clinical expression varies from mild localized lesions to extreme cases with severe limb, organ, and central nervous system defects.[17] Nail involvement is not exceptional and may present as paronychia, periungual hyperkeratosis, and nail dystrophy; hypophalangism may occur.[18] The treatment of choice is a combination of topical statin and cholesterol.[19–21]

6.1.1 Histopathology

The nail in trachyonychia is wavy with innumerable small impressions on its surface. Polarization microscopy makes the wavy aspect even more obvious. The epidermis in ADIV exhibits a very thin or absent granular layer with very small crumbly keratohyalin granules.[22] Filaggrin is markedly reduced or almost absent.[23]

X-linked ichthyosis is characterized by an orthohyperkeratosis and a well-preserved granular layer, which may even be thickened. Electron microscopy reveals persistent corneodesmosomes as evidence of a retention hyperkeratosis.

(a)   (b)

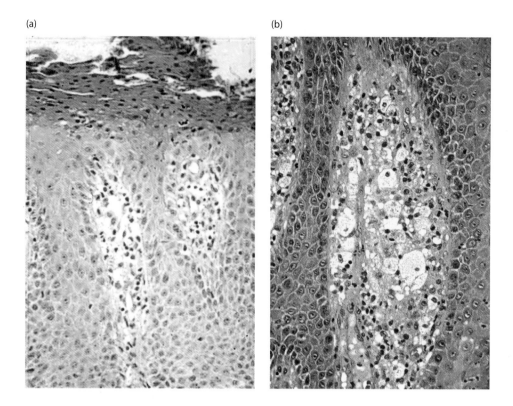

Figure 6.1 (a,b) Verruciform xanthoma in the proximal nail fold of a girl with CHILD nevus. (Courtesy of Prof. Dr. R. Happle, Freiburg, Germany.)

The skin around the nails in lamellar autosomal recessive congenital ichthyosis is slightly acanthotic with a thick homogeneously eosinophilic orthokeratotic stratum corneum and an unremarkable granular layer. There is no inflammatory infiltrate in the dermis. The cornified envelope in transglutaminase 1-negative lamellar ichthyosis is defective after detergent extraction as seen by light and electron microscopy.[24] Ultrasonography of the nails shows a thickened compact nail without the so-called interplate space, a hypoechoic zone between the dorsal and ventral layers of the nail plate.[25]

Epidermolytic hyperkeratosis is the hallmark of epidermolytic ichthyosis of Brocq, which is a keratinopathic ichthyosis.[26] The entire skin is involved although the nails are usually normal. Histologically, the epidermis shows conspicuous alterations starting with clumping of the tonofibrils in the suprabasal layer that becomes more and more obvious toward the granular layer. This results in eosinophilic granules in the keratinocyte cytoplasm of the suprabasal and spinous cells. In the stratum granulosum, they appear basophilic as the keratohyalin spreads along the tonofibrils that are clumped to granules in this condition (hence the historical term of granular degeneration, which has nothing to do with the granular layer).

Multiple binucleate cells are seen in ichthyosis hystrix.[27] Immunostaining reveals decreased intensity but normal distribution of keratin 1 and abnormal distribution of loricrin with frequent clumping at the bottom of the papillae.[28]

Histopathology of CHILD syndrome is diagnostic when the skin lesion shows features of verruciform xanthoma: The connective tissue papillae are filled with foam cells (Figure 6.1). In other cases, the histopathological changes may mimic those of psoriasis. The epidermis is acanthotic and shows alternating areas of orthohyperkeratosis and parakeratosis and is slightly papillomatous. There is exocytosis of neutrophils, and the stratum corneum may even contain accumulations similar to microabscesses of Munro.[29] Nail dystrophy is secondary to disturbed keratinization of the involved nail matrix and bed structures.

6.1.2 Differential diagnosis

The histologic changes do not allow the various ichthyoses to be differentiated by their nail changes. Verruciform xanthoma is identical with the skin lesions of CHILD syndrome.

6.2 PALMAR AND PLANTAR KERATOSES

The classification of palmar and plantar keratoses (PPK) is still mostly clinical. Non-syndromic and syndromic types are differentiated, diffuse from localized and non-transgredient from transgredient forms. The most common types are the epidermolytic PPK of Vörner and Thost (OMIM 144200), often with stubby nails and many hangnails, and non-epidermolytic PPK of Unna. More rarely occurring types are PPK of Buschke–Brauer–Fischer (OMIM 148600) as well as the recessive PKKs of the transgredient Meleda type (OMIM 248300) and the

Papillon-Lefèvre syndrome (OMIM 245000),[30] which is virtually identical to the Haim–Munk syndrome (OMIM 245010) that has nail changes in addition.[31]

6.2.1 Histopathology

The histopathology of the nails in epidermolytic PPK has only once been described.[32] An own case, a 50-year-old woman, presented with markedly thickened, dull, opaque nails, some of which exhibited a huge subungual hyperkeratosis giving the aspect of pachyonychia congenita that disturbed and embarrassed her in her profession and social life. The nail thickening had started roughly 5 years prior to consultation. A lateral longitudinal nail biopsy revealed involvement of all epithelial structures of the nail unit though to a variable degree (Figure 6.2). The matrix was slightly papillomatous whereas the nail bed demonstrated a very pronounced papillomatosis. The basal and immediate suprabasal cell rows of the matrix epithelium were normal. There was mild keratin clumping in the cells of the prekeratogenous zone that became more obvious in the keratogenous zone where the cells also appeared to be lighter. These cells abruptly turned into nail plate cells. The nail bed changes were very pronounced. Keratin filament clumping started in the suprabasal cells as evidenced by small eosinophilic granules and eosinophilic perinuclear shells. Both these granules as well as the keratinocytes continuously enlarged in the upper spinous layers with the cells exhibiting a vacuolated appearance. Keratohyalin granules were observed in the uppermost layers and were of different size and perfectly round shape. Thus, the changes are different from the palmoplantar skin although the characteristic pattern of this type of keratosis is retained. A compact eosinophilic hyperkeratosis developed in the nail bed. Serum and lymphocyte inclusions

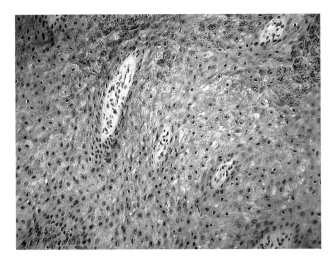

Figure 6.2 Epidermolytic keratosis palmaris et plantaris with classical changes in the nail bed: The suprabasal keratinocytes show clumps of eosinophilic keratin filaments, which is more and more pronounced to the upper spinous layer. There is no cell membrane rupture. Perfectly round keratohyaline granules are seen in some areas of the uppermost spinous layer.

were seen above the tips of the papillae of the hyperplastic nail bed. A band-like lymphocytic infiltrate was present under the matrix and proximal nail bed. The epidermis of the proximal nail fold was acanthotic and thickened with pronounced alterations identical to those of epidermolytic PPK. The nail plate appeared compact. In PAS stained sections, fungal hyphae were seen prompting the assumption that the fungal infection may have triggered the nail changes as is known from Köbner's phenomenon.

Electron microscopy shows marked tonofibril aggregation causing clumps and perinuclear shells leading to loss of the orderly cytoskeleton with disturbance of the tonofibril-desmosome association rendering the cells susceptible to cell membrane rupture.[33]

6.2.2 Differential diagnosis

Epidermolytic hyperkeratosis in small foci is an occasional accidental finding in many biopsies and apparently without pathologic relevance. Further, it is the hallmark of solitary and disseminated epidermolytic acanthoma, epidermolytic epidermal nevus, and bullous ichthyosiform erythroderma, the former being a mosaic form of the latter.[34] Ichthyosis hystrix may look similar at the first glance.

6.3 PACHYONYCHIA CONGENITA

Pachyonychia congenita (PC) is a group of rare autosomal dominant keratin disorders. Historically divided into type I of Jadassohn-Lewandowski[35] (OMIM 167200) and type II of Jackson-Lawler[36] (OMIM 167210) and two more debated types, these disorders are now molecular genetically defined by the International Pachyonychia Congenita Consortium. It was shown that the clinical classification is unreliable and imprecise and often does not correspond to the molecular typing.[37] Mutations in five keratin genes are known to cause PC: *KRT6A*, *KRT6B*, *KRT6C*, *KRT16*, and *KRT17*. The nomenclature has now been changed to PC-K6a, PC-K6b, PC-K6c, PC-K16, and PC-K17, with *KRT6C* mutations exhibiting little nail involvement but painful focal palmoplantar hyperkeratoses. The latter are the most pertinent signs of PC often in combination with blistering followed by the characteristic nail changes of huge subungual hyperkeratosis being covered by a horseshoe-like nail plate, less pronounced palmar hyperkeratoses again mainly on mechanically exposed areas, and white oral mucosal lesions without a tendency to undergo malignant degeneration. Further signs are multiple vellus hair cysts and/or steatocystomas, follicular keratoses, natal teeth, most of them reflecting the keratins present in these cutaneous structures, as well as hoarseness and hair changes.[38,39] However, there is a great variability of signs among pachyonychia congenita patients and the classical subtypes may overlap phenotypically.[40] Mutation analysis is therefore requested to determine the type of pachyonychia congenita.[41] So-called mixed types[42] have to be defined by gene analysis.

Pachyonychia congenita type 1 is defined by mutations in the genes for keratin 6a/16, and type 2 displays keratin 6b/17 mutations. Although keratin 6a/16 mutations cause type 1 PC, the clinical phenotype appears to be more severe in subjects with a keratin 6a mutation as compared to those with a keratin 16 mutation.[43] Double homozygous negative mutation of keratin 17 leads to a particularly severe phenotype of pachyonychia congenita with alopecia.[44,45]

The nail lesions are the most consistent signs, but exhibit great variations in lesion character and severity.[35] Usually, all 20 nails are involved. They are hard, thickened, and discolored. Many patients are already born with these unsightly nails, but birth with complete anonychia was also observed.[46] However, close inspection reveals that in most cases there is a tremendous subungual hyperkeratosis progressively elevating the nail in distal direction. In typical cases, the nail plate looks like a horse-shoe filled with keratin. Some nails taper off distally before they reach the tip of the digit. These nail changes can severely interfere with manual dexterity. Trauma or infection easily leads to nail loss. Treatment has been surgical in the past,[47] but recently rapamycin,[48] statins,[49] and mutant-specific small interfering (si) RNAs for pachyonychia congenita mutations have been developed and proven to have unprecedented specificity and potency.[50–52]

6.3.1 Histopathology

There are surprisingly few histologic examinations of the nails in pachyonychia congenita. Most histopathologic studies including immunohistochemistry of different keratins comprise the palmo-plantar hyperkeratoses,[53,54] which probably, but not necessarily, are similar to what one might expect to see in the nail bed.

Independent from the type, there is prominent hyperkeratosis with admixed parakeratosis surmounting an acanthotically thickened epithelium. Keratins 6a/16 are physiologically expressed in the nail bed, but not in the matrix explaining why the nail plate itself is relatively mildly altered. Keratins 6b/17 are also expressed in the matrix, but apparently to a degree that their mutation does not markedly alter the nail plate. A biopsy of the proximal nail fold, matrix, and proximal portion of the nail bed showed normal histologic structures. One report described an absent granular layer in the nail bed like in the normal nail.[55] However, in another case, there was hyperkeratosis, a granular layer, irregular acanthosis, and papillomatosis in the distal nail bed. Focal areas of dyskeratosis with ovoid eosinophilic bodies were seen within the hyperkeratosis. The keratohyalin granules varied markedly in size and there were focal areas of keratinocyte vacuolization.[56] This may also be an explanation why nail bed ablation in some cases improved the condition, whereas in others complete nail ablation was necessary.[54,57]

6.3.2 Differential diagnosis

Virtually all conditions causing subungual hyperkeratosis have to be considered. Special stains will exclude nail bed mycosis although it has not been investigated whether fungi may colonize or infect the nails in pachyonychia congenita. Massively hyperkeratotic nail bed psoriasis may clinically mimic pachyonychia congenita; however, the microabscesses and columnar parakeratosis so typical for psoriasis are not seen in pachyonychia congenita. Subungual warts do not affect virtually all nails, and the tiers of parakeratotic nuclei over the tips of the papillae are not seen in pachyonychia congenita. A family with two members affected by hystrix-like keratosis exhibiting a cornoid lamella, plantar hyperkeratosis, and considerable nail thickening was described; however, no nail histopathology was performed.[11] Hyperplastic subungual Bowen's disease affects only one nail and shows marked cellular atypia.

6.4 POROKERATOSES

Porokeratoses comprise a group of clinically different skin conditions that are all defined by the presence of a so-called cornoid lamella. Most are autosomal dominant although sporadic cases and an actinically caused disseminated superficial actinic porokeratosis (DSAP) are also seen. Except for the punctate porokeratosis, they are characterized by a unique keratotic rim representing the cornoid lamella.

Porokeratosis of Mibelli (OMIM 175800) is defined by one or a few plaques of up to several centimeters in diameter with a slightly atrophic, but keratotic center and a peripheral ridge of keratin material. It grows by peripheral extension and may involve the nail that first exhibits a segmental dystrophy potentially as a type 2 segmental manifestation, ridging and fissuring until the entire nail is involved and becomes severely dystrophic.[58,59]

Linear porokeratosis is aligned along the Blaschko lines and often involves the tips of the digits leading to nail dystrophy;[60] however, this is no longer accepted as an entity but thought to be a "superimposed linear manifestation."[34] Bone involvement was observed.[61] As in the Mibelli variant, it may be seen as longitudinal ridging and pterygium.[62] Topical all-*trans* retinoic acid was highly effective in one case.[63]

Porokeratosis palmaris, plantaris et disseminata (OMIM 175850) starts with papular lesions on the palms and soles in adolescence that may later extend on other body areas.[64]

The type 2 segmental manifestations in the form of superimposed linear porokeratoses have a higher risk to develop basal cell carcinoma, Bowen's disease, and squamous cell carcinoma in their lesions.[65]

6.4.1 Histopathology

The biopsy for the diagnosis of any porokeratosis must be taken from the peripheral raised keratotic rim. This shows an oblique epidermal invagination that points outward and is filled with a parakeratotic plug called the cornoid lamella. It appears homogenously eosinophilic with pycnotic nuclei. At the base of the cornoid lamella, the epidermis shows an irregular arrangement of the keratinocytes with dense chromatin and a perinuclear edema or even vacuolization. Some may be dyskeratotic. A granular layer is lacking here (Figure 6.3). The adjacent epidermis is often atrophic. There may be a mild inflammatory infiltrate in the upper dermis.

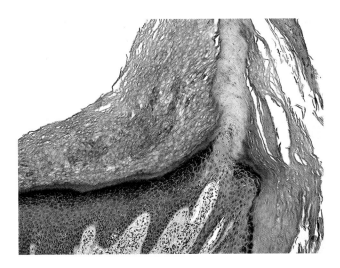

Figure 6.3 Cornoid lamella in a case of porokeratosis Mibelli mimicking a spike formation instead of the cuticle.

In the nail, structures reminiscent of a cornoid lamella may be seen. When they derive from the matrix and extend into the nail plate, a band-like parakeratosis is seen in the nail plate.

6.4.2 Differential diagnosis

A cornoid lamella may be an incidental finding in a variety of inflammatory dermatoses, seborrheic keratosis, verruca vulgaris, and cutaneous carcinomas. However, in porokeratosis, PAS positive globules may be seen that are not observed in accidental cornoid lamellae.

6.5 ACANTHOLYTIC DISORDERS

Two well-defined genodermatoses are characterized by acantholysis and variable degree of dyskeratoses.

6.5.1 Darier disease

Darier disease (OMIM 124200) is an autosomal dominant trait with high penetrance and variable expressivity.[66] It is due to a mutation of the ATP2A2 gene encoding the sarcoplasmic endoplasmic reticulum calcium pumping ATPase SERCA2 on chromosome 12q24.11. Slowly progressive keratotic papules are distributed mostly on the so-called "seborrheic" areas of the body. They tend to coalesce and may cause crusted and verrucous areas. Mucosal membrane involvement may occur as white papules on the lingual and buccal mucosae, palate, and gingiva with a cobblestone appearance. Palms and soles show characteristic pits. Nail involvement is common and is characterized by V-shaped nicking of the free nail margin, longitudinal red and white alternating bands, and subungual hyperkeratosis at the distal aspect of the nail bed.[67] The nail itself may be thin or thick. Isolated nail involvement was described.[68–70] Keratotic papules also occur on the proximal nail fold. A large vegetating tumor developed on the dorsal aspect of the distal thumb in a pregnant woman with known Darier disease.[71]

6.5.1.1 Histopathology

A peculiar abnormal keratinization resulting in so-called corps ronds and grains as well as many dyskeratoses, loss of intercellular keratinocyte adhesion by acantholysis leading to suprabasal clefts and lacunae, irregular upward projection of the papillae into the cleavage thus forming villi lined with a single layer of basal cells, and irregular hyperkeratosis with nucleated cells that often exhibit features of acantholysis are seen in skin biopsies. The corps ronds (round bodies) occur in the upper spinous and particularly the granular layer and can be followed into the stratum corneum. They have a central homogenously basophilic dark nucleus surrounded by a clear halo. The grains are isolated acantholytic parakeratotic cells. The histopathologic changes of the nail alterations[72] are more subtle. Acantholysis and suprabasal clefting are often not observed, but may be focally pronounced (Figure 6.4). Corps ronds and grains are rarely seen if at all. However, binucleated and multinucleated cells occur (Figure 6.5). A clear-cut identification of the red or white stripes in the nail is not possible on histologic grounds, but the red lines are attributed to nail thinning due to matrix involvement whereas the whitish lines are thought to represent nail thickening due to epithelial hyperplasia in the matrix. There is no inflammatory infiltrate in the nail bed dermis.

Ultrastructurally, the basal cells have a decreased number of desmosomes that are separated from the tonofibrils, which show perinuclear circular aggregates in suprabasal location. Corps ronds display many lamellar bodies resembling apoptotic cells.[73,74]

Secondary infection with dermatophytes is not uncommon.

6.5.1.2 Differential diagnosis

The most important differential diagnosis is Hailey–Hailey disease as it also causes longitudinal striation of many if

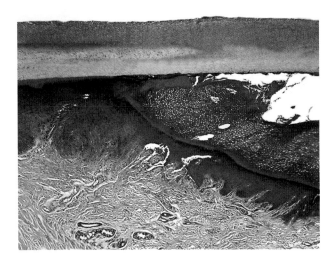

Figure 6.4 Darier disease with marked acantholysis in the hyponychium area.

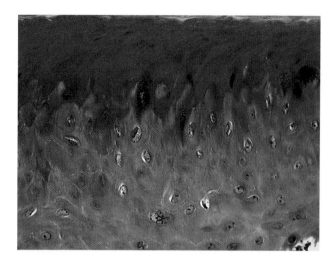

Figure 6.5 Darier disease with multinucleated cell in the mid-nail bed.

not all nails; however, the lines are mainly whitish. An isolated distal subungual striate hyperkeratosis was described as localized multinucleate distal subungual keratosis.[75] A red subungual streak is also caused by subungual warty dyskeratoma.[76,77] Onychopapilloma is a fairly common condition usually occurring in one nail only. Its histopathology is different from Darier disease. Subungual filamentous tumor is a rare lesion characterized by a narrow longitudinal whitish, yellowish, or light brown band due to a keratotic rim under the nail. It is not yet well-defined histopathologically. Acantholytic dyskeratotic acanthoma exhibits much more pronounced changes and is a solitary lesion.[78] Lichen planus of the nail also causes striated nails and a particular challenge is its association with onychopapilloma.[79] Subungual Bowen's disease, squamous cell carcinoma, and amelanotic melanoma may also cause a reddish or whitish line.

6.5.2 Pemphigus familiaris benignus of Hailey-Hailey

Hailey-Hailey disease (OMIM 169600) is a rare autosomal dominant acantholytic disease caused by mutations in the gene encoding the endoplasmic reticulum and Golgi apparatus calcium channels ATP2C1 on chromosome 3q22.1.[80] Clinically, it is characterized by fissured and crusted erosions, blisters, and plaques usually beginning in the third or fourth decade in the axillae, groins, perianally, perigenitally, and in large body folds. Nail lesions are found in approximately three-quarters of the patients, mainly as whitish lines.[81–83] These lines remain asymptomatic. Dermatoscopy makes them even better visible.[84]

6.5.2.1 Histopathology

Skin biopsies demonstrate extensive suprabasal acantholysis reaching into the spinous layer and giving the epidermis the aspect of a delapidated brick wall. Corps ronds and grains are usually lacking. As in Darier disease, the histopathologic alterations in the nail are subtle and consist of occasional incomplete acantholysis. The subungual keratosis is unremarkable. Multinucleate cells are absent.

6.5.2.2 Differential diagnosis

The main differential diagnosis is Darier disease. Pemphigus vulgaris often shows oral mucosal involvement and intercellular antibodies in immunofluorescence studies.

6.6 ACROKERATOSIS VERRUCIFORMIS OF HOPF

Acrokeratosis verruciformis (AKV) (OMIM 101900) is a very rare condition thought to be an autosomal dominant or sporadic genodermatosis; it is now widely held to be a manifestation of Darier disease. The gene defect is located on chromosome 12q24.11. Patients demonstrate flat-topped, skin-colored, asymptomatic papules on the dorsa of their hands, feet, and digits.[85] An occasional palmar pit may occur. The nails may be affected and show mild longitudinal ridging and onychorrhexis. The clinical differential diagnosis comprises flat warts, acral localization of Darier disease, lichen planus, epidermodysplasia verruciformis, acrokeratoelastoidosis, and other acrokeratoses as well as stuccokeratoses.[86] Darier disease can usually be diagnosed due to its more common occurrence of palmar and plantar pits, common nail involvement with whitish and reddish striations leading to distal notch formation, the greasy lesions in so-called seborrheic areas, and its frequent superinfection particularly of the intertriginous areas, mucosal papules, and neuropsychiatric abnormalities. However, acrokeratosis verruciformis and Darier disease were also described as occurring together in the same family.[87] Acral lesions of Darier disease may appear early in childhood, and rarely, patients with AKV-like lesions may later develop classic lesions of Darier disease elsewhere.[67] Coincidences of Darier disease and acrokeratosis verruciformis of Hopf were also described.[88]

Finally, mutations in the ATP2A gene characteristic of Darier disease have recently been described in two families with acrokeratosis verruciformis,[89,90] but were not found in other cases.[91]

No standard treatment exists for acrokeratosis verruciformis. Superficially ablative methods such as keratolytics, peels, cryotherapy, CO_2, or neodymium:YAG laser were tried. Retinoids were reported to be beneficial.[92,93]

6.6.1 Histopathology

Acrokeratosis verruciformis exhibits marked compact orthokeratosis with hypergranulosis, mild regular acanthosis, and variable "church spire" papillomatosis (Figure 6.6). Viral cytopathic changes, parakeratosis, acantholysis, or dyskeratosis are not seen.

6.6.2 Differential diagnosis

Acrokeratosis verruciformis may be similar to the acrokeratoses discussed in the acrokeratoelastoidosis paragraphs although it is mainly located on the dorsa of hands, feet, and digits. It has to be stressed that it does not display viral cytopathic effects allowing it to be

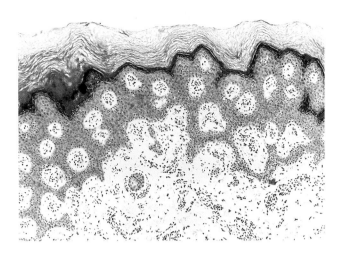

Figure 6.6 Acrokeratosis verruciformis of Hopf displaying marked acanthopapillomatosis and hyperkeratosis. There are no cytopathic effects and no similarity with Darier disease.

differentiated from flat warts. There are no elastic tissue alterations. The lack of dyskeratoses allows its differentiation from Darier disease.

6.7 DYSKERATOSIS CONGENITA

Dyskeratosis congenita (DC) of Zinsser-Cole-Engman (OMIM 305000) is an inherited bone marrow failure and cancer predisposition syndrome characterized by germline mutations in telomere biology. It can be inherited as an X-linked, autosomal dominant (AD) (on chromosome Xq28), or autosomal recessive (AR) type (OMIM 615190, 224239). De novo germline mutations are rather frequent in DC. About 70% of DC patients have an identifiable germline mutation.[94] It is clinically heterogeneous and usually diagnosed by the mucocutaneous triad of progressively dystrophic nails, abnormal pigmentation, and leukoplakias of the oral mucosa, often associated with severe periodontitis. Hoyeraal–Hreidarsson syndrome (HH) is a clinically severe variant of DC also including cerebellar hypoplasia, immunodeficiency, and intrauterine growth retardation.[95] The germline mutation is in one of nine genes, the products of which are all involved in telomere biology. DC is very rare with an annual incidence of <1 per million. Patients with DC show considerable disease diversity in terms of age at onset, symptoms, and severity. Even with the same gene mutation, the disease manifestations are variable making it sometimes difficult to reach a correct diagnosis.[96] Due to the heredity pattern, females may have less severe clinical features.[97] Approximately 90% of patients suffer from nail dystrophy affecting the fingernails first and then the toenails. It begins with ridging and longitudinal splitting and gradually progresses, resulting in small, rudimentary, or absent nails.

In childhood, bone marrow failure, and in adults, lung fibrosis are the most common causes of premature death. Hemopoietic stem cell transplantation is the treatment of choice, but androgens may also improve the bone marrow failure.

6.7.1 Histopathology

Whereas skin biopsies show a pigmentary incontinence of variable degree and mucosal biopsies a premalignant leukoplakia or even squamous cell carcinoma,[98] nail biopsies are not performed.[99] One case showed a short nail pocket with an epidermis-like matrix producing keratin lamellae instead of a nail plate.

6.7.2 Differential diagnosis

A similar matrix alteration is seen in postlichen nail changes and in amyloidosis.

6.8 ROTHMUND–THOMSON SYNDROME

The main clinical characteristics of Rothmund–Thomson syndrome (OMIM 268400, chromosome 8q24.3) are universal skin changes consisting of striae, atrophy, and abnormal, often reticular pigmentation, short stature, variable cataract, hypogonadism, sparse hair, marked hypogonadism, dystrophic nails, and developmental abnormalities of the teeth. Some cases developed carcinomas early;[100] these have to be differentiated from dyskeratosis congenita.[101]

6.8.1 Histopathology

Skin biopsies in the early phase show hydropic degeneration of the basal layer with pigmentary incontinence and melanophages in the upper dermis. There may be a mild band-like lymphocytic infiltrate close to the epidermis. Later, there are a flattened epidermis, dilated capillaries, and melanophages in the upper dermis.[102] The dermis may show fragmentation of elastic fibers.[103] These changes can also be found on the dorsa of the fingers.

6.8.2 Differential diagnosis

Dyskeratosis congenita does not exhibit an inflammatory infiltrate.

Poikiloderma with neutropenia of the Clericuzio type (OMIM 604371) is a recently described entity associated with nail dystrophy, palmoplantar hyperkeratosis, chronic neutropenia, and recurrent infections; molecular biologically, it has nothing to do with Rothmund–Thomson syndrome.[104]

6.9 ECTODERMAL DYSPLASIAS

Ectodermal dysplasias (EDs) represent a very large group of different conditions that share a dysplasia of cutaneous appendages such as the hair, nails, teeth, and sweat glands. Non-ectodermal manifestations are frequent and thus more than 200 different EDs are now known. For a more simple classification, the EDs are subdivided into hidrotic and hypohidrotic forms. In the strict sense of the terminology, at least two skin appendages must be involved; epidermal changes are not considered. The clinical classification denoting hair (1), teeth (2), nail (3), and sweat gland (4) dysplasias has now been abandoned in favor of molecular biologic results.[105, 106] Thus, Clouston type was also called tricho-onychotic ectodermal dysplasia (1–3).

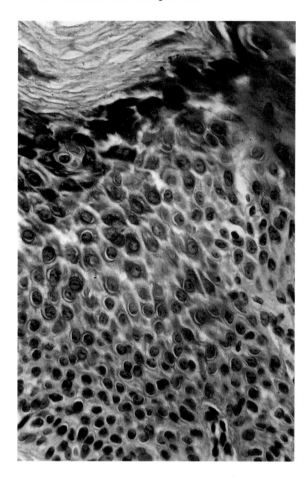

Figure 6.7 Proximal nail fold biopsy from a child with ectodermal dysplasia—skin fragility syndrome.

Many of the hidrotic EDs as well as hypohidrotic EDs present with nail changes, which in general, are rather unspecific. Hypoplasia and even aplasia can be found, but also very slowly growing, plicated nails.[107,108]

6.9.1 Histopathology

The nail changes in the onychotic types vary from almost normal to near absence. There are no specific changes in the nail unit allowing a particular ED diagnosis to be made.

In the ectodermal dysplasia-skin fragility syndrome, a plakophilin-1 mutation leads to hair and teeth abnormalities. The nails become thickened. Histologically a widening of the intercellular spaces between the keratinocytes from the suprabasal to the granular layer is observed (Figure 6.7).[109]

6.10 EPIDERMOLYSIS BULLOSA GROUP

Although the classification and terminology have been changed in recent time,[110] this large and genetically heterogeneous group of skin fragility diseases is commonly divided into three groups:

- Epidermolysis bullosa hereditaria (EBH) simplex
- Epidermolysis bullosa hereditaria junctionalis
- Epidermolysis bullosa hereditaria dystrophica

Whereas most simplex types are due to defects in keratins 4, 5, and 14[111] and show a cytolytic blister formation in the basal cells between the nuclei and the basal cell membrane, junctional EBHs form blisters within the lamina lucida of the basal lamina complex. The dystrophic EBHs are further subdivided into autosomal dominant and recessive affecting the anchoring fibers or collagen 7A1, respectively.[112] These changes are best seen by electron microscopy.[113]

The most common and mildest form of epidermolysis bullosa simplex is the Weber–Cockayne type (EBSWC; OMIM 131800) where blistering is limited to the hands and feet. Blisters are not present at birth, but develop later after an identifiable traumatic event. Secondary infections of blistering lesions on the feet are the most common complication. Nail changes are not a common feature, but periungual blisters and erosions may occasionally be seen. The Köbner type (EBS-K; OMIM 131900) manifests after birth with generalized, but relatively mild blistering also affecting hands and feet. The Dowling-Meara form (EBS-DM; OMIM 131760) is the most severe simplex subtype presenting with extensive grouped blistering, called "herpetiform" pattern. It is already present at birth with erosions and areas of denuded skin. Serous and hemorrhagic blisters develop on the entire skin, but most frequently on palms and soles, around the mouth, on the trunk, and neck. Oral mucosal involvement, progressive palmoplantar keratosis, and nail dystrophies are common. Usually the lesions heal without scarring; however, inflammation especially of hemorrhagic blisters may be followed by milia formation. EBS-DM with extensive involvement may be fatal in the neonatal period. Ultrastructural examination of skin biopsies shows characteristic clumps of keratin intermediate filaments in the cytoplasm of basal keratinocytes. These three EBS forms are due to keratin 5 and 14 mutations. EBS with mottled pigmentation is another rare subtype that may be associated with punctate palmar and plantar keratoses.[114] Blistering is usually more pronounced in childhood. Nail changes may develop in later age. Bart's syndrome (OMIM 132000) is also thought to be an EBS with predominant blistering in the neonatal phase and later nail dystrophy.[115] Further rare simplex types are due to mutations of the genes encoding plectin, the 230-kDa bullous pemphigoid antigen, β4 integrin, plakophilin-1, desmoplakin,[116] plakoglobin, transglutaminase 5, and exophilin-5.[117]

The junctional epidermolyses are characterized by a molecular defect of laminin 332 (laminin 5) (Herlitz type: lethal, generalized) (OMIM 226700), type XVII collagen (non-Herlitz) OMIM 226050,[118] or α6β4 integrin (junctional EB with pyloric atresia, OMIM 226730). Particularly the generalized types show blistering in the nail region, often with complete loss of the nail. The digital tips are round and covered with extremely fragile thin skin.[119] Shabbir's syndrome, also called laryngo-onychocutaneous syndrome (OMIM 245660), stands out by excessive formation of granulation tissue and marked nail involvement. The defect was localized in the laminin-332 α3 chain.

The dystrophic epidermolyses are either autosomal dominant or autosomal recessive.[120] The main molecular mutation results in a defect of collagen VII (COL7A1) permitting splitting in the sublamina densa level. The dominant and recessive types were found to differ in electron microscopy. In the severe forms of dystrophic EBs, the nails get lost leaving a denuded, very fragile tip of the digit. The risk of skin cancer is not significantly increased.

Three types of localized dystrophic EBs stand out by their nail involvement: EBD nails only, pretibial EBD, and EBD pruriginosa (OMIM 604129). These types are often diagnosed very late and therefore a number of them might never have been diagnosed.[121,122] It is not clear whether these three forms really represent clear-cut entities. The nails become dystrophic and are lost with time. Whereas the risk of skin cancer is not increased in the dominant EBD types of Pasini and Cockayne-Touraine, invasive squamous cell carcinomas often develop in the recessive types and may be fatal, particularly in the Hallopeau-Siemens subtype.[123]

Kindler's syndrome (OMIM 173650), originally described as poikiloderma with blistering and photosensitivity, is now generally described as an EB with trauma-induced acral blisters. It is autosomal recessive clinically mimicking severe EB types. The molecular defect is in a protein called kindlin-1 encoded by FERMT1, which enables contacts with actin filaments in basal keratinocytes.[124] However, this is the only mechanobullous genodermatosis with different cleavage levels. Finger webbing, pseudosyndactyly, marked atrophy of the skin of the fingers, and nail dystrophy are observed.[125] The cuticles may be extremely long and cover up to one half of the nails.[126] Several publications have described invasive cutaneous and extracutaneous squamous cell carcinomas.[127]

6.10.1 Histopathology

Biopsies of the nails are usually not performed in hereditary epidermolyses. They might, however, occasionally be done under another clinical diagnosis. It has to be stressed that light microscopic histopathology cannot make an accurate diagnosis of any one of the many EBs. Clinical information is crucial, not only concerning the biopsied patient but also his or her family history.

Occasionally, the plane of blistering may be suggested in the simplex types as the split is at a supra-basal lamina level when stained with PAS and the sections are thin enough or in plastic embedded semithin sections (Figure 6.8). Semithin sections may also reveal the tonofibril clumping in EBS Dowling-Meara.[128] Further subtyping is not possible histologically. The desmoplakin mutation shows plantar and periungual hyperkeratosis and thickened nails. Immunohistochemically, a complete lack of desmoplakin staining is observed and electron microscopy shows clumping of the tonofibrils that do not anchor in the desmosomes.[107]

An amputation specimen of a case of Herlitz type junctional EB revealed scarring of the tip of the digit with very thin epidermis and without any trace of the nail unit (unpublished observation).

Autosomal recessive severe dystrophic EBs cannot be distinguished.

A lateral longitudinal nail biopsy was performed in a case of pruriginous dystrophic EB with severe nail dystrophy in a 62-year-old woman. The rudimentary nail plate was partially torn off the nail bed. There was a split formation between the matrix and nail bed epithelium and the scarred nail dermis. No inflammatory infiltrate was present. Immunofluorescence mapping using collagen VII

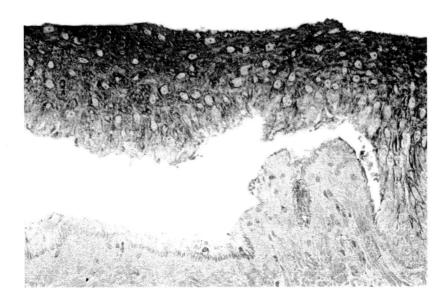

Figure 6.8 Periungual blister in a 28-year-old man with epidermolysis bullosa simplex of Weber–Cockayne. This semithin section shows the cytolytic blister to be above a narrow zone of basal cytoplasm of the basal cells.

antibodies revealed a sublamina densa split characteristic for dystrophic EB.[129]

6.10.2 Differential diagnosis

All blistering diseases have to be considered. Complete lack of inflammation is characteristic for hereditary epidermolyses without infectious complications although acquired bullous epidermolysis may also remain without an inflammatory infiltrate.[130] Immunomapping helps to precisely define the plane of split formation and also to identify the target antigen. Molecular genetic analyses are able to subtype many of the hereditary EBs.

6.11 INCONTINENTIA PIGMENTI

Incontinentia pigmenti (IP) (OMIM #308300) is an X-linked dominant disorder usually lethal to male offspring. It is due to a mutation in the NEMO gene causing loss-of-function of NEMO/IKKgamma.[131–133] Surviving males harbor either a postzygotic new mutation or a karyotype 46,XXY. Due to the lyonization effect, the lesions are distributed along Blaschko lines.[134] They typically start as small blisters on an erythematous base that undergo a papillomatous-hyperkeratotic change until they develop into light-brown spattered, whorled, or linear lesions. After several years, they diminish insidiously and finally subtle faintly hypochromic or atrophic lesions remain, best visible on the calves. Bald patches in Blaschko-linear distribution may be seen on the scalp. Central nervous system, eye and tooth abnormalities occur in approximately 80%. Nail involvement is mainly seen in the first and second stages as periungual blisters and verrucous lesions, the latter sometimes causing linear nail ridging. This may resolve spontaneously.[135] Nail dystrophy may even be the sole manifestation of IP[136] or occur at a late age.[137,138] The most characteristic nail lesions are seen as painful subungual tumors in females from the age of 15 to approximately 35 years,[139–145] and very rarely in prepubertal girls.[146] They may be associated with scalloped bony deformations of the distal phalanges.[147,148] The subungual

tumors respond well to retinoid treatment.[149,150] They may be confused with subungual keratoacanthoma or squamous cell carcinoma.[151,152]

6.11.1 Histopathology

There are no reports on nail dystrophy in children with stage 1 and 2 IP. Periungual lesions, however, are characteristic. In the early inflammatory lesions, intraepidermal spongiotic vesicles filled with numerous eosinophils are seen (Figure 6.9a). They are also abundant in the surrounding epidermis yielding the pattern of eosinophilic spongiosis. There may be single apoptotic cells and whorls of squamous cells with occasional central keratinization. The dermal infiltrate is also rich in eosinophils. The second stage demonstrates an acanthotic epidermis with papillomatosis and hyperkeratosis. There are many dyskeratotic cells and again whorls of keratinocytes with dyskeratoses. The basal cells exhibit vacuolar degeneration and an increase in melanin. The dermal infiltrate is mild with melanophages.

The subungual tumors of IP are unique. The nail bed is verrucous or grossly hyperplastic often displaying a pseudoepitheliomatous pattern. Dyskeratotic cells abound and in some levels make up for almost 100% of the cells (Figure 6.9b). Thus, this pattern is an exaggeration of what is seen in the second stage (see Chapter 8).

6.11.2 Differential diagnosis

Warts, fibromas, subungual epidermoid inclusions, and squamous cell carcinoma have to be excluded. The most difficult differential diagnoses are subungual keratoacanthoma[153] and proliferating onycholemmal tumor, which may be indistinguishable if the entire architecture of the keratoacanthoma is not available for evaluation. Eosinophilia is a characteristic feature of incontinentia pigmenti and not as pronounced in keratoacanthoma and proliferating onycholemmal tumor. We observed a man in his late fifties with a huge subungual horn entirely composed of acantholytic dyskeratotic cells looking like an exaggerated subungual keratosis of IP (unpublished observation).

(a)

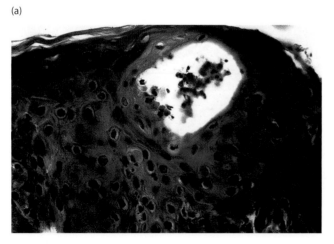

(b)

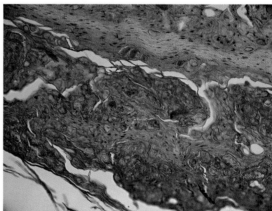

Figure 6.9 (a) Vesicular stage of incontinentia pigmenti with eosinophilic intraepidermal abscesses and many dyskeratotic cells. (b) Subungual keratotic tumor of incontinentia pigmenti with masses of dyskeratoses.

6.12 PACHYDERMOPERIOSTOSIS

Pachydermoperiostosis (OMIM#167100) is also referred to as primary hypertrophic osteoarthropathy (HOP) or Touraine-Solente-Golé syndrome. Pachydermia with cutis verticis gyrata, ptosis of the eyelids,[154] skin thickening of the palms and soles with hyperhidrosis, productive periostitis, and clubbing are the main signs.[155] Although many cases are isolated, it is assumed that the autosomal dominant cases are due to a mutation of the 15-hydroxy-prostaglandin dehydrogenase gene encoding the major prostaglandin PGE_2 catabolizing enzyme.[156-159] In autosomal recessive HOP (OMIM'614441), the transporter gene SCLO2A1 is mutated.[160,161] Twenty-three cases of pachydermoperiostosis had myelofibrosis in addition.[162,163]

Secondary HOP is mainly seen in patients with lung carcinoma, lung metastases, pleural tumors, and other intrathoracic neoplasms (see Sections 5.1.1 and 5.2.4).[164]

6.12.1 Histopathology

Clubbing in pachydermoperiostosis is identical with clubbing due to chronic hypoxemia and other conditions. Dermal edema, mucin deposition, and elastic fiber degeneration are present in all cases of pachydermoperiostosis.[165]

6.12.2 Differential diagnosis

Psoriatic onychopachydermoperiostitis may be clinically similar although usually only the big toes are involved.[166-168] In most cases, it shows psoriatic features in the nail and no clubbing although one case of a combination was described.[169]

6.13 FOCAL DERMAL HYPOPLASIA

Focal dermal hypoplasia (OMIM 305600) was first described by Goltz in 1962.[170] It is a rare meso-ectodermal syndrome due to a mutation of the PORCN gene mapped on chromosome Xp11.23.[171] PORCN encodes an enzyme that allows membrane targeting and secretion of several Wnt proteins critical for normal tissue development.[172] It is lethal for hemizygous male embryos. About 10% of the patients, however, are male because males with a postzygotic new mutation or with Klinefelter syndrome can survive.[173] The clinical expression is very variable and may even be hemicorporal.[174-176] The developmental skin defects are characterized by widespread lesions distributed along the Blaschko lines and affecting mainly the dermis and cutaneous fat. There are also dental[177] and osseous lesions, the latter being visible as striation of the long bones on X-rays.[178] Multiple organ defects may be present.[177,179] The skin lesions are characterized by telangiectasia, hypo- or hyperpigmentation, herniation of fatty tissue, thin hair in the affected scalp regions, and varying degree of nail hypoplasia. Nails may also be striated, ridged, dysplastic, hypoplastic, or absent.[174,176]

6.13.1 Histopathology

The histopathological changes depend on the severity of the skin lesions. In classical lesions, the dermis is thin, displays telangiectasiae, and fat may protrude as herniations. The overlying epidermis is thinned with loss of rete ridges.

6.13.2 Differential diagnosis

Cutaneous lesions of focal dermal hypoplasia associated esophageal papillomatosis were reported in females of four generations of the same family. The disorder was misdiagnosed as "angioma serpiginosum"[178] but later reclassified as familial Goltz syndrome.[181] Aplasia cutis congenita manifests with open wounds at birth that heal with typical atrophic scars.

6.14 APLASIA CUTIS CONGENITA

Aplasia cutis congenita (OMIM 107600) is a rare condition caused by a heterozygous mutation of the BMS1 gene on chromosome 11q21. However, most cases are not identical with OMIM 107600 but represent other entities.[182]

It is characterized by localized absence of skin at birth or with a thin transparent membrane, through which the underlying structures are visible. In most cases, the scalp is involved, but rarely the distal extremities. In 20%–30%, the underlying bone is also affected.[183] Both autosomal dominant as well as recessive inheritance have been reported. Bart syndrome (OMIM132000) is the association of epidermolysis bullosa of various types with skin aplasia and absence or deformity of the nails; it belongs into the epidermolysis bullosa group.[184-186] Some other rare syndromes may also be associated with aplasia cutis congenita such as the scalp-ear-nipple syndrome Finlay-Marks (OMIM 181270),[187] Adams-Oliver syndrome (OMIM 100300), Johanson-Blizzard syndrome (OMIM 243800), Fryns syndrome (OMIM 194190), dominant deafness and onychodystrophy (OMIM 124480), and nail dystrophy.[188-191] The nail itself is not affected by aplasia.

6.14.1 Histopathology

The histopathology of aplasia cutis congenita depends on the time of biopsy. Fresh lesions exhibit a complete lack of the dermis and epidermis or just contain a flat epidermis with hyperkeratosis. With time there is scar tissue that develops into fibrosis and later sclerosis. The nail dystrophy itself has not yet been examined histopathologically. Immunohistochemical examination shows that collagen IV is localized at the roof of blistered skin.[192] Electron microscopy demonstrates that the anchoring fibrils are poorly developed.

6.14.2 Differential diagnosis

Usually the clinical diagnosis is evident.

6.15 EHLERS–DANLOS SYNDROME

Ehlers–Danlos syndrome (OMIM#130000) is a group of collagen diseases classified into types I (severe classic type), II (mild classic type), and III (mitis) as well as several other types. They share loose joints with hyperextensibility and fragile bruisable skin with healing with cigarette-paper like scars. Type IV is characterized by vessel fragility and excessive bruising due to deficiency in collagen III.[193]

Narrow long nails are often associated with Ehlers–Danlos syndrome, but also with Marfan syndrome.[194]

6.15.1 Histopathology

Specific nail histopathology examinations have not been performed.[195,196] In the vascular type, a microangiopathy with leakage of fluorescent dyes, microaneurysms, and microbleedings was observed.

6.15.2 Differential diagnosis

Histopathologic alterations are not sufficiently different to allow a specific diagnosis to be made without clinico-pathologic correlation.

6.16 TUBEROUS SCLEROSIS COMPLEX (SEE CHAPTER 9)

Tuberous sclerosis is a fairly common autosomal dominant disease, of which approximately half of the cases are due to new mutations either in the chromosome 9q34.13 termed tuberous sclerosis complex (TSC) 1 (OMIM 191100), or 12q15/16p13.3 in TSC 2 (OMIM 613254). The clinical features are virtually identical. Apart from the very characteristic peri- and subungual fibromas or Koenen tumors, a number of other dermatological and organ manifestations may be observed.

6.17 BLOOM'S SYNDROME

Bloom's syndrome (OMIM 210900) is a classical chromosomal instability syndrome due to mutations of the DNA helicase RecQ protein-like 2 gene on chromosome 15q26.1. It is autosomal recessive and associated with pre- and postnatal growth retardation, telangiectasiae, hypo- and hyperpigmentation of the skin, and a propensity to develop infections and cancers. Photosensitivity is the leading symptom. The skin shows a telangiectatic erythema that begins in the face and slowly extends to the arms and hands. Café au lait macules may appear. Specific nail changes have not been observed.

6.17.1 Histopathology

The epidermis is thin and may show vacuolar degeneration of the basal cells. Capillary dilatation is characteristic. A perivascular infiltrate may be present but is not mandatory. These changes are not pronounced around the nails.

6.17.2 Differential diagnosis

Lupus erythematosus has to be ruled out in case of hydropic degeneration of basal cells, but no lupus band is seen in Bloom syndrome. Pigmentary incontinence is more a feature of congenital poikiloderma.

6.18 ATAXIA-TELANGIECTASIA (LOUIS–BAR SYNDROME)

Ataxia-telangiectasia (OMIM 208900, 11q22.3) is a very rare autosomal recessive disorder characterized by cerebellar ataxia developing in infancy, telangiectasiae, immune defects, and predisposition to malignancy. Ionizing radiation easily kills the cells of these patients due to chromosomal breakage. The telangiectasiae first occur on the conjunctivae and then extend to the face, ears, neck, extremities, and oral mucosa. Telangiectasiae may also develop in the nail bed.[197] Death usually occurs in the third to fourth decade due to infections and lymphoma or leukemia.[198]

6.18.1 Histopathology

There are abundant dilated vessels in the upper dermis. Inflammatory infiltrates are not seen.[199]

6.19 XERODERMA PIGMENTOSUM

Xeroderma pigmentosum represents a group of autosomal recessive disorders of DNS repair rendering the affected individuals highly prone to develop skin cancers in sun-exposed skin. At least seven complementation groups (A–G) and a variant are differentiated.[200] They differ in the chromosomal location of the gene defects, severity of ultraviolet sensitivity, frequency, and age of onset of malignancies. Xeroderma pigmentosum with mental deficiency, progressive neurologic deterioration, dwarfism, and gonadal hypoplasia was first described by A. Neisser in Breslau.[201] Other syndromes were described, such as a combination with trichothiodystrophy features.[202] From early infancy on, the skin develops diffuse erythema, scaling, and freckle-like hyperpigmentation. Within a few years, the skin becomes atrophic with mottled pigmentation and telangiectasiae resembling radiodermatitis and develops actinic keratoses. As early as in adolescence, skin cancers, mainly of the squamous cell type, but also basal cell carcinomas, melanomas,[203] and rarely fibrosarcomas develop in sun-exposed skin, that is, also the dorsa of the hands, feet, and digits. Complete avoidance of sunlight prevents these changes ("moon-light children").

6.19.1 Histopathology

Hyperkeratosis, thinning of the spinous layer, atrophy, or elongation of rete ridges, irregular melanin distribution, and inflammatory infiltrates in the upper dermis are seen in the early stage making the skin appear older. Later, thickening of the horny layer and pigmentation are more marked with irregular epidermal acanthosis and atrophy often similar to actinic keratoses. Solar degeneration of the upper dermal connective tissue is already present in childhood. In early adolescence, malignant skin tumors develop, such as squamous cell carcinomas, basal cell carcinomas, melanomas, and fibrosarcomas. These changes and malignant tumors may also develop around the nail.

6.19.2 Differential diagnosis

Premature aging due to excessive sun exposure is not uncommon in fair-skinned Caucasians. It is common in other DNA excision repair disorders[204] that also may show nail dystrophy.[205] The cutaneous malignancies are microscopically indistinguishable from those of unaffected persons.

6.20 WERNER SYNDROME

Werner syndrome (OMIM #277700) is a very rare autosomal recessive genetic instability and progeroid ("premature aging") syndrome, which is associated with an elevated risk of cancer.[206] It is caused by loss-of-function mutations in the WRN gene on chromosome 8p12 encoding a RecQ type helicase. Dermatologic signs are graying and loss of hair, scleroderma-like skin hardening due to loss of subcutaneous fat, and lower leg ulcers. Mottled and diffuse pigmentation may give the aspect of poikiloderma. The fingers may become sclerotic with glistening shiny atrophic tips.[207,208] The nails become dystrophic or lost.[209,210] Systemic alterations include cataracts, muscle atrophy, post-pubertal growth arrest, hoarseness, high-pitched voice, diabetes mellitus type 2, osteoporosis, hypogonadism, and severe atherosclerosis usually leading to death between the age of 40 and 60 years.[211,212] Clinically, progeria may be mistaken for scleroderma.[213] Severe acroosteolysis and nail dystrophy were also seen in another progeroid syndrome.[214]

6.20.1 Histopathology

The epidermis is atrophic and the dermis appears thick with hyalinization of the collagen fibers. The pilosebaceous structures are lacking.[215]

6.20.2 Differential diagnosis

Scleroderma is the main differential diagnosis, but the diagnosis requires a clinicopathologic correlation.

6.21 FOXN1 DEFICIENCY

When the nude mouse was identified in 1966, it was detected that the hair follicles could not enter the epidermis and that there was an inborn dysgenesis of the thymus making this animal an excellent model for the study of primary immunodeficiency and xenotransplantation.[216] Although mentioned in the original publication, the nail changes found little attention and were only investigated late. A mutation in the winged-helix-nude gene *Whn* encoding a highly conserved transcription factor now called FOXN1 is responsible for the nude phenotype. Although the exact function of FOXN1 remained long unclear, it is now thought to play a key role in the early stages of keratinocyte differentiation. It directly activates keratin 1 synthesis.[217] In nude mice, Krt 3 and other keratins are absent in the hair.[218] Although nude mice have the same number of hair follicles[219] and show an active cyclical growth pattern,[220] the hair shafts have no normal cuticle and break.[221] It was shown that the FOXN1 mRNA and acidic hair keratin 3 are co-expressed both in the hair follicles and the nails.[220] Less than 20 years ago, the human phenotype of severe functional T cell impairment and congenital alopecia with nail dystrophy was observed.[222–227] As was shown recently,[228] there are considerable analogies between mouse and human nails and the study of the nail in the nude mouse and other mutant and transgenic mice with nail abnormalities[229] may help us understand human nail physiology and pathology.[230,231] Nail dystrophy occurs both in homozygous and heterozygous FOXN1 mutant humans whereas hair alterations are not seen in the heterozygous carriers.[232]

6.21.1 Histopathology

The nails in FOXN1-deficient humans are dystrophic and leukonychotic, some show koilonychia. In the nude mice, the nails are markedly shortened with a blunt tip ending at the hyponychium. The nails are very thin with smaller onychocytes on their surface. The matrix is thinner and extends farther distally without a sharp border between matrix and nail bed. The superficial matrix cells are larger, do not flatten, and contain keratohyalin granules, which are still visible in the nail plate. This is thin and basophilic as compared to the light plate in normal mice. The sulfur content is lower. Keratin 1 is absent and filaggrin is demonstrable. Keratin 5, several integrins, and Ki67 proliferation marker are unaltered. The nail bed is not altered.[233]

6.21.2 Differential diagnosis

Thin, epidermis-like nails are seen in late lichen planus, graft-versus-host disease, dyskeratosis congenita, amyloidosis, and a variety of other inflammatory diseases involving the matrix. All irritations of the matrix epithelium may lead to keratohyalin granule formation in the matrix.[234–236] Leukonychia shows nail plate cells with an eosinophilic cytoplasm.

REFERENCES

1. Mori MA, Lapunzina P, Delicado A, Nunez G, Rodriguez JI, de Torres ML, Herreo F, Valverde E, Lopez-Pajares I. A prenatally diagnosed patient with full monosomy 21: Ultrasound, cytogenetic, clinical, molecular, and necropsy findings. *Am J Med Genet* 2004;127A:69–73.
2. Schmuth M, Martinz V, Janecke AR, Fauth C, Schossig A, Zschocke J, Gruber R. Inherited ichthyoses/generalized Mendelian disorders of cornification. *Eur J Hum Gen* 2013;21:123–133.
3. Oji V, Tadini G, Akiyama M, Blanchet Bardon C, Bodemer C, Bourrat E, Coudiere P et al. Revised nomenclature and classification of inherited ichthyoses: Results of the First Ichthyosis Consensus Conference in Sorèze 2009. *J Am Acad Derematol* 2010;63:607–641.
4. Thyssen JP, Godoy-Gijon E, Elias PM. Ichthyosis vulgaris: The filaggrin mutation disease. *Br J Dermatol* 2013;168:1155–1166.
5. James WD, Odom RB, Horn RT. Twenty-nail dystrophy and ichthyosis vulgaris. *Arch Dermatol* 1981;117:316.
6. Rand RE, Baden HP. The ichthyoses—A review. *J Am Acad Dermatol* 1983;8:285–305.
7. Hoeger PH, Adwani SS, Whitehead BF, Finlay AY, Harper JI. Ichthyosiform erythroderma and cardiomyopathy: Report of two cases and review of the literature. *Br J Dermatol.* 1998;139:1055–1059.
8. Irvine AD, McLean WH. Human keratin diseases: The increasing spectrum of disease and subtlety of the phenotype-genotype correlation. *Br J Dermatol* 1999;140:815–828.

9. Al Fahaad H. Keratosis-ichthyosis-deafness syndrome: First affected family described in the Middle East. *Int Med Case Rep J* 2014;7:63–66.

10. Biswas P, De A, Sendur S, Nag F, Saha A, Chatterjee G. A case of ichthyosis hystrix: Unusual manifestation of this rare disease. *Ind J Dermatol* 2014;59:82–84.

11. Schulz-Kiesow M, Metze D, Traupe H. Hystrix-like keratosis with nail and joint-involvement: A new genodermatosis? *Dermatology* 1996;192:321–324.

12. Wang HJ, Tang ZL, Lin ZM, Dai LL, Chen Q, Yang Y. Recurrent splice-site mutation in MBTPS2 underlying IFAP syndrome with Olmsted syndrome-like features in a Chinese patient. *Clin Exp Dermatol* 2014;39:158–161.

13. Matsumoto T, Sakura N, Ueda K. Steroid sulfatase activity in nails: Screening for X-linked ichthyosis. *Pediatr Dermatol* 1990;7:266–269.

14. Happle R, Koch H, Lenz W. The CHILD syndrome: Congenital hemidysplasia with ichthyosiform erythroderma and limb defects. *Eur J Pediatr* 1980;134:27–33.

15. Happle R. Ptychotropism as a cutaneous feature of the CHILD syndrome. *J Am Acad Dermatol* 1990;23:763–766.

16. König A, Happle R, Bornholdt D, Engel H, Grzeschik KH. Mutations in the NSDHL gene, encoding a 3beta-hydroxysteroid dehydrogenase, cause CHILD syndrome. *Am J Med Genet* 2000;90:339–346.

17. Gantner S, Rütten A, Requena L, Gassenmaier G, Landthaler M, Hafner C. CHILD syndrome with mild skin lesions: Histopathologic clues for the diagnosis. *J Cutan Pathol* 2014;41:787–790.

18. Liu T, Qian G, Wang XX, Zhang YG. CHILD syndrome: Effective treatment of ichthyosiform naevus with oral and topical ketoconazole. *Acta Derm Venereol* 2015;95:91–92.

19. Paller AS, van Steensel MA, Rodriguez-Martín M, Sorrell J, Heath C, Crumrine D, van Geel M, Cabrera AN, Elias PM. Pathogenesis-based therapy reverses cutaneous abnormalities in an inherited disorder of distal cholesterol metabolism. *J Invest Dermatol* 2011;131:2242–2248.

20. Merino De Paz N, Rodriguez-Martin M, Contreras-Ferrer P, Garcia Bustinduy M, Gonzalez Perera I, Virgos Aller T, Martin Herrera A, Noda Cabrera A. Topical treatment of CHILD nevus and Sjögren-Larsson Syndrome with combined lovastatin and cholesterol. *Eur J Dermatol* 2011;21:1026–1027.

21. Kiritsi D, Schauer F, Wölfle U, Valari M, Bruckner-Tuderman L, Has C, Happle R. Targeting epidermal lipids for treatment of Mendelian disorders of cornification. *Orphanet J Rare Dis* 2014 Mar 7;9:33, doi: 10.1186/1750-1172-9-33

22. Fartasch M, Haneke E, Anton-Lamprecht I. Ultrastructural study on the occurrence of autosomal dominant ichthyosis vulgaris in atopic eczema. *Arch Dermatol Res* 1987;279:270–272.

23. Haneke E, Vigneswaran N, Gruschwitz M. Immuno-histochemical study of keratinocyte maturation and differentiation markers in atopic dermatitis and different types of ichthyosis. *Ped Dermatol News* 1987;6:339–341.

24. Rice RH, Crumrine D, Hohl D, Munro CS, Elias PM. Cross-linked envelopes in nail plate in lamellar ichthyosis. *Br J Dermatol* 2003;149:1050–1054.

25. Wortsman X, Aranibar L, Morales C. Postnatal 2- and 3-dimensional sonography of the skin and nail in congenital autosomal recessive ichthyosis correlated with cutaneous histologic findings. *J Ultrasound Med* 2011;30:1437–1439.

26. Traupe H, Fischer J, Oji V. Nonsyndromic types of ichthyoses—An update. *J Dtsch Dermatol Ges* 2014;12:109–121.

27. Fleckman P, Digiovanna JJ. The Ichthyoses. Disorders of epidermal differentiation and keratinization. In: Wolff K, Goldsmith LA, Katz S, Gilchrest BA, Paller AS, Leffell DJ, eds. *Fitzpatrick's Dermatology in General Medicine*, 7th edn. NY: McGraw-Hill Division, 2008; 414.

28. Sprecher E, Ishida-Yamamoto A, Becker OM, Marekov L, Miller CJ, Steinert PM, Neldner K, Richard G. Evidence for novel functions of the keratin tail emerging from a mutation causing ichthyosis hystrix. *J Invest Dermatol* 2001;116:511–519.

29. Happle R, Mittag H, Küster W. The CHILD nevus: A distinct skin disorder. *Dermatology* 1995;191:210–216.

30. Haneke E. The Papillon-Lefèvre syndrome: Keratosis palmoplantaris with periodontopathy. *Hum Genet* 1979;51:1–35.

31. Hart TC, Hart PS, Michalec MD, Zhang Y, Firatli E, Van Dyke TE, Stabholz A, Zlotogorski A, Shapira L, Soskolne WA. Haim-Munk syndrome and Papillon-Lefèvre syndrome are allelic mutations in cathepsin C. *J Med Genet* 2000;37:88–94.

32. Tosti A, Fanti PA, Piraccini BM, Bardazzi F, Misciali C. Epidermolytic hyperkeratosis of the nails in keratosis palmoplantaris nummularis. *Acta Derm Venereol* 1995;75:405–406.

33. Haneke E. Keratosis palmaris et plantaris cum degeneratione granulosa Vörner. *Hautarzt* 1982;33:654–656.

34. Happle R. *Mosaicism in Human Skin. Understanding Nevi, Nevoid Skin Disorders, and Cutaneous Neoplasia*. Heidelberg: Springer, 2014.

35. Jadassohn J, Lewandowsky F. Pachyonychia congenita: Keratosis disseminata circumscripta (follicularis). Tylomata. Leucokeratosis linguae. In: Neisser A, Jacobi E, eds. *Iconographia Dermatologica*, Berlin: Urban und Schwarzenberg, 1906; 29–31.

36. Jackson ADM, Lawler SD. Pachyonychia congenita: A report of six cases in one family with a note on linkage data. *Ann Eugen* 1951;16:142–146.

37. Van Steensel MAM, Coulombe PA, Kaspar RL, Milstone LM, McLean IWH, Roop DR, Smith FJD,

Sprecher E, Schartz ME. Report of the 10th Annual International Pachyonychia Congenita Consortium Meeting. *J Invest Dermatol* 2014;134:588–591.

38. Smith FJD, Kaspar RL, Schwartz ME, McLean WHI, Leachman SA. Pachyonychia congenita. In: Pagon RA, Bird TD, Dolan CR, Stephens K, eds. *GeneReviews [Internet]*. Seattle (WA): University of Washington, 1993–2006.

39. Eliason MJ, Leachman SA, Feng BJ, Schwartz ME, Hansen CD. A review of the clinical phenotype of 254 patients with genetically confirmed pachyonychia congenita. *J Am Acad Dermatol* 2012;67:680–686.

40. Smith FJD, Liao H, Cassidy AJ, Stewart A, Hamill KJ, Wood P, Joval I et al. The genetic basis of pachyonychia congenita. *J Investig Dermatol Symp Proc* 2005;10:21–30.

41. Leachman SA, Kaspar RL, Fleckman P, Florell SR, Smith FJ, McLean WH, Lunny DP et al. Clinical and pathological features of pachyonychia congenita. *J Investig Dermatol Symp Proc* 2005;10:3–17.

42. Cardinali C, Torchia D, Caproni M, Petrini N, Fabbri P. Case study: Pachyonychia congenita: A mixed type II-type IV presentation. *Skinmed* 2004;3:233–235.

43. Spaunhurst KM, Hogendorf AM, Smith FJ, Lingala B, Schwartz ME, Cywinska-Bernas A, Zeman KJ, Tang JY. Pachyonychia congenita patients with mutations in KRT6A have more extensive disease compared with patients who have mutations in KRT16. *Br J Dermatol* 2012;166:875–878.

44. Wilson NJ, Pérez ML, Vahlquist A, Schwartz ME, Hansen CD, McLean WH, Smith FJ. Homozygous dominant missense mutation in keratin 17 leads to alopecia in addition to severe pachyonychia congenita. *J Invest Dermatol* 2012;132:1921–1924.

45. Irvine AD. Double trouble: Homozygous dominant mutations and hair loss in pachyonychia congenita. *J Invest Dermatol* 2012;132:1757–1759.

46. Duarte GV, Cunha R. Syndrome in question. Steatocystoma multiplex as a manifestation of pachyonychia congenita type 2. *An Bras Dermatol* 2011;86:1222–1232.

47. Milstone LM, Fleckman P, Leachman SA, Leigh IM, Paller AS, van Steensel MA, Swartling C. Treatment of pachyonychia congenita. *J Investig Dermatol Symp Proc* 2005;10:18–20.

48. Hickerson RP, Leake D, Pho LN, Leachman SA, Kaspar RL. Rapamycin selectively inhibits expression of an inducible keratin (K6a) in human keratinocytes and improves symptoms in pachyonychia congenita patients. *J Invest Dermatol* 2009;56:82–88.

49. Zhao Y, Gartner U, Smith FJD, McLean WHI. Statins downregulate K6a promoter activity: A possible therapeutic avenue for pachyonychia congenita. *J Invest Dermatol* 2011;131:1045–1052.

50. Hickerson RP, Leachman SA, Pho LN, Gonzalez-Gonzalez E, Smith FJ, McLean WH, Contag CH, Leake D, Milstone LM, Kaspar RL. Development of quantitative molecular clinical end points for siRNA clinical trials. *J Invest Dermatol* 2011;131:1029–1036.

51. Hickerson RP, Flores MA, Leake D, Lara MF, Contag CH, Leachman SA, Kaspar RL. Use of self-delivery siRNAs to inhibit gene expression in an organotypic pachyonychia congenita model. *J Invest Dermatol* 2011;131:1037–1044.

52. McLean WH, Moore CB. Keratin disorders: From gene to therapy. *Hum Mol Genet* 2011;20(R2):R189–R197.

53. Su WP, Chun SI, Hammond DE, Gordon H. Pachyonychia congenita: A clinical study of 12 cases and review of the literature. *Pediatr Dermatol* 1990;7:33–38.

54. Wollina U, Schaarschmidt H, Fünfstück V, Knopf B. Pachyonychia congenita. Immunohistologic findings. *Zentralbl Pathol* 1991;137:372–375.

55. Kelly EW, Pinkus H. Report of a case of pachyonychia congenita. *Arch Dermatol* 1958;77:724.

56. Thomsen RJ, Zuehlke RL, Beckman BI. Pachyonychia congenita. Surgical management of the nail changes. *J Dermatol Surg Oncol* 1982;8:24–28.

57. Cosman B, Symonds FC Jr, Crikelair GF. Plastic surgery in pachyonychia congenita and other dyskeratoses. Case report and review of the literature. *Plast Reconstr Surg* 1964;33:226–326.

58. Respighi E. Di una ipercheratosi non ancora descritta. *G It Dermatol Venereol* 1893;28:356.

59. Karthikeyan K, Thappa DM, Udayashankar C. Porokeratosis of Mibelli with nail dystrophy. *J Dermatol* 2003;30:420–422.

60. Chen HH, Liao YH. Onychodystrophy in congenital linear porokeratosis. *Br J Dermatol* 2002;147:1272–1273.

61. Tseng SS, Levit EK, Ilarda I, Garzon MC, Grossman ME. Linear porokeratosis with underlying bony abnormalities. *Cutis* 2002;69:309–312.

62. Dervis E, Demirkesen C. Generalized linear porokeratosis. *Int J Dermatol* 2006;45:1077–1079.

63. Venkatarajan S, LeLeux TM, Yang D, Rosen T, Orengo I. Porokeratosis of Mibelli: Successful treatment with 5% topical imiquimod and topical 5% 5-fluorouracil. *Dermatol Online J* 2010;16(12):10.

64. Brasch J, Scheuer B, Christophers E. Porokeratosis palmaris, plantaris et disseminata. *Hautarzt* 1985;36:456–461.

65. Guenova E, Hoetzenecker W, Metzler G, Röcken M, Schaller M. Multicentric Bowen disease in linear porokeratosis. *Eur J Dermatol* 2007;17:439–440.

66. Munro CS. The phenotype of Darier's disease: Penetrance and expressivity in adults and children. *Br J Dermatol* 1992;127:126–130.

67. Burge SM, Wilkinson JD. Darier-White disease: A review of the clinical features of 163 patients. *J Am Acad Dermatol* 1992;27:40–50.

68. Ronchese F. The nail in Darier's disease. *Arch Dermatol* 1965;91:617–618.

69. Bingham EA, Burrow D. Darier's disease. *Br J Dermatol* 1984;111(Suppl 26):88–89.

70. Munro CS, MacLeod RI. Variable expression of the Darier's disease gene. *Br J Dermatol* 1991;125(Suppl 38):37.

71. De la Rosa Carillo D. Vegetating Darier's disease during pregnancy. *Acta Derm Venereol* 2006;86:259–260.

72. Zaias N, Ackerman AB. The nail in Darier–White disease. *Arch Dermatol* 1973;107:193–197.

73. Caulfield J, Wilgren G. An electron microscopic study of dyskeratosis and acantholysis in Darier's disease. *J Invest Dermatol* 1963;41:57–61.

74. Burge SM, Schomberg KH. Adhesion molecules and related proteins in Darier's disease and Hailey–Hailey disease. *Br J Dermatol* 1992;127:335–343.

75. Baran R, Perrin C. Localized multinucleate distal subungual keratosis. *Br J Dermatol* 1995;133:77–82.

76. Isonokami M, Higashi N. Focal acantholytic dyskeratosis. *Hifu* 1990;32:507–510.

77. Baran R, Perrin C. Focal subungual warty dyskeratoma. *Dermatology* 1997;195:278–280.

78. Sass U, Kolivras A, Richert B, Moulonguet I, Goettmann-Bonvallot S, Anseeuw M, Theunis A, André J. Acantholytic tumor of the nail: Acantholytic dyskeratotic acanthoma. *J Cutan Pathol* 2009;36:1308–1311.

79. Richert B, Iorizzo M, Tosti A, André J. Nail bed lichen planus associated with onychopapilloma. *Br J Dermatol* 2007;156:1071–1072.

80. Dhitavat J, Fairclough RJ, Hovnanian A, Burge SM. Calcium pumps and keratinocytes: Lessons from Darier's disease and Hailey-Hailey disease. *Br J Dermatol* 2004;150:821–828.

81. Burge SM. Hailey-Hailey disease: The clinical features, response to treatment and prognosis. *Br J Dermatol* 1992;126:275–282.

82. Kirtschig G, Effendy I, Happle R. Leukonychia longitudinalis as the primary symptom of Hailey-Hailey disease. *Hautarzt* 1992;43:451–452.

83. Kostaki D, Castillo JC, Ruzicka T, Sárdy M. Longitudinal leuconychia striata: Is it a common sign in Hailey-Hailey and Darier disease? *J Eur Acad Dermatol Venereol* 2014;28:126–127.

84. Bel B, Jeudy G, Vabres P. Dermoscopy of longitudinal leukonychia in Hailey-Hailey disease. *Arch Dermatol.* 2010;146:1204.

85. Panja RK. Acrokeratosis verruciformis (Hopf)—A clinical entity? *Br J Dermatol* 1977;96:643–652.

86. Waisman M. Verruciform manifestations of keratosis follicularis. *Arch Dermatol* 1960;81:1–14.

87. Herndon J, Wilson J. Acrokeratosis (Hopf) and Darier's disease. *Arch Dermatol* 1966;93:305–310.

88. Piskin S, Saygin A, Doganay L, Kircuval D, Gurkan E. Coexistence of Darier's disease and acrokeratosis verruciformis of Hopf. *Yonsei Med J* 2004;45:956–959.

89. Dhitavat J, Macfarlane S, Dode L, Leslie N, Sakuntabhai A, MacSween R, Saihan E, Hovnanian A. Acrokeratosis verruciformis of Hopf is caused by mutation in ATP2A2: Evidence that it is allelic to Darier's disease. *J Invest Dermatol* 2003;120:229–232.

90. Berk DR, Taube JM, Bruckner AL, Lane AT. A sporadic patient with acrokeratosis verruciformis of Hopf and a novel ATP2A2 mutation. *Br J Dermat* 2010;163:641–666.

91. Wang PG, Gao M, Lin GS Yang S, Lin D, Liang YH, Zhang GL et al. Genetic heterogeneity in acrokeratosis verruciformis of Hopf. *Clin Exp Dermatol* 2006;31:558–563.

92. Farro P, Zalaudek I, Ferrara G Fulgione E, Cicale L, Petrillo G, Zanchini R, Ruocco E, Argenziano G. Unusual association between acrokeratosis verruciformis of Hopf and multiple keratoacanthomas. Successful therapy with acitretin. *J Dtsch Dermatol Ges* 2004;2:440–442.

93. Serarslan G, Balci DD, Homan S. Acitretin treatment in acrokeratosis verruciformis of Hopf. *J Dermatol Treat* 2007;18:123–125.

94. Fernández García MS, Teruya-Feldstein J. The diagnosis and treatment of dyskeratosis congenita: A review. *J Blood Med* 2014 21;5:157–167.

95. Kocak H, Ballew BJ, Bisht K, Eggebeen R, Hicks BD, Suman S, O'Neil A et al. NCI DCEG Cancer Genomics Research Laboratory; NCI DCEG Cancer Sequencing Working Group. Hoyeraal–Hreidarsson syndrome caused by a germline mutation in the TEL patch of the telomere protein TPP1. *Genes Dev* 2014;28:2090–2102.

96. Beier F, Foronda M, Martinez P, Blasco MA. Conditional TRF1 knockout in the hematopoietic compartment leads to bone marrow failure and recapitulates clinical features of dyskeratosis congenita. *Blood* 2012;120:2990–3000.

97. Mason PJ, Bessler M. The genetics of dyskeratosis congenita. *Cancer Genet* 2011;204:635–645.

98. Anil S, Beena VT, Raji MA, Remani P, Ankathil R, Vijayakumar T. Oral squamous cell carcinoma in a case of dyskeratosis congenita. *Ann Dent* 1994;53:15–18.

99. Kawaguchi K, Sakamaki H, Onozawa Y, Koike M. Dyskeratosis congenita (Zinsser-Cole-Engman syndrome). An autopsy case presenting with rectal carcinoma, non-cirrhotic portal hypertension, and Pneumocystis carinii pneumonia. *Virchows Arch A Pathol Anat Histopathol* 1990;417:247–253.

100. Haneke E, Gutschmidt E. Warty hyperkeratoses, cellular immune defect, and tapetoretinal degeneration in poikiloderma congenitale. *Dermatologica* 1976;152:331–336.

101. Haneke E, Gutschmidt E. Premature multiple Bowen's disease in poikiloderma congenitale with warty hyperkeratoses. *Dermatologica* 1979;158:384–388.

102. Rook A, Davis R, Stevanovic D. Poikiloderma congenitale: Rothmund–Thomson syndrome. *Acta Derm Venereol* 1959;39:392–420.

103. Kerr B, Ashcroft GS, Scott D, Horan MA, Ferguson MW, Donnai D. Rothmund–Thomson syndrome: Two case reports show heterogeneous cutaneous abnormalities, an association with genetically

programmed ageing changes, and increased chromosomal radiosensitivity. *J Med Genet.* 1996;33:928–934.

104. Chantorn R, Shwayder T. Poikiloderma with neutropenia: Report of three cases including one with calcinosis cutis. *Pediatr Dermatol.* 2012;29:463–472.

105. Lamartine J. Towards a new classification of ectodermal dysplasias. *Clin Exp Dermatol* 2003;28:351–355.

106. Itin PH, Fistarol SK. Ectodermal dysplasias. *Am J Med Genet C Semin Med Genet* 2004;131C:45–51.

107. Wilsch L, Haneke E, Hornstein OP. Über die trichoonychotische Subgruppe der hidrotischen ektodermalen Dysplasie. *Klin Pädiat* 1977;189:343–345.

108. Haneke E. Hidrotic ectodermal dysplasias. In: Happle R, Grosshans E, eds. *Pediatric Dermatology. Advances in Diagnosis and Treatment*, Berlin–Heidelberg–New York–London–Paris–Tokyo: Springer, 1987;46–54.

109. McGrath JA, Hoeger PH, Shemanko CS, Runwick SK, Leigh IM, Lane EB, Garrod DR, Eady RA. Mutations in the plakophilin 1 gene result in ectodermal dysplasia/skin fragility syndrome. *Nat Gen* 1997;17:240–244.

110. Fine JD, Bruckner-Tuderman L, Eady RA, Bauer EA, Bauer JW, Has C, Heagerty A et al. Inherited epidermolysis bullosa: Updated recommendations on diagnosis and classification. *J Am Acad Dermatol* 2014;70:1103–1106.

111. Jantke M, Has C, Haenssle HA, Schön MP, Emmert S. Epidermolysis bullosa simplex: Greater penetrance due to a keratin 5 gene variant. *Clin Exp Dermatol* 2014;39:80–81.

112. Fine J-D, Eady RAJ, Bauer EA, Bauer JW, Bruckner-Tuderman L, Heagerty A, Hintner H et al. The classification of inherited epidermolysis bullosa (EB): Report of the Third International Consensus Meeting on Diagnosis and Classification of EB. *J Am Acad Dermatol* 2008;58:931–950.

113. Haneke E, Anton-Lamprecht I. Ultrastructure of blister formation in epidermolysis bullosa hereditaria: V. Epidermolysis bullosa simplex localisata type Weber–Cockayne. *J Invest Derm* 1982;78:219–223.

114. Moog U, de Die-Smulders CE, Scheffer H, van der Vlies P, Henquet CJ, Jonkman MF. Epidermolysis bullosa simplex with mottled pigmentation: Clinical aspects and confirmation of the P24L mutation in the *KRT5* gene in further patients. *Am J Med Genet* 1999;86:376–379.

115. Sirota L, Dulitzky F, Metzker A. Bart's syndrome: A mechanobullous disease of the newborn. Report of five cases and review. *Clin Pediatr (Phila)* 1986;25:252–254.

116. Vahlquist A, Virtanen M, Hellström-Pigg M, Dragomir A, Ryberg K, Wilson NJ, Östman-Smith I, Lu L, McGrath JA, Smith FJD. A Scandinavian case of skin fragility, alopecia and cardiomyopathy caused by *DSP* mutations. *Clin Exp Dermatol* 2014;39:30–34.

117. Liu L, Mellerio JE, Martinez AE, McMillan JR, Aristodemou S, Parsons M, McGrath JA. Mutations

in *EXPH5* result in autosomal recessive inherited skin fragility. *Br J Dermatol* 2014;170:196–199.

118. Guerriero C, De Simone C, Venier A, Rotoli M, Patrizia P, Zambruno G, Amerio P. Non-Herlitz junctional epidermolysis bullosa without hair involvement associated with BP180 deficiency. *Dermatology* 2001;202:58–62.

119. Anton-Lamprecht I, Schnyder UW. Zur Ultrastruktur der Epidermolysen mit junktionaler Blasenbildung. *Dermatologica* 1979;159:377–382.

120. Anton-Lamprecht I, Schnyder UW. Epidermolysis bullosa dystrophica dominans. Ein Defekt der anchoring fibrils? *Dermatologica* 1973;147:289–298.

121. Pruneddu S, Castiglia D, Floriddia G, Cottoni F, Zambruno G. COL7A1 recessive mutations in two siblings with distinct subtypes of dystrophic epidermolysis bullosa: Pruriginosa versus nails only. *Dermatology* 2011;222:10–14.

122. Coronado Cha C, Samorano LP, Motta Dacache F, da Matta Rivitti-Machado MC, Prado de Oliveira ZN. Underrecognition of epidermolysis bullosa pruriginosa. *J Dtsch Dermatol Ges* 2015;13:1035–1038.

123. Storbeck K, Hausser I, Haneke E. Squamous cell carcinoma in dystrophic epidermolysis bullosa: Successful treatment with a mesh graft. *J Eur Acad Dermatol Venereol* 1998;11:S163.

124. Jobard F, Bouadjar B, Caux F, Hadj-Rabia S, Has C, Matsuda F, Weissenbach J, Lathrop M, Prud'homme JF, Fischer J. Identification of mutations in a new gene encoding a FERM family protein with a pleckstrin homology domain in Kindler syndrome. *Hum Mol Genet* 2003;12:925–935.

125. El Hachem M, Diociaiuti A, Proto V, Fortugno P, Zambruno G, Castiglia D, Naim M. Kindler syndrome with severe mucosal involvement in a large Palestinian pedigree. *Eur J Dermatol* 2015;25:14–19.

126. Gupta V, Dogra D, Gupta N, Parveen S. Kindler's syndrome with long thick cuticles and mottled hyperpigmentation. *Indian J Dermatol Venereol Leprol* 2011;77:66–68.

127. Mizutani H, Masuda K, Nakamura N, Takenaka H, Tsuruta D, Katoh N. Cutaneous and laryngeal squamous cell carcinoma in mixed epidermolysis bullosa, Kindler syndrome. *Case Rep Dermatol* 2012;4:133–138.

128. Häberle M, Haneke E. Epidermolysis bullosa simplex herpetiformis Dowling-Meara. Jahrestagung der fränkisch-oberpfälzischen Dermatologen in Verbindung mit dem Tumorzentrum Erlangen, Erlangen, Nov 9, 1985, *Zbl Haut GeschlKr* 152:1–11.

129. Duarte AF, Correia O, Haneke E, Azevedo R, Jonkman MF. Pretibial epidermolysis bullosa—Case report. P0494. 22nd World Cong Dermatol, Seoul, May 24–29, 2011.

130. Chen M, Kim GH, Prakash L, Woodley DT. Epidermolysis bullosa acquisita: Autoimmunity to anchoring fibril collagen. *Autoimmunity* 2012;45:91–101.

131. Smahi A, Courtois G, Vabres P, Yamaoka S, Heuertz S, Munnich A, Israël A et al. Genomic rearrangement in NEMO impairs NF-kappaB activation and is a cause of incontinentia pigmenti. The International Incontinentia Pigmenti (IP) Consortium. *Nature* 2000;405:466–472.

132. Thakur S, Puri RD, Kohli S, Saxena R, Verma IC. Utility of molecular studies in incontinentia pigmenti patients. *Indian J Med Res* 2011;133: 442–445.

133. Conte MI, Pescatore A, Paciolla M, Esposito E, Miano MG, Lioi MB, McAleer MA et al. Insight into IKBKG/NEMO locus: Report of new mutations and complex genomic rearrangements leading to incontinentia pigmenti disease. *Hum Mutat* 2014;35:165–177.

134. Happle R. Lyonization and the lines of Blaschko. *Hum Genet* 1985;70:200–206.

135. Landy SJ, Donnai D. Incontinentia pigmenti (Bloch-Sulzberger syndrome). *J Med Genet* 1993;30:53–59.

136. Nicolaou N, Graham-Brown RA. Nail dystrophy, an unusual presentation of incontinentia pigmenti. *Br J Dermatol* 2003;149:1286–1288.

137. Bittar M, Danarti R, König A, Gal A, Happle R. Late-onset familial onychodystrophy heralding incontinentia pigmenti. *Acta Derm Venereol* 2005; 85:274–275.

138. Chun SR, Rashid RM. Delayed onychodystrophy of incontinentia pigmenti: An evidence-based review of epidemiology, diagnosis and management. *J Drugs Dermatol* 2010;9:350–354.

139. Hartman DL. Incontinentia pigmenti associated with subungual tumors. *Arch Dermatol* 1966;94:632–635.

140. Pinol Aguadé J, Mascaro JM, Herrero C, Castel T. Painful and spontaneously healing subungual dyskeratotic tumors; their relation to incontinentia pigmenti. *Ann Dermatol Syphiligr (Paris)* 1973;100: 159–168.

141. Mascaro JM, Palou J, Vives P. Painful subungual keratotic tumors in incontinentia pigmenti. *J Am Acad Dermatol* 1985;13:913–918.

142. Adeniran A, Townsend PL, Peachey RD. Incontinentia pigmenti (Bloch-Sulzberger syndrome) manifesting as painful periungual and subungual tumours. *J Hand Surg Br* 1993;18:667–669.

143. Montes CM, Maize JC, Guerry-Force ML. Incontinentia pigmenti with painful subungual tumors: A two-generation study. *J Am Acad Dermatol.* 2004;50(2 Suppl):S45–S52.

144. Young A, Manolson P, Cohen B, Klapper M, Barrett T. Painful subungual dyskeratotic tumors in incontinentia pigmenti. *J Am Acad Dermatol* 2005;52:726–729.

145. Lamb RC, Milne AW, Tavadia S. A subungual lesion on the finger of a young woman. *Int J Dermatol* 2012; 51:1177–1779.

146. Abimelec P, Rybojad M, Cambiaghi S, Moraillon I, Cavelier-Balloy B, Marx C, Morel P. Late, painful, subungual hyperkeratosis in incontinentia pigmenti. *Pediatr Dermatol* 1995;12:340–342.

147. Simmons DA, Kegel MF, Scher RK, Hines YC. Subungual tumors in incontinentia pigmenti. *Arch Dermatol* 1986;122:1431–1434.

148. Doyle TC, Nurse DS. Tuft erosion in incontinentia pigmenti. *Australas Radiol* 1987;31:304–305.

149. Malvehy J, Palou J, Mascaró JM. Painful subungual tumour in incontinentia pigmenti. Response to treatment with etretinate. *Br J Dermatol* 1998;138: 554–555.

150. Donati P, Muscardin L, Amantea A, Paolini F, Venuti A. Detection of HPV-15 in painful subungual tumors of incontinentia pigmenti: Successful topical therapy with retinoic acid. *Eur J Dermatol.* 2009;19:243–247.

151. Mahmoud BH, Zembowicz A, Fisher E. Controversies over subungual tumors in incontinentia pigmenti. *Dermatol Surg* 2014;40:1157–1159.

152. Pena ZG, Brewer JD. Multiple subungual squamous cell carcinomas in a patient with incontinentia pigmenti. *Dermatol Surg* 2014;40:1159–1161.

153. Baran R, Goettmann S. Distal digital keratoacanthoma: A report of 12 cases and a review of the literature. *Br J Dermatol* 1998;139:512–515.

154. El Aoud S, Frikha F, Snoussi M, Ben Salah R, Bahloul Z. Bilateral ptosis as a presenting feature of primary hypertrophic osteoarthropathy (pachydermoperiostosis): A case report. *Reumatismo* 2014;66: 249–253.

155. Lubach D, Freyschmidt J, Bolten D. Pachydermoperiostosis (Touraine-Solente-Golé syndrome). Clinical and radiological differential diagnosis. *Z Hautkr* 1981;56:175–186.

156. Uppal S, Diggle CP, Carr IM, Fishwick CW, Ahmed M, Ibrahim GH, Helliwell PS et al. Mutations in 15-hydroxyprostaglandin dehydrogenase cause primary hypertrophic osteoarthropathy. *Nat Genet* 2008;40:789–793.

157. Bergmann C, Wobser M, Morbach H, Falkenbach A, Wittenhagen D, Lassay L, Ott H, Zerres K, Girschick HJ, Hamm H. Primary hypertrophic osteoarthropathy with digital clubbing and palmoplantar hyperhidrosis caused by 15-PGHD/HPGD loss-of-function mutations. *Exp Dermatol* 2011;20:531–533.

158. Nakazawa S, Niizeki H, Matsuda M, Nakabayashi K, Seki A, Mori T, Tokura Y. Involvement of prostaglandin E2 in the first Japanese case of pachydermoperiostosis with HPGD mutation and recalcitrant leg ulcer. *J Dermatol Sci* 2015;78:153–155.

159. Wang L, Yu J, Li Y, Liu X, Zhang Z. Genetic diagnosis for a Chinese Han family with primary hypertrophic osteoarthropathy. *Zhonghua Yi Xue Yi Chuan Xue Za Zhi* 2015;32:213–217.

160. Zhang Z, Xia W, He J, Zhang Z, Ke Y, Yue H, Wang C et al. Exome sequencing identifies SLCO2A1 mutations as a cause of primary hypertrophic osteoarthropathy. *Am J Hum Genet* 2012;90:125–132.

161. Busch J, Frank V, Bachmann N, Otsuka A, Oji V, Metze D, Shah K et al. Mutations in the prostaglandin transporter SLCO2A1 cause primary hypertrophic osteoarthropathy with digital clubbing. *J Invest Dermatol* 2012;132:2473–2476.

162. Li S, Li Q, Wang Q, Chen D, Li J. Primary hypertrophic osteoarthropathy with myelofibrosis and anemia: A case report and review of literature. *Int J Clin Exp Med* 2015;8(1):1467–1471 eCollection 2015.

163. Kelle B, Yıldız F, Paydas S, Bagır EK, Ergin M, Kozanoglu E. Coexistência de osteoartropatia hipertrófica e mielofibrose. *Rev Bras Reumatol* 2015. pii: S0482-5004(14)00247-2, doi: 10.1016/j.rbr.2014.11.003. [Epub ahead of print]

164. Coury C. Hippocratic fingers and hypertrophic osteoarthropathy: Study of 350 cases. *Br J Dis Chest* 1960;54:202–209.

165. Tanese K, Niizeki H, Seki A, Otsuka A, Kabashima K, Kosaki K, Kuwahara M et al. Pathological characterization of pachydermia in pachydermoperiostosis. *J Dermatol* 2015;42:710–714.

166. Fournie B, Viraben R, Durroux R, Lassoued S, Gay R, Fournie A. Psoriatic onycho-pachydermo-periostitis of the big toe. Anatomo-clinical study and physiopathogenic approach apropos of 4 cases. *Rev Rhum Mal Osteoartic* 1989;56:579–582.

167. Schröder K, Goerdt S, Sieper J, Krasagakis K, Almond-Roesler B, Orfanos CE. Psoriatic onycho-pachydermo-periostitis (POPP). *Hautarzt* 1997;48:500–503.

168. Boisseau-Garsaud AM, Beylot-Barry M, Doutre MS, Beylot C, Baran R. Psoriatic onycho-pachydermo-periostitis. A variant of psoriatic distal interphalangeal arthritis? *Arch Dermatol* 1996;132:176–180.

169. Fietta P, Manganelli P. Pachydermoperiostosis and psoriatic onychopathy: An unusual association. *J Eur Acad Dermatol Venereol* 2003;17:73–76.

170. Goltz RW. Focal dermal hypoplasia. *Arch Dermatol* 1962;86:708–717.

171. Grzeschik KH, Bornholdt D, Oeffner F, König A, del Carmen Boente M, Enders H, Fritz B et al. Deficiency of *PORCN*, a regulator of Wnt signaling, is associated with focal dermal hypoplasia. *Nat Genet* 2007;39:833–835.

172. Clements SE, Wessagowit V, Lai-Cheong JE, Arita K, McGrath JA. Focal dermal hypoplasia resulting from a new nonsense mutation, p.E300X, in the PORCN gene. *J Dermatol Sci* 2008;49:39–42.

173. Alkindi S, Battin M, Aftimos S, Purvis D. Focal dermal hypoplasia due to a novel mutation in a boy with Klinefelter syndrome. *Pediatr Dermatol* 2013;30:476–479.

174. Kilmer SL, Grix AW Jr, Isseroff RR. Focal dermal hypoplasia: Four cases with widely varying presentations. *J Am Acad Dermatol* 1993;28:839–843.

175. Nagalo K, Laberge JM, Nguyen VH, Laberge-Caouette L, Turgeon J. Focal dermal hypoplasia (Goltz syndrome) in the neonate: Report of a case presenting with cleft lip and palate. *Arch Pédiatr* 2012;19:160–162.

176. Denis-Thely L, Cordier MP, Cambazard F, Misery L. Unilateral focal dermal hypoplasia. *Ann Dermatol Vénéréol* 2002;129:1161–1163.

177. Greer RO Jr, Reissner MW. Focal dermal hypoplasia. Current concepts and differential diagnosis. *J Periodontol* 1989;60:330–335.

178. Hardman CM, Garioch JJ, Eady RA, Fry L. Focal dermal hypoplasia: Report of a case with cutaneous and skeletal manifestations. *Clin Exp Dermatol* 1998;23:281–285.

179. Lopez-Porras RF, Arroyo C, Soto-Vega E. Focal dermal hypoplasia with uterus bicornis and renal ectopia: Case report and review of the literature. *Case Rep Dermatol* 2011;3:158–163.

180. Sutton VR, Van den Veyver IB. Focal dermal hypoplasia. In: Pagon RA, Bird TD, Dolan CR, Stephens K, Adam MP, eds. *GeneReviews™ [Internet]*, Seattle (WA): University of Washington, 1993–2008 May 15.

181. Happle R. Angioma serpiginosum is not caused by *PORCN* mutations. *Eur J Hum Genet* 2009;17:881–882.

182. Frieden IJ. Aplasia cutis congenita: A clinical review and proposal for classification. *J Am Acad Dermatol* 1986;14:646–660.

183. Elliott AM, Teebi AS. Further examples of autosomal dominant transmission of nonsyndromic aplasia cutis congenita. *Am J Med Genet* 1997;73:495–496.

184. Bart BJ. Epidermolysis bullosa and congenital localized absence of skin. *Arch Dermatol* 1970;101:78–81.

185. Medenica L, Lens M. Recessive dystrophic epidermolysis bullosa: Presentation of two forms. *Dermatol Online J* 2008;14(2):2.

186. Pfendner EG, Lucky AW. Junctional epidermolysis bullosa. In: Pagon RA, Bird TD, Dolan CR, Stephens K, Adam MP, eds. *GeneReviews™ [Internet]*, Seattle (WA): University of Washington, 1993–2008 Feb 22.

187. Marneros AG, Beck AE, Turner EH, McMillin MJ, Edwards MJ, Field M, de Macena Sobreira NL et al. Mutations in KCTD1 cause scalp-ear-nipple syndrome. *Am J Hum Genet* 2013;92:621–626.

188. Rodrigues RG. Aplasia cutis congenita, congenital heart lesions, and frontonasal cysts in four successive generations. *Clin Genet* 2007;71:558–560.

189. Naik P, Kini P, Chopra D, Gupta Y. Finlay-Marks syndrome: Report of two siblings and review of literature. *Am J Med Genet A* 2012;158A:1696–1701.

190. Bilginer B, Onal MB, Bahadir S, Akalan N. Aplasia cutis congenita of the scalp, skull and dura associated with Adams-Oliver syndrome. *Turk Neurosurg* 2008;18:191–193.

191. White SM, Fahey M. Report of a further family with dominant deafness-onychodystrophy (DDOD) syndrome. *Am J Med Genet A* 2011;155A:2512–2515.

192. Zelickson B, Matsumura K, Kist D, Epstein EH Jr, Bart BJ. Bart's syndrome: Ultrastructure and genetic linkage. *Arch Dermatol* 1995;131:663–668.

193. Superti-Furga A, Saesseli B, Steinmann B, Bollinger A. Microangiopathy in Ehlers–Danlos syndrome type IV. *Int J Microcirc Clin Exp* 1992;11:241–247.

194. Cohen PR, Milewicz DM. Dolichonychia in women with Marfan syndrome. *South Med J.* 2004;97:354–358.

195. Miescher G, Storck H. Abortive Ehlers–Danlos syndrome combined with abnormality of the nails. *Dermatologica* 1951;102:381–382.

196. Laugier P, Bulte C. Ehlers–Danlos syndrome and nail lesions. *Bull Soc Fr Dermatol Syphiligr* 1961;68:978–979.

197. Chakravarthi S, Goyal MK. Spontaneous pneumothorax in ataxia telangiectasia. *Indian J Med Res* 2014;140:321–322.

198. Swift M, Morrell D, Massey RB, Chase CL. Incidence of cancer in 161 families affected by ataxia-telangiectasia. *N Engl J Med* 1991;325:1831–1836.

199. Gschnait F, Grabner G, Brenner W, Tappeiner J. Ataxia telangiectasia (Louis–Bar syndrome). *Hautarzt* 1979;30:527–531.

200. Masutani C, Kusumoto R, Yamada A, Dohmae N, Yokoi M, Yuasa M, Araki M, Iwai S, Takio K, Hanaoka F. The XPV (xeroderma pigmentosum variant) gene encodes human DNA polymerase eta. *Nature* 1999;399(6737):700–704.

201. Kraemer KH, Lee MM, Scotto J. Xeroderma pigmentosum: Cutaneous, ocular, and neurologic abnormalities in 830 published cases. *Arch Dermatol* 1987;123:241–250.

202. Rebora A, Crovato F. PIBI(D)S syndrome–trichothiodystrophy with xeroderma pigmentosum (group D) mutation. *J Am Acad Dermatol* 1987;16:940–947.

203. Tullis GD, Lynde CW, McLean DI, Stewart WD. Multiple melanomas occurring in a patient with xeroderma pigmentosum. *J Am Acad Dermatol* 1984;11:364–367.

204. Krieger L, Berneburg M. Pigmentary lesions in patients with increased DNA damage due to defective DNA repair. *Ann Dermatol Venereol* 2012;139(Suppl 4):S130–S134.

205. Frouin E, Laugel V, Durand M, Dollfus H, Lipsker D. Dermatologic findings in 16 patients with Cockayne syndrome and cerebro-oculo-facial-skeletal syndrome. *JAMA Dermatol* 2013;149:1414–1418.

206. Monnat RJ Jr. "…Rewritten in the Skin": Clues to skin biology and aging from inherited disease. *J Invest Dermatol* 2015;135:1484–1490.

207. Tanenbaum MH. Werner's syndrome. Progeria of the adult. *Arch Intern Med* 1965;116:499–504.

208. Mansur AT, Elçioglu NH, Demirci GT. Werner syndrome: Clinical evaluation of two cases and a novel mutation. *Genet Couns* 2014;25:119–127.

209. Hallaji Z, Barzegari M, Kiavash K. Werner syndrome in an Iranian family. *Skinmed* 2010;8:184–186.

210. Duvic M, Lemak NA. Werner's syndrome. *Dermatol Clin* 1995;13:163–168.

211. Epstein CJ, Martin GM, Schultz AL, Motulsky AG. Werner's syndrome: A review of its symptomatology, natural history, pathologic features, genetics and relationship to the natural aging process. *Medicine (Baltimore)* 1966;45:177–221.

212. Goto M. Hierarchical deterioration of body systems in Werner's syndrome: Implications for normal ageing. *Mech Ageing Dev* 1997;98:239–254.

213. Gonullu E, Bilge NS, Kaşifoğlu T, Korkmaz C. Werner's syndrome may be lost in the shadow of the scleroderma. *Rheumatol Int* 2013;33:1309–1312.

214. Welsh O. Study of a family with a new progeroid syndrome. *Birth Defects Orig Artic Ser* 1975;11(5):25–38.

215. Fleischmajer R, Nedwich A. Werner's syndrome. *Am J Med* 1973;54:111–118.

216. Flanagan SP. "Nude," a new hairless gene with pleiotropic effects in the mouse. *Genet Res* 1966;8:295–309.

217. Lee D, Prowse DM, Brissette JL. Association between mouse nude gene expression and the initiation of epithelial terminal differentiation. *Dev Biol* 1999;208:362–374.

218. Schorpp M, Schlake T, Kreamalmeyer D, Allen PM, Boehm T. Genetically separable determinants of hair keratin gene expression. *Dev Dyn* 2000;218:537–543.

219. Koepf-Maier P, Mboneko VF, Merker HJ. Nude mice are not hairless. *Acta Anat* 1990;138:178–190.

220. Militzer K. Hair growth pattern in nude mice. *Cells Tissues Organs* 2001;168:285–294.

221. Mecklenburg L, Nakamura M, Sundberg JP, Paus R. The nude mouse skin phenotype: The role of Foxn1 in hair follicle development and cycling. *Exp Mol Pathol* 2001;71:171–178.

222. Pignata C, Fiore M, Guzzetta V, Castaldo A, Sebastio G, Porta F, Guarino A. Congenital Alopecia and nail dystrophy associated with severe functional T-cell immunodeficiency in two sibs. *Am J Med Genet* 1996;65:167–170.

223. Frank J, Pignata C, Panteleyev AA, Prowse DM, Baden H, Weiner L, Gaetaniello L et al. Exposing the human nude phenotype. *Nature* 19993;98:473–474.

224. Pignata C. A lesson to unraveling complex aspects of novel immunodeficiencies from the human equivalent of the nude/SCID phenotype. *Journal of Hematotherapy and Stem Cell Research* 2002;11:409–414.

225. Adriani M, Martinez-Mir A, Fusco F, Busiello R, Frank J, Telese S, Matrecano E, Ursini MV, Christiano AM, Pignata C. Ancestral founder mutation of the nude (FOXN1) gene in congenital severe combined immunodeficiency associated with alopecia in southern Italy population. *Ann Hum Genet* 2004;68:265–268.

226. Amorosi S, D'Armiento M, Calcagno G, Russo I, Adriani M, Christiano AM, Weiner L, Brissette JL, Pignata C. FOXN1 homozygous mutation associated with anencephaly and severe neural tube defect in human athymic Nude/SCID fetus. *Clin Genet* 2008;73:380–384.

227. Levy E, Neven B, Entz-Werle N, Cribier B, Lipsker D. Post-thymus transplant vitiligo in a child with Foxn1 deficiency. *Ann Dermatol Venereol* 2012;139:468–471.

228. Fleckman P, Jaeger K, Silva KA, Sundberg JP. Comparative anatomy of mouse and human nail units. *Anat Rec (Hoboken)* 2013;296:521–532.

229. Morita K, Hogan ME, Nanney LB, King LE, Manabe M, Sun TT, Sundberg JP. Cutaneous ultrastructural features of the flaky skin (fsn) mouse mutation. *J Dermatol* 1995;22:385–395.

230. Fleckman P. Current and future nail research—Areas ripe for study. *Skin Pharmacol Appl Skin Physiol* 1999;12:146–153.

231. Paus R, Peker S. Biology of hair and nail. In: Bologna JL, Jorizzo JL, Rapini RP, eds. *Dermatology*, London: Mosby, 2003; 1007–1032.

232. Auricchio L, Adriani M, Frank J, Busiello R, Christiano A, Pignata C. Nail dystrophy associated with a heterozygous mutation of the Nude/SCID human FOXN1 (WHN) gene. *Arch Dermatol* 2005;141:647–648.

233. Mecklenburg L, Paus R, Halata Z, Bechtold LS, Fleckman P, Sundbergy JP. FOXN1 is critical for onycholemmal terminal differentiation in nude (Foxn1nu) mice. *J Invest Dermatol* 2004;123:1001–1011.

234. Fanti PA, Tosti A, Cameli N, Varotti C. Nail matrix hypergranulosis. *Am J Dermatopathol* 1994;16:607–610.

235. Krebsova A, Hamm H, Karl S, Reis A, Hennies HC. Assignment of the gene for a new hereditary nail disorder, isolated congenital nail dysplasia, to chromosome 17p13. *J Invest Dermatol* 2000;115:664–667.

236. Fleckman P, Omura EF. Histopathology of the nail. *Adv Dermatol* 2001;17:385–406.

Nail specific conditions

This chapter intends to describe lesions that are not observed elsewhere in the body. They comprise specific nail plate alterations and therapeutic and cosmetic effects on the nail.

7.1 ANONYCHIA AND HYPONYCHIA

Anonychia is the absence of nail. It may be hereditary or acquired. Isolated anonychia has been described as an autosomal dominant as well as a recessive trait.[1–4] Sporadic cases occur.[5] Often, some nails are lacking and others are hypoplastic or the nails of some fingers, such as the thumb, are absent.[6] The association of both nail aplasia and hypoplasia suggests that the development of the nail anlage was arrested at different time points.[7] Aplastic anonychia is observed when the distal phalanx is absent.[8–10] Here a tiny keratotic spicule may be seen at the tip in prolongation of the finger axis, which may be taken as evidence that the nail development starts at the most distal point and not at the dorsum of the digit.[11] Anonychia keratodes is a condition where the nail field does not have a nail plate and only some keratosis is present instead of a nail. Many congenital syndromes are associated with anonychia or hyponychia.[12] The onychotic types of ectodermal dysplasias usually have a hypoplastic nail. Progressive loss of the nail is commonly seen in hereditary epidermolysis bullosa, particularly in the dystrophic forms. Acquired anonychia or hyponychia may be due to trauma or drugs.

Clinically, either the nail is completely lacking with a smooth tip of the digit as in anonychia aplastica, or the nail field may be barely discernable and show some keratosis as in anonychia keratodes. In many ectodermal dysplasias, the nails are usually small or malformed and brittle. In the various forms of epidermolsysis bullosa hereditaria that affect the nail, children may be born with normal nails as in most cases of the simplex types, but they may already show some damage at birth in the severe junctional and dystrophic types. Particularly in epidermolysis bullosa hereditaria dystrophica of Hallopeau-Siemens, the nails become progressively atrophic until they are lost completely.

7.1.1 Histopathology

In complete anonychia, normal or atrophic skin is seen. Anonychia keratodes shows a rudimentary proximal nail fold and matrix and the nail bed exhibits a metaplastic acanthotic epidermis with a marked horny layer and a stratum lucidum, or the matrix is lacking.[13] No histopathologic criteria of hypoplastic nails have been studied. In acquired anonychia, whether due to epidermolysis bullosa, trauma, or drug, the skin is usually atrophic. Until now, no attempt has been made to characterize the nails in the different forms of anonychia, hyponychia, ectodermal dysplasias, and other malformation syndromes.

7.1.2 Differential diagnosis

In rudimentary polydactyly, the digital tip was covered with a stratum corneum instead of an accessory nail.[14]

7.2 LEUKONYCHIA

White nail coloration is called leukonychia. Three types of white nails are distinguished: true leukonychia where the white color originates from the matrix and hence is in the nail, apparent leukonychia, which is due to pale or whitish subungual tissue, and pseudoleukonychia, mainly due to (superficial) fungal infection.

There are different types of true leukonychia, both morphologically as well as etiologically. The most common type is called leukonychia vulgaris, or gift spots, which may be congenital or acquired. Leukonychia may be punctate, striate, macular, or total. Particularly the punctate and striate leukonychias are due to minor trauma, most commonly to overzealous manicure. The white color is thought to be due to light reflection by nucleated cells that are not correctly keratinized. The idea of small air blisters in the nail as cause of leukonychia has been rejected.[15] When looking through a leukonychotic spot it appears dark. Total leukonychia is seen isolated and as part of various syndromes.[16,17] Probably another mechanism of development as the reason for acquired total leukonychia is prolonged contact with salt solutions.[18,19] Subtotal diffuse leukonychia is characterized by a pink distal margin; it may be a phase of total leukonychia. Half-and-half nails or Lindsay's nails are characteristic for chronic kidney disease where it is seen in 20%–50% of the cases.[20] They show a proximal white zone and a distal brownish area; their proportion is roughly 20%–60%.[21] Transverse leukonychia may occur as a white band parallel to the lunula border and usually occurs in all nails at the same site. Different acute systemic diseases may be the cause. The leukopathias described in the older literature, which were due to thallium, arsenic or antimonium intoxication, or infections as in tuberculosis or typhoid, most probably belong to this group. Repeated white bands may reflect courses of chemotherapy or menstruation.[22] However, spontaneous resolution of leukonychia during late pregnancy was also observed.[23] White bands were seen in proximal white subungual onychomycosis thought to be due to fungal spread via local blood or lymph vessels.[24] Superficial white onychomycosis[25,26] is a so-called pseudo-leukonychia, but subungual onychomycosis may also appear as white spots.[27] They are due to *Trichophyton* species as well as some molds, particularly *Fusarium* spp.[28]

7.2.1 Histopathology

Although there are only a few studies on the histopathology of common leukonychia, it appears that most types are due to incomplete (par)onychotization, or in another term, parakeratosis in the nail plate.[15,29]

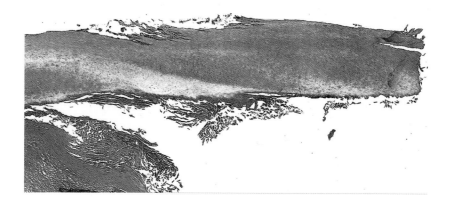

Figure 7.1 Leukonychia exhibits nail cells with an eosinophilic cytoplasm. These cells are arranged in an oblique manner from proximal-superficial to distal-deep.

Most transverse banded leukonychias are characterized by large areas of onychocytes in the nail containing nuclei, exhibiting a markedly eosinophilic cytoplasm in contrast to the normal very pale or clear appearance, and having cell membranes visible both in H&E as well as PAS stains (Figure 7.1). This is also seen in multiple transverse bands. The area of nucleated nail plate cells is arranged in a distal-deep direction and usually does not affect the nail plate surface. The former reflects the way of nail regeneration. In the old literature, leukonychotic cells were found to stand out after gold impregnation and seen in dark-field illumination.[30]

An increase in vessel wall thickness and melanin deposition were seen in the distal nail bed of half-and-half nails.[21]

In a family with hereditary diffuse (sub)total leukonychia, both the proximal and distal nail matrix had a broad granular layer. The nail plate was markedly parakeratotic and its superficial layer had a loose, lamellar appearance. The upper plate appeared to shed packages of horny cells at the surface and rapidly decreased in thickness, finally disappearing at two-thirds of the total nail length. The nail bed was normal without a granular layer.[31] Electron microscopy showed abnormal keratinization of the proximal matrix with abundant keratohyaline-like, electron-dense granules in the cytoplasm of the uppermost keratinocytes of the matrix. The most striking features were numerous intracellular nonmembrane-bound lipid-like droplets that appeared in the proximal matrix and grew in size by coalescence in the cornifying cells of the upper nail plate. These electron-lucent inclusions displayed amorphous contents.

In longitudinal leukonychia, a mound of keratinocytes results in loss of transparency thus making the nail appear whitish;[27] most cases were either subungual filamentous tumors or onychopapillomas.

7.2.2 Differential diagnosis

A PAS or Grocott stain is necessary to rule out fungal pseudoleukonychia. Longitudinal white to grayish bands are seen in Darier's and Hailey-Hailey disease, in epidermal hamartoma[32] due to nevoid matrix changes,[33] or in Bowen's disease.

7.3 ERYTHRONYCHIA

Red nails occur as two distinct signs: longitudinal erythronychia as a red streak from the lunula to the hyponychium[34] and red lunula.[35]

Longitudinal erythronychia is seen in Darier's and Hailey-Hailey's disease, in warty dyskeratoma of the nail bed, in lichen planus, in subungual filamentous tumor, localized multinucleate distal subungual keratosis, onychopapilloma, acantholytic dyskeratotic acanthoma, Bowen's disease, and celiac disease. In many cases of glomus tumors, a broad violaceous-red streak is seen extending distally from the tumor. Except for dyskeratosis follicularis of Darier, pemphigus familiaris benignus of Hailey-Hailey, amyloidosis, celiac disease,[36] and graft-versus-host disease,[37] the other conditions cause monodactylous lines. An idiopathic polydactylous erythronychia associated with[38] or without[39-41] pain and nail fragility was also described.

Red lunulae may be seen in a great number of different dermatologic,[42] cardiovascular, gastrointestinal, endocrine, hematologic, infectious, neoplastic, pulmonary, and rheumatologic disorders and were also observed in proteinuria, cerebrovascular accident, liver cirrhosis, and due to repeated trauma. The causal relationship is not always clear. The red color may be diffuse or punctuate.

7.3.1 Histopathology

There are distinct histopathologic features in Darier's and Hailey-Hailey's disease (see Chapter 6) as well as warty dyskeratoma, which however may be difficult to distinguish from each other. Subungual filamentous tumor, localized multinucleate distal subungual keratosis, and onychopapilloma can also be differentiated although it is not yet clear whether distal subungual keratosis is a variant of onychopapilloma. In idiopathic longitudinal erythronychia, a longitudinal thinning of the nail plate due

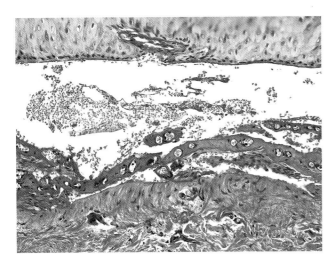

Figure 7.2 Capillary proliferation in the superficial dermis of the distal matrix caused a reddish spot in the lunula. In such a case, blood may be degraded to hemosiderin and blood droplets may also be included in the nail.

to a localized defective nail formation in the distal matrix may cause a vascular phenomenon of decompression with hyperemia along the nail thinning whereas the rest of the nail compresses the matrix and nail bed vessels keeping them pale.[43] In Bowen's disease, atypical keratinocytes allow the correct diagnosis to be made. We have seen a capillary proliferation in the proximal nail bed causing a red spot in the lunula (Figure 7.2). Another red spot was seen in the lunula that turned out to be a traumatic matrix cyst.

Red lunulae may reveal the features of the basic dermatosis although this is not always the case.[44]

7.3.2 Differential diagnosis

There are many different causes, some of which can be ascribed to a specific diagnosis. Keratotic debris containing large amounts of round single necrotic keratinocytes is found in subungual squamous cell carcinoma.

7.4 GREEN NAILS

Green nails, also called chloronychia, are a common sign of *Pseudomonas aeruginosa* colonization or infection of onycholytic nails. In most cases, the lateral margin of one or more fingernails is greenish ranging from light to almost black-green. The color is most intense at the margin and fades off toward the center of the plate. However, almost the entire nail may be green depending on the degree of onycholysis and its underlying pathology. Usually, there is a concomitant paronychia when the green color extends under the proximal nail fold.[45] Chloronychia may also develop after a subungual hematoma.[46] A green color in the middle of the nail is either a sign of marked onycholysis with heavy *Pseudomonas aeruginosa* colonization or even of a subungual *Pseudomonas* abscess. The green color results from the production of the soluble pigments pyocyanin and pyoverdin.[47]

Figure 7.3 Pseudomonas biofilm at the undersurface of the nail plate with faint yellowish-green staining of the nail plate.

The treatment is either with a disinfective solution, brushing with diluted vinegar, ciprofloxacin, nadifloxacin, or tobramycin.[48–50]

7.4.1 Histopathology

Clippings from *Pseudomonas* nails may show a slightly dark tinge, but in most cases there is also a bacterial biofilm at the undersurface of the nail plate (Figure 7.3). The nature of the bacteria cannot be clarified by histopathology. PAS stain may show fungal invasion in addition as this may facilitate *Pseudomonas* colonization.

In *Pseudomonas* abscess, the undersurface of the nail is tinted greenish. Under it, a lake of pus is seen, and the bottom is formed by superficial granulation tissue in the center and severely infiltrated matrix epithelium at the margin that may even show spongiform pustule formation.

7.4.2 Differential diagnosis

All dark pigmentations have to be considered. In the histologic slides, the green color is not seen.

7.5 BROWN AND BLACK NAILS (EXCLUDING MELANIN-INDUCED MELANONYCHIA)

A variety of microorganisms, dark substances, dirt, and chemicals can stain the nail brown to black.

Pigmentation due to *Proteus* spp. and *Klebsiella* spp. is usually seen either at the lateral margin or coming out from under the proximal nail fold that shows a mild but chronic paronychia.[51,52] The nail plate is often irregularly and transversely ridged.

Fungal melanonychia is frequently shaped like a spike or wedge with the base at the distal end of the nail plate. Superficial black onychomycosis is due to *Scytalidium dimidiatum*, rarely also to *Trichophyton rubrum*, but altogether 21 dematiaceous and 8 nondematiaceous fungi were identified as causing fungal melanonychia.[53–56] Among molds, *Aspergillus niger* may cause black discoloration often surrounded by a milky white nail.[57,58] Yeasts may cause brown nails.[59–61]

Tar stains the skin and nails, but it can easily be removed with a fatty ointment or an organic solvent. Brown nail staining from excessive smoking is common, but has not yet been studied histopathologically.

A diffuse brown stain of the nails is often seen when potassium permanganate baths were used for a longer period. The surrounding skin also shows a dirty brown. The nail grows out with normal color from the proximal nail fold. The brown stain is due to manganese dioxide, which is produced from the potassium permanganate. It can be reduced to colorless manganese oxide: Rubbing the nail surface with gauze that was soaked in ascorbic acid 5%–10% makes the unsightly nail look almost normal again.

The most obvious black nail stain is by silver nitrate, either as a solution or by applying a stick, called *lapis infernalis*. It is still often used to cauterize granulation tissue and oozing lesions. First being white it rapidly turns black under the influence of light. The nail may be colored black when silver nitrate solution spills over on the nail or the nail is rubbed with the silver nitrate stick. The nail plate grows out normally with a border parallel to that of the proximal nail fold. We have seen twice that an oozing amelanotic melanoma had been cauterized without a diagnosis and the black color from the silver finally made the surgeon refer the patient to us for the diagnosis of melanoma.

7.5.1 Histopathology

Clippings from *Proteus* or *Klebsiella* nails with a dirty gray color, either coming out from under the proximal nail fold or at the lateral margin, give a slightly grayish tinge of the nail surface when this is stained lightly with hematoxylin and eosin. The nail plate itself shows multiple transverse furrows. The nature of the pigment cannot be clarified. It develops because these enterobacteria produce hydrogen sulfide that reacts with heavy metals contaminating the environment. The metal sulfides precipitate on the nail surface giving it the dirty stain.[50]

In Central Europe, onychomycosis nigricans is seen due to some strains of *Trichophyton rubrum* var. *nigricans* that produce a soluble melanin-type pigment, whereas molds are more common in hot climate.[62] The soluble fungal melanin is seen as a diffuse yellow color both in H&E and PAS stained nails. One case of melanonychia was seen due to Medlar bodies.[63] These are sclerotic or muriform cells of several dematiaceous pigmented fungi and are characterized by three-dimensional septation; common causes of chromoblastomycosis are *Fonsecaea pedrosoi*, *Fonsecaea compacta*, *Cladosporium carrionii*, *Phialophora verrucosa*, *Rhinocladiella aquaspersa*, and *Aureobasidium pullulans*. The fungi are identified by PAS or Grocott stains. We have seen thick-walled pigmented spores in a wooden splinter under the nail in a female patient without the history of travel to subtropical or tropical regions (Figure 4.22). Darkly pigmented spores and hyphae were also seen in a patient with onychogryphosis (Figure 4.20).

Tar is not seen in histologic slides of nails as it is fat soluble and removed during the processing.

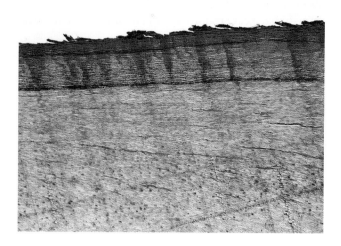

Figure 7.4 Silver nitrate imbibition of the superficial layers of the nail plate shows jet-black granules in the plate.

Silver nitrate stains between one-third to one-half of the superficial portion of the nail plate. In H&E sections, it is seen as relatively large round jet-black granules several times larger than human melanin granules (Figure 7.4).

Greenish-brown chromonychia was seen due to hemosiderin from a proliferation of markedly dilated capillaries and showed small Prussian blue positive granules in the nail plate over the distal matrix.[64] However, hemosiderin in the nail is an exceptional finding that can only be explained by hemosiderin getting into the matrix epithelium from the dermis as blood of hematomas is not degraded by macrophages.

7.5.2 Differential diagnosis

All dark pigmentations have to be considered in the differential diagnosis of brown and black nails. Whatever the cause of melanin in the nail, human melanin is intracellular, finely granular, and can be stained with the argentaffin reaction of Fontana-Masson. Blood is included in the nail between the nail cells as large accumulations. Fungal melanonychia is usually identified by fungal stains. Some clinically evident nail pigmentations cannot be seen on histopathologic slides. Brown pigmentation due to human melanin is dealt with in Chapter 15 on melanocytic lesions.

7.6 SUBUNGUAL HEMATOMA

Two types of subungual hematoma can be distinguished: acute due to a more or less heavy trauma, and chronic due to repeated minor trauma such as friction. Most hematomas appear as black areas under the nail; however, dermatoscopy usually shows a reddish tinge and an irregular distal border often corresponding to the rete ridges of the nail bed, or globules of variable size are seen. Frictional hematoma is most commonly seen on the big toe[65] whereas acute hematoma may be due to the blow of a hammer or a car door crush injury hitting the fingernail or fall of a heavy object on the toes.[66] Particularly a blow or crush injury often causes a small leukonychia over the hematoma. Acute traumatic hematomas occupying more than 50% of the visible nail are often associated with a fracture of the terminal phalanx requiring an X-ray and nail bed repair.[67] Frictional hematomas are often oval with their long axis in longitudinal direction; most are located on the lateral aspect of the big toenail as a result of rubbing of the first to the second toe. They frequently have a yellow margin either from the perilesional onycholysis or from blood decomposition. Subungual hematomas never involve the free margin of the nail in contrast to longitudinal melanonychia. Treatment of acute hematomas is by trephination of the overlying nail plate as long as the blood is still liquid so that it can escape and the pain, which is mainly due to the pressure of the hematoma squeezed between the nail plate and bed, almost instantaneously disappears.

7.6.1 Histopathology

Hematomas are not commonly biopsied, but after a heavy trauma with a large area of hematoma the nail may dissolve from the bed and can be clipped and examined. In an H&E stained section, the blood is seen as a flat oval eosinophilic mass included in the regrown nail by a thin deep nail lamella. Blood invariably remains extracellular (Figure 7.5). The hematoma is always oriented with its proximal part being more superficial thus allowing even the nail growth direction to be determined from a longitudinal section. Under polarized light, the nail plate shows a bright birefringence around the dark blood accumulation (Figure 7.5c). In the beginning, the hematoma is delimited by matrix epithelium and the overlying nail plate, later by the nail also at its deep border and therefore has no contact with the body's phagocytic system. Hence, blood of the hematoma is not degraded to hemosiderin and the Prussian blue reaction remains negative. Blood can, however, be specifically demonstrated with the pseudocatalase reaction (benzidine reaction)[68,69] and also with patent blue, which is a less specific and completely different agent staining hemoglobin an intense blue-green.[70]

7.6.2 Differential diagnosis

All dark pigmentations have to be considered in the differential diagnosis of brown and black nails. Melanin is finely granular, is intracellular, and can be stained with the argentaffin reaction of Fontana-Masson. Blood can also be demonstrated by scraping the dark pigment into a small test tube, adding a few drops of distilled water, agitating it for some minutes, and immersing a test strip for blood as used for the diagnosis of hematuria or fecal blood.[68]

7.7 ONYCHOLYSIS

The separation of the nail from the hyponychium and distal nail bed is called onycholysis. It is a frequent phenomenon that is in most cases nonspecific. It may be of traumatic, inflammatory, or neoplastic origin or drug-induced with the first being the most frequent.[71] Once the firm physiologic attachment of the distal nail with the hyponychium is lost, the nail plate—nail bed attachment—is easily damaged by simple procedures such as cleaning the nail. Dirt is accumulating under the detached nail inciting the patient to clean even more, and this vicious cycle of dirt accumulation—cleaning—detachment of the nail aggravates the onycholysis. This condition is called onycholysis semilunaris and almost invariably due to manicure. The nail overlying the onycholysis is usually white to ivory to yellowish depending on the original condition and some other factors such as profession or nail adornments. Onycholysis is often seen on one edge of the big toenail and probably due to friction, but it is clinically often misdiagnosed as an onychomycosis.[72–74] Onycholysis is a very frequent feature of nail psoriasis and is due to the loose attachment of the parakeratotic cells. However, any process leading to nail bed keratinization will eventually cause onycholysis. In taxane-induced onycholysis, there is often a hemorrhagic component. Oozing onycholysis is usually a sign of an advanced subungual malignancy, most commonly a squamous cell carcinoma or ulcerated melanoma.

The "disappearing nail bed" is shrinkage of the nail bed[75] due to long-standing onycholysis or loss of the nail,

(a)

(b)

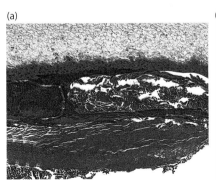
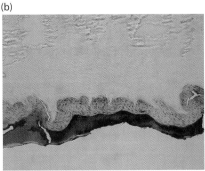

(c)

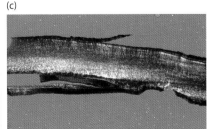

Figure 7.5 A subungual frictional hematoma is squeezed between the nail plate and subungual keratin. There is a dark eosinophilic parakeratotic layer under the nail plate, then blood inclusions and keratotic debris, then an orthokeratotic nail bed keratosis. (a) H&E stain. (b) PAS stain. (c) Traumatic subungual hematoma, already being included in the nail by a thin nail layer at its bottom. Giemsa stain, 50% polarization.

the latter most commonly on the big toenail. It is stage V in the grading system of onycholysis.[76]

7.7.1 Histopathology

Onycholysis is histopathologically characterized by a split formation between the nail plate and nail bed that may, depending on its severity, reach almost to the matrix. The nail bed shows an epidermal type of keratinization, which may be mild or very thick elevating the nail from the bed. Usually, no specific diagnosis can be made except in onychomycosis, psoriasis, and sometimes nail bed lichen planus. The nail plate often shows a thick bacterial biofilm at its undersurface that stains basophilic in H&E and PAS stains (Figure 7.3). In onycholysis semilunaris, the nail plate undersurface may have lost its characteristic wavy relief as it is maniacally scraped off by some patients.

Immunohistochemically, nail bed keratinocytes express a nonspecific cross-reacting antigen of the carcinoembryonic antigen (CEA) family in the central cells of the nail bed; this was believed to be linked to nail plate adhesion to the nail bed.[77]

The disappearing nail bed of the big toe is characterized by an extremely short nail bed and the development of a false distal nail fold. Histopathology shows that the hyponychium is still present but dislocated dorso-proximally. The nail bed exhibits a granular layer and orthohyperkeratosis and the distal nail fold is normal ridged skin of the tip of the toe.

7.7.2 Differential diagnosis

The origin of the onycholysis can often not be determined by histopathology. Except for specific nail diseases, just the diagnosis of onycholysis can be made. A PAS stain should always be made to rule out a mycotic pathogenesis. A nail clipping is often adequate to rule out onychomycosis and psoriasis.[78]

7.8 SUBUNGUAL HYPERKERATOSIS

Hyperkeratosis of the nail bed is one of the very common signs of a variety of nail diseases, among which psoriasis and onychomycosis are the most frequent ones. As such, subungual hyperkeratosis is a nonspecific sign, but biopsy can often clarify the nature of the underlying cause.[79] Further nail disorders characterized by subungual hyperkeratosis are pityriasis rubra pilaris,[80] subungual epidermoid inclusions,[81] acrokeratosis paraneoplastica of Bazex,[82] Sézary's syndrome, and it is often grotesque in pachyonychia congenita.[83] Painful subungual hyperkeratosis is characteristic for incontinentia pigmenti of Bloch–Sulzberger. In most nail conditions, the hyperkeratosis slowly extends proximally and one of the most consistent sequels is onycholysis as the subungual keratosis and the overlying nail plate are not firmly attached to each other. Subungual hyperkeratosis can also be associated with drug intake,[84] nail hardeners,[85] systemic malignancies,[86] ectodermal dysplasia,[87] punctate keratoderma,[88] and many more conditions.

Unilateral subungual hyperkeratosis is exceptional and may be a hint at a cerebrovascular accident.[89]

7.8.1 Histopathology

In contrast to normal skin, the nail bed epithelium most commonly reacts to irritation with epidermization, develops a granular layer and produces keratin, in most instances orthokeratosis, even in severe inflammation.[90] In psoriasis, the subungual hyperkeratosis may contain serum and neutrophils and often obliquely arranged columns of parakeratosis are seen. They commonly contain pycnotic neutrophils in the manner of Munro's microabscesses (see Section 3.1). In distal subungual onychomycosis, parakeratotic columns are rare. The subungual hyperkeratosis contains most of the pathogenic fungi, often in huge amounts. Collections of dried neutrophils are also seen in subungual onychomycosis; however, a PAS or Grocott stain will reveal fungi, and it has repeatedly been shown that histomycology is approximately double as sensitive as mycologic cultures.[91–93] Other causes of subungual hyperkeratosis usually only show epidermization and require more material for a specific histopathologic diagnosis. Portions of the subungual hyperkeratosis may contain areas of granular parakeratosis, particularly in the big toe; this is usually a sign of trauma.

7.8.2 Differential diagnosis

There are many different causes, some of which can be ascribed to a specific diagnosis. Keratotic debris containing large amounts of round single necrotic keratinocytes is found in subungual squamous cell carcinoma and seen in subungual tumors of incontinentia pigmenti.

7.9 ONYCHOGRYPOSIS

Onychogryposis, usually misspelled as onychogryphosis, is an extremely thick nail in the shape of a ram's horn.* In most cases, the big toenail is affected, but lesser toes and very rarely fingernails may also be involved. The nail grows up instead of out, is transformed into a hard keratin mass, is usually curved upward or to one side and may reach the toe again where it may cause a pressure ulcer. The patients are often debilitated or neglected elderly persons, but peripheral neuropathy may also be a reason. Ichthyosis and psoriasis as well as a variety of other diseases have been observed in association with onychogryposis; however, it is not always clear whether this was a causal relationship or a chance association. Congenital malalignment of the big toenail when left untreated may develop into onychogryposis even in persons between 20 and 30 years of age. Syndromic onychogryposis is seen in the Haim-Munk variant of Papillon–Lefèvre syndrome.[94,95] Clinically, the nail field is small and triangular and covered with a parchment-like keratinous membrane, a distal nail fold is

---

* Grypos (γρυπος Greek) is horn; gryphos (γρυφος), Latin gryphus, is a mythic animal with the head of a bird and the body of a lion, thus the correct term is onychogryposis and not onychogryphosis.

seen, and the nail pocket is very short as felt when inserting a nail elevator under the proximal nail fold.

7.9.1 Histopathology

Onychogrypotic nails require a long time of softening in order to be cut and to get reasonably good sections; we immerse them for 8–10 days in cedar oil before processing them. The nail looks like a pile of keratin lamellae one above the other that tend to split at irregular distances. The nail pocket is reduced to a tiny invagination (Figure 7.6). Parakeratosis is a common finding.[96] Sometimes, some fungal hyphae or spores in irregular arrangement may be seen (Figure 4.20). When the onychogryposis is turned plantarly, huge masses of keratin debris are seen at its undersurface. The nail bed is covered with a thick, mostly orthokeratotic horny layer.

7.9.2 Differential diagnosis

The most important differential diagnosis is pachyonychia congenita. However, tremendous subungual hyperkeratoses can also develop in ungual psoriasis and onychomycosis.

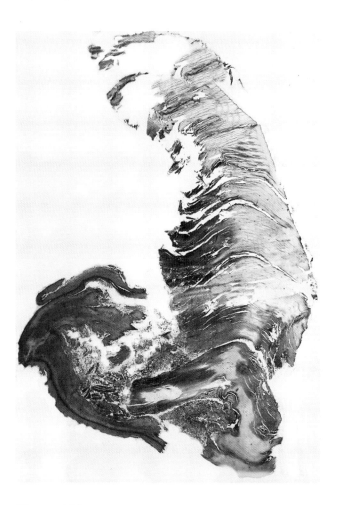

Figure 7.6 Onychogryposis is characterized by an enormously thick nail made up of many stacks of nail lamellae. The matrix is seen on the lower left corner. The nail pocket is very shallow and contains keratotic debris.

7.10 PTERYGIUM INVERSUM

The distal extension of the hyponychium is called pterygium inversum or ventral pterygium.[97] No distal groove is seen anymore. The congenital type was called painful aberrant hyponychium.[98] Some cases were familiar.[99] Systemic acral scleroderma and lupus erythematosus are other common causes,[100,101] but other conditions were also described.[102,103] Recently, new nomenclature was proposed: (1) Congenital aberrant hyponychium, (2) acquired pterygium inversum, and (3) acquired reversible extended hyponychium.[104] The chief complaint is pain when trimming the nails.

7.10.1 Histopathology

There is epidermal hyperplasia and considerable hyperkeratosis that is firmly attached to the nail plate. Some parakeratosis may be present.[104,105] The distal groove is no longer discernable. The nail plate is completely normal. In one case, there seemed to be an increase in the number of glomus bodies and nerve fibers thought to be responsible for the pain.[104] The pterygium inversum may be seen as an abnormal nail isthmus.[106,107]

7.10.2 Differential diagnosis

Any hyperkeratosis of the hyponychium has to be considered. It is useful to differentiate secondary pterygium inversum due to systemic scleroderma, systemic lupus erythematosus, and ischemia from the primary type.

7.11 PTERYGIUM

A pterygium is a wing-like structure obliterating the proximal nail fold. In most cases, this dorsal pterygium is due to a cicatricial process. It may be caused by a trauma or a scarring dermatosis; congenital pterygium is very rare. This process usually starts in the central or paramedian matrix area and may slowly extend causing a split in the nail, then dividing it into two parts until the nail disappears completely when the entire matrix is involved. In most cases, the fingers are affected.[108–110] The most common causes are lichen planus and trauma, but pterygium formation was also observed with a variety of other conditions.

7.11.1 Histopathology

An excisional biopsy of a dorsal pterygium shows scar tissue covered with a smooth epidermis (Figure 7.7). One biopsy showed a mild inflammation.[111] In lichen planus, some lichenoid lymphocytic infiltrate may be seen at the margin of the pterygium.

7.11.2 Differential diagnosis

All scars stretching from the proximal nail fold to the matrix are in fact a pterygium.

7.12 OVERCURVATURE (PINCER NAIL)

Transverse overcurvature is a very common condition. In most cases, the curvature increases from proximal to distal and pinches the distal part of the nail bed. This gives

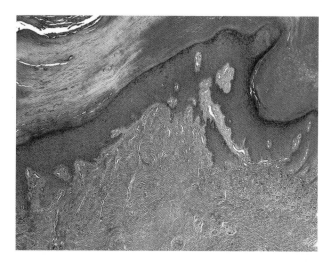

Figure 7.7 Cicatricial pterygium in an old ungual lichen planus. No inflammation is seen.

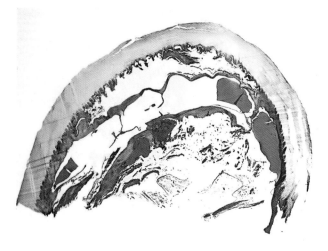

Figure 7.8 Transversely cut overcurved nail shows crenellated subungual keratin with plasma inclusions and subungual frictional hematoma.

the nail the appearance of a trumpet or omega, and in very marked cases, the form of a closed roll.[112] There are several etiopathogenetic variants:

1. The most common is hereditary, develops often around the age of 30, and is symmetrical with involvement of the big toenails, which show a lateral deviation of their long axis. When the lesser toenails are involved, they are medially deviated. The condition often remains painless, but may lead to excruciating pain. The cause of this overcurvature is an underlying bone deformity with a large medial exophyte distal to the base of the terminal phalanx of the great toe and a smaller one on the lateral condylus. This unrolls the curved nail proximally leading to an aggravation of the curvature distally.[113] Systematic X-ray examinations have shown that there is also a traction osteophyte on the distal dorsal tuft of the terminal phalanx and a lateral deviation of the terminal big toenail phalanx.[113]

2. Acquired transverse overcurvature may be associated with foot deformity. This is not symmetrical and the lesser toes are either not or also not symmetrically involved.

3. Some dermatoses, such as psoriasis or onychomycosis, may cause transverse overcurvature.[114] The nail in pachyonychia congenita covers the huge nail bed keratosis like a horseshoe.

4. Fingernail overcurvature is usually associated with degenerative distal interphalangeal osteoarthritis with Heberden nodes.

The treatment of pincer nails is either conservative with nail softening, braces, and clips,[115,116] or surgical with either phenolization of the lateral matrix horns or nail narrowing plus a nail bed plasty.[113,117,118]

7.12.1 Histopathology

Transverse sections of an avulsed overcurved nail show a marked curvature of the thick nail plate and massive subungual hyperkeratosis that is crenellated reflecting the hypertrophy of the nail bed (Figure 7.8). This

hyperkeratosis is produced by the nail bed as a response to the nail plate tending to lift up; the nail bed produces a reactive hyperkeratosis to fill the potential space under the curvature. Nail bed sections also demonstrate a papillomatosis and massive hyperkeratosis of the nail bed. The hyperkeratosis is usually orthokeratotic, but may contain small and large plasma globules that are homogeneously eosinophilic in H&E and violet in PAS sections. Demonstration of fungi is surprisingly rare. Longitudinal sections of the lateral nail when cut almost tangentially may mimic onychomatricoma.

7.12.2 Differential diagnosis

The nails in pachyonychia congenita are commonly horseshoe-like and cover a huge hyperkeratosis of the nail bed. In contrast, the nail plate itself is not thickened.

7.13 BEAU'S LINES

Described as early as 1846 after typhoid fever,[119] Beau's lines are seen as a retrospective sign of a previous serious systemic disease. Reil's lines,[120] which are white transverse bands observed after high fever, are probably a mild version of Beau's lines. Beau's lines run transverse with a convex curvature exactly parallel to the distal lunula border. They are superficial grooves more pronounced in the median portion of the nail. Thumb and big toe nails are most commonly affected. Asymmetric Beau's lines give a hint at a unilateral event, Beau's lines of one hand or foot only suggest an incident concerning this extremity,[121] and a single-digit Beau's line is almost invariably seen after nail surgery. Beau's lines are due to a temporary reduction or arrest of nail matrix activity and are thus analogous to the Pohl-Pincus lines of hair. In newborns, Beau's lines are physiologic, growing out within several weeks. In addition, they may be due to serious infections with high fever, Kawasaki's disease, zinc deficiency, but also antimitotic chemotherapy. Repeated Beau's lines may reflect the

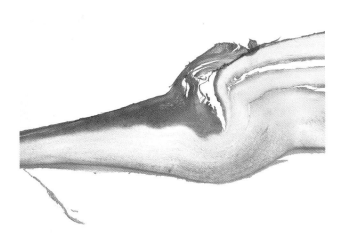

Figure 7.9 A Beau's line is characterized by an indentation of the nail plate.

repetitions of chemotherapy courses.[122-124] Whereas Beau's lines after a serious systemic disease tend to be symmetrical, those recently described after hand-foot-mouth disease are irregularly distributed on the digits and probably due to a direct involvement of the matrix by this Coxsackie virus infection.[125] Onychomadesis can be seen as an exaggerated Beau's line.[126]

7.13.1 Histopathology

Only longitudinal sections of the nail plate containing the transverse groove are contributory. Depending on the acuity of the lesion and its depth, the changes may be subtle or more pronounced. Usually a circumscribed depression of the nail surface is seen with the nail plate cells also being arranged wavy (Figure 7.9). No inflammatory changes are seen. Splits may occur.

7.13.2 Differential diagnosis

A variety of mechanical factors may also cause transverse grooves. More or less regularly arranged multiple transverse depressions giving the nail an oyster shell-like appearance is common in congenital malalignment of the big toenail and in "compression nails," also called horseshoe-crab like onychodystrophy,[127] a condition that may be defined as a noninflammatory precursor of retronychia. Here, sharply delimited splits are seen extending from the depression into distal-deep direction of the nail plate.

7.14 ONYCHOMADESIS

Proximal detachment of the nail from the matrix and nail bed is called onychomadesis. It may lead to shedding of the nail plate. Its pathogenesis is very similar to Beau's lines;[128] however, a much longer complete arrest of nail formation is needed to produce onychomadesis. As in Beau's lines, severe general diseases, but also erythema multiforme, toxic epidermal necrolysis, bullous diseases, systemic lupus erythematosus, some drugs, particularly anticancer agents,[129] are known to cause onychomadesis. Few cases

were idiopathic.[130,131] In recent years, onychomadesis of several fingernails was seen some 4–6 weeks after hand-foot-mouth disease.[125,132] Usually, normal nails regrow after a lag time of 4–6 months, except in alopecia areata where pitted rough nails may grow out.[133]

7.14.1 Histopathology

No longitudinal nail biopsy study has been reported showing the anatomic relation of the matrix and the nail plate. The latter when cut longitudinally shows a proximal smooth end. No search for virus particles in the nail was performed in hand-foot-mouth disease.

7.14.2 Differential diagnosis

Any traumatic temporary nail arrest may cause an identical histologic picture.

7.15 NAIL DEGLOVING

Shedding of the skin of the digital tip including the nail is called nail degloving. Three types were differentiated: the thimble like degloving involving the entire tip of the digit, a partial shedding of the nail with its surrounding skin, and the total shedding of the nail with its matrix, nail bed, ventral surface of the proximal nail fold, and the hyponychium.[134] Particular trauma mechanisms,[135-137] lichen planus of the nail,[132] toxic epidermal necrolysis,[138] Stevens–Johnson syndrome,[139] gangrene,[140] acute peripheral gangrene in the newborn,[141] and a variety of drugs are responsible for nail degloving.[132] The nails may later regrow normally or become dystrophic.

7.15.1 Histopathology

Examination of biopsies from a lichen planus-induced nail degloving exhibited a naked dermis with a superficial band of lymphocytic infiltrate in the proximal nailfold and the matrix[134] thus closely resembling the dermal portion of lichen planus. The degloved part was examined in three portions. The proximal piece of degloved tissue demonstrated an epidermis with keratohyalin granules, and virtually no attached dermis. The epithelium was thin and had a basket-weave orthokeratotic horny layer. The basal layer was almost straight with no epithelial pegs. In contrast, the epithelium of the lower transverse section was thick and remnants of the keratogenous zone were noted in a few areas of the matrix. The stratum corneum of the lower transverse sections was compact, had a homogenous texture, and no affinity for eosin stain, demonstrating a continuing synthesis of the nail plate. This was interpreted as a pseudonail. It was surmounted by a compact cornified layer. The upper portion of this pseudonail was undulated with depressions filled by the compact horny layer. These histologic characteristics suggested that the upper transverse layers were the middle and distal ventral portion of the proximal nailfold and that the inferior sections were the nail matrix with a modified nail plate and the horny layer of the proximal ventral portion of the proximal nailfold. Both samples showed a lichenoid dermatitis with the basal cell layer being infiltrated by lymphocytes and demonstrating vacuolar interface change as well as keratinocyte necrosis. An irregular epidermal hyperplasia with a triangular, saw-tooth configuration was seen in the lower portion. The longitudinal sections of the nail bed and hyponychium lacked the dermis except for rare tiny remnants of dermal papillae that adhered to the epithelium. These papillae exhibited a relatively dense lymphocytic infiltrate. Hydropic degeneration of the basal cells was diffuse. Basal necrosis and a dense lymphocytic infiltrate obscured the dermo-epidermal interface. The nail bed had a marked granular layer. These histologic changes were interpreted as a hyperkeratotic and pseudobullous nail lichen planus.[134] The pathogenesis of nail degloving is a loss of adherence of the epithelial nail unit component to the underlying connective tissue by widespread liquefaction degeneration of the basal layer, for example, in lichen planus, Stevens–Johnson syndrome, and toxic epidermal necrolysis, by massive edema and necrosis of the basal epidermis in gangrene, detachment of the epidermis at the basal lamina level in bullous pemphigoid, and acantholysis in pemphigus.

7.15.2 Differential diagnosis

Nail degloving is a sign of various conditions as outlined in the clinical features. These conditions also have to be ruled out histopathologically.

7.16 PITS

Pits are regular small depressions in the nail surface usually due to a disturbance in the nail formation. They are most common in psoriasis; when there are more than 10 pits in a single nail or more than 60 pits in all nails, they are held to be pathognomonic. However, there are many other conditions that occasionally give rise to pits, such as eczema or even onychomycosis.[142] They are also seen in early onset juvenile arthritis, particularly when this is located distally.[143] The pits may be arranged randomly or in longitudinal or transverse direction. The process leading to pits is limited both in time and space. The severity of the lesion that causes the defect in nail production defines the depth of the pit whereas the width and the duration of the lesion are responsible for the width and length of the pit, respectively. As the pits are on the nail plate surface, they must arise from the most proximal matrix. Pitted nails may grow faster than normal nails.[144] Atomic force microscopy of lesional hair in psoriatics shows similar pits in the hair as seen in nails.[145] Superficial pits may be a sign of generalized lichen nitidus,[146] twenty-nail dystrophy,[147] and alopecia areata.[148,149]

Larger surface defects are called elkonyxis. This may be due to some diseases[150] as well as retinoids.[151,152]

7.16.1 Histopathology

The depression of the nail in pits is easily seen in a nail clipping (Figure 7.10). The more distal the clipping the less likely a specific diagnosis is. Psoriatic pits, however, are usually deeper than those seen in alopecia areata, twenty-nail dystrophy, or lichen nitidus, but in all these conditions they are of relatively even size within their diagnosis. In eczema and onychomycosis, they may vary considerably in size. Psoriatic pits develop from small mounds of parakeratosis, and this can often be seen in the more proximal portion of the plate (Figure 7.10b). Toluidine blue clearly stains the nuclear remnants in the parakeratosis of psoriatic pits. This can also be seen in scanning electron microscopy,[153,154] where a whorled arrangement of the nail cells is evident.[155]

7.16.2 Differential diagnosis

Mechanically induced nail plate depressions can often, but by far not always, be distinguished from disease-induced ones by their sharp delimitation and often also the damage involving single onychocytes.

7.17 TRACHYONYCHIA

Trachyonychia means rough nail. It is a sign of various nail conditions, both congenital as well as acquired

(a)

(b)

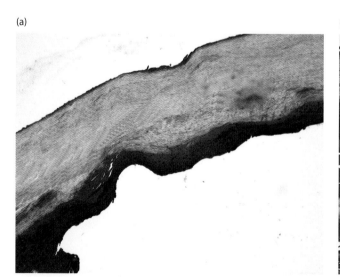
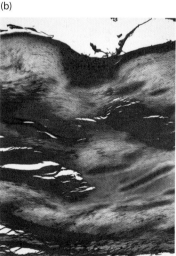

Figure 7.10 Nail pits and spots. (a) Nail pit in a patient with ungual lichen planus. This pit does not permit a diagnosis to be made from the nail plate. (b) Psoriatic pit. This pit contains still parakeratosis and is clinically seen as a slightly depressed whitish spot.

inflammatory.[156–158] The nail plate surface is rough through a multitude of tiny depressions, it is gray and opaque tending to split at its free margin. When virtually all nails are involved, the diagnosis is twenty-nail dystrophy.[159,160] A rare clinical variant is the shiny trachyonychia. It has been reported as an autosomal dominant trait.[161,162] Lichen planus,[163,164] alopecia areata,[165–167] psoriasis,[158] immunoglobulin A deficiency,[168] and ichthyosis vulgaris[169] were the most common underlying diseases. Association with vitiligo was also observed;[170,171] however, trachyonychia is histologically not uniform.[172] Twenty-nail dystrophy of childhood usually runs a self-limited course.

7.17.1 Histopathology

In hereditary trachyonychia observed in four generations, no signs of lichen planus, psoriasis, or alopecia areata were found.[7] There was epidermal thickening with acanthosis, a broad granular layer, and splitting of the stratum lucidum. The nail bed epithelium, in contrast, was thin with flat epithelial ridges. There was mild vascular proliferation and mild connective tissue degeneration. In a second case, there was an inflammatory infiltrate in the superficial dermis, however, without any lichenoid features.[7]

In acquired trachyonychia, nail biopsies show a spongiotic dermatitis[173] with serum exudation and some lymphocytic exocytosis, which are finally included into the nail and are the reason for the loss of nail transparency, its often mild thickening, and brittleness.[174,175] In the shiny variant, there is much less serum inclusion.

A case of twenty-nail dystrophy in an 11-year-old boy with an atopic family history showed dense lymphocytic infiltrates with marked epidermotropism and several areas of spongiosis. This mimicked a lichenoid pattern but there was no vacuolar basal layer change; thus, the diagnosis was lichenoid eczema. Immunophenotyping showed that all intraepithelial lymphocytes as well as the overwhelming majority of subepithelial cells were CD3-positive, of which approximately two-thirds were CD4+ and one-third CD8+. Only about 5% of the dermal lymphocytes were CD20+ B lymphocytes (Figure 7.11).[176]

7.17.2 Differential diagnosis

Lichen planus and nail psoriasis have to be excluded; they usually exhibit their characteristic features in the nail when being the cause of trachyonychia. Alopecia areata and nail eczema as spongiotic dermatitides may be indistinguishable.

7.18 PSEUDO-MYCOTIC ONYCHIA

Pseudo-mycotic nail dystrophy is a term for a specific nail condition mimicking a fungal infection. In the four cases observed in Japan, all finger and toe nails were affected demonstrating longitudinal striations, fissuring, scaling of the surface, and occasionally a yellow-brown discoloration.[177] Erythrasma of the nails of the toes was also called a pseudomycotic onychosis.[178]

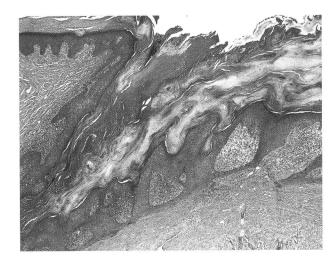

Figure 7.11 Trachyonychia in a patient with atopic dermatitis showing severe spongiotic dermatitis. Both the irregular surface and the inclusion of inflammatory cells and plasma make the nail intransparent.

7.18.1 Histopathology

The matrix epithelium displays hyperplasia with development of a stratum granulosum and projections similar to the crest of a wave. There is an inflammatory infiltrate in the upper matrical dermis. The nail plate consists of regularly keratinized and abnormal layers in a stratiform pattern. In the study on nail erythrasma, hyperkeratosis and onycholysis were observed. Giemsa stained preparations of KOH-treated nail specimens showed gram-positive, acid-fast organisms with a tendency to form filaments with short lateral branches.

7.18.2 Differential diagnosis

Pseudo-mycotic onychia requires exclusion of a fungal infection, of the asymmetric gait nail unit syndrome,[73,179,180] and of long-standing alopecia areata.[181] However, the significance of this condition as an entity is disputed.[182]

7.19 RETRONYCHIA

Retronychia describes retrograde ingrowing of the nail.[183] Most cases were observed on toes although it is occasionally observed on fingers.[184,185] The cause is either a single acute trauma where the patient falls on the free margin of the nail pushing it forcefully proximally, or repeated trauma detaching the nail from the nail bed and allowing it to be repeatedly pushed back.[186] This leads to shearing of the nail plate from the matrix causing almost horizontally running splits in the proximal plate when a new layer of nail is produced while the distal three-quarters of the nail remain joined.[186] With more and more new nail layers produced proximally, the oldest and uppermost layer develops a very hard and sharp margin, which is pushed back into the nail pocket and cuts into the ventral layer of the proximal nail fold.[186] The nail plate does not grow out any more, and some patients report that the nail even receded in the last weeks to months. Finally, granulation tissue is produced by the continuous traumatization of

(a)

(b)

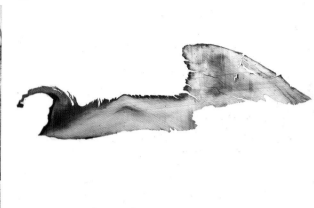

Figure 7.12 In retronychia, the proximal margin of the nail plate is (a) split like an asymmetric Y or (b) shows a step.

the proximal nail fold's ventral surface that is easily seen when gently pressing on the nail fold.[186,187] This inflammation may be misdiagnosed as paronychia.[188–191] Ultrasound confirms the diagnosis.[192,193] Whereas in the early reports a tight attachment of the nail plate to the nail bed was postulated, we have seen that in all our cases there was a severe onycholysis allowing the nail plate to be moved back and forth.[186,194] The treatment of choice is nail avulsion; however, it requires consistent taping to avoid the development of a distal nail fold.[195]

7.19.1 Histopathology

Longitudinal sections of the avulsed nail show that the proximal part of the nail plate has two, three, or even four ends, one above the other. From their junction, splits reach into the nail plate for a certain distance until they disappear in an intact nail plate (Figure 7.12).[191] The nail bed is hyperkeratotic and detached from the nail.

7.19.2 Differential diagnosis

A non-inflammatory variant described under the term of horseshoe-crab like nail or compression nail is relatively commonly seen on the big toes. In contrast to retronychia, the nail plate continues to move forward so that the onychomadetic part does not cut into the ventral surface of the proximal nail fold.

7.20 INGROWN NAIL (UNGUIS INCARNATUS, ONYCHOCRYPTOSIS)

Ingrown nails are observed in all ages from newborns to the old (Table 7.1). Most cases demonstrate lateral ingrowing, but distal and proximal ingrowing are also seen. Whereas ingrown nails in little children are not treated surgically, the adolescent type is often operated.

In the juvenile type, the nail plate is large and markedly curved. Its distal lateral edge may hurt, particularly when its corner is cut too short and the tip of the toe can be compressed by the shoes. Often, the edge is not cut smooth, but a tiny hook-like spicule is left, which pierces into the distal lateral groove, causes granulation tissue with oozing, and finally infection with pus secretion. The treatment of choice in early cases is conservative with taping, packing, gutter treatment, or a combination of them.[196] The overcurvature can be treated with orthonyxia braces or a shape memory alloy clip. When this is not successful, a selective lateral matrix horn resection is indicated. This can be done by careful dissection from the lateral condylus of the base of the distal phalanx, by laser vaporization, or by chemocautery with either liquefied phenol, 10% sodium hydroxide, or trichloroacetic acid.[197] In our experience, wedge excisions and other radical methods lead to mutilation of the toes and they have an extremely high recurrence rate;[198] however, they give specimens for histopathologic examination.

Table 7.1 Types of ingrown nails

Type of ingrown nail	Site of ingrowing	Histopathology
Neonatal	Distal	Granulation tissue
Neonatal-infantile	Medial distal	Abnormal nail structure with splits in the nail running from
Congenital malalignment of the big toenail		proximal-superficial to distal-deep
Hypertrophic lateral lip	Medial nail groove	Fibrotic lateral nail fold, there may be many small myelinated nerves
Juvenile type	Distal lateral and medial	Granulation tissue, hyperplastic epidermis, frayed nail margin
Adult type	Medial and lateral groove	Hyperkeratosis in the depth of the lateral groove
Overcurvature	Medial and lateral groove	Hypertrophic hyperkeratotic nail bed
Distal type	False distal nail fold	Dorsally dislocated pulp skin
Retronychia	Proximal nail fold	Granulation tissue, thick and Y-shaped to serrated proximal nail

Ingrown nails due to overcurvature of the nails have been described (see Section 7.12).

7.20.1 Histopathology

The histopathology of ingrown nails depends on the stage of development and the type of excision or biopsy specimen. The granulation tissue is loose with proliferation of thin-walled vessels and capillaries, edematous stroma, and variable amounts of lymphocytes, plasma cells, and neutrophils. There is often a stratification of the infiltrate with the neutrophils being the outermost, the lymphocytes at the inner margin, and the plasma cells in between. This histological feature is definitely different from pyogenic granuloma. When more of the lateral nail fold has been excised, the epidermis is seen lacking in the most severely inflamed areas and markedly acanthotic at the margins.[199] Under the epidermis, there is a mainly plasmocytic infiltrate with variable amounts of lymphocytes, which may sometimes even form small follicles. The expression of CD10 and CD34 is preserved in ingrown nail specimens.[200] In case the lateral ingrown nail plate is left in the specimen, it is seen to pierce into the nail groove, which has completely lost its epidermis. This is substituted by an inflammatory infiltrate consisting of neutrophils, plasma cells, lymphocytes, and histiocytes of which some may form giant cells. The nail plate is sliced and neutrophils are seen to digest the nail keratin (Figure 7.13).[201]

7.20.2 Differential diagnosis

The differential diagnosis comprises all chronic inflammations of the nail folds. The epidermal hyperplasia may look like squamous cell carcinoma, but proliferation marker studies can rule this out.[200]

7.21 NAIL KERATIN GRANULOMA

Keratin displaced into dermal and subcutaneous tissue may elicit a granulomatous reaction as it is seen as a foreign substance by the body. Whereas keratin granulomas are very common in glabrous skin, e.g. after rupture of follicular cysts of the acroinfundibular and rarely the isthmus-catagen type it is relatively rare in the nail region. A highly inflammatory

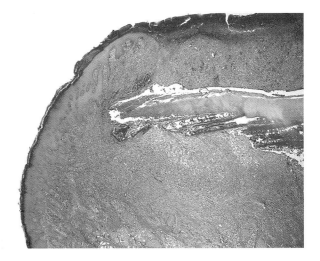

Figure 7.13 Wedge excision specimen of an ingrown big toenail. The lateral margin of the nail is frayed, blood and neutrophils are seen in the splits of the nail, and the lateral nail fold is severely inflamed.

reaction may develop when the nail pierces through the epidermis into the dermis or subcutis as in ingrown nails. However, other types of nail keratin inclusions often form a slowly enlarging, slightly red lesion with or without acute inflammation. However, this is a surprisingly rare event.[202] A whole plethora of clinical differential diagnoses is possible ranging from chronic paronychia, gout, cysts, or inflammatory pseudotumors to malignancies.

An experimental study with rat nails implanted into skin showed that nail material first elicits an inflammatory reaction which subsides after several months and leaves the nail material embedded in a stable fibrous tissue.[203]

7.21.1 Histopathology

Isolated nail granulomas are rare. There is a broad range of reactive changes, from an almost completely acellular, slightly fibrotic lesion (Figure 7.14) to a mild to pronounced granulomatous reaction (Figure 7.15) to a highly inflammatory response as seen in ingrown nails (see

(a)

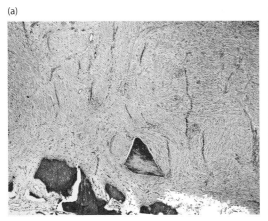

(b)

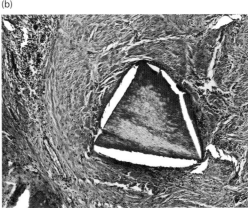

Figure 7.14 A triangular piece of nail is seen in the deep dermis of the distal nail bed in a patient with *in situ* melanoma. This was a chance observation after removal of the entire nail organ for an *in situ* melanoma. (a) Scanning magnification and (b) close-up.

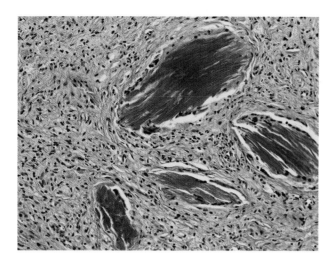

Figure 7.15 Nail granuloma in a patient after incorrect ingrown nail surgery by a wedge excision.

Chapter 7.20). The degree of inflammation may change in the same specimen at different section levels. Most nail granulomas occur after surgery when pieces of nail plate material without epithelial remnants are enclosed in the dermis. Polarization microscopy may help to identify the nature of this type of foreign body.

7.21.2 Differential diagnosis

The correct diagnosis depends on the demonstration of nail keratin in the granuloma. This is facilitated by using polarization microscopy. However, plant materials such as wood or cactus spines (Figure 7.16) and sea-urchin spines are also birefringent, but their internal structure is different from nail substance.[204] Granuloma formation is also seen when epithelial remnants are left behind during tumor surgery of the nail (Figure 7.17). Periungual interstitial granulomatous dermatitis involved all nails and other skin areas.[205]

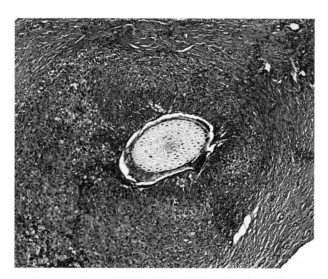

Figure 7.16 Subungual cactus spine with granuloma formation and a rim of caseation necrosis immediately around the spine.

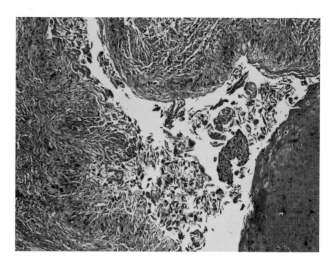

Figure 7.17 Buried part of Bowen carcinoma, which induced a granulomatous reaction. This apparently prevented further invasive growth of the carcinoma.

7.22 DOUBLE (ACCESSORY) FIFTH TOENAIL

The little toenail is the smallest of all nails and rarely gets attention. A peculiar condition is the rudimentary double or accessory small toenail first described in the medical literature more than 45 years ago.[206] According to our experience, it is not uncommon and occurs in all races.[207,208] Usually, the little toenail is too wide and demonstrates a paramedian longitudinal sulcus on its lateral side. Here the cuticle protrudes a little bit more distally. Most cases were just chance observations although in individuals with a splay foot and outward rotation of the little toe, this may cause discomfort similar to a corn at the lateral side of the little toe. Both men and women are affected, but there are more female than male patients. Genetic studies have not yet been published, but some of our more than 60 cases were familiar. Treatment is by complete excision of the accessory nail with its matrix and nail bed or selective phenolization of the corresponding matrix.[209]

7.22.1 Histopathology

Histologically, the changes vary from a saucer-like depression of the skin with hyperkeratosis that in its center resembles a nail plate to a small but otherwise normally structured nail with matrix, proximal nail fold, nail bed, and hyponychium. No inflammation is seen (Figure 7.18).

7.22.2 Differential diagnosis

The most important differential diagnosis is an ungual heloma or corn. It is characterized by a cone-shaped hyperkeratosis with a central parakeratotic column. Warts have the characteristic cytopathic effects. Hyperplastic Bowen's disease is a carcinoma *in situ* that stands out by its cellular atypia. A nail spicule after insufficient ingrown nail surgery and post-traumatic double nail[210] may be virtually indistinguishable. Acquired ungual fibrokeratoma may exhibit an accessory nail matrix.[211–213]

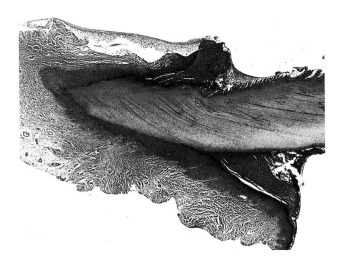

Figure 7.18 Excision specimen of a fully developed double little toenail.

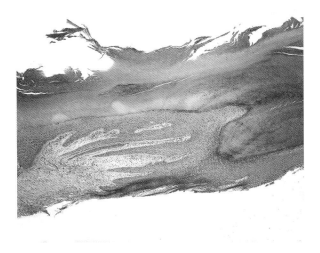

Figure 7.19 Onychotillomania exhibits an acanthotic and hyperkeratotic distal matrix and nail bed and often some minute accumulations of neutrophils and/or lymphocytes.

7.23 ONYCHOTILLOMANIA

Onychotillomania is one of several different types of a self-destructive behavior where the patient pulls the nails out or files them with a variety of instruments. This results in partial to complete loss of the nail, often associated with lack of the cuticle and a hypertrophy of the proximal nail bed—matrix region. The proximal nail fold may show alterations comparable to chronic rubbing trauma such as in lichen simplex chronicus. Other types of self-injurious nail behaviors are onychophagia (nail "eating"), periony-chotillomania (habitual picking of the periungual skin including hangnails), onychoteiromania (chronic rubbing of the nail), and onychotemnomania (maniacal removing of the nail with sharp instruments) whereas onychoda-knomania (biting on the nail root in order to elicit pain) is a frankly psychotic trait. Except for the last, the other habits usually leave a damaged nail unit. Longitudinal mela-nonychia may also be caused by onychophagia.[214,215] Most patients are either not aware of their self-destructive habit or are vigorously rejecting this assumption.[216] The clinical diagnosis can be difficult as a large variety of other diseases causing nail dystrophy have to be considered.

7.23.1 Histopathology

Onychotillomania has very rarely been biopsied. Its histopathologic features are not specific and mainly show epithelial hyperplasia of the nail bed characterized by acanthosis, hypergranulosis, and hyperkeratosis (Figure 7.19).[217] The proximal fold may exhibit alterations comparable to lichen simplex chronicus with acanthosis, hyperkeratosis, and mild hyperpigmentation.[218] Importantly, an inflammatory infiltrate is lacking.

7.23.2 Differential diagnosis

The diagnosis is mainly made by the absence of an inflammatory infiltrate ruling out psoriasis or lichen planus and by the lack of fungal elements in PAS stained slides.

7.24 NAIL LACQUER

Nail lacquer or nail varnish is one of the most commonly applied cosmetics nowadays even seen in female babies. All colors and designs are possible.

7.24.1 Histopathology

Nail lacquer is usually a chance observation and may easily be overlooked if one is not familiar with its appearance in a histologic slide. On top of the nail plate, there is a layer of finely granular material that in most cases appears grayish in H&E stained sections; its original color is no more identifiable in most cases.[219] It may penetrate splits of the nail surface, but it does not induce any further tissue reaction (Figure 7.20).

7.24.2 Differential diagnosis

No other material gives a similar aspect and stays on the nail during processing of the specimen.

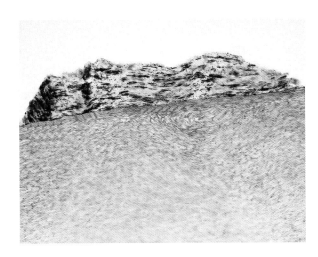

Figure 7.20 Nail lacquer is seen as a granular material on top of the nail plate.

(a)   (b)

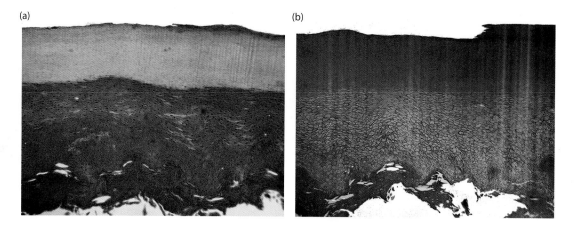

Figure 7.21 Effect of high-concentration urea paste on the nail. The upper half of the nail plate remains almost normal, the lower half is densely eosinophilic in H&E (a) and appears to have empty cells in PAS stain (b); the subungual keratin has a slightly dark-pink hue in H&E and is compact bluish-violet in PAS stain.

7.25 EFFECT OF HIGH-CONCENTRATION UREA PASTE

Atraumatic avulsion of mycotic nails has become a treatment option when 40% urea paste became available. The periungual skin is protected with tape, a thick layer of the urea paste is applied on the nail, and covered with an occlusive tape. This is left in place for a few days and removed. The infected nail portion becomes very soft and can be cut away easily with normal scissors and the underlying subungual hyperkeratosis scraped off. Provided this is done correctly, it is a very effective adjunct to other topical and systemic antifungal therapies of onychomycoses.[220–222] One case of acute dermatitis of the periungual skin was described after 40% urea paste.[223]

7.25.1 Histopathology

The nail and subungual keratin show unique changes. The superficial half of the nail thickness remains almost normal whereas the deep half exhibits large, usually empty appearing or slightly eosinophilic cells that stain bluish gray with PAS (Figure 7.21). They may contain fungal elements. The subungual keratosis stains another red compared to the lower half of the nail plate and remains compact with no plant-cell like changes.

7.25.2 Differential diagnosis

Some repeated microtraumas such as friction may cause large keratinocytes with a very light cytoplasm. Leukonychia shows a dense eosinophilic cytoplasm of the nail plate cells.

REFERENCES

1. Salamon T. Vererbung von Haar- und Nagelkrankheiten. In: Jadassohn J, ed. *Handbuch der Haut- und Geschlechtskrankheiten*, vol. 7, ErgWerk, Berlin: Springer, 1963:363–439.
2. Timerman I, Museteanu C, Simionescu NN. Dominant anonychia and onychodystrophy. *J Med Genet* 1969;6: 105–106.
3. Mahloudji M, Amidi M. Simple anonchia. Further evidence for autosomal recessive inheritance. *J Med Genet* 1971;8:478.
4. Afsar FS, Karakuzu A. Total congenital anonychia. *Pediatr Dermatol* 2014;31:743–744.
5. Baran R, Juhlin L. Bone dependent nail formation. *Br J Dermatol* 1986;114:371–375.
6. Strandskov HH. Inheritance of absence of thumb nails. *J Hered* 1939;30:53.
7. Alkiewicz J, Pfister R. *Atlas der Nagelkrankheiten. Pathohistologie, Klinik und Differentialdiagnose.* Stuttgart New York: Schattauer, 1976:70.
8. Cooks RG, Hertz M, Katznelson MB, Goodman RM. A new nail dysplasia syndrome with anonychia and absence and/or hypoplasia of distal phalanges. *Clin Genet* 1985;27:85–91.
9. Nevin NC, Thomas PS, Eedy DJ, Shepherd C. Anonychia and absence/hypoplasia of distal phalanges (Cooks syndrome): Report of a second family. *J Med Genet* 1995;32:638–641.
10. Chatterjee D. Congenital anonychia and brachydactyly of the left foot—Cooks syndrome variant: Case report and review of literature. *Indian J Hum Genet* 2014;20:206–208.
11. Alkiewicz J. On the original location of the germ of human nails. *Bull Soc Amis Sci Poznan, Sér C* 1951;2:56–57.
12. Sequeiros J, Sack GH Jr. Linear skin atrophy, scarring alopecia, anonychia, and tongue lesion: A "new" syndrome? *Am J Med Genet* 1985;21:669–680.
13. Berge A, Weissenbach RJ. Absence congénitale complète des ongles de tous les doigts—Biopsie. *Ann Dermatol Syph (Paris)* 1912;3:244.
14. Baden HP, Alper JC, Lee LD. Rudimentary polydactyly presenting as a claw. *Arch Dermatol* 1976;112: 1006–1007.
15. Alkiewicz J. Leucopathie des ongles. *Del IX Congr Int Dermatol, Budapest* 1935;1:750.

16. Marinho FS, Pirmez R, Nogueira R, Cuzzi T, Sodré CT, Silva M. Cutaneous manifestations in POEMS syndrome: Case report and review. *Case Rep Dermatol* 2015;7:61–69.

17. Lin Z, Zhao J, Nitoiu D, Scott CA, Plagnol V, Smith FJ, Wilson NJ et al. Loss-of-function mutations in CAST cause peeling skin, leukonychia, acral punctate keratoses, cheilitis, and knuckle pads. *Am J Hum Genet* 2015;96:440–447.

18. Thal M. Leukonychie als Berufsschaden im Fleischergewerbe. *Dermatol Wschr* 1956;134:1178–1183.

19. Frenk E, Leu F. Leukonychie durch beruflichen Kontakt mit gesalzenen Därmen. *Hautarzt* 1966;17:233–235.

20. Stewart WK, Raffle EJ. Brown nail-bed arcs and chronic renal disease. *Br Med J* 1972;1:784–786.

21. Lindsay PG. The half-and-half nail. *Arch Intern Med* 1967;119:583–587.

22. Robert C, Sibaud V, Mateus C, Verschoore M, Charles C, Lanoy E, Baran R. Nail toxicities induced by systemic anticancer treatments. *Lancet Oncol* 2015;16:e181–e189.

23. Chaudhry SI, Black MM. True transverse leuconychia with spontaneous resolution during pregnancy. *Br J Dermatol* 2006;154:1212–1213.

24. Hay RJ, Baran R. Deep dermatophytosis: Rare infections or common, but unrecognised, complications of lymphatic spread? *Curr Opin Infect Dis* 2004;17:77–79.

25. Jessner M. Über eine neue Form von Nagelmykosen (Leukonychia trichophytica). *Arch Dermatol Res* 1922;141:1–8.

26. Zaias N. Superficial white onychomycosis. *Sabouraudia* 1966;5:99–103.

27. Stühmer A. Nageltrichophytie. *Arch Dermatol Syph (Berlin)* 1957;193:527.

28. van Gelderen de Komaid A, Borges de Kestelman I, Durán EL. Etiology and clinical characteristics of mycotic leukonychia. *Mycopathologia* 1996;136:9–15.

29. Alkiewicz J. Klinik und Histopathologie der Leukonychie. *Przegl Dermatol* 1935;30:1–36.

30. Alkiewicz J, Pfister R. *Atlas der Nagelkrankheiten. Pathohistologie, Klinik und Differentialdiagnose.* Stuttgart: FK Schattauer, 1976: 130–133.

31. Norgette EE, Wolf F, Balme B, Leigh IM, Perrot H, Kelsell DP, Haftek M. Hereditary "white nails": A genetic and structural study. *Br J Dermatol* 2004;151:65–72.

32. Moulin G, Baran R, Perrin C. Epidermal hamartoma presenting as longitudinal pachyleukonychia: A new nail génodermatoses. *J Am Acad Dermatol* 1996;35:675–677.

33. Higashi N, Sugai T, Yamamoto T. Leukonychia striata longitudinalis. *Arch Dermatol* 1971;104:192–196.

34. Jellinek NJ. Longitudinal erythronychia: Suggestions for evaluation and management. *J Am Acad Dermatol* 2011;64:167e1–167e11.

35. Cohen PR. Red lunulae: Case report and literature review. *J Am Acad Dermatol* 1992;26:292–294.

36. Zali MR, Rostami Nejad M, Al Dulaimi D, Rostami K. Nail changes: Unusual presentation of celiac disease. *Am J Gastroenterol* 2011;106:2202–2204.

37. Baran R. The red nail—Always benign? *Acta Dermosifiligr* 2009;100(Suppl 1):106–113.

38. Baran R, Dawber RP, Perrin C, Drapé JL. Idiopathic polydactylous longitudinal erythronychia: A newly described entity. *Br J Dermatol* 2006;155:219–221.

39. Cohen PR. Longitudinal erythronychia: Individual or multiple linear red bands of the nail plate—A review of clinical features and associated conditions. *Am J Clin Dermatol* 2011;12:217–231.

40. Cohen PR. Idiopathic polydactylous longitudinal erythronychia. *J Clin Aesthet Dermatol* 2011;4(4):22–28.

41. Cohen PR. Multiple linear red bands on the fingernails: Idiopathic polydactylous longitudinal erythronychia. *Dermatolgy Online J* 2012;18(2):6.

42. Bergner T, Donhauser G, Ruzicka T. Red lunulae in severe alopecia areata. *Acta Derm Venereol* 1992;72:203–205.

43. De Berker DA, Perrin C, Baran R. Localized longitudinal erythronychia: Diagnostic significance and physical explanation. *Arch Dermatol* 2004;140:1253–1257.

44. Wilkerson MG, Wilkin JK. Red lunulae revisited: A clinical and histopathologic examination. *J Am Acad Dermatol* 1989;20:453–457.

45. Maes M, Richert B, de la Brassine M. Le syndrome des ongles verts ou chloronychie. *Rev Med Liege* 2002;57:233–235.

46. Matheson N, Weekes M, Coggle S. Skier's toe: Traumatic onycholysis complicated by *Pseudomonas chloronychia*. *BMJ Case Rep* 2009;2009: ii, bcr07.2009.2074.

47. Pier GB, Ramphal R. *Pseudomonas aeruginosa*. In: Mandell GL, Bennett JE, Dolin R, eds. *Principles and Practice of Infectious Diseases*, 6th edn. Philadelphia: Chirchill Livingstone, 2004: 2587–2615.

48. Nenoff P, Paasch U, Handrick W. Infections of finger and toe nails due to fungi and bacteria. *Hautarzt* 2014;65:337–348.

49. Müller S, Ebnöther M, Itin P. Green nail syndrome (*Pseudomonas aeruginosa* nail infection): Two cases successfully treated with topical nadifloxaxin, an acne medication. *Case Rep Dermatol* 2014;6:180–184.

50. Bae Y, Lee GM, Sim JH, Lee S, Lee SY, Park YL. Green nail syndrome treated with the application of tobramycin eye drop. *Ann Dermatol* 2014;26:514–516.

51. Zuehlke RL, Taylor WB. Black nails with Proteus mirabilis. *Arch Dermatol* 1970;102:154–155.

52. Qadripur SA, Schauder S, Schwartz P. Ungues nigri durch Proteus mirabilis. *Hautarzt* 2001;52:658–661.

53. de Carvalho LM, Mendonça I, de Oliveira JC, Val A, Hering B, Stallone C, Jimenez PA. Melanoníquia: A propósito de um caso de micotização ungueal simulando melanoma. *Dermatol Online J* 2010;16(3):6.

54. Hamasaka E, Akiyama M, Hata H, Aoyagi S, Shimizu H. Melanonychia caused by *Stenotrophomonas maltophilia*. *Clin Exp Dermatol* 2009;34:242–243.

55. Finch J, Arenas R, Baran R. Fungal melanonychia. *J Am Acad Dermatol* 2012;66:830–841.

56. Schiavo AL, Gambardella A, Caccavale S. Fungal melanonychia and Exophiala dermatitidis. *Mycoses* 2012 Jun 8. doi: 10.1111/j.1439-0507.2012.02217.x. [Epub ahead of print]

57. Tosti A, Piraccini BM. Proximal subungual onychomycosis due to *Aspergillus niger*: Report of two cases. *Br J Dermatol* 1998;139:156–157.

58. Kim DM, Suh MK, Ha GY, Sohng SH. Fingernail onychomycosis due to *Aspergillus niger*. *Ann Dermatol* 2012;24:459–463.

59. Vélez A, Fernández-Roldán JC, Linares M, Casal M. Melanonychia due to *Candida humicola*. *Br J Dermatol* 1996;134:375–376.

60. Parlak AH, Goksugur N, Karabay O. A case of melanonychia due to *Candida albicans*. *Clin Exp Dermatol* 2006;31:398–400.

61. Cho E, Lee YB, Park HJ, Cho BK. Fungal melanonychia due to *Candida albicans*. *Int J Dermatol* 2013;52:1598–1600.

62. Cursi IB, Freitas LB, Neves M de L, Silva IC. Onychomycosis due to *Scytalidium* spp.: A clinical and epidemiologic study at a University Hospital in Rio de Janeiro, Brazil. *An Bras Dermatol* 2011;86: 689–693.

63. Ko CJ, Sarantopoulos GP, Pai G, Binder SW. Longitudinal melanonychia of the toenails with presence of Medlar bodies on biopsy. *J Cutan Pathol* 2005;32:63–65.

64. Lee YB, Cho E, Park HJ, Cho BK. Proximal and lateral chromonychia with capillary proliferation on the distal nail matrix. *Ann Dermatol* 2012;24:240–241.

65. Chang P, Haneke E, Borjas Leiva CA, Pellecer D. Hematoma friccional subungueal. *Dermatología CMQ* 2012;10(1):48–50.

66. Schöffl V, Küpper T. Feet injuries in rock climbers. *World J Orthop* 2013;4:218–228.

67. Patel L. Management of simple nail bed lacerations and subungual hematomas in the emergency department. *Pediatr Emerg Care* 2014;30:742–745.

68. Haneke E, Baran R. Subunguale Tumoren. *Z Hautkr* 1982;57:355–362.

69. Baran R, Haneke E. Diagnostik und Therapie der streifenförmigen Nagelpigmentierung. *Hautarzt* 1984;35:359–365.

70. Hafner J, Haenseler E, Ossent P, Burg G, Panizzon RG. Benzidine stain for the histochemical detection of hemoglobin in splinter hemorrhage (subungual hematoma) and black heel. *Am J Dermatopathol* 1995;17:362–367.

71. Alkiewicz J, Majewski C. Clinical features and histopathology of onycholysis. *Przegl Dermatol* 1956;41:437–441.

72. Baran R, Badillet G. Primary onycholysis of the big toenails: A review of 113 cases. *Br J Dermatol* 1982;106:529–534.

73. Zaias N, Rebell G, Casal G, Appel J. The asymmetric gait toenail unit sign. *Skinmed* 2012;10:213–217.

74. Zaias N, Escobar SX, Zaiac MN. Finger and toenail onycholysis. *J Eur Acad Dermatol Venereol* 2015;29:848–853.

75. Daniel CR 3rd, Tosti A, Iorizzo M, Piraccini BM. The disappearing nail bed: A possible outcome of onycholysis. *Cutis* 2005;76:325–327.

76. Daniel CR 3rd, Iorizzo M, Piraccini BM, Tosti A. Grading simple chronic paronychia and onycholysis. *Int J Dermatol* 2006;45:1447–1448.

77. Egawa K, Kuroki M, Inoue Y, Ono T. The nail bed keratinocytes express an antigen of the carcinoembryonic antigen (CEA) family. *Br J Dermatol* 2000;143:79–83.

78. Baran R, Hay R, Haneke E, Tosti A. *Onychomycosis. The Current Approach to Diagnosis and Therapy*, 2nd edn. Abingdon: Taylor & Francis, 57–68.

79. Haneke E. Fungal infections of the nail. *Sem Dermatol* 1991;10:41–53.

80. Sonnex TS, Dawber RP, Zachary CB, Millard PR, Griffiths AD. The nails in adult type 1 pityriasis rubra pilaris. A comparison with Sézary syndrome and psoriasis. *J Am Acad Dermatol* 1986;15: 956–960.

81. Fanti PA, Tosti A. Subungual epidermoid inclusions: Report of 8 cases. *Dermatologica* 1989;178:209–212.

82. von Hintzenstern J, Kiesewetter F, Simon M Jr, Schell H, Hornstein OP. Paraneoplastische Akrokeratose Bazex—Verlauf unter palliativer Therapie eines Zungengrundkarzinoms. *Hautarzt* 1990;41:490–493.

83. Fitzgerald BJ, Sanders LJ. Pachyonychia congenita: A four generation pedigree. *Cutis* 1990;46:435–439.

84. Dixit VB, Chaudhary SD, Jain VK. Clofazimine induced nail changes. *Indian J Lepr* 1989;61:476–478.

85. Norton AL. Common and uncommon reactions to formaldehyde-containing nail hardeners. *Sem Dermatol* 1991;10:29–33.

86. Timpatanapong P, Hathirat P, Isarangkura P. Nail involvement in histiocytosis X. A 12-year retrospective study. *Arch Dermatol* 1984;120:1052–1056.

87. Witkop CJ Jr, Brearley LJ, Gentry WC Jr. Hypoplastic enamel, onycholysis, and hypohidrosis inherited as an autosomal dominant trait. A review of ectodermal dysplasia syndromes. *Oral Surg Oral Med Oral Pathol* 1975;39:71–86.

88. Tosti A, Morelli R, Fanti PA, Cameli N. Nail changes of punctate keratoderma: A clinical and pathological study of two patients. *Acta Derm Venereol* 1993;73:66–68.

89. Badger J, Banerjee AK, McFadden J. Unilateral subungual hyperkeratosis following a cerebrovascular incident in a patient with psoriasis. *Clin Exp Dermatol* 1992;17:454–455.

90. Haneke E. Pathology of inflammatory nail diseases. 7th International Dermatopathology Colloquium, Graz, May 23–25, 1986, Book of Abstracts.

91. Haneke E. Nail biopsies in onychomycosis. *Mykosen* 1985;28:473–480.

92. Haneke E. Differentialdiagnose von Onychomykosen. In: Hay RJ, Hrsg. *Fortschritte in der lokalen antimykotischen Therapie.* Berlin: Springer, 1988:99–106.

93. Lawry M, Haneke E, Storbeck K, Martin S, Zimmer B, Romano P. Methods for diagnosing onychomycosis: A comparative study and review of the literature. *Arch Dermatol* 2000;136:1112–1126.

94. Haim S, Munk J. Keratosis palmo-plantaris congenita, with periodontosis, arachnodactyly and peculiar deformity of the terminal phalanges. *Br J Dermatol* 1965;77:42–54.

95. Janjua SA, Iftikhar N, Hussain I. Dermatologic, periodontal, and skeletal manifestations of Haim-Munk syndrome in two siblings. *J Am Acad Dermatol* 2008;58:339–344.

96. Freiberg A, Dougherty S. A review of management of ingrown toenails and onychogryphosis. *Can Fam Physician* 1988;34:2675–2681.

97. Caputo R, Prandi B. Pterygium inversum unguis. *Arch Dermatol* 1973;108:817–818.

98. Odom RB, Stein KM, Maibach HI. Congenital painful, aberrant hyponychium. *Arch Dermatol* 1974;110: 89–90.

99. Christophers E. Familiäre subunguale Pterygien. *Hautarzt* 1975;26:543–544.

100. Patterson JW. Pterygium inversum unguis-like changes in scleroderma. Report of four cases. *Arch Dermatol* 1977;113:1429–1430.

101. Caputo R, Cappio F, Rigoni C, Scarabelli G, Toffolo P, Spinelli G, Crosti C. Pterygium inversum unguis. Report of 19 cases and review of the literature. *Arch Dermatol* 1993;129:1307–1309.

102. Paley K, English JC 3rd, Zirwas MJ. Pterygium inversum unguis secondary to acrylate allergy. *J Am Acad Dermatol* 2008;58(2 Suppl):S53–S54.

103. Huang JT, Duncan CN, Boyer D, Khosravi H, Lehmann LE, Saavedra A. Nail dystrophy, edema, and eosinophilia: Harbingers of severe chronic GVDH of the skin in children. *Bone Marrow Transplant* 2014;49:1521–1527.

104. Zaias N, Escovar SX, Zaiac MN, del Rio E, Dou N, Ricotti C, Karai L, Florez-White M. Hyponychium abnormalities. Congenital aberrant hyponychium vs. acquired *Pterygium unguis* inversum vs. acquired extended hyponychium: A proposed classification based on origin, pathology and outcome. *J Eur Acad Dermatol Venereol* 2015;29:1427–1431.

105. Vadmal M, Reyter I, Oshtory S, Hensley B, Woodley DT. Pterygium inversum unguis associated with stroke. *J Am Acad Dermatol* 2005;53:501–503.

106. Oiso N, Narita T, Tsuruta D, Kawara S, Kawada A. Pterygium inversum unguis: Aberrantly regulated keratinization in the nail isthmus. *Clin Exp Dermat* 2009;34:e514–e515.

107. Oiso N, Kurokawa I, Kawada A. Nail isthmus: A distinct region of the nail apparatus. *Dermatol Res Pract* 2012;2012:925023.

108. Lembo G, Montesano M, Balato N. Complete *Pterygium unguis. Cutis* 1985;36:427–429.

109. Erdogan AG, Karahacloglu FB, Kavak A. *Pterygium unguis* in leprosy. *Int J Dermatol* 2013;52:1621–1623.

110. Haneke E, Borradori L. *Pterygium unguis*: A new sign of bullous pemphigoid. Submitted.

111. Nallegowda M, Yadav SL, Singh U, Singh MK, Tejaswi T. An unusual nail presentation in Marfan's syndrome. *J Dermatol* 2002;29:164–167.

112. Cornelius CE 3rd, Shelley WB. Pincer nail syndrome. *Arch Surg* 1968;96:321–322.

113. Haneke E. Etiopathogénie et traitement de l'hypercourbure transversale de l'ongle du gros orteil. *J Méd Esthét* 1992;29:123–127.

114. Higashi N. Pincer nail due to tinea unguium. *Hifu* 1990;32:40–44.

115. Effendy I, Ossowski B, Happle R. Pincer nail. Conservative correction by attachment of a plastic brace. *Hautarzt* 1993;44:800–802.

116. Lee JM, Baek SR, Kim YJ. Complication after pincer nail treatment using a shape memory alloy device. *Dermatol Surg* 2013;39:1520–1526.

117. Baran R, Haneke E, Richert B. Pincer nails: Definition and surgical treatment. *Dermatol Surg* 2001;27:261–266.

118. Haneke E. Nail surgery. *Clin Dermatol* 2013;31:516–525.

119. Beau JHS. Note sur certains caractères de séméiologie rétrospective présentés par les ongles. *Arch Gén Méd* 1846;11:447–458.

120. Reil JC. Unguium vitia in convalescentibus a febre maligna observata. In: *Memorabilia Clinica Medicinae Practicae*, vol. III. Halle, 1792.

121. Gönül M, Cakmak SK, Yayla D, Oguz ID, Mungan S, Sivas F. Unilateral Beau's lines in a case of complex regional pain syndrome (reflex sympathetic dystrophy). *Indian J Dermatol Venereol Leprol* 2012;78:775.

122. Naumann R, Wozel G. Transverse leukonychia following chemotherapy in a patient with Hodgkin's disease. *Eur J Dermatol* 2000;10:392–394.

123. Piraccini BM, Iorizzo M, Starace M, Tosti A. Drug-induced nail diseases. *Dermatol Clin* 2006;24: 387–391.

124. Kim IS, Lee JW, Park KY, Li K, Seo SJ, Hong CK. Nail change after chemotherapy: Simultaneous development of Beau's lines and Mees' lines. *Ann Dermatol* 2012;24:238–239.

125. Haneke E. Onychomadesis and hand, foot and mouth disease—Is there a connection? *Euro Surveill* 2010;15(37):19664.

126. Hardin J, Haber RM. Onychomadesis: Literature review. *Br J Dermatol* 2014 Aug 16. Doi: 10.1111/bjd.13339 (Epub ahead of print).

127. Kowalzik L, Schell B, Eickenscheidt L, Ziegler H. Pfeilschwanzkrebs-Onychodystrophie. *Akt Dermatol* 2008;34:26–28.

128. Fleming CJ, Hunt MJ, Barnetson R. Mycosis fungoides with onychomadesis. *Br J Dermatol* 1996;135:1012.

129. Kochupillai V, Bhide NK, Prabhu M. Cancer chemotherapy and nail loss (onychomadesis). *Acta Haematol* 1983;70:137.

130. Oliver WJ. Recurrent onychoptosis occurring as a familial disorder. *Br J Dermatol Syph* 1927;39:297–299.

131. Mehra A, Murphy RJ, Wilson BB. Idiopathic familial onychomadesis. *J Am Acad Dermatol* 2000;43:349–350.

132. Bernier V, Labrèze C, Bury F, Taieb A. Nail matrix arrest in the course of hand, foot and mouth diseases. *Eur J Pediatr* 2001;160:649–651.

133. Tosti A, Morelli R, Bardazzi F, Peluso AM. Prevalence of nail abnormalities in children with alopecia areata. *Pediatr Dermatol* 1994;11:112–115.

134. Baran R, Perrin C. Nail degloving, a polyetiologic condition with 3 main patterns: A new syndrome. *J Am Acad Dermatol* 2008;58:232–237.

135. Frederiks E. Treatment of degloved fingers. *Hand* 1973;5:140–144.

136. Tajima T. Treatment of open crushing type of industrial injuries of the hand and forearm: Degloving, open circumferential, heat press, and nail bed injuries. *J Trauma* 1974;14:995–1011.

137. Krishnamoorthy R, Karthikeyan G. Degloving injuries of the hand. *Indian J Plast Surg* 2011;44:227–236.

138. Baran R, Roujeau J. New millenium, new nail problems. *Dermatol Ther* 2002;15:64–70.

139. Fellahi A, Zouhair K, Amraoui A, Benchikhi H. Séquelles cutanéomuqueuses et oculaires des SJS et de Lyell. *Ann Dermatol Vénéréol* 2011;138:88–92.

140. Manios SG, Kanakoundi F, Miliaras-Ulachakis M. Gangrene of lower extremities in a newborn infant, associated with intravascular coagulation (recession of gangrene after heparin therapy). *Helv Paediat Acta* 1972;27:187–192.

141. Wollina U, Verma SB. Acute digital gangrene of a newborn. *Arch Dermatol* 2007;143:121–122.

142. Haneke E. Non-infectious inflammatory disorders of the nail apparatus. *J Dtsch Dermatol Ges* 2009;7:787–797.

143. Stoll ML, Nigrovic PA, Gotte AC, Punaro M. Clinical comparison of early-onset psoriatic and non-psoriatic oligoarticular juvenile idiopathic arthritis. *Clin Exp Rheumatol* 2011;29:582–588.

144. Samman PD. *The Nails in Disease*, 3rd edn. London: Heinemann Med Books, 1978.

145. Shin MK, Kim KS, Ahn JJ, Kim NI, Park HK, Haw CR. Investigation of the hair of patients with scalp psoriasis using atomic force microscopy. *Clin Exp Dermatol* 2012;37:156–163.

146. Bettoli V, De Padova MP, Corazza M, Virgili A. Generalized lichen nitidus with oral and nail involvement in a child. *Dermatology* 1997;194:367–369.

147. Balci S, Kanra G, Aypar E, Son YA. Twenty-nail dystrophy in a mother and her 7-year-old daughter associated with balanced translocation 46, XX, t(6q13;10p13). *Clin Dysmorphol* 2002;11:171–173.

148. Dotz WI, Lieber CD, Vogt PJ. Leukonychia punctata and pitted nails in alopecia areata. *Arch Dermatol* 1985;121:1452–1454.

149. Gandhi V, Baruah MC, Bhattacharaya SN. Nail changes in alopecia areata: Incidence and pattern. *Indian J Dermatol Venereol Leprol* 2003;69:114–115.

150. Caputo R, Gelmetti C, Cambiaghi S. Severe self-healing nail dystrophy in a patient on peritoneal dialysis. *Dermatology* 1997;195:274–275.

151. Cannata G, Gambetti M. Elconyxis, une complication inconnue de l'étrétinate. *Nouv Dermatol* 1990;9:251.

152. Yung A, Johnson P, Goodfield MJ. Isotretinoin-induced elkonyxis. *Br J Dermatol* 2005;153:671–672.

153. Orfanos CE, Mahrle G. Psoriasis (Haut, Nägel, Haare) im Stereomikroskop. *Arch Dermatol Forsch* 1973;244:606–608.

154. Mauro J, Lumpkin LR, Dantzig PI. Scanning electron microscopy of psoriatic nail pits. *N Y State J Med* 1975;75:339–342.

155. Pfister R. Die Psoriasis des Nagels. *Schweiz Rundschau Med* 1981;70:1967–1973.

156. Alkiewicz J. Trachyonychie. *Ann Dermatol Syphiligr* 1950;10:136–140.

157. Achten G, Wanet-Rouard J. Nail atrophy and trachyonychia. *Arch Belge Dermatol* 1974;30:201–207.

158. Samman PD. Trachyonychia (rough nails). *Br J Dermatol* 1979;101:701–705.

159. Hazelrigg DE, Duncan WC, Jarratt M. Twenty-nail dystrophy of childhood. *Arch Dermatol* 1977;113:73–75.

160. Wilkinson JD, Dawber RP, Bowers RP, Fleming K. Twenty-nail dystrophy of childhood. Case report and histopathological findings. *Br J Dermatol* 1979;100:217–221.

161. Arias AM, Yung CW, Rendler S, Soltani K, Lorincz AL. Familial severe twenty-nail dystrophy. *J Am Acad Dermatol* 1982;7:349–352.

162. Pavone L, Li Volti S, Guarneri B, La Rosa M, Sorge G, Incorpora G, Mollica F. Hereditary twenty-nail dystrophy in a Sicilian family. *J Med Genet* 1982;19:337–340.

163. Scher RK, Fischbein R, Ackerman AB. Twenty-nail dystrophy: A variant of lichen planus. *Arch Dermatol* 1978;114(4):612–613.

164. Silverman RA, Rhodes AR. Twenty-nail dystrophy of childhood: A sign of localized lichen planus. *Pediatr Dermatol* 1984;1:207–210.

165. Baran R, Dupré A, Christol B, Bonafé JL, Sayag J, Ferrère J. Vertical striated sand-papered twenty-nail dystrophy. *Ann Dermatol Venereol* 1978;105:387–392.

166. Horn RT Jr, Odom RB. Twenty-nail dystrophy of alopecia areata. *Arch Dermatol* 1980;116:573–574.

167. Kanwar AJ, Ghosh S, Thami GP, Kaur S. Twenty-nail dystrophy due to lichen planus in a patient with alopecia areata. *Clin Exp Dermatol* 1993;18:293–294.

168. Leong AB, Gange RW, O'Connor RD. Twenty-nail dystrophy (trachyonychia) associated with selective IgA deficiency. *J Pediatr* 1982;100:418–420.

169. James WD, Odom RB, Horn RT. Twenty-nail dystrophy and ichthyosis vulgaris. *Arch Dermatol* 1981;117:316.

170. Peloro TM, Pride HB. Twenty-nail dystrophy and vitiligo: A rare association. *J Am Acad Dermatol* 1999;40:488–490.

171. Khandpur S, Reddy BS. An association of twenty-nail dystrophy with vitiligo. *J Dermatol* 2001;28:38–42.

172. Tosti A, Bardazzi F, Piraccini BM, Fanti PA. Idiopathic trachyonychia (twenty-nail dystrophy): A pathological study of 23 patients. *Br J Dermatol* 1994;131:866–872.

173. Tosti A, Fanti PA, Morelli R, Bardazzi F. Trachyonychia associated with alopecia areata: A clinical and pathologic study. *J Am Acad Deramtol* 1991;25:266–270.

174. Jerasutus S, Suvanprakorn P, Kitchawengkul O. Twenty-nail dystrophy. A clinical manifestation of spongiotic inflammation of the nail matrix. *Arch Dermatol* 1990;126:1068–1070.

175. Ohta Y, Katsuoka K. A case report of twenty-nail dystrophy. *J Dermatol* 1997;24:60–62.

176. El Kehdy J, Perruchoud D, Haneke E. Trachyonychia. *Poster, Swiss Soc Dermatol Venereol, Zürich*, Aug 26–28, 2015.

177. Higashi N, Kume A, Ueda K. Clinical and histopathologic study of pseudo-mycotic onychia. *Hifu* 1997;39:469–474.

178. Negroni P. Erythrasma of the nails. *Med Cutan Ibero Lat Am* 1976;4:349–357.

179. Zaias N, Rebell G, Escovar S. Asymmetric gait nail unit syndrome: The most common worldwide toenail abnormality and onychomycosis. *Skinmed* 2014;12:217–223.

180. Zaias N, Escovar SX, Rebell G. Opportunistic toenail onychomycosis. The fungal colonization of an available nail unit space by nondermatophytes is produced by the trauma of the closed shoe by an asymmetric gait or other trauma. A plausible theory. *J Eur Acad Dermatol Venereol* 2014;28:1002–1006.

181. Demis DJ, Weiner MA. Alopecia unversalis, onychodystrophy, and total vitiligo. *Arch Dermatol* 1963;88:195–201.

182. Rubin AI, Baran R. Physical signs. In: Baran R, de Berker DAR, Holzberg M, Thomas L. *Baran & Dawber's Diseases of the Nails and Their Management.* Chichester: Wiley-Blackwell, 2012: 51–99.

183. De Berker DA, Rendall JRS. Retronychia: A proximal ingrowing nail. *J Eur Acad Dermatol* 1999;12:S126.

184. de Berker DA, Richert B, Duhard E, Piraccini BM, André J, Baran R. Retronychia: Proximal ingrowing of the nail plate. *J Am Acad Dermatol* 2008;58:978–983.

185. Dahdah MJ, Kibbi AG, Ghosn S. Retronychia: Report of two cases. *J Am Acad Dermatol* 2008;58:1051–1053.

186. Baumgartner M, Haneke E. Retronychia: Diagnosis and treatment. *Dermatol Surg* 2010;36:1610–1614.

187. Chang P, Haneke E. Retroniquia. Reporte de un caso. *Dermatología CMQ* 2012;10:46–47.

188. Chiheb S, Richert B, Belyamani S, Benchikhi H. Ingrown nail: A new cause of chronic perionyxis. *Ann Dermatol Venereol* 2010;137:645–647.

189. Zaraa I, Kort R, Mokni M, Ben Osman A. Retronychia: A rare cause of chronic paronychia. *Dermatol Online J* 2012;18(6):9.

190. Reigneau M, Pouaha J, Truchetet F. Retronychia: Four new cases. *Eur J Dermatol* 2013;24:882–884.

191. Cabete J, Lencastre A. Recognizing and treating retronychia. *Int J Dermatol* 2015;54:e51–e52.

192. Wortsman X, Wortsman J, Guerrero R, Soto R, Baran R. Anatomical changes in retronychia and onychomadesis detected using ultrasound. *Dermatol Surg* 2010;36:1615–1620.

193. Wortsman X, Calderon P, Baran R. Finger retronychias detected early by 3D ultrasound examination. *J Eur Acad Dermatol Venereol* 2012;26:254–256.

194. Ventura F, Correia O, Barros AM, Haneke E. Retronychia. A study of 20 cases. *J Eur Acad Dermatol* 2016;30:16–19.

195. Piraccini BM, Richert B, de Berker DA, Tengatti V, Sgubbi P, Patrizi A, Stinchi C, Savoia F. Retronychia in children, adolescents and young adults: A case series. *J Am Acad Dermatol* 2014;70:388–390.

196. Arai H, Arai T, Nakajima H, Haneke E. Formable acrylic treatment for ingrowing nail with gutter splint and sculptured nail. *Int J Dermatol* 2004;43:759–765.

197. Haneke E. Controversies in the treatment of ingrown nails. *Dermatol Res Pract* 2012;2012:1–12 Article ID 783924.

198. Mitchell S, Jackson CR, Wilson-Storey D. Surgical treatment of ingrown toenails in children: What is best practice? *Ann R Coll Surg Engl* 2011;93:99–102.

199. Fernandez-Flores A, Martínez-Nova A, Salgado-Fernandez S. Ingrown toenail: Histopathologic and immunohistochemical study. *Am J Dermatopathol* 2009;31:439–445.

200. Fernandez-Flores A, Martínez-Nova A. The use of immunohistochemistry in the evaluation of the nail matrix in biopsies of ingrown toenails. *Rom J Morphol Embryol* 213;54:253–259.

201. Heller J. *Die Krankheiten der Nägel.* Berlin: A Hirschwald, 1900: 100–104, 251–252.

202. Vanhooteghem O, Henrijean A, André J, Richert B, de la Brassine M. Un ongle d'inclusion: une complication de la cure chirurgicale d'ongle incarné selon la technique de Zadik. *Ann Dermatol Venereol* 2006;133:1009–1010.

203. Taylor P, Kaakedjian G. Preliminary studies of the use of nail as a material for reconstructive or cosmetic surgery. *Plast Reconstr Surg* 1998;101:1276–1279.

204. Haneke E, Tosti A, Piraccini BM. Sea urchin granuloma of the nail apparatus: Report of 2 cases. *Dermatology* 1996;192:140–142.

205. Nakamura N, Asai J, Daito J, Takenaka H, Katoh N. Interstitial granulomatous dermatitis? An unusual presentation in the mucosa and periungual skin. *J Dermatol* 2011;38:382–385.

206. Hundeiker M. Hereditäre Nageldysplasie der 5. *Zehe Hautarzt* 1969;20:281–282.

207. Haneke E. Therapie von Nagelfehlbildungen. In: Landthaler M, Hohenleutner U, eds. *Fortschritte der Operativen Dermatologie*, vol. 12. Berlin Wien: Blackwell Wiss-Verl, 1997:180–187.

208. Chi CC, Wang SH. Inherited accessory nail of the fifth toe cured by surgical matricectomy. *Dermatol Surg* 2004;30:1177–1179.

209. Haneke E. Double nail of the little toe. *Skin Appendage Disord* 2016;1:163–167.

210. Mahdi S, Beardsmore J. Post-traumatic double fingernail deformity. *J Hand Surg Br* 1997;22:752–753.

211. Shelley WB, Phillips E. Recurring accessory "fingernail": Periungual fibrokeratoma. *Cutis* 1985;35: 451–454.

212. Perrin C, Baran R. Invaginated fibrokeratoma with matrix differentiation: A new histological variant of acquired fibrokeratoma. *Br J Dermatol* 1994;130: 654–657.

213. Saito S, Ishikawa K. Acquired periungual fibrokeratoma with accessory germinal matrix. *J Hand Surg Br* 2002;27:549–555.

214. Baran R. Nail biting and picking as a possible cause of longitudinal melanonychia: A study of 6 cases. *Dermatologica* 1990;181:126.

215. Anolik RB, Shah K, Rubin AI. Onychophagia-induced longitudinal melanonychia. *Pediatr Dermatol* 2012;29:488.

216. Haneke E. Autoaggressive nail disorders. Trastornos de autoagresión hacia las uñas (Engl & Span). *Dermatol Rev Mex* 2013;57:225–234.

217. Reese JM, Hudacek KD, Rubin AI. Onychotillomania: Clinico-pathologic correlations. *J Cut Pathol* 2013;40:419–423.

218. Kouskoukis CE, Scher RK, Ackerman AB. The problem of features of lichen simplex chronicus complicating the histology of diseases of the nail. *Am J Dermatopathol* 1984;6:45.

219. Anolik RB, Elenitsas R, Minakawa S, Nguyen J, Rubin AI. Histologic features of nail cosmetics. *Am J Dermatopathol* 2012;34:412–415.

220. Hay RJ, ed. *Fortschritte in der lokalen antimykotischen Therapie*. Berlin-Heidelberg-New York-London-Paris Tokyo: Springer, 1988.

221. Baran R, Hay R, Haneke E, Tosti A. *Onychomycosis*, 2nd edn. Oxon: Taylor & Francis, 2006.

222. Abeck D, Haneke E, Nolting S, Reinel D, Seebacher C. Onychomykose. *Dtsch Ärztebl* 2000;97: A-1984–A-1986.

223. Piraccini BM, Alessandrini A, Bruni F, Starace M. Acute periungueal dermatitis induced by application of urea-containing cream under occlusion. *J Dermatol Case Rep* 2012;6:18–20.

Epithelial and fibroepithelial tumors

8

Virtually all tissues comprising the tip of the digit can be the origin of a tumor affecting the nail. Not only are the types of the tumor but also the very structure of the digital tip involved are responsible for the macroscopic appearance of the nail apparatus. In contrast to the hair follicle with its many presumed follicular tumors, specific nail apparatus neoplasms are rare and have only been described recently.[1,2]

Epithelial, fibroepithelial, fibrous and other mesenchymal, vascular, neurogenic, hematogenous, melanocytic, and metastatic tumors plus a variety of reactive and degenerative pseudotumorous lesions occur in and around the nail unit. Whereas their clinical diagnosis often poses difficulties, their histopathology is commonly sufficiently characteristic to allow them to be diagnosed. However, secondary changes due to trauma or infection may alter the histological pattern and a thorough personal history of the patient is therefore mandatory.

There are some general rules concerning the effect of a tumor on nail growth and appearance and vice versa. Any swelling of the nail bed usually leads to lifting of the nail plate often associated with subungual hyperkeratosis; a tumor of the matrix may cause pseudoclubbing or nail dystrophy whereas a circumscribed neoplasm in the proximal nail fold exerts pressure on the matrix causing a longitudinal groove in the nail plate. Lesions obliterating the nail pocket or cul-de-sac frequently give rise to a pterygium and those interfering with the integrity of the matrix epithelium may cause a split nail. Malignant neoplasms may lead to nail destruction whereas slow-growing benign tumors commonly cause nail deformation.

Another potential source of error is pigmentation of a tumor that is usually not pigmented. Hence it may be useful for the nail pathologist to know the skin type of the patient as darkly pigmented individuals tend to present with pigmented epithelial lesions. A peroxidase reaction, which can often be performed by the clinician, can diagnose blood; however, any bleeding tumor including melanomas may be positive with the benzidine reaction.[3,4]

Various types of tumors can affect the subungual space, including benign solid tumors (glomus tumor, subungual exostosis, soft-tissue chondroma, keratoacanthoma, hemangioma, lobular capillary hemangioma), benign cystic lesions (epidermal and myxoid cysts), and malignant tumors (squamous cell carcinoma, malignant melanoma). Modern-day imaging plays an important role in the detection and differentiation of subungual tumors because of their small size, nonspecific clinical manifestations, and functional significance. Ultrasonography (US)—in particular, high-resolution US with color Doppler studies—provides useful information regarding tumor size, location, shape, and internal characteristics (cystic, solid, or mixed), but it is limited in the further characterization of tissue.

Magnetic resonance imaging (MRI) has an important role in categorizing tumors according to their anatomic location, pathologic origin, and signal characteristics. There is some overlap between the US and MR imaging features of subungual tumors; however, certain features can allow accurate diagnosis and expedite management when correlated with clinical and pathologic findings.[5]

8.1 BENIGN EPITHELIAL AND FIBROEPITHELIAL TUMORS

As there are very few purely epithelial tumors and the differentiation between epithelial and fibroepithelial neoplasms is often arbitrary, these neoplasms will be dealt with in this subsection.

8.1.1 Viral warts

Warts are certainly the most frequent reactive tumors of the nail apparatus. They are often observed in children though adults may also be infected. Most are due to common benign human papillomavirus (HPV) types such as types 1, 2, 4, and 7, with the latter being commonly observed in butchers. Warts are slowly growing, weakly contagious fibroepithelial growths and said to have a natural lifespan of 2–5 years. Their clinical appearance depends on their localization within the nail apparatus: those on the proximal nail fold are not different from other body sites, those on the lateral nail folds are usually more oval and often fissured, those at the hyponychium may appear as a deeply fissured keratotic horn or a slightly hyperkeratotic rim, which swells and becomes white more rapidly than the surrounding skin after immersion in water. Subungual warts may raise the nail plate. The most important differential diagnoses in adults are subungual Bowen disease and squamous cell carcinoma. Warts on the ridged skin of the tip of the digit look like palmar or plantar warts, respectively.

The major clinical challenge of subungual and periungual warts is their treatment as they often persist longer than the predicted 2–5 years and may be a source of spread during this period.[3,6]

8.1.1.1 Histopathology

In typical cases that are very rarely biopsied, ungual verrucae vulgares do not differ from warts elsewhere. They present a marked acanthosis, irregular hyperkeratosis, and broad granular layer with clumped keratohyalin granules and marked cytopathic effects though infrequently as strong as in classical plantar warts. There may be long connective tissue papillae with dilated capillaries, the tips of which are often thrombosed. Frequently, parakeratotic columns overlie these papillae and they contain small blood clots, probably due to transepidermal elimination of the thrombosed tips of the capillary loops. Koilocytes are present in the uppermost spinous layer and the granular layer. Trichilemmal differentiation is commonly seen in old warts. The fan-like architecture seen in cutaneous warts is rare in ungual warts.

Verrucae of the hyponychium may only show considerable thickening of the epidermis, vacuolization of the granular layer, and a thick, but loose basket weave-like horny layer.

As many subjects tend to traumatize their ungual warts, some bleeding and inflammation may be seen. A lichenoid infiltrate is assumed to be a sign of wart regression.

8.1.1.2 Differential diagnosis

The differential diagnosis comprises all potentially verrucous lesions, the most important of which are squamous cell carcinoma, Bowen's disease, and verrucous melanoma. However, there are many more infectious and benign lesions such as tuberculosis cutis verrucosa, also called prosector's wart or butcher's nodule, onychopapilloma, onycholemmal horn,[1] subungual corn (heloma subunguale), subungual warty hyperkeratoses in incontinentia pigmenti, subungual keratoacanthoma, subungual vegetations in amyloidosis, inflammatory linear verrucous epidermal nevus, or lichen striatus. Multicentric reticulohistiocytosis may cause a rim of small verrucous nodules along the free margin of the proximal nail fold. Onychophosis is a painful keratotic lesion in the lateral nail groove of the toenails. Mucinous eccrine metaplasia may clinically appear like a subungual wart.[7] Vacuolization of keratinocytes, also called pagetoid dyskeratosis, of the tip of the toe is a frequent chance observation without pathologic relevance (Figure 8.1) and must be differentiated from the flat wart type at the hyponychium.

8.1.2 Seborrheic keratosis

Whereas seborrheic keratoses (SKs) are probably the most frequent benign tumors of humankind, they are exceedingly rare in the subungual location. Clinically, SKs may resemble onychopapilloma or subungual linear keratotic melanonychia,[8] but white keratin inclusions are seen by dermatoscopy.[9]

8.1.2.1 Histopathology

Mainly in the matrix region, an acanthoma-like thickening of the epithelium is seen that appears to be made up of basaloid cells. The architecture is regular with some keratin inclusions. There are no mitoses, cellular atypias, nor dyskeratoses (Figure 8.2). Pigmentation is not very pronounced.

We observed a case of subungual irritated seborrheic keratosis with less regular architecture and some squamous eddies that were made up of nail-like keratin (Figure 8.3).

8.1.2.2 Differential diagnosis

Acanthosis of the nail bed epithelium is also found in onychopapilloma and Bowen's disease. Subepithelial keratin inclusions are seen in the so-called subungual epidermal inclusion cysts and onychopapilloma. Basal cell carcinoma

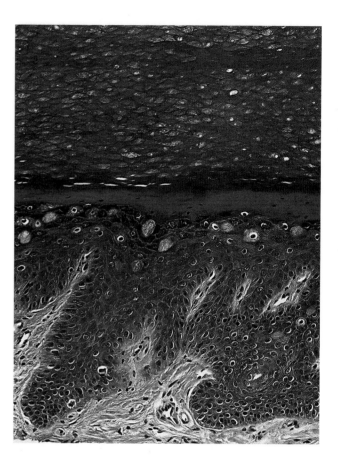

Figure 8.1 Pagetoid dyskeratosis of the tip of the toe in a patient with a distal nail fold. H&E.

may also be very similar. Onychocytic matricoma[10] is histologically very similar, if not identical.

8.1.3 Subungual linear keratotic melanonychia

Two cases of this particular lesion have been described. Clinically, a narrow brown streak in the nail was seen running from the distal lunula to the hyponychium but not involving the nail's free margin.[8]

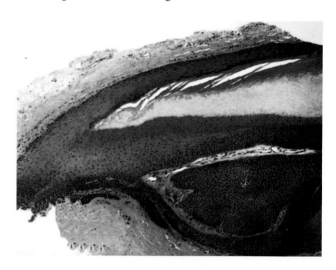

Figure 8.2 Subungual seborrheic keratosis. H&E. (Courtesy of Dr. C. Treewittayapoom, Bangkok.)

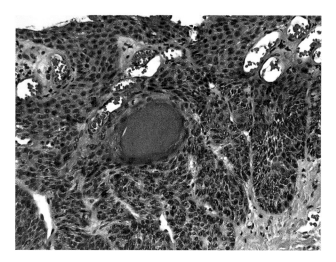

Figure 8.3 So-called irritated subungual seborrheic keratosis. The cells are all small basophilic cuboid cells, the horn pearl is orthokeratotic but without a keratogenous zone. H&E.

8.1.3.1 Histopathology

There is only one report of the nail plate with adherent pigmented basaloid keratinocytes in two patients. The nail plate is slightly indented and heavily pigmented keratinocytes undergoing cornification are attached to its undersurface. The lesions are similar to seborrheic keratoses.[8]

8.1.3.2 Differential diagnosis

Onychopapilloma and onychocytic acanthoma are the main differential diagnoses, but the former is usually not or only slightly pigmented.

8.1.4 Onychocytic acanthoma

Onychocytic acanthoma was recently described as an entity of its own; a relation to subungual seborrheic keratosis (SK) was dismissed as SKs are said to be only observed on hairy skin. Clinically, a dark brown longitudinal streak with slight thickening of the nail plate is seen[10,11] that appears as a keratotic lesion at the undersurface of the free margin. Thus, the lesion is very similar, if not identical, to subungual seborrheic keratosis and linear keratotic melanonychia. In the meantime, a hypopigmented variant was also described. On partial nail avulsion, a yellow-white nodule was seen in the matrix and held to be responsible for the production of the thickened yellowish nail streak.[12]

8.1.4.1 Histopathology

The matrix epithelium shows an acanthoma-like thickening due to predominantly basaloid cells with basophilic nuclei. They tend to form whorls of cells of the prekeratogenous and keratogenous zones with central keratinization giving rise to pearl-like structures (Figure 8.4). A mild inflammatory infiltrate may be present in the upper dermis. Melanin stains such as Fontana as well as immunohistochemical demonstration of melanocytes clearly show the pigment and melanocytes.

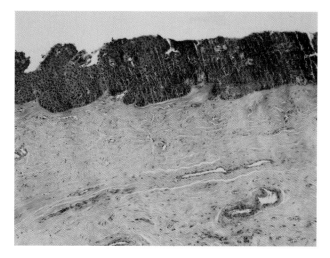

Figure 8.4 Onychocytic matricoma showing great similarity with the subungual seborrheic keratosis. H&E.

8.1.4.2 Differential diagnosis

Subungual SK and subungual linear keratotic melanonychia are probably identical lesions. Onychopapilloma is not made up of basaloid cells only.

8.1.5 Subungual filamentous tumor

Originally described by Samman in 1972,[13] subungual filamentous tumor is now thought by some authors to be a narrow onychopapilloma. However, we believe that these two lesions are sufficiently different both on clinical as well as histological grounds to consider them to be entities of their own.

Subungual filamentous tumor is seen as a 1–1.5 mm wide streak in the nail running from the distal matrix to the free end of the nail plate. The color is whitish to yellowish, rarely light brown or reddish. It forms a small keratotic rim at the undersurface of the free margin that can be easily and painlessly pared off. Growth is slow and the duration of the lesion is often not remembered. Frequently, a small V-shaped notch is present in the free margin, which is often the reason to consult the dermatologist. Careful nail plate avulsion shows it as a very narrow keratotic rim running all along the undersurface of the nail plate that causes a slight longitudinal depression in the nail bed. Its origin in the matrix is barely seen, even when using a head magnifier lens.

8.1.5.1 Histopathology

A transverse section through the nail plate with the attached subungual filamentous tumor reveals a rim of keratin with a somewhat whorled structure. There is no pigmentation.

The biopsy of the lesion in the matrix reveals a tiny hood-like structure covered with a thin epidermis with a relatively pronounced granular layer on top (Figure 8.5).

8.1.5.2 Differential diagnosis

Onychopapilloma and other longitudinal keratotic structures have to be considered.

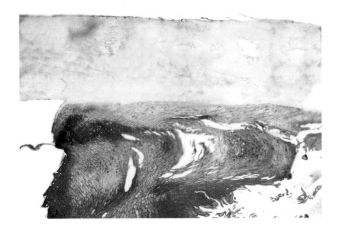

Figure 8.5 Subungual filamentous tumor. There is no alteration of the nail plate. PAS stain.

8.1.6 Onychopapilloma

The term of onychopapilloma was first coined in 2000 for longitudinal erythronychia with distal subungual keratosis; the authors proposed to use this term instead of localized, distal, subungual keratosis with multinucleate cells.[14] The existence of onychopapilloma was first disputed,[15] but is now generally accepted.[16,17] Onychopapillomas are not identical with the ungual papillomas mentioned by Heller more than 100 years ago;[18,19] he had already stressed that this term designates a potpourri of different entities. However, he had cited another observation of a painful subungual papilloma,[20] the nature of which is not clear.

Onychopapilloma is a fairly common lesion of the nails. Most occur on fingers although some were also seen on toes. They commonly present as a longitudinal whitish, yellowish, reddish, or sometimes light brown streak in the nail that originates from the distal matrix as a pink band with a cuneiform beginning.[21,22] Its width is usually 3–4 mm and does not exceed 5–6 mm. Splinter hemorrhages occur in about one-quarter of the cases. Looking at the undersurface of the free nail margin reveals a keratosis of variable thickness and a circumscribed thinning of the nail plate. There is often a wedge-shaped area of distal onycholysis and also a distal fissure in the nail plate. This may be embarrassing, but other signs and symptoms are usually not present. Our treatment of choice is horizontal excision along its entire length, which leads to normal nail growth without recurrence. In contrast, simple nail avulsion or traumatic nail abrasion is followed by nail regrowth with the same appearance of the onychopapilloma (unpublished observation).

8.1.6.1 Histopathology

The histopathological picture varies according to the type of biopsy or excision and to the level and direction of sectioning.[23]

In transverse sections of a full-thickness excision specimen, at its most proximal level in the distal matrix, there is a circumscribed acanthosis of the matrix epithelium with finger-like rete ridges that spread a bit outward to the depth like a fan. A tendency to premature keratinization is seen; however, the keratinized cells remain identifiable as single cells and differ from normal maturing cells of the matrix. The overlying nail plate exhibits a slight but well-circumscribed indentation, which remains visible all along the nail plate until its free margin. At the level of the nail bed, the acanthosis becomes more obvious. The prematurely keratinized cells are still discernable, but are more condensed. The cells of the acanthotic rete ridges take on a peculiar fusiform shape in vertical to oblique arrangement, which is also seen very distally. Their cytoplasm exhibits keratin fibers that usually run up vertically or slightly obliquely. Occasional binucleate and multinucleated keratinocytes are seen in the mid-nail bed level. In the hyponychium area, the hyperkeratosis is compact to verruciform but still adheres to the nail plate. Splinter hemorrhages may be seen as small lakes of blood either at the border between the epithelium and the keratosis or in the hyperkeratosis.

When the lesion was removed tangentially after partial nail avulsion, only the lower epithelial portion is commonly seen. The more the section is distal, the more the cells take on a fusiform shape; the cells are often oriented vertically and the unique fibers are more clearly seen. The hyperkeratosis tends to get more compact.

Occasionally, the cells of the acanthotic proximal portion may have a light cytoplasm and resemble sebaceous cells (Figure 8.6). In the nail bed, there may be some large

(a) (b)

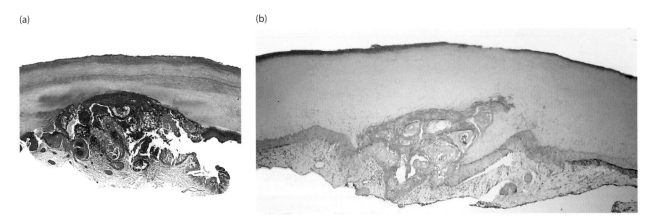

Figure 8.6 (a,b) Onychopapilloma, transverse section at the level of the distal matrix. H&E.

(a) (b) (c)

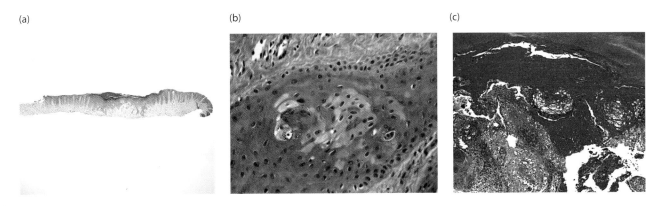

Figure 8.7 Onychopapilloma demonstrating large clear cells with some keratohyaline-like granules in the depth of a deep tumor peg, mid- to distal nail bed. H&E. (a) Scanning magnification of a longitudinal tangential excision from the distal matrix to the hyponychium. (b) Bottom of a proliferated rete ridge at the level of the mid-nail bed with large light cells and small round keratohyalin-like granules. (c) Transverse section of a full-thickness excision specimen with clear cells in the papillomatous portion.

clear cells in the depth of the acanthotic rete ridges that exhibit small round keratohyalin granules (Figure 8.7). Some multinucleate cells may be present, but dyskeratoses and mitoses do not occur. Association with ungual lichen planus has also been observed (Figure 8.8). Pigmentation is possible.[24]

The keratin deriving from the onychopapilloma has different staining properties and is more eosinophilic than that of the nail plate. It is apparently prone to fungal invasion. Up to now, no human papillomavirus DNA has been found by immunohistochemistry.

Immunohistochemistry shows a cytokeratin pattern of the onychopapilloma like that of the surrounding epithelium as well as an identical CD10 and CD34 staining.

8.1.6.2 Differential diagnosis

As has been mentioned before, seborrheic keratosis and linear acanthotic melanonychia have to be ruled out in case of a brown onychopapilloma. Bowen's disease may also appear as an erythronychia[25,26] and is thus an important differential diagnosis. However, a variety of other circumscribed lesions originating in the distal matrix or proximal nail bed may cause a similar band-like appearance, such as subungual acantholytic dyskeratotic acanthoma and warty dyskeratoma.

8.1.7 Localized multinucleate distal subungual keratosis

Distal subungual multinucleate keratosis is a circumscribed lesion said to originate from the distal nail bed. Clinically, it exhibits a wart-like hyperkeratosis under the free margin of the nail plate indenting the hyponychial skin. It may look like a subungual fibrokeratoma with a particularly hyperkeratotic tip. The authors later joined this lesion to onychopapilloma.

8.1.7.1 Histopathology

There is an acanthosis with occasional dyskeratotic cells and a marked hyperkeratosis between the lesional nail bed and the nail plate. Extirpation of the entire lesion reveals that its origin is the distal matrix. It is most probably an onychopapilloma variant.[14,27]

8.1.7.2 Differential diagnosis

As the first authors later clarified, they assume it to be an onychopapilloma (variant). Apart from it, the most

(a) (b)

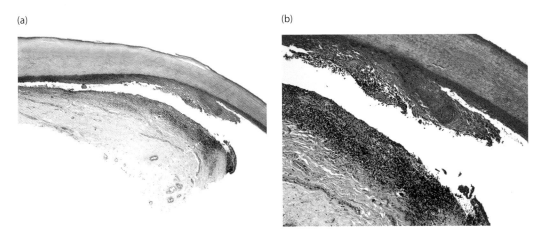

Figure 8.8 (a,b) Onychopapilloma with lichen planus. Longitudinal section from matrix till hyponychium. H&E.

important clinical and histological differential diagnoses are Bowen's disease and subungual squamous cell carcinoma.

8.1.8 Subungual acantholytic dyskeratotic acanthoma

This lesion was recently described in the subungual location. All three cases were clinically diagnosed as onychopapillomas, 3–5 mm in width. The time of evolution was about 6–9 months. Clinically, the lesions were yellowish over the nail bed and reddish over the matrix. One case presented splinter hemorrhages.[28] We have observed another three cases.

8.1.8.1 Histopathology

The histopathological changes involve the distal matrix, nail bed, hyponychium, and digital pulp. The epithelium is acanthotic with pronounced subungual parakeratotic hyperkeratosis that lifts the nail plate up. Sometimes, many neutrophils are found in the hyperkeratosis. Abundant suprabasal acantholytic clefts and dyskeratotic cells are demonstrated in the nail bed. They remain either polygonal or resemble corps ronds and grains. An occasional atypical cell and mitosis may be seen (Figure 8.9).

8.1.8.2 Differential diagnosis

The unique coexistence of acantholysis and dyskeratosis is only found in subungual warty dyskeratoma, which shows a pronounced villous structure and numerous multinucleate cells. The histopathologic changes in Darier's dyskeratosis follicularis and pemphigus familiaris of Hailey-Hailey are much less pronounced.

8.1.9 Subungual warty dyskeratoma

Warty dyskeratoma is an uncommon benign tumor usually found in hairy skin. Its location in the distal matrix is exceedingly rare. Clinically it causes a longitudinal red streak with fine splinter hemorrhages and slight fissuring of the free nail plate margin. At the hyponychium, a small keratin-filled crater is seen.[29]

8.1.9.1 Histopathology

As its counterpart in other locations, subungual warty dyskeratoma is histologically characterized by an endophytic proliferation of squamous epithelium with prominent acantholytic dyskeratosis resulting in suprabasal clefting. There is a circumscribed acanthosis with digitiform rete ridges that tend to spread out and run almost horizontally under the nail bed epithelium.[29] Numerous multinucleate keratinocytes, prominent suprabasal acantholysis, and many dyskeratotic cells are found. Often, mitoses are observed.

8.1.9.2 Differential diagnosis

The main differential diagnosis is subungual acantholytic dyskeratotic acanthoma. Nail involvement in dyskeratosis follicularis of Darier exhibits similar changes but much less pronounced.[29] Benign familial pemphigus of Hailey-Hailey commonly causes whitish longitudinal bands but its histologic appearance is similar if not almost identical to ungual Darier's disease. In the publication on subungual warty dyskeratoma, subungual focal acantholytic dyskeratosis was interpreted as another case of warty dyskeratoma.[30]

8.1.10 Epidermal nevi

There are a variety of different types of epidermal nevi though involvement of the distal dorsal digit and the nail is only described in verrucous epidermal nevi. Most are present since birth, but they may also occur in later life. Depending on their localization in the nail apparatus, they may cause wart-like lesions on the proximal nail fold, ridging of the nail plate when its undersurface is affected, or nail splitting in case of matrix and/or nail bed involvement.[31] A clinically similar condition was observed in a little girl with a porokeratotic eccrine duct and hair follicle nevus.[32]

8.1.10.1 Histopathology

The histology is identical with verrucous epidermal nevi elsewhere. There is marked epidermal papillomatosis with hyperorthokeratosis, but acanthosis is usually not very pronounced. When it occurs in the matrix, no normal nail formation is observed. There is no inflammatory infiltrate and cytopathic effects as seen in viral warts are not present.

So-called epidermolytic epidermal nevi as sometimes observed in family members of patients with bullous ichthyosiform erythroderma have, to our knowledge, not

(a)

(b)

(c)

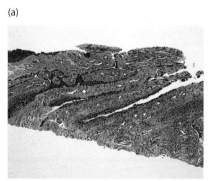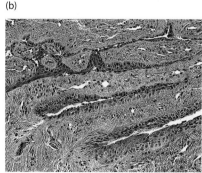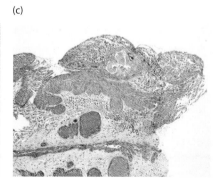

Figure 8.9 (a,b,c) Subungual acantholytic dyskeratotic acanthoma.

been observed in the nail apparatus although bullous ichthyosiform erythroderma may involve the nail (see Chapter 6).

8.1.10.2 Differential diagnosis

Epidermal nevi cannot be distinguished from widespread lesions of the same type.

8.1.11 Subungual verrucous proliferations of incontinentia pigmenti

Incontinentia pigmenti of Bloch-Sulzberger is an X-linked dominant syndrome, which is usually lethal for male offspring. Many different organs may be involved, but the skin typically undergoes a development in stages: the first stage is seen at birth or shortly thereafter as multilocular intraepidermal blisters with characteristic eosinophilia, the second stage is verrucous with almost identical changes as seen in young women with subungual lesions, and the third stage is characterized by linear hyperpigmentations that with time may become hypopigmented and are sometimes referred to as stage 4. All these lesions are distributed along the Blaschko lines.[33,34] The underlying molecular defect is a mutation of the NEMO gene, which is required for nuclear factor κB (NFκB) activation.[35]

Nail involvement is observed between the ages of 15 and 35 years (3 and 45 years[36]) and may be the sole manifestation.[37] It mainly occurs on fingers, but big toenail involvement has been described.[38,39] They are usually painful warty or tumorous lesions elevating the nail from its bed.[40–42] Marginal erythema may be observed. Matrix involvement leads to nail destruction. Bone erosion may be responsible for the pain. Spontaneous resolution followed by recurrence was observed in a patient during her two pregnancies. In one case, human papillomavirus type 15 was detected.[43]

Many cases have finally resolved, but retinoids appear to be the treatment of choice.[44]

8.1.11.1 Histopathology

The nail bed and/or matrix are acanthotic with a very pronounced, irregularly arranged, and even whorled hyperkeratosis. There are many clusters of dyskeratotic cells in all levels of the epithelium and particularly within the hyperkeratosis, which is diagnostic for these lesions (Figure 8.10).

8.1.11.2 Differential diagnosis

Keratoacanthoma, which is also characterized by pain and often shows many single dyskeratoses, may be almost indistinguishable. Warts, acantholytic dyskeratotic acanthoma, subungual epidermoid inclusions, subungual fibroma, Bowen's disease, and squamous cell carcinoma have to be considered.[45,46]

8.1.12 Epidermal cysts

Epidermal cysts of the nail apparatus are usually due to trauma, which may, however, not always be remembered by the patient. A heavy trauma may even lead to intraosseous implantation of squamous epithelium.[47–50] Postoperative epidermal cysts are found in the very vicinity of the

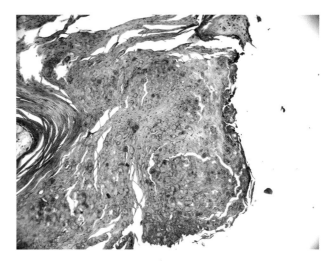

Figure 8.10 Painful subungual tumor of incontinentia pigmenti showing masses of dyskeratotic cells within parakeratosis. H&E.

scar.[51,52] Most epidermal cysts are slow-growing, symptomless lesions.[53] Rapidly enlarging cysts may cause discomfort and pain and lead to nail loss.[54] When localized in the matrix connective tissue, transverse overcurvature or clubbing may develop. Radiograph may show indentation of the bone.[55] Ultrasound is said to have a high sensitivity.[56]

8.1.12.1 Histopathology

The cyst is lined with a regular thin epidermis with a normal stratum granulosum. The keratin is usually layered in an onion-shell like manner. However, rupture is frequent and may lead to partial disappearance of the epidermal lining with formation of a keratin granuloma (Figure 8.11).

8.1.12.2 Differential diagnosis

All space occupying lesions may clinically mimic an ungual epidermal cyst. Histologically, other cysts and cystic tumors have to be considered. Matrix and onycholemmal cysts develop mainly when the corresponding part of

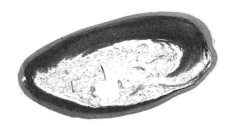

Figure 8.11 Subungual traumatic epidermal cyst. H&E.

the nail apparatus was buried due to a heavy trauma or during surgery, most commonly for ingrown nails.

8.1.13 Matrix cysts

Matrix cysts are clinically indistinguishable from epidermal inclusion cysts, but they are usually due to a surgical intervention in the matrix region.

8.1.13.1 Histopathology

This cyst type is characterized by a lining that at least in part consists of matrix epithelium and may show true nail formation within its lumen. In addition, there may also be a structure similar to the nail bed, to which the intracystic nail is attached. The roof is then composed of epidermis similar to the ventral surface of the proximal nail fold (Figure 8.12).

Matrix cysts may also be histologically diagnosed when a nail spicule is cut horizontally giving the appearance of a nail completely surrounded (in 2 dimensions!) by matrix epithelium. However, hybrid matrix-epidermis cysts are not rare and are mainly seen after matrix tissue was left in the depth of the lateral matrix horn after wedge excision for an ingrown nail. This type of cyst imitates the nail unit in that its cyst lining consists of matrix epithelium producing nail and of epidermis producing layered compact eosinophilic keratin.

8.1.13.2 Differential diagnosis

All other cysts, particularly epidermal cysts, have to be considered in the histopathologic differential diagnosis. So-called subungual epidermoid inclusions are much smaller and often occur as multiple lesions.

8.1.14 Subungual epidermoid inclusions-onycholemmal cysts

Subungual epidermoid inclusions usually do not cause signs or symptoms; however, in some cases they have led to subungual hyperkeratosis or were observed in association with finger clubbing.[57,58] In our experience, they are a frequent incidental finding in nail biopsies commonly without pathognomonic significance. They are thought to derive from epidermal buds of the rete ridges.[59] Trauma has been assumed to play an etiological role.[60] We have also seen them in several subungual melanomas; whether this is a sign of irritation of the nail bed is not yet clear.

8.1.14.1 Histopathology

Subungual epidermoid inclusions are found in the distal matrix and above all in the nail bed dermis. They are small round to oval epithelial structures. In contrast to epidermal cysts, they do not grow bigger than approximately 1 mm in diameter. An elongation of the rete ridges with pinching off of the lower parts may be seen thus giving rise to free-lying cysts in the nail bed dermis. They are filled with concentric orthokeratotic keratin, but often do not develop a granular layer and their cells do not flatten toward the lumen, hence they were also called multiple subungual onycholemmal cysts.[61] They may occur singly or as multiple lesions (Figures 8.13 and 8.14), often in association with an onychopapilloma. We have seen several cases of subungual melanoma with underlying onycholemmal cysts (unpublished observation). Calcification has been described;[61] this is not a rare phenomenon and sometimes there is no epithelium left around it. Possibly, at least a part of the so-called subungual calcifications develop by this mechanism.

Another variant with marked subungual hyperkeratosis, hyperplasia of the nail bed, and short and dystrophic nails was described; a traumatic origin was assumed.[62]

8.1.14.2 Differential diagnosis

All conditions causing subungual hyperkeratosis, particularly nail psoriasis, eczema, and onychomycosis have to be ruled out. Epidermoid inclusions were assumed to mimic miniature trichilemmal cysts.[61]

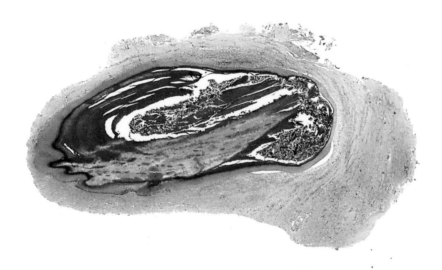

Figure 8.12 Subungual postoperative matrix cyst with all elements of a nail including matrix, nail plate formation, nail bed, and isthmus. H&E.

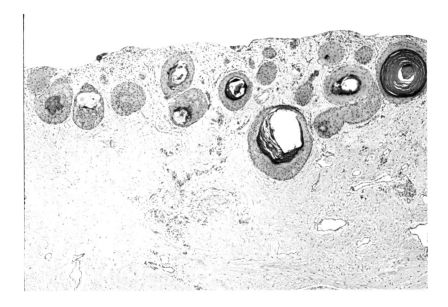

Figure 8.13 Multiple small onycholemmal cysts in the nail bed dermis. H&E.

8.1.15 Subungual trichoadenoma

Trichoadenoma is a rare tumor that mainly develops in the face or on the buttocks,[63] rarely on the neck, arm, or thigh.[64,65] One report described a subungual trichoadenoma as a very tender, hyperkeratotic nodule under a fingernail.[66] There was neither bone destruction nor ossification in the distal phalanx. It was mentioned that the origin of this "trichoadenoma" remains unclear as there are no hair follicles in the nail region; whether this can be seen as another hint at the developmental similarity between the hair and nail[1] or was just a case of multiple small subungual epidermoid inclusions in a very distal location is not clear.

8.1.15.1 Histopathology

Numerous small keratin-filled cysts, longitudinal cystic structures, and solid tumor islands were scattered in the nail bed dermis. There was no continuity between the nail bed epithelium and the tumor. Keratin-filled cysts were surrounded by a proliferation of eosinophilic epidermoid cells. Most of the cyst linings contained a granular layer with keratohyaline granules. Solid tumor islands consisted only of epithelial cells without keratinization. Cytokeratin antibodies exhibited a staining pattern similar to epidermis (CK1-8, CK1, CK10), to suprabasal cells of the follicular infundibulum (CK1, CK10), and to the lower part of follicular epithelium (CK17). Antibodies marking secretory cells of sweat glands (CK7, CK8, CK18, CK19) and the outermost cells of the hair bulge (CK19) were negative.[66]

8.1.15.2 Differential diagnosis

Trichoadenoma is believed to differentiate toward infundibular epithelium. The most important histopathologic differential diagnosis is subungual epithelial inclusions, which, however, do not display a granular layer.

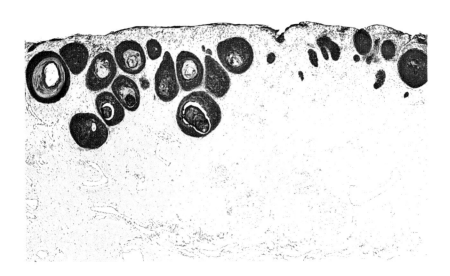

Figure 8.14 The onycholemmal cysts are clearly demonstrated using a pancytokeratin antibody.

8.1.16 Onycholemmal horn

Onycholemmal horn is a rare lesion originating from the nail bed, mostly its lateral part. It is a slow-growing symptomless lesion and clinically resembles a wart or another hyperkeratotic tumor including keratoacanthoma and squamous cell carcinoma.[1] The term "onycholemmal horn" was coined as it architecturally and cytologically closely resembles a trichilemmal horn.[67–69] The nail bed is analogous to the outer root sheath of the hair follicle in its way of keratinization.[70] Also Ackerman considered the nail bed to be similar to the outer root sheath.[71]

8.1.16.1 Histopathology

The lesion is markedly hyperkeratotic and acanthotic. The epithelium resembles that of a trichilemmal horn with large pale cells becoming larger toward the surface and keratinizing abruptly without flattening, often without forming a granular layer, although this may in part be present. There may be multiple apoptoses. The basal layer consists of one or two rows of small cuboid cells. Mitoses and cell atypias are not seen.[1] Another such lesion that was clinically considered to be a squamous cell carcinoma had a more verrucous aspect and again enlarging cells toward the surface. Here, keratohyalin granules were present in many of these large round keratinocytes, which often dissolved from the acanthotic epithelium and freely "floated" in the markedly eosinophilic orthokeratin (Figure 8.15). No cytopathic effects were seen (unpublished observation).

8.1.16.2 Differential diagnosis

Depending on the architecture, a common wart, a keratoacanthoma, or a squamous cell carcinoma may have to be considered.

8.1.17 Proliferating onycholemmal tumor

Proliferating onycholemmal tumor is a very rare lesion deriving from the nail bed. It grows slowly without causing symptoms. Clinically it may resemble a wart, onycholemmal horn, Bowen's disease, keratoacanthoma, or squamous cell carcinoma.

8.1.17.1 Histopathology

Proliferating onycholemmal tumor presents as an exophytic lesion with striking cytologic and architectural resemblance with a proliferating trichilemmal tumor. It is a solid growth with small and regularly arranged basal cells with round basophilic nuclei. The cells gradually enlarge and become paler until they abruptly keratinize. Cyst formation is not seen though small keratinized areas may appear. There are no mitoses and cellular atypias. The border to the neighboring epidermal and nail bed keratinocytes is clearly discernable. Dyskeratoses are absent or very few (Figure 8.16). As the lesion originates from the nail bed, the nail plate itself is not involved.

8.1.17.2 Differential diagnosis

The main histological differential diagnoses are onycholemmal horn, proliferating onycholemmal cyst, and subungual tumors of incontinentia pigmenti, but keratoacanthoma may also have to be considered.

8.1.18 Proliferating onycholemmal cyst

Proliferating onycholemmal cyst is an exceedingly rare lesion of the nail bed with insidious symptomless growth. Clinically it resembles a wart, Bowen's disease, or squamous cell carcinoma; it can be distinguished from keratoacanthoma due to its very slow progression and absence of pain.

8.1.18.1 Histopathology

Proliferating onycholemmal cyst is morphologically very similar to proliferating trichilemmal cyst, hence its designation. It appears solid and mainly exophytic, though many small and medium-sized cyst-like formations are seen. The peripheral cells are relatively small with dense nuclei, but their arrangement is not as regular as in a

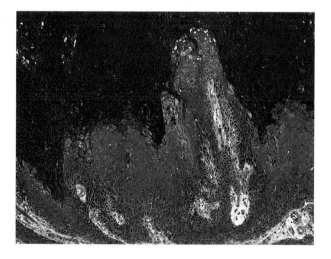

Figure 8.15 Onycholemmal horn with small cuboidal basal cells and large cells of the spinous layer that abruptly keratinize. H&E.

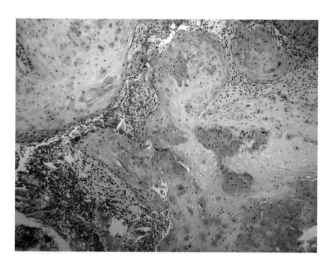

Figure 8.16 Proliferating onycholemmal tumor with large-cell tumor conglomerates.

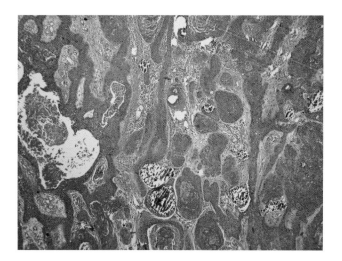

Figure 8.17 Proliferating onycholemmal cyst displaying great similarity with a proliferating trichilemmal cyst.

trichilemmal cyst. Toward the center of the tumor formations, the cells increase in size to finally keratinize abruptly without a granular layer. Again, the keratin is not as regular as in a trichilemmal cyst and often has the appearance as if it were rather the result of keratinocyte necrosis than of regular keratinization. Long slender digitiform epithelial extensions are seen between the tumor islands (Figure 8.17).

The lesion shows strong nuclear labeling with p63, but MIB1 stains more cells of the normal digitiform epithelial strands than of the lesion itself.

8.1.18.2 Differential diagnosis

Onycholemmal horn and proliferating onycholemmal tumor have to be differentiated. Careful evaluation of the different criteria will allow onycholemmal horn to be distinguished.[1] Malignant onycholemmal cyst exhibits cellular atypias and pathological mitoses.

8.1.19 Onychomatricoma

Onychomatricoma is probably an underdiagnosed benign tumor of the nail matrix. Since its first description by Baran and Kint in 1992,[72] roughly 200 cases have been described but certainly more were observed.[73–77] Men and women are equally affected. By far, most patients are middle-aged Caucasians, but one patient was black[78] and one case occurred in a child.[79] Fingers are twice as frequently involved as toes.[80] Clinically, it is an insidiously growing, painless tumor characterized by a funnel-shaped, yellow streaky, thickened nail with transverse overcurvature and splinter hemorrhages in its proximal portion.[81] Usually, only a segment of the nail is involved, but also the entire matrix may be affected.[82] End-on dermatoscopy exhibits tiny holes in the nail plate. On cutting such a nail, it may bleed from such a hole[83] as the long filiform projections of the tumor may extend to the free margin of the nail and dilated capillaries may remain patent although this is very rare. Pigmented variants of onychomatricoma and onychomatricomas leading to a pterygium-like appearance have been described.[84–86] Depending on their main location, they may also cause nail fold swelling.[63] In rare occasions, a cutaneous horn may be formed.[87] A polypoid variant was also reported.[88] Onychomycosis may be a complicating additional factor.[84]

Magnetic resonance imaging shows the same characteristics as normal matrix tissue, but the characteristic channels in the nail plate are clearly visible.[89,90] They can also be visualized by confocal laser scanning microscopy.[91] Ultrasound may help to make the correct diagnosis.[92] The bone is not involved.

8.1.19.1 Histopathology

Onychomatricoma has quite a distinctive histological appearance allowing the diagnosis to be made both from the nail plate as well as the tumor itself. It is a benign fibro-epithelial neoplasm, the stroma of which consists in its more superficial portion of densely packed, but mainly fine, wavy collagen fibers and many fibroblasts with a relatively well pronounced cytoplasm (Figure 8.18). The deeper part of the stroma has coarser collagen fibers. The stroma is characteristically positive for both CD10 and CD34.[93] Mucin may be abundant in the stroma (Figure 8.19).[94]

The epithelial component is identical to normal matrix epithelium and apparently produces nail substance at a normal rate.[73]

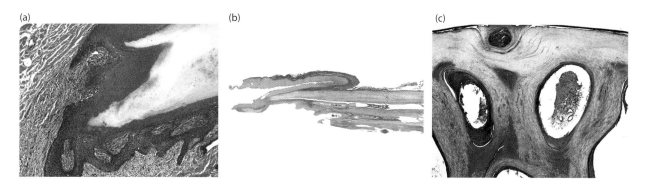

Figure 8.18 Onychomatricoma. (a) There is a papillomatous matrix epithelium and a characteristic cell-rich stroma. (b) Longitudinal section of an early onychomatricoma with the overlying nail exhibiting long channels with edematous stroma. (c) A transverse section of the nail shows the typical holes lined by matrix epithelium and appearing almost empty. H&E.

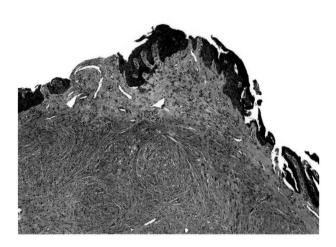

Figure 8.19 Mucinous onychomatricoma with papillomatous matrix epithelium and a strongly mucinous stroma. H&E.

The peculiarity of this tumor is, however, its unique architecture. It forms long slender filiform digitations both outward as well as inward into the connective tissue stroma. This leads to a tremendous increase in matrix epithelium surface, which is the reason for the circumscribed nail thickening.[73] Both on longitudinal as well as transverse sections of the tumor, these features are clearly seen. In sections containing both the tumor together with its nail, the filiform projections are seen to extend into the nail substance and to form channels in the nail plate. These are lined by normal matrix epithelium undergoing normal onychotization and at their base they contain the densely cellular stroma that gradually "degenerates" to highly edematous, cell-poor tissue with capillary vessels (Figure 8.18). These tend to become thrombosed distally seen as splinter hemorrhages, but may remain patent, which gives rise to the bleeding nail on cutting its free margin.

The nail plate reveals characteristic changes.[95] On transverse cuts, round to oval holes are seen in the nail plate, which particularly in the more proximal portion of the nail plate are lined by the superficial compartment of the matrix epithelium. This epithelial lining is seen to gradually degenerate toward the distal margin of the nail (Figure 8.18b,c).

There are several variants of onychomatricoma. Most cases are broad based, but some are polypoid. When there is clinically a pterygium, the undersurface of the proximal nail fold is partially or completely transformed into onychomatricoma.

We have seen also a polypoid onychomatricoma with a heavily mucinous stroma (unpublished) (Figure 8.19). Pigmentation is a rare event. Melanocyte markers show a moderate number of melanocytes.

Electron microscopy was performed on two onychomatricomas. There is a normal basal lamina separating the epithelial portion from the stroma. The hemidesmosomes are normal. The basal cells exhibit a variable morphology ranging from lacunar to cytoplasm-poor cells that are rich in mitochondria. The nuclei are large and chromatin-dense.

As a whole, tonofilaments appear to be rather rare, both in basal as well as suprabasal cells. Toward the keratinizing columns of the epithelium, the cells elongate and develop distinct tonofibrils running parallel to the oval nuclei. The tonofibrils anchor in many desmosomes. The cells finally undergo parakeratinization.[74]

Immunohistochemistry has shown a normal pattern of nuclear Ki67 (MiB1)[73] and pancytokeratin such as A1/A3, keratins 4, 5, 6, 14, 16, 17, and 75 staining of the epithelial component,[96] but is negative for CD99 and epithelial membrane antigen.[97] The stroma also shows a normal nuclear Ki67 staining[73] and is positive for CD34[74] and CD10 underlining its origin from the matrix connective tissue.[98,99]

Comparative genomic hybridization has shown 34 genomic alterations in one onychomatricoma; they were mostly genomic losses on chromosome 11.[100]

Several variants such as onychoblastoma,[101,102] unguioblastic fibroma, and unguioblastoma[103,104] have been described the independence of which remains, however, disputed.[105] They are most probably just variants of onychomatricoma with variable amounts of connective tissue stroma or epithelial component.

8.1.19.2 Differential diagnosis

The histological features are sufficiently characteristic to allow a correct diagnosis to be made both from a surgical biopsy as well as from nail clippings. Onychocytic matricoma[10] may be considered when there is merely an epithelial component with little digitiform projections. Papillomatous Bowen's disease of the matrix may exhibit a similar architecture. We have seen three cases of a collision of onychomatricoma with onychopapilloma (Haneke E, Oral Communication, Vars Dermatopathol Seminar, 2016, Vars, France).

8.1.20 Syringoma

Syringomas are small benign tumors thought to arise from the excretory ducts of eccrine sweat glands. Their stroma is sclerotic. They are almost always multiple. Subungual hyperkeratosis and onycholysis were observed in the nail bed of the big toe of a middle-aged woman after trauma.[106]

8.1.20.1 Histopathology

There were round to oval islands of mainly cuboid eosinophilic tumor cells that were either solid or showed small (duct) lumina filled with keratin. The morphology was deemed to be similar to a syringoma. Syringomas are positive for protein S 100 and CEA.

8.1.20.2 Differential diagnosis

The histological differential diagnosis is mainly subungual epidermoid inclusions and trichoadenoma.

8.1.21 Chondroid syringoma

Chondroid syringoma, previously also called cutaneous mixed tumor, is a benign adnexal tumor composed of epithelial and connective tissue elements. There appears

(a)

(b)

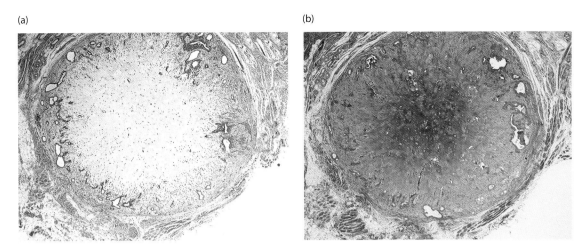

Figure 8.20 (a,b) Chondroid syringoma exhibiting sweat duct structures at the margin of a hyaline-chondroid stroma. H&E.

to be an analogy to mixed tumors of the salivary glands although they do not tend to recur after local excision. The case of a 25-year-old black woman was described with a deformed big toe and osteolytic changes in the distal phalanx.[107]

8.1.21.1 Histopathology

Histological examination of the amputation specimen exhibited a typical chondroid syringoma penetrating and permeating the bone. Low-power microscopy revealed a well-circumscribed lesion composed of anastomosing epithelial strands that were embedded in a myxoid, fibrous, and chondroid metachromatic stroma (Figure 8.20). Immunohistochemistry was positive for S-100 and vimentin in the outer cell layer and stains with antibodies against cytokeratin; carcinoembryonic antigen (CEA) and epithelial membrane antigen (EMA) were positive.[108]

8.1.21.2 Differential diagnosis

When the epithelial component prevails, syringoma and hidradenoma have to be considered. In cases with predominant myxoid stroma, a myxoma or chondroma has to be ruled out.

8.1.22 Eccrine syringofibroadenoma and eccrine syringofibroadenomatosis

Syringofibroadenoma is a rare benign neoplasm of eccrine ductal differentiation. Its clinical appearance is variable, but its histology is characteristic. Most lesions develop on acral skin of elderly persons and present as solitary nodules, which may be verrucous. In contrast, eccrine syringofibroadenomatosis is often seen as large plaques with an irregular papillomatous or verrucous surface on the foot and may be a reactive lesion to chronic (lymph)edema, long-standing ulcers, burn scars, squamous cell carcinoma, and even pincer nail.[109] This may also involve the periungual skin, but solitary eccrine syringofibroadenoma of the nail is exceptional.[110,111] It may present as a whitish longitudinal band similar to onychopapilloma.[112]

8.1.22.1 Histopathology

Eccrine syringofibroadenoma is composed of long slender anastomosing strands of mostly cuboid cells and abundant fibrovascular stroma.[113] Multiple narrow cords and strands of uniformly cuboid cells often forming a small lumen between their two cell rows extend from the epithelium into the dermis.[109,112] The cells have round basophilic nuclei. The tumor strands are often interlacing similar to the way fibroepithelioma of Pinkus does. In between them, marked fibrovascular stroma is seen. In the nail, the rare clear-cell variant was described containing considerable amounts of mucopolysaccharides.[112] The luminal cells are positive for carcinoembryonic antigen[112] as is the excretory duct of eccrine sweat glands. There is a strong p63 positivity (Figure 8.21).

One case of syringofibrocarcinoma due to malignant degeneration of a preexisting syringofibroadenoma on the foot extending to the little toe was observed in an

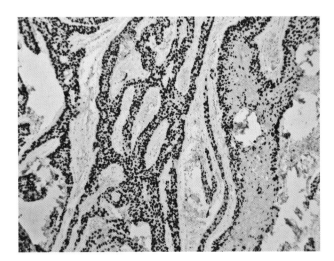

Figure 8.21 Reactive syringofibroadenoma of the distal phalanx of the great toe. P63 demonstration. (Courtesy of Prof. M. Landthaler, Regensburg, Germany.)

80-year-old patient with Clouston's hidrotic ectodermal dysplasia.[114]

8.1.22.2 Differential diagnosis

The clinical appearance of eccrine syringofibroadenoma is uncharacteristic and any potentially papular hyperkeratotic or verrucous lesion may be considered. Histologically, fibroepithelioma of Pinkus may be similar though, to our knowledge, it has not been observed in the nail apparatus.

8.1.23 Eccrine poroma

Eccrine poroma is a benign neoplasm thought to derive from terminal eccrine sweat gland ducts. They are usually solitary neoplasms although multiple poromas were also observed on palms and soles. They usually appear as small dome-shaped nodules not exceeding 10 mm in diameter, rarely bigger. Nail bed involvement may cause elevation of the nail plate,[59] whereas periungual localization led to an enlarged distal phalanx with destroyed nail.[115] Subungual poromas may look like a pyogenic granuloma.[116] One case each was observed on the nail fold[117] and one at the hyponychium mimicking an angiofibroma.[118]

8.1.23.1 Histopathology

Eccrine poroma is usually a well-circumscribed basophilic tumor with cuboid basaloid cells and small regular nuclei. The cytoplasm may stain positive with PAS as it often contains glycogen. When ductal structures are present, they display a diastase resistant PAS positive cuticle. One case also displayed clear cells.[118] Poromas may be connected to the overlying epidermis or lie in the mid- to deep dermis; the latter are often called dermal duct tumor. Keratin 77 expression is limited to luminal cells of intact ductal structures within the tumors.[119]

8.1.23.2 Differential diagnosis

Clinically, seborrheic keratosis and basal cell carcinoma may be considered. Histologically, again these neoplasms have to be ruled out.

8.1.24 Eccrine angiomatous hamartoma

Eccrine angiomatous hamartoma, also called angio-eccrine hamartoma, is a rare nevoid lesion composed of mature eccrine sweat glands and a variable amount of mostly capillary vessels among and around the eccrine glands. Clinically, it may appear as an induration, plaque or nodule, single or multiple. Tenderness or pain, itching, localized hypertrichosis and hyperhidrosis are the most common symptoms and signs.[120] Nail involvement is rare[121] and may cause nail destruction.[122] Misdiagnosis may lead to unnecessary amputation.[123] One case of mucinous eccrine nevus involving four toes including the periungual skin was described.[124]

8.1.24.1 Histopathology

In the typical case, there is a proliferation of otherwise normal sweat glands and small blood vessels, mostly

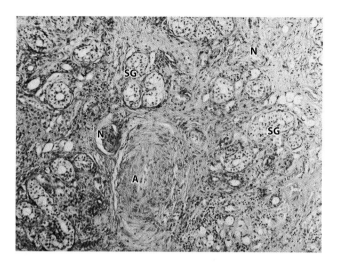

Figure 8.22 Neuro-arterio-syringeal hamartoma with large eccrine sweat glands (SG), multiple myelinated nerves (N) and thick-walled arteries (A). H&E.

capillaries, in the deep dermis. The stroma may be myxoid and/or lipomatous. Staining for epithelial membrane antigen reveals excessive surface extensions and narrow intercellular canaliculi. The secretory coils of the eccrine sweat glands are positive for protein S100, carcinoembryonic antigen, and cytokeratines, which are also present in normal eccrine glands. The endothelial cells of the vessels are positive for CD34 and factor VIII-related antigen.[125]

A peculiar painful subungual lesion of the big toe was described consisting of a well-circumscribed proliferation of densely packed eccrine sweat glands, thick-walled arterial vessels, and thick myelinated nerves; it was termed neuro-arterio-syringeal hamartoma (Figure 8.22).[126]

8.1.24.2 Differential diagnosis

Any painful ungual lesion has to be considered clinically. Histologically, eccrine nevus on one side and a capillary malformation on the other side have to be ruled out. Sudoriparous angioma exhibits vessels of large caliber and dilated eccrine sweat glands.[127] In contrast, congenital hemangioma of sweat glands is characterized by abundant wide capillary vessels with prominent endothelial cells located around the secretory portion of the sweat glands; this lesion slowly regresses spontaneously.[128]

8.1.25 Ungual keratoacanthoma

Keratoacanthoma (KA) is a relatively common tumor of chronically sun-exposed hair-bearing skin of elderly persons. Particularly in the United States, it is considered a variant of (verrucous) squamous cell carcinoma. Its localization in the nail apparatus is rare, but not exceptional.[129,130] It grows rapidly and often aggressively, most commonly under the free edge of the nail, in the distal nail bed or the lateral nail groove.[131] Localization in the proximal nail fold causes a paronychia-like chronic swelling.[132] Multiple subungual keratoacanthomas of the nail are exceedingly rare.[133,134] One subungual KA was observed in a patient with Muir-Torre syndrome and a germline mutation in the MSH mismatch repair gene.[135] Keratoacanthoma is characteristically painful probably due to its rapid growth and frequent bone erosion. Clinically, a keratotic nodule is commonly seen that may be tender on palpation. Pressure from the sides may make the central keratotic plug emerge from the tumor crater. Metastases have not been observed. Total excision is the treatment of choice as spontaneous involution of ungual keratoacanthomas is rare. In case of recurrence, Mohs micrographic surgery may be indicated.[136]

8.1.25.1 Histopathology

Keratoacanthomas show characteristic evolution stages in their development, which are, however, rarely seen in ungual lesions.[137] (Sub)ungual keratoacanthomas are more endophytic than exophytic. Their growth direction is more vertical or oblique in proximal-deep direction whereas keratoacanthomas of the skin tend to grow more horizontally and are exo-endophytic. A narrow central keratin plug is regularly seen extending deep into the dermis under the nail bed. Lip formation is pronounced though there is usually no overhanging shoulder. The tumor cells are large and pale and some may contain keratohyalin granules. The blunt tumor downgrowths have an irregular lower border. The peripheral cells are basaloid. There may be mitoses that are normal, which is said to be an important differential diagnostic criterion between keratoacanthoma and squamous cell carcinoma. There is often a mixed inflammatory infiltrate including neutrophils and eosinophils at the base of the tumor, and even abscess formation may be observed. Bone erosion is often seen in specimens large and deep enough and this is thought to be the reason of the pain caused by KA. Exceptionally large portions of the distal phalanx may be resorbed (Figure 8.23). Perineural invasion often seen in skin is not a prominent feature of ungual keratoacanthomas. Immunohistochemically, keratoacanthomas stain with a cytokeratin cocktail. The proliferation markers p53 and Ki67 (MIB1) are positive with

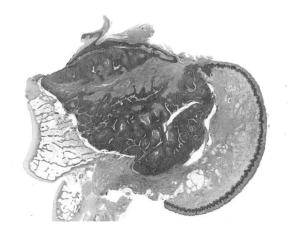

Figure 8.23 Giant subungual keratoacanthoma with major lytic changes of the terminal phalanx. H&E. (Courtesy of Dr. J. J. Sullivan, Brisbane.)

a relatively regular distribution from the basal cell layers gradually decreasing to the more superficial tumor cells.

8.1.25.2 Differential diagnosis

There are many attempts to safely distinguish subungual keratoacanthoma from SCC.[138–140] Clinically, KA patients are usually younger, the tumor grows faster, the duration of symptoms is shorter, bone invasion is more rapid and more common, and multiple KAs do occur though rarely. Many distinguishing histological criteria have already been mentioned. In skin, hypertrophic lichen planus may pose some difficulties.

Whereas the clinical differential diagnosis comprises virtually all painful nail lesions, squamous cell carcinoma, onycholemmal horn, subungual hyperkeratosis of incontinentia pigmenti, hypertrophic lichen planus and, depending on the particular case, a variety of other lesions have to be differentiated from keratoacanthoma. First, the classical architecture of keratoacanthoma with its relatively well-circumscribed oval shape, lateral superficial lip formation, and central keratin plug are usually typical enough to make the correct diagnosis, provided the biopsy/excision specimen allows the entire architecture to be evaluated. Atypical mitoses and infiltration or single cell formations are a feature of squamous cell carcinoma. Although the proliferation index in keratoacanthomas is higher than in hypertrophic lichen planus, this is not statistically significant, but penetrating elastic fibers are very rare in hypertrophic lichen planus as compared to keratoacanthoma.[141] Verrucous (hyperkeratotic) lupus erythematosus may be clinically similar to keratoacanthoma and SCC,[142] and SCC development on it has been observed.[143] The differential diagnosis may be particularly difficult when there is a sequence of wart-keratoacanthoma-verrucous carcinoma at the same site.[144]

Immunohistochemistry has often claimed to be of discriminative value; however, the differences are usually only quantitative. There is no difference in p16 expression.[145] Compared to SCC, keratoacanthoma demonstrates a more regular peripheral p53, PCNA, and MiB1 (Ki67) staining than SCC. The same is true for the nuclear factor kappa B p50 subunit and cortactin that shows a peripheral pattern in keratoacanthoma and a more scattered pattern in SCC.[146] Also, p63 does not reliably distinguish KA from SCC.[147] Whereas tumor necrosis factor-like weak inducer of apoptosis (TWEAK) is negative in keratoacanthoma, it is from strong to absent in SCC.[148] SCC expresses more caspase[149] and apoptosis inducing factor than KA.[150] However, SCC also expresses more Bcl-x, which is a member of the Bcl-2 antiapoptosis protein family.[151,152] Ezrin, a cytoskeleton linker protein actively involved in regulating the growth and metastatic capacity of cancer cells, is markedly expressed in the cytoplasm of SCC, whereas KA shows only cellular membrane expression.[153]

Keratoacanthoma is usually distinct from follicular (infundibular) and infundibulocystic squamous cell carcinoma,[154,155] but there is no infundibular structure around the nail.

8.2 MALIGNANT EPITHELIAL NAIL TUMORS

There are a variety of malignant neoplasms of the nail apparatus with melanoma, Bowen's disease, and squamous cell carcinoma being the most common. As a whole, they are relatively rare and a high amount of clinical suspicion is necessary to make an early correct diagnosis, which in many cases is the prerequisite for a good prognosis. On the other hand, virtually all tissues of the tip of the digit may give rise to malignant tumors and also metastases are occasionally seen.

New or recurrent swellings and lesions that do not respond to treatment based on an initial clinical impression should be subjected to biopsy.[156]

8.3 KERATINOCYTIC PRECANCERS, *IN SITU* CARCINOMA, AND CARCINOMAS

By definition, carcinomas are malignant epithelial (keratinocytic) neoplasms. Particularly squamous cell carcinomas may be preceded by so-called precanceroses, a term now more and more abandoned in favor of *in situ* carcinoma.

8.3.1 Actinic keratosis

Actinic keratosis or solar keratosis used to be called senile keratosis. It is the most common precancerous alteration of the skin and seen in almost two-thirds of light-skinned Caucasians over the age of 65 years. Patients with actinic keratoses are more likely to develop other nonmelanoma skin cancers.[157,158] They may be found by the hundreds in the face, on the scalp, and the dorsa of the hands although other regions with chronic sun damage may also develop actinic keratoses; this phenomenon is now known as field cancerization. Progression to invasive squamous cell carcinoma is estimated to be between 0.025% and 16% per year, but approximately one-quarter of the lesions can disappear spontaneously. The problem is that up to now there is no possibility to identify which lesion may involute, persist, or degenerate into an invasive squamous cell carcinoma.[159,160] Most commonly, they present as hyperkeratotic or crusted rough lesions on an erythematous base with telangiectasiae. Sometimes the hyperkeratosis may be exaggerated giving rise to a cutaneous horn. In the nail organ, actinic keratoses are surprisingly rare and occur mainly on the proximal nail fold. As the nail plate is an efficient ultraviolet radiation filter,[161,162] subungual actinic keratoses have not been reported. The clinical differential diagnosis comprises warts, chronic radiodermatitis, arsenical keratosis, keratoacanthoma, Bowen's disease, squamous cell carcinoma, other carcinomas, other cutaneous horns, and a variety of other lesions that may occasionally develop a hyperkeratosis.

8.3.1.1 Histopathology

Actinic keratosis is now also called keratinocytic intraepidermal neoplasia (KIN) or dermal intraepithelial neoplasia (DIN)[163] and is graded from I to III. There are different types of solar keratoses but in the nail region it is either hyperkeratotic or atrophic. The earliest changes often not yet noted clinically are crowding of the basal cells and loss of their polarity. These changes extend to the suprabasal and spinous layers and become more pronounced with hyperchromatic and large nuclei, an occasional binucleate or giant cell. Later, atypical mitoses and dyskeratoses are observed. Whereas the atrophic variant of actinic keratosis is quite common in the head and neck area, those on the dorsa of the hand, fingers, and proximal nail fold tend to be covered by a thick and very compact hyperkeratosis that contains a major proportion of parakeratosis. The hyperkeratosis is often located in a slightly deepened or even saucer-shaped depressed epidermis. In the immediate vicinity of the nail where no hair follicles occur any more, the formation of parakeratotic columns often seen elsewhere is not pronounced. There is no invasion although some papillomatosis and downward proliferations of the epidermis may be seen. Where the sweat ducts penetrate an actinic keratosis the epidermis retains its normal appearance and keratinization. Actinic elastosis is always present. An inflammatory infiltrate may be present, which may be lichenoid and lead to some liquefaction degeneration of the basal cells. Patients with certain syndromes characterized by insufficient DNA repair, for example, xeroderma pigmentosum, are prone to develop hundreds of actinic keratoses including on the distal phalanx that tend to degenerate to invasive squamous cell carcinoma.

8.3.1.2 Differential diagnosis

The histopathological differential diagnosis may be difficult in very early lesions. It comprises arsenical keratosis, Bowen's disease, and squamous cell carcinoma.[164] However, some authors called them all superficial squamous cell carcinoma and vehemently rejected the terms carcinoma *in situ* or KIN.[165,166] When there is a lichenoid inflammatory infiltrate, it may be similar to lichen planus-like keratosis. This, however, shows rather dissolution of the basal cell layer than atypical cells. The keratoses seen in organ transplant recipients are histologically often different in that they are characterized by epithelial proliferations of large cells that initially show surprisingly little atypia but once they transform, they rapidly progress to invasive squamous cell carcinoma. They exhibit early keratin 17 expression.[167]

8.3.2 Arsenical keratosis

Arsenical keratoses are now mainly seen in regions with a high content of arsenic in the drinking water[168] or after professional exposure.[169] This may be associated with arsenical melanosis.[170] The use of arsenical insecticides in the wine-growing industry was forbidden in Europe in the late 1920s/early 1930s and the therapeutic administration of arsenical compounds such as Fowler's solution or Asiatic pills, was declared obsolete many decades ago although there are still countries in which they are used to treat psoriasis and lichen planus. With the advent of Ayurvedic medicine, a new source of chronic arsenicism has appeared.[171] Patients with arsenical keratoses have a very high risk of developing internal cancers in various organs. The diagnosis must therefore prompt a general checkup of the patient. Clinically, arsenical keratoses appear as small hard keratotic papules that develop anywhere on the skin, but particularly on the palms and soles. They are said to exhibit a higher autofluorescence with ultraviolet light than the surrounding epidermis of the palms and soles. Around and under the nails, keratotic papules and plaques develop that may eventually degenerate to Bowen's disease and/or squamous cell carcinoma.[172] It is not yet clear whether superficial basal cell carcinoma is more frequently arsenic-induced than Bowen's disease.[173] Nail dystrophy is an unspecific sign.

8.3.2.1 Histopathology

The microscopic picture resembles that of actinic keratosis or even Bowen's disease with loss of polarity of the basal cells, large hyperchromatic nuclei, clumping, atypical mitoses, and dyskeratoses, but there are often larger areas of hyperkeratosis without obvious nuclear atypia.[174] Some lesions may progress to basal cell carcinoma, but often there is a mixture of Bowen's disease and basal cell carcinoma.[171] However, actinic elastosis is usually absent.

8.3.2.2 Differential diagnoses

Actinic keratosis, Bowen's disease, squamous cell carcinoma, and basal cell carcinoma are the most important differential diagnoses, but they are also induced by chronic arsenicosis. The latter may contain squamous metaplasia.[175]

8.3.3 Bowen's disease

Bowen's disease is an *in situ* carcinoma or intraepithelial neoplasia grade IV; others call it superficial squamous cell carcinoma. In the skin, it is mainly located on chronically sun-exposed areas although those cases due to chemical carcinogens and high-risk human papilloma viruses also, if not predominantly, occur in non sun-damaged skin. Arsenic, other potential carcinogenic compounds, chronic X-irradiation[176] and high-risk human papillomaviruses are accepted etiologic agents. It is mainly seen in middle-aged to elderly persons with a peak incidence between 50 and 70 years. Males predominate. The diagnosis is very often delayed for many months or years, particularly in ungual Bowen's disease.[177,178] On glabrous skin, Bowen's disease forms a slightly elevated, reddish plaque covered with a characteristic scale crust. When localized on palms and soles, it may be even more obvious and localization in the webspace of the toes often shows a macerated white keratosis. Ulceration may be a sign of beginning invasion. On the finger pulp and at the hyponychium, it usually looks like a flat, fissured wart. On the proximal nail fold, its clinical appearance is often that of a red, flat hyperkeratotic, or verrucous plaque,[179] but it may also present as a reddish macule, particularly in association with an erythematous plaque. In the lateral groove, apparently the most frequent nail localization, it may be verrucous, macerated, or even fibrokeratoma-like.[180] Where it affects the cuticle it appears whitish. Longitudinal leukonychia[59] and

nail dystrophy[181] are the result of matrix involvement.[59] Erythronychia, either as a single red line or several lines, may be observed.[182] Subungual localization often presents as onycholysis.[183] Marked hyperkeratosis may result in a pachyonychia congenita-like appearance[184] or even a cutaneous horn.[185] Pigmented Bowen's disease of the nail may cause regular or irregular longitudinal melanonychia or pigmentation of the skin surrounding the nail.[186–190] Multiple digits may be affected by ungual Bowen's disease.[191,192] In the last two decades, more and more cases of ungual Bowen's disease were proven to be due to high-risk human papillomaviruses such as HPV 16, 18, 26, 33, 34, 35, 45, 51, 53, 73, and more,[193–200] which are also often found in genital lesions thus indicating a genital-to-digital infection or auto-inoculation.[201] Co-infection of different HPV types was also described.[202] HPV 56-induced ungual Bowen's disease was found to be associated with longitudinal melanonychia in a Japanese group.[203] Longitudinal melanonychia was also seen in a patient with epidermodysplasia verruciformis of Lewandowsky-Lutz and subungual Bowen's disease.[204] Bowen's disease is very rare in toes. Bowen's disease of the nail is more likely to progress to invasive carcinoma,[205] but this is less likely to metastasize. The treatment of choice of ungual Bowen's disease is Mohs micrographic surgery,[206] but a variety of surgical[207,208] and non-surgical methods have also been described.[209–212] Clinical differential diagnoses depending on the localization in the nail apparatus are viral warts, paronychia, psoriasis, onychomycosis and other infections, arsenical keratosis, actinic keratosis, subungual exostosis, onychomatricoma,[213] squamous cell carcinoma, and many more.

8.3.3.1 Histopathology

Bowen's disease is a classical *in situ* carcinoma. However, as it is possible that another section plane would show an invasive component some authors prefer the term of epidermoid carcinoma for both Bowen's disease and invasive squamous cell carcinoma.[214,215]

Depending on where the lesion is located within the nail organ there are some differences in the histopathologic pattern although the diagnosis is always obvious. Around the nail, the lesion is characterized by an acanthotic thickening of the epidermis that lacks an orderly architecture in its entire thickness. Papillomatosis and hyperkeratosis are common. There is crowding and loss of polaritiy of the basal cells, and the stratification into basal, spinous, and granular layers is absent. There are large and pleomorphic, often hyperchromatic nuclei, some cells have more nuclei or clumped nuclei, and all stages of mitoses including many pathologic ones are seen in all layers. Dyskeratoses and necrotic keratinocytes in mitosis are a frequent finding; dyskeratosis may in some areas be the only sign. Keratinization is irregular and mainly parakeratotic, but usually without flattening of the nuclei (Figure 8.24). In many cases, perinuclear vacuolization is seen suggesting a viral cause (Figure 8.25). Subungual Bowen's disease is similar but its hyperkeratosis is usually much less pronounced. When the nail is clipped

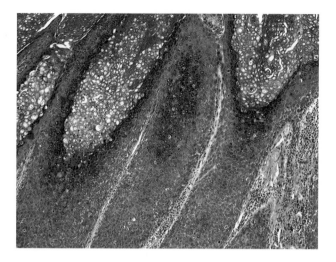

Figure 8.24 Ungual Bowen's disease with masses of atypical cells, pathological mitoses, nuclear clumping, and dyskeratoses.

with the nail bed keratosis this is often seen containing dyskeratoses and some large nuclei allowing the diagnosis of Bowen's disease to be suspected. Clear-cell Bowen's disease has been described, both with large round Paget-like and trichilemmal sheath-like cells.[181] Bowen's disease of the matrix results in inclusion of dyskeratotic cells into the nail plate clinically appearing as leukonychia. Papillomatous-hyperplastic Bowen of the matrix may be similar to onychomatricoma. In pigmented Bowen's disease, dendritic melanocytes may be seen populating the lesion. Immunohistochemistry for HPV is positive in HPV-related Bowen's disease.[201] Immunohistochemically, keratin 17 is expressed suprabasally in all dysplastic lesions and panepithelially in cancer.[168]

8.3.3.2 Differential diagnosis

As outlined above, when diagnosing Bowen's disease one has to be aware that another section plane of the same

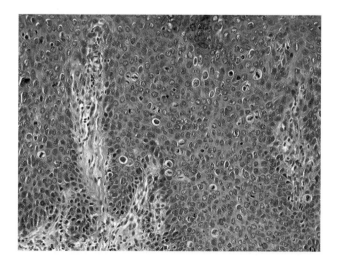

Figure 8.25 Characteristic koilocytes of HPV-16 associated ungual Bowen's disease. H&E.

surgical specimen might show invasive Bowen's carcinoma, hence the term epidermoid carcinoma. Most of the differential diagnoses of Bowen's disease are not relevant, as the nail apparatus does not contain hair follicles and apocrine glands; eccrine sweat glands do, however, occur around the nail. Freezing artifacts may simulate Bowen's disease.[216] Pagetoid dyskeratosis, characterized by clear cells arranged singly or in clusters and described as mainly occurring in the head and neck area,[217] is a relatively frequent accidental finding on the tip of the toe in little children and sometimes also adults, but it is very rare in the nail matrix.

Subungual seborrheic keratosis may be similar but does not exhibit cellular atypia and pathologic mitoses.[9] When there is regular psoriasiform acanthosis and pronounced parakeratosis, psoriasis can be excluded by the mitoses in all layers of the lesion, the lack of suprapapillary thinning, and oval to round nuclei in the parakeratosis.

8.3.4 Squamous cell carcinoma

Squamous cell carcinoma (SCC) is very frequent in light-skinned Caucasians but much less in dark-skinned individuals. Most cases develop in sun-exposed skin as hard keratotic nodules with a tendency to ulcerate. In contrast to the pinna of the ear, lips, and genitalia,[218] they tend to metastasize late if at all. They are extremely common in organ transplant recipients[219] and other immunodeficiency states such as epidermodysplasia verruciformis;[220] in the former, they make up almost two-thirds of all nonmelanoma skin cancers and have a specific mortality rate of 25%.[221,222] SCC together with Bowen's disease is the most frequent nail malignancy.[223] In the nail apparatus, they occur in the subungual location, rarely on the proximal or lateral nail folds, and are exceptional in the hyponychium-finger pulp region.[224] The most common sign of subungual squamous cell carcinoma is onycholysis with oozing—a sign shared with subungual Bowen's and rarely other subungual diseases. Bleeding and formation of a nodule or ulceration indicate an invasive carcinoma. Bone invasion is rare[225] and metastases have been observed mainly in SCC patients with ectodermal dysplasia,[226,227] but more recently also independently.[228–231] Removal of the overlying onycholytic nail plate is essential to make the clinical diagnosis. Treatment of choice of subungual SCC is microscopically controlled surgery.

8.3.4.1 Histopathology

Periungual SCC does not differ from SCC in other locations.[232] Large atypical epithelial proliferations extend into the dermis. A variable degree of keratinization and superficial ulceration is present. The basal as well as spinous-appearing cells display a high degree of atypia with large and hyperchromatic nuclei. Atypical mitoses are seen in the entire tumor thickness. There is no orderly stratification of the epithelium although in most cases, the origin from squamous epithelium can be suggested (Figure 8.26). There is often irregular and incomplete keratinization, but

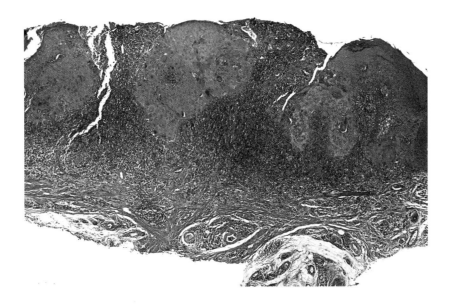

Figure 8.26 Common type of subungual squamous cell carcinoma with large keratinocytes and without koilocytes. H&E.

keratohyalin granule containing cells are rare. In long-standing SCC, there may be deep invasion down to the bone, but this is surprisingly rare subungually. This type of ungual SCC is negative for HPV DNA.[221]

Bowen's carcinoma derives from Bowen's disease and commonly retains some similarity with *in situ* Bowen's lesions (Figure 8.27).[233] Clear cells are more often observed.[234]

Immunohistochemistry is positive for almost all cutaneous SCC markers. Some markers have a prognostic value.[235] Whereas p16 is positive in *in situ* carcinoma, it is negative in most invasive ones.[236]

8.3.4.2 Differential diagnosis

As outlined above, Bowen's disease is generally seen as an *in situ* carcinoma and as long as the entire specimen

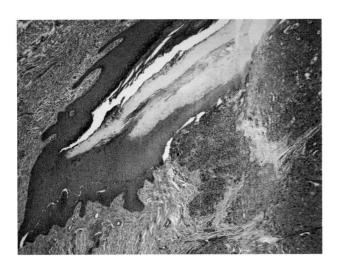

Figure 8.27 Bowen's-type subungual invasive carcinoma.

is not cut there is always a remote possibility that another area would show invasive Bowen's carcinoma, hence the term of epidermoid carcinoma for both Bowen's disease and invasive SCC. However, Bowen's carcinoma retains the cytologic characteristics of Bowen's disease whereas the common type of SCC exhibits the typical squamous epithelial morphology. One of the most pertinent differential diagnoses is subungual keratoacanthoma. The main differential diagnostic points have been mentioned in the section on keratoacanthoma: SCC demonstrates a very irregular stratification if at all, but there is more or less normal maturation of the epithelial cells from the peripheral basal layer to the center in keratoacanthoma, the cells may exhibit a ground glass appearance and often form a granular layer; lip formation is virtually always seen in subungual keratoacanthoma but not in SCC; proliferation markers are more positive in the periphery and decrease toward the center whereas they are more irregularly distributed in SCC; keratoacanthoma often shows intratumoral elastic fibers as a sign of its rapid growth, which is not seen in SCC. Tumor necrosis factor-like weak inducer of apoptosis (TWEAK) is absent in keratoacanthoma and from absent to strongly expressed in SCC.[140] Serpin peptidase inhibitor clade A member 1 (SerpinA1) is upregulated in SCC as compared to normal skin and actinic keratosis.[237] Comparative genomic hybridization has shown statistically significant differences between the two entities: Less than 40% of keratoacanthomas and more than 80% of SCC have shown genomic aberrations, and gains and losses of genetic material were mostly different between the two, which points to different genetic mechanisms involved in their developments.[238] Verrucous Bowen's disease of the matrix has to be differentiated from onychocytic carcinoma.

8.3.5 Carcinoma cuniculatum

Carcinoma cuniculatum, because of its very slow growth and virtual absence of metastases, also called epithelioma cuniculatum, is a variant of verrucous carcinoma, which is considered to be a low-grade squamous cell carcinoma. Its main localization is the webspace of the foot where it may cause channels and sinuses—hence the term carcinoma cuniculatum—often releasing a smelly material upon pressure. Few cases were observed in the nail apparatus causing distal-lateral onycholysis and paronychia, nail bed inflammation, and discharge of a foul-smelling yellow-white paste-like material from the nail bed with loss of the nail plate,[239] verrucous tumor of the distal part of the thumb,[240,241] and subungual tumor with deep holes in the nail bed.[242] The big and the little toes were involved with loss of the nail.[243–248] Despite the fact that metastases do not occur except when the carcinoma was treated with radiotherapy,[249] bone erosion is frequent probably because of the long duration before treatment.[250] The etiology of this particular type of low-grade carcinoma is not known, but one patient was an internist who had performed X-ray screening examinations over a period of more than 20 years.[238] Clinical differential diagnosis includes warts and keratoacanthoma, papillomatosis, eccrine porocarcinoma, and a variety of sinus-forming and fistulating processes.

8.3.5.1 Histopathology

The diagnostic biopsy has to be large and deep and may have to be repeated. The localization and the architecture are important keys to the diagnosis. There is a proliferation of squamous cells with epithelium-lined sinuses and tracts containing keratinous debris. The deep border is pushing rather than invasive. There is a well-organized stratification of the epithelium, often with marked focal hypergranulosis. Cellular atypia is absent to mild. Mitoses are very rare and usually not pathologic. Dyskeratoses are also rare.

Immunohistochemistry with antibodies to a variety of different cytokeratins, involucrin, and filaggrin as well as lectin histochemistry with peanut agglutinin suggests a high degree of differentiation.[251] Filaggrin is present where keratohyalin can be seen in H&E stained sections and also involucrin is expressed by the majority of the tumor cells. PNA binding is variable with both completely positive and negative areas. Neuraminidase digestion unmasks the Friedreich–Thomsen antigen, thus rendering all tumor cells positive (E. Haneke, unpublished data).

8.3.5.2 Differential diagnosis

Differential diagnosis includes verrucae (even histologically) and keratoacanthoma, which exhibits rapid growth and clinically aggressive behavior. Squamous cell carcinoma is less verrucous and shows considerable dysplasia. Pseudoepitheliomatous hyperplasia is even more regular, does not form epithelium-lined channels, and has a very irregular papillomatous and jagged deep border. However, sometimes several biopsies are necessary to make the correct diagnosis.[252]

8.3.6 Basal cell carcinoma

Apart from actinic keratoses plus squamous cell carcinoma, basal cell carcinoma is the most frequent malignant neoplasm of humans.[253] Less than 25 cases have been described in the nail region.[254,255] Commonly, basal cell carcinoma presents as a periungual eczema or chronic paronychia that may be associated with granulation tissue, erosion or ulceration, and pain.[256–259] Jagged border was observed in superficial basal cell carcinoma.[260] One case in a white patient presented as an acquired longitudinal melanonychia.[261] Fingers are the most common localization, ten of them in the thumb,[262] only seven basal cell carcinomas were observed in the ungual region of the toes.[59,263–265] Multiple small periungual basal cell carcinomas were seen as pearl-like transparent papules in an 8-month-old baby[266] and two more children[267]. The diagnostic delay ranges from 1 to 40 years.[268] The treatment of choice is microscopically controlled surgery. The clinical differential diagnosis comprises trauma, onychomycosis, bacterial infection, eczema, chronic paronychia, pyogenic granuloma, squamous cell carcinoma, and amelanotic melanoma.

Molecular and genetic anomalies were found in sporadic and syndromic basal cell carcinomas. An inappropriate activation of the hedgehog signaling pathway is now thought to be responsible, but mutations of the tumor-suppressor gene p53 may also play a role. The sonic hedgehog protein links with the tumor suppressing protein patched homologue 1 (PTCH1) that arrests the intracellular signal inhibitor smoothen (SMO), this regulates the glioma-associated oncogene (GLI) family of transcription factors. A mutation inactivating PTCH1 was found in Gorlin's syndrome and in 30%–40% of sporadic cases of basal cell carcinoma. SMO is thus constitutionally active and is responsible for a permanent activation of the target genes. This is the basis for the new chemotherapy of basal cell carcinoma with the hedgehog pathway inhibitor vismodegib.

8.3.6.1 Histopathology

Basal cell carcinoma is an adnexal carcinoma probably arising from the outer root sheath of the hair follicle.[269] Histopathologic examination shows a basophilic tumor with palisaded basal cells and small cuboid cells in the center. There is often a split formation between the epithelial carcinomatous component and its surrounding soft tissue. Mitoses are rare.

Immunohistochemistry showed an identical cytokeratin profile in the hair follicle and basal cell carcinoma[270] and confirmed the relation of basal cell carcinoma with embryonal hair follicle formation by the demonstration of the epithelial adhesion molecule Ep-CAM in all basal cell carcinomas, the human embryonic hair follicle, the secondary hair germ, and the outer root sheath of the vellus hair follicle, but not the adult anagen hair follicles. In contrast, the embryonic nail organ completely lacks Ep-CAM reactivity.[271] This may be an explanation why basal cell carcinoma is so exceptional in the nail region. Ep-CAM demonstrated with the antibody Ber-EP4 allows the differentiation of basal cell carcinomas from actinic keratoses and squamous cell carcinoma, which are negative.[272,273]

8.3.6.2 Differential diagnosis

All tumors composed of relatively small basophilic cells have to be considered. These comprise subungual seborrheic keratosis, sometimes also onychopapilloma, eccrine poroma, subungual epidermoid inclusions, and above all small-cell amelanotic melanoma and Merkel cell carcinoma. The antibody Ber-EP4 allows reliably differentiating basal cell carcinoma and microcystic adnexal carcinoma, which to our knowledge has not yet been observed in the nail apparatus.[274]

8.3.7 Onychocytic carcinoma

Longitudinal band-like thickening of the nail with yellow color was the presenting sign of this tumor in two cases. End-on examination revealed minute holes in the nail's free margin.[275,276]

8.3.7.1 Histopathology

Onychocytic carcinoma is a fairly well-delimited tumor of the matrix and sometimes the adjacent nail bed. There is an *in situ* carcinoma component with striking small epithelial projections into the nail plate, which in contrast to onychomatricoma, do not have a connective tissue papilla. In continuation of the digitations, there are small cavities in the nail plate, again without capillaries and a lining epithelium. The basal compartment of the lesion is basophilic similar to the prekeratogenous zone, but the cells are reminiscent of Bowen's disease with nuclear atypia, often round clear cells, and some mitoses (Figure 8.28). Invasion into the matrix dermis is possible.[277]

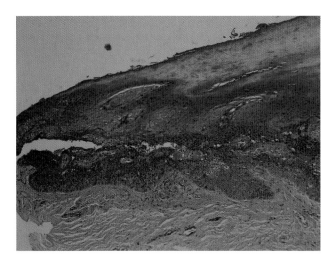

Figure 8.28 Onychocytic carcinoma with digitiform projections into the nail and atypical cells in the basophilic prekeratogenous zone and basal compartment.

Immunohistochemically, the tumor focally expresses hair and nail keratins including K31, K85, and K86.[278]

8.3.7.2 Differential diagnosis

The histological differential diagnosis depends on the structure available for microscopic examination. The epithelial matrix portion resembles Bowen's disease whereas the digitiform projections may be mistaken for onychomatricoma. However, the characteristic stroma of onychomatricoma is lacking and the cavities in the nail plate are not lined with classical matrix epithelium.

8.3.8 Onycholemmal carcinoma

Onycholemmal carcinoma is a rare malignancy originating from the nail bed epithelium. Few cases have been described.[279–281] Clinically, they may be warty, crusted, or ulcerated lesions or appear as a cracked nail and onychodystrophy with an insidious history. Pain is associated in about half of the cases. Patient age ranges from the fourth to the eighth decade of life. There is no gender predilection. Fingers are more frequently involved than toes. Treatment ranged from radiation, excision with curettage of the nail bed, nail unit ablation, and Mohs surgery to amputation, but no recurrences occurred with any of these methods.[282]

8.3.8.1 Histopathology

The tumor is made up of invasive cell complexes with mostly eosinophilic round squamoid cells without flattening. Abrupt keratinization is seen centrally in the tumor lobules without a granular layer. The cells are often highly atypical with markedly hyperchromatic nuclei (Figure 8.29a). One of our onycholemmal carcinomas also had a large area of clear cells similar to that of outer root sheath cells (Figure 8.29b). Another case described exhibited features of apocrine and sebaceous differentiation prompting the authors to speculate that this might be a microcystic nail bed carcinoma.[283] HPV DNA could not be demonstrated.

8.3.9 Aggressive digital papillary adenocarcinoma

This lesion used to be called aggressive digital papillary adenoma but due to its propensity to recur and metastasize it is now considered to be a malignant sweat gland neoplasm; the distinction into aggressive digital papillary adenoma and adenocarcinoma[284] is no longer thought to be justified.[285] Aggressive digital papillary adenocarcinoma occurs almost exclusively on the fingers, palms, toes, and soles, with preponderance of the hands. The patients are generally men between 40 and 70 years of age,[286] but this carcinoma may also occur in adolescents.[287–289] In most cases, there is an insidiously growing, firm, tan-gray to white-pink, rubbery, sometimes cystic, deep-seated nodule or infiltration in an upper extremity digit, specifically on the volar surface or between the nail bed and the distal interphalangeal joint. It may be ulcerated. Despite its diameter up to several centimeters, it usually does not impede joint mobility. Nail bed involvement is rare.[290,291] One case mimicked an acquired digital fibrokeratoma.[292]

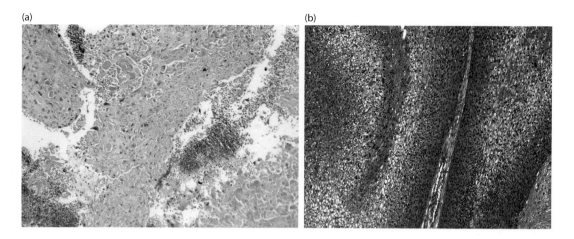

Figure 8.29 Onycholemmal carcinomas (a) with islands of atypical cells and (b) large complexes of clear cells. H&E.

The nail apparatus is secondarily affected in most cases. Pain may be a sign of extension to the bone, joint, or nerves. Metastasis as the presenting sign is rare. Radiographs are unremarkable as long as the bone is not invaded. Almost 50% of the carcinomas recur after initial surgical removal and 40% metastasize with the lung being the most frequent site followed by lymph nodes, brain, kidneys, bone, and retroperitoneum.[263] Although sentinel lymph node biopsy may detect metastases earlier, the survival benefit of this procedure is not clear.[293] Radical excision or preferably amputation of the digit is the treatment of choice.[294] The clinical differential diagnoses comprise various cysts and pseudocysts, calluses, pyogenic and foreign body granulomas, squamous cell carcinomas, hemangiomas, giant cell tumors, osteomyelitis, soft tissue infections, or gout.[284,285,289]

8.3.9.1 Histopathology

The neoplasm is made up of multilobular aggregates of cuboid to low columnar basophilic cells with round to oval nuclei. Often, spaces are formed into which tumor cell proliferations protrude giving the appearance of a papillary lesion. Sometimes a cribriform pattern is noted. A fibrovascular core may be seen in some areas whereas other projections lack stromal support. There is little cytologic atypia, but mitoses and necrotic areas are frequent. Sebaceous differentiation and focal decapitation secretion were reported.[276,284,285] Cysts contain necrotic debris or eosinophilic material similar to secretory material. There are both well-circumscribed tumors as well as those with an infiltrative border. Lymphatic invasion may be seen. Immunohistochemically, it is often positive for ferritin, S-100 protein, polyclonal keratin mix, CAM 5.2, and cytokeratin 7 and negative for cytokeratin 20, carcinoembryonic antigen, prostate-specific antigen, alpha-fetoprotein, synaptophysin, and chromogranin.[295]

On the basis of 57 patients, a distinction into either aggressive digital papillary adenoma or aggressive digital papillary adenocarcinoma was made because 40 were found to have aggressive digital papillary adenoma and

17 had aggressive digital papillary adenocarcinoma.[284] The carcinomas were differentiated from the adenomas by poor glandular differentiation, cellular atypia, necrosis, pleomorphism, and invasion of bone, soft tissue, and vasculature. A retrospective analysis of these tumors later found that of the 30 cases initially diagnosed as aggressive digital papillary adenoma, 9 recurred and 3 developed metastases.[284] It was therefore concluded that a histological diagnosis of adenoma could not accurately be made and that all lesions suspected to be adenomas should be treated as if they were aggressive digital papillary adenocarcinoma. This was also confirmed by other authors.[285]

8.3.9.2 Differential diagnosis

Aggressive digital papillary adenocarcinoma is thought to derive from eccrine sweat glands.[296] Hence an important differential diagnosis is papillary eccrine adenoma. This is a well-delimited lesion with dilated ducts with distinct two-layered epithelial walls and only delicate papillae. The immunohistochemical demonstration of ferritin is also in favor of an eccrine sweat gland origin. Other histologic differential diagnoses are eccrine acrospiroma, hidradenoma, chondroid syringoma, and, rarely, metastatic papillary adenocarcinoma of the breast, lung, thyroid, or ovary.[290] No specific histologic features have been identified to predict recurrence or metastasis.[284] Occasionally, decapitation secretion was observed and this was used as an argument for classifying this lesion as being of apocrine derivation. However, this phenomenon can also be seen in occluded eccrine glands[297] and should not be an argument to classify aggressive digital papillary adenocarcinoma as being apocrine despite exclusively occurring in an apocrine-devoid area.

8.3.10 Eccrine porocarcinoma

Eccrine porocarcinoma is a rare tumor mainly seen in the palms and soles of elderly persons.[298,299] It is exceptional in the tip of the digit.[300] One case was apparently induced by chronic exposure to Roentgen rays as the ulcerating tumor developed in the middle finger of a chronic radiodermatitis of both hands.[301] When it occurs in the lateral nail fold, it may simulate squamous cell carcinoma.[302] We have

(a)

(b)

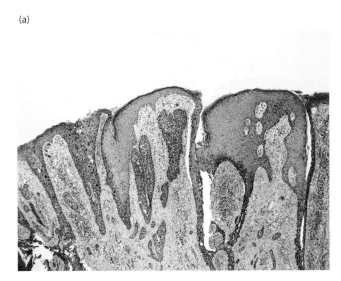
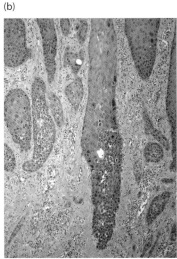

Figure 8.30 (a,b) Eccrine porocarcinoma with strands of atypical cells, duct formation, and pathological mitoses. H&E.

seen a large eccrine porocarcinoma of the fifth metatarsal-fifth toe area completely overgrowing the nail of the little toe with a massively hyperkeratotic verrucous growth (Haneke, unpublished). Most porocarcinomas appear to arise de novo although one-fifth to one-half of them may develop by malignant transformation of a benign pre-existing poroma.[303,304]

8.3.10.1 Histopathology

Eccrine porocarcinoma originates from the eccrine sweat ducts. It grows as intraepidermal and dermal, mostly solid cords and nests of cuboid to polygonal cells with pale cytoplasm. It may grow to large, well-circumscribed tumor masses although this is not seen in the distal phalanx. The cell nuclei are pleomorphic with irregular shape, prominent nucleoli, and multiple mitoses (Figure 8.30). Intraepithelial tumor cells are sharply demarcated from the adjacent keratinocytes. They form nests or are seen as single cells in the epidermis in a pagetoid pattern.[305] Despite the occasional clinically verrucous appearance, keratinization is commonly lacking. The tumor cells may contain glycogen,[306] which may make the cytoplasm appear pale. Lymphatic invasion in the deep dermis is probably the reason for the sometimes catastrophic course.[307] Immunohistochemistry shows positivity for pancytokeratin; intraepithelial porocarcinoma cells are usually weaker stained than the surrounding epithelium.[308,309] Ductal formations in the tumor stain with antibodies to carcinoembryonic antigen and epithelial membrane antigen.[290,292] Whereas p53 is expressed in both eccrine poroma as well as porocarcinoma,[310,311] p16 is negative throughout eccrine porocarcinoma.[312]

8.3.10.2 Differential diagnosis

The main differential diagnoses are benign eccrine poroma, hidracanthoma simplex, and Paget's disease.[313] Although eccrine poroma and hidracanthoma simplex may show some focal atypicality, they are symmetrical and well delimited. Apart from the fact that the tip of the

digit is not a region with apocrine glands, Paget's disease has more intraepithelial round cells that are positive for mucin and stain with PAS even after diastase digestion.

8.3.11 Adenocystic sweat gland carcinoma

Adenocystic sweat gland carcinoma is a rare neoplasm of which one case of a mucinous variant was observed in the tip of the great toe of a 30-year-old black female. The tumor was tender and movable.[314] Its relation to adenoid cystic carcinoma and microcystic adnexal carcinoma is not entirely clear.

8.3.11.1 Histopathology

The lesion demonstrates an adenoid, tubular, or cribriform differentiation with abundant small epithelial islands. Round spaces imitating lumina are lined by carcinoma cells and contain an amphophilic material similar to basement membrane substance. Mucin accumulation may transform the lumina into cystic appearing spaces that are lined by a flattened epithelium. The adenocystic sweat gland carcinoma of the nail was composed of solid, papillary, and trabecular tumor cell aggregates focally exhibiting abundant mitoses.[295]

Immunohistochemically, the tumor cells are positive for amylase, cytokeratin AE1/3, CK34BE12, CK5/6, CK7, CK14, p63, alpha-smooth muscle actin (ASMA), S100 protein, p53, Ki-67 (labeling 85% in one case), KIT, PDGFRA, and CD56, but negative for cytokeratin CAM5.2, CK8, CK18, CK19, CK20, epithelial membrane antigen, desmin, carcinoembryonic antigen in one study, HMB45, CD10, CD34, neuron-specific enolase, chromogranin, synaptophysin, CDX2, MUC1, MUC2, MUC5AC, and MUC6.[315] HMB45- and S100-positive melanocytes may be seen in a very few areas.

8.3.11.2 Differential diagnosis

Microcystic adnexal carcinoma, adenoid cystic carcinoma, aggressive digital papillary adenocarcinoma, and eccrine porocarcinoma are all thought to derive from eccrine sweat glands and may, at least focally, show some similarities. Immunohistochemistry is usually not helpful as these carcinomas display the same antigen profile. However, the characteristic cribriform pattern of the tumor, the epithelial and myoepithelial markers (CD14, p63, ASMA, S100 protein), and KIT suggest the diagnosis of adenoid cystic carcinoma.

8.3.12 Spiradenocarcinoma

Spiradenocarcinoma is considered to result from malignant degeneration of a benign spiradenoma. It is an extremely rare neoplasm. Middle-aged persons are mainly affected. Upper and lower extremities, trunk, head, and neck are involved in decreasing order. There is no sex predilection.[316,317] This carcinoma usually develops from a long-standing lesion that abruptly enlarges to a neoplasm of 8 mm to 10 cm, ulcerates, changes its color, and becomes tender. Spiradenocarcinoma is an aggressive tumor that may metastasize into lymph nodes, lung, and bones.[318,319] A history of multiple eccrine spiradenomas may be present.[320] A single case was described in the big toe involving the nail bed that had developed over a period of approximately 10 years from a benign spiradenoma of the dorsolateral aspect of the toe after multiple cauterizations and a local excision.[321] Another case showed a huge spiradenocarcinoma of the distal and middle phalanx occupying the whole dorsal region including the proximal nail fold.[322]

8.3.12.1 Histopathology

All spiradenocarcinomas consist of well-circumscribed nodules of typical benign eccrine spiradenoma with its characteristic two cell types of peripheral cuboid basal cells and luminal cells. The carcinomatous change is seen as a gradual transition to a malignant area in the tumor where the two-layered spiradenoma architecture changes to monomorphous carcinoma with ill-defined nests and cords of tumor cells. Duct-like structures may be completely missing and glandular components as well as hyaline globules are decreased. The other type usually presents as a spiradenocarcinoma adjacent to the benign tumor without transition. There may be bowenoid, squamous, ductal carcinoma-like, tubular, histiocytoid, and carcinosarcomatous changes with rhabdomyoblastic and osteosarcomatous differentiation.[323–325] Necrosis and hemorrhage are found in advanced spiradenocarcinoma.

Many cytokeratins, carcinoembryonic antigen, epithelial membrane antigen, and p53 overexpression have been found in spiradenocarcinoma.[326–328]

8.3.12.2 Differential diagnosis

The most important differential diagnosis is benign spiradenoma as the diagnosis of malignant transformation may be missed in case of an insufficient biopsy.

8.3.13 Hidradenocarcinoma

Hidradenocarcinoma is a rare neoplasm that has been described under various terms, such as clear-cell papillary carcinoma,[329] clear-cell hidradenocarcinoma,[330,331] malignant clear-cell hidradenoma,[332,333] malignant clear-cell acrospiroma,[334] malignant eccrine acrospiroma,[335] nodular hidradenocarcinoma, clear-cell eccrine carcinoma,[336] mucoepidermoid hidradenocarcinoma,[337] and malignant nodular clear-cell hidradenoma;[338] whether the term primary mucoepidermoid carcinoma of the skin[339,340] is justified remains disputed. Most patients are around 50 years of age. There may be a slight female preponderance. There is no characteristic appearance allowing a clinical diagnosis to be made. It is a slow growing, asymptomatic solitary tumor. Two cases were described in the nail apparatus. One was that of a 77-year-old black man with a slowly growing mass on the right middle finger nail bed, which had begun as a pigmented band rapidly enlarging in size in the last months prior to consultation. Clinically, there was an ulcerated dome-shaped red nodule involving most of the nail proximally to the proximal nail fold. The nail plate was destroyed and partially lost. The remaining nail plate on both sides of the lesion was hyperpigmented.[341] Another hidradenocarcinoma of the nail apparatus appeared clinically as a recurrent onychomycosis in a 72-year-old man.

8.3.13.1 Histopathology

There are one or several tumor nodules of variable shape and size, often with tubular and ductal structures as well as mass necrosis. Although the overlying epithelium may be eroded or ulcerated, there is no connection with the epidermis. The tumor proliferations are made up of pale to clear-cells with a distinct cytoplasmic membrane, pleomorphic nuclei, and many mitoses. Nuclear atypia may be absent, but was described in the ungual hidradenocarcinoma.

Immunohistochemistry is positive for low molecular weight cytokeratin CAM 5.2 and cytokeratin 19. The luminal border and ductal structures stain for carcinoembryonic antigen and epithelial membrane antigen. Scattered cells may be protein S100 positive.

8.3.13.2 Differential diagnosis

Benign clear-cell hidradenoma with focal degenerative changes has to be differentiated. Other differential diagnoses depend on the cytologic criteria and include other clear-cell tumors such as clear-cell Bowen's carcinoma, but also tumors with rhabdoid cells and a granular cytoplasm.

8.3.14 Sebaceous carcinoma

Sebaceous carcinoma is a malignant neoplasm with sebocytic differentiation. Originally subdivided into ocular and extraocular sebaceous carcinomas, this has now been abandoned as there is no biologic or histopathologic difference.[342-346] Most patients are between 55 and 70 years of age. Women are affected twice as often as men. Prior radiotherapy was observed to be complicated by eyelid sebaceous carcinoma in Asians.[347] Clinically, sebaceous carcinomas present as painless, sometimes multifocal nodules in the eyelids. They are frequently mistaken for chalazions, blepharitis, or conjunctivitis.[348-350] There is one report of a sebaceous gland carcinoma of the lateral aspect of the right index finger in a 46-year-old man. It presented as a painless swelling without bony alterations on X-ray. The excision was carried out under the clinical diagnosis of an epidermoid cyst and showed an irregular, well-circumscribed lesion with a pseudocapsule. The lesion was finally treated by amputation.[351]

8.3.14.1 Histopathology

Vacuolated and multivesicular clear cells characterize sebaceous carcinoma. It is an organoid proliferation of dermal lobules of atypical polygonal cells. The fibrovascular stroma characteristically lacks desmoplasia. Central tumor portions often show necrosis giving it a comedo-like growth pattern. There are relatively highly and poorly differentiated carcinomas. Well-differentiated sebaceous carcinomas have cells with abundant cytoplasm, oval vesicular nuclei with distinct nucleoli, and variable numbers of mitoses.

The poorly differentiated neoplasms have a high nuclear to cytoplasmic ratio, prominent nucleoli, high mitotic activity, and often less intracellular vacuoles. Sebaceous carcinomas are graded in I to III: Grade I carcinomas are well demarcated with approximately equally sized cell lobules; grade II neoplasms exhibit an admixture of well-defined areas with infiltration or confluent cell groups; grade III tumors demonstrate a highly invasive growth pattern or medullary sheet-like pattern. Independent of their grade, they may show overlying carcinoma *in situ* or extramammary Paget disease of the sebaceous type.[352,353] They are thought to be rather marker lesions representing a field cancerization than precursors or extensions of sebaceous carcinomas.[354] The periungual sebaceous carcinoma had many atypical mitoses and the nuclei were hyperchromatic and pleomorphic.[338] Immunohistochemically, sebaceous carcinoma is positive for pankeratin, epithelial membrane antigen, CD15, CA15.3, CU 18, Thomsen-Friedreich antigen, human milk fat globule protein-2, and androgen receptor protein.[355–357] EMA staining makes the vacuolar cell changes stand out even more clearly although this is not seen in all sebaceous carcinomas.

8.3.14.2 Differential diagnosis

Whereas well-differentiated sebaceous carcinoma has to be differentiated from sebaceous adenoma and sebaceoma, less well-differentiated ones must be differentiated from squamous cell and basal cell carcinoma.[358] Basaloid sebaceous carcinoma may resemble basal cell carcinoma, as the cells are small, have scant cytoplasm, and often show peripheral palisading. Squamoid sebaceous carcinoma develops squamous metaplasia with many keratin pearls and sometimes spindle cells, the latter leading to a sarcomatoid appearance. Neuroendocrine-like structures have also been observed.[359]

REFERENCES

1. Haneke E. "Onycholemmal" horn. *Dermatologica* 1983;167:155–158.
2. Baran R, Kint A. Onychomatrixoma. Filamentous tufted tumour in the matrix of a funnel-shaped nail: A new entity. *Br J Dermatol* 1992;126:510–515.
3. Haneke E. Differentialdiagnose und Therapie von Schwielen, Hühneraugen und Plantarwarzen. *Z Hautkr* 1982;57:263–272.
4. Poudyal S, Elpern DJ. Simple diagnostic tests for subungual pigmentation. *Dermatol Res Pract* 2009;2009:278040.
5. Baek HJ, Lee SJ, Cho KH, Choo HJ, Lee SM, Lee YH, Suh KJ et al. Subungual tumors: Clinicopathologic correlation with US and MR imaging findings. *Radiographics* 2010;30:1621–1636.
6. Haneke E, Baran R. Subunguale tumoren. *Z Hautkr* 1982;57:355–362.
7. Scully C, Assad A. Mucinous syringometaplasia. *J Am Acad Dermatol* 1984;11:503–508.
8. Baran R, Perrin C. Linear melanonychia due to subungual keratosis of the nail bed: A report of two cases. *Br J Dermatol* 1999;140:730–733.
9. Bon Mardion M, Poulalhon N, Balme B, Thomas L. Ungual seborrheic keratosis. *J Eur Acad Dermatol Venereol* 2010;24:1102–1104.
10. Perrin C, Cannata GE, Bossard C, Grill JM, Ambrossetti D, Michiels J-F. Onychocytic matricoma presenting as pachyonychia longitudinal. A new entity. *Am J Dermatopathol* 2012;34:54–59.
11. Wanat KA, Reid E, Rubin AI. Onychocytic matricoma: A new, important nail-unit tumor mistaken for a foreign body. *JAMA Dermatol* 2014;150:335–337.
12. Spaccarelli N, Wanat KA, Miller CJ, Rubin AI. Hypopigmented onychocytic matricoma as a clinical mimic of onychomatricoma: Clinical, intraoperative and histopathologic correlations. *J Cutan Pathol* 2013;40:591–594.
13. Samman PD. *The Nails in Disease*, 3rd ed. London: Heinemann, 1978;153.
14. Baran R, Perrin C. Longitudinal erythronychia with distal subungual keratosis. Onychopapilloma of the nail bed and Bowen's disease. *Br J Dermatol* 2000;143:132–135.
15. Gee BC, Millard PR, Dawber RP. Onychopapilloma is not a distinct clinicopathological entity. *Br J Dermatol* 2002;146:156–157.
16. Criscione V, Telang G, Jellinek NJ. Onychopapilloma presenting as longitudinal leukonychia. *J Am Acad Dermatol* 2010;63:541–542.
17. Cohen PR. Longitudinal erythronychia: Individual or multiple linear red bands of the nail plate: A review of clinical features and associated conditions. *Am J Clin Dermatol* 2011;12:217–231.
18. Heller J. *Die Krankheiten der Nägel*. Berlin: A Hirschwald, 1900;106.
19. Heller J. Die Krankheiten der Nägel. In: Jadassohn J, ed. *Handbuch der Haut- und Geschlechtskrankheiten. Spezielle Dermatologie vol VIII/2*. Berlin: Springer 1927.
20. Lebouc L. Etude clinique et anatomique sur quelques tumeurs sous-unguéales. *Thèse*, Paris 1889.
21. Higashi N, Sugai T, Tamamoto T. Leukonychia striata longitudinalis. *Arch Dermatol* 1971;104:192.

22. de Berker D, Perrin C, Baran R. Localized longitudinal erythronychia: Diagnostic significance and physical explanation. *Arch Dermatol* 2004;140:1253–1257.

23. Haneke E, Gutierrez Mendoza D, Borradori L. Subungual filamentous tumor and onychopapilloma. Submitted.

24. Miteva M, Fanti PA, Romanelli P, Zaiac M, Tosti A. Onychopapilloma presenting as longitudinal melanonychia. *J Am Acad Dermatol* 2012;66:e242–243.

25. Criscione V, Telang G, Jellinek NJ. Onychopapilloma presenting as longitudinal leukonychia. *J Am Acad Dermatol* 2010;63:541–542.

26. Jellinek NJ. Longitudinal erythronychia: Suggestions for evaluation and management. *J Am Acad Dermatol* 2011;64:167.e1–11.

27. Baran R, Perrin C. Localised multinucleate distal subungual keratosis. *Br J Dermatol* 1995;133:77–82.

28. Sass U, Kolivras A, Richert B, Moulonguet I, Goettmann-Bonvallot S, Anseeuw M, Theunis A, André J. Acantholytic tumor of the nail: Acantholytic dyskeratotic acanthoma. *J Cutan Pathol* 2009;36:1308–1311.

29. Baran R, Perrin C. Focal subungual warty dyskeratoma. *Dermatology* 1997;195:278–280.

30. Higashi N. Focal acantholytic dyskeratosis. *Hifu* 1990;32:507–510.

31. Atherton DJ. Naevi and other developmental defects. In Champion RH, Burton JL, Burns DA, Breathnach SM, eds. *Textbook of Dermatology*, Oxford: Blackwell Science, 1998;523–526.

32. Vicente MA, Baselga E, García Pig R, Zamora E, Cusí V, Vilá J, González Enseñat MA. Porokeratotic eccrine duct and hair follicle naevus. A familial case with systematized involvement. *Ann Dermatol Vénéréol* 1998;125(Suppl 1):S176.

33. El-Benhawi MO, George WM. Incontinentia pigmenti. *A review. Cutis* 1988;41:259–262.

34. Hadj-Rabia S, Rimella A, Smahi A, Fraitag S, Hamel-Teillac D, Bonnefont JP, de Prost Y, Bodemer C. Clinical and histologic features of incontinentia pigmenti in adults with nuclear factor-κB essential modulator gene mutations. *J Am Acad Dermatol* 2011;64:508–515.

35. Fusco F, Bardaro T, Fimiani G, Mercadante V, Miano MG, Falco G, Israël A, Courtois G, D'Urso M, Ursini MV. Molecular analysis of the genetic defect in a large cohort of IP patients and identification of novel NEMO mutations interfering with NF-kappaB activation. *Hum Mol Genet* 2004;13:1763–1773.

36. Chun SR, Rashid RM. Delayed onychodystrophy of incontinentia pigmenti: An evidence-based review of epidemiology, diagnosis and management. *J Drugs Dermatol* 2010;9:350–354.

37. Nicolaou N, Graham-Brown RA. Nail dystrophy, an unusual presentation of incontinentia pigmenti. *Br J Dermatol* 2003;149:1286–1288.

38. Piñol-Aguadé JP, Mascaró JM, Herrero C, Castel T. Tumeurs sous-unguéales dyskératosiques douloureuses et spontanément résolutives: Ses rapports avec l'incontinentia pigmenti . *Ann Dermatol Syphiligr* 1973;100:159–168.

39. Hartman DL, Danville PA. Incontinentia pigmenti associated with subungual tumours . *Arch Dermatol* 1976;112:535–542.

40. Mascaró JM, Palou J, Vives P. Painful subungual keratotic tumors in incontinentia pigmenti. *J Am Acad Dermatol* 1985;13:913–918.

41. Simmons DA, Kegel MF, Scher RK, Hines YC. Subungual tumors in incontinentia pigmenti. *Arch Dermatol* 1986;122:1431–1434.

42. Montes CM, Maize JC, Guerry-Force ML. Incontinentia pigmenti with painful subungual tumors: A two-generation study. *J Am Acad Dermatol* 2004; 50(Suppl):S45–S52.

43. Donati P, Muscardin L, Amantea A, Paolini F, Venuti A. Detection of HPV-15 in painful subungual tumors of incontinentia pigmenti: Successful topical therapy with retinoic acid. *Eur J Dermatol* 2009;19:243–247.

44. Malvehy J, Palou J, Mascaró JM. Painful subungual tumour in incontinentia pigmenti. Response to treatment with etretinate. *Br J Dermatol* 1998; 138:554–555.

45. Mahmoud BH, Zembowicz A, Fisher E. Controversies over subungual tumors in incontinentia pigmenti. *Dermatol Surg* 2014;40:1157–1159.

46. Pena ZG, Brewer JD. Multiple subungual squamous cell carcinomas in a patient with incontinentia pigmenti. *Dermatol Surg* 2014;40:1159–1161.

47. Drewes J, Günther D, Nolden HH. Intraossäre Epidermiszysten der Finger und Zehen. *Akt Chir* 1985;20:171–177.

48. Challier L, Binet O, Baran R, Levy A, Beltzer-Garelly E, Revol M. Kystes épidermoides d'implantation intra-osseuse de la phalange distal des deux gros orteils. *Ann Dermatol Vénéréol* 1996;123:203–204.

49. Berghs B, Feyen J. Intraosseous epidermal inclusion cyst following surgery for ingrowing toenail. *Foot* 1998;8:138–140.

50. Connolly JE, Ratcliffe NR. Intraosseous epidermoid inclusion cyst presenting as a paronychia of the hallux. *J Am Podiatr Med Ass* 2010;100:133–137.

51. Puhaindran ME, Cordeiro PG, Disa JJ, Mehrara BJ, Athanasian EA. Full-thickness skin graft after nail complex resection for malignant tumors. *Tech Hand Up Extrem Surg* 2011;15:84–86.

52. Wadhams PS, McDonald JF, Jenkin WM. Epidermal inclusion cysts as a complication of nail surgery. *J Am Podiatr Med Ass* 1990;80:610–612.

53. Baran R, Bureau H. Two postoperative epidermoid cysts following realignment of the hallux nail. *Br J Dermatol* 1989;119:245–247.

54. Chavallaz O, Borradori L, Haneke E. Subungual epidermoid cyst: Report of a case with rapid growth and nail loss mimicking a malignant tumor. *J Clin Dermatol* 2010;1(2):73–75.

55. Vanhoenacker FM, Eyselbergs M, Van Hul E, Van Dyck P, De Schepper AM. Pseudotumoural soft tissue lesions of the hand and wrist: A pictorial review. *Insights Imaging* 2011;2:319–333.

56. Kuwano Y, Ishizaki K, Watanabe R, Nanko H. Efficacy of diagnostic ultrasonography of lipomas, epidermal cysts, and ganglions. *Arch Dermatol* 2009;145:761–764.

57. Lewin K. Subungual epidermoid inclusion. *Br J Dermatol* 1969;81:671–675.

58. Bukhari IA, Al-Mugharbel R. Subungual epidermoid inclusions. *Saudi Med J* 2004;25:522–523.

59. Zaias N. *The Nail in Health and Disease.* Norwalk, CT: Appleton and Lange, 1990.

60. Samman PD. The human toenail, its genesis and blood supply. *Br J Dermatol* 1959;71:296–302.

61. Telang GH, Jellinek N. Multiple calcified subungual epidermoid inclusions. *J Am Acad Dermatol* 2007;56:336–339.

62. Fanti PA, Tosti A. Subungual epidermoid inclusions: Report of 8 cases. *Dermatologica* 1989;17:209–212.

63. Nikolowski W. Tricho-Adenom (Organoides Follikel-Hamartom). *Arch Klin Exp Dermatol* 1958;207:34–45.

64. Yazaki K, Sakai K, Ueda H. Solitary trichoepithelioma. *Nishinihon J Dermatol* 1978;40:662–667.

65. Bonvalet D, Duerque M, Ducret JP. Trichoadénome de Nikolowski. *Ann Dermatol Venereol* 1988;115:1186–1188.

66. Miyazaki-Nakajima K, Hara H, Terui T. Subungual trichoadenoma showing differentiation toward follicular infundibulum. *J Dermatol* 2011;38:1118–1121.

67. Brownstein MH. Trichilemmal horn: Cutaneous horn showing trichilemmal keratinization. *Br J Dermatol* 1979;100:303–309.

68. Kudo M, Uchigasaki S, Baba S, Suzuki H. Trichilemmal horn on burn scar tissue. *Eur J Dermatol* 2002;12:77–78.

69. Baran R, Dawber RPR, Richert B. Physical signs. In: Baran R, Dawber RPR, de Berker D, Haneke E, Tosti A, eds. *Diseases of the Nails and Their Management,* 3rd edn. Oxford: Blackwell Science Ltd 2001; 48–103.

70. Achten G, André J, Parent D, Laporte M. Le poil et l'ongle. *Dermatologica* 1985;171:494–495.

71. Ackerman AB. *Histologic Diagnosis of Inflammatory Skin Diseases.* Philadelphia: Lea & Febiger 1978;83.

72. Baran R, Kint A. Onychomatrixoma. Filamentous tufted tumour in the matrix of a funnel-shaped nail: A new entity (report of three cases). *Br J Dermatol* 1992;126:510–515.

73. Haneke E, Fränken J. Onychomatricoma. *Dermatol Surg* 1995;21:984–987.

74. Kint A, Baran R, Geerts ML. The onychomatricoma: An electron microscopic study. *J Cutan Pathol* 1997;24:183–188.

75. Goettmann S, Drapé JL, Baran R, Perrin C, Haneke E, Belaïch S. Onychomatricome: Deux nouveaux cas. Intérêt de la resonance magnétique nucléaire. *Ann Dermatol Venereol* 1994;121(Suppl 1):145.

76. Perrin C, Goettmann S, Baran R. Onychomatricoma: Clinical and histopathologic findings in 12 cases. *J Am Acad Dermatol* 1998;39:560–564.

77. Thomas L, Baran R, Haneke E, Drapé J-L, Zook EG. Tumors of the nail apparatus and adjacent tissues. In Baran R. *Diseases of the Nails and Their Management,* 4th edn. Wiley 2012:637–743.

78. Tosti A, Piraccini BM, Calderoni O, Fanti PA, Cameli N, Varotti E. Onychomatricoma: A report of three cases, including the first recognized in a colored man. *Eur J Dermatol* 2000;10:604–606.

79. Piraccini BM, Antonucci A, Rech G, Starace M, Misciali C, Tosti A. Onychomatricoma: First description in a child. *Pediatr Dermatol* 2007;24:46–48.

80. Cloetingh D, Helm KF, Ioffreda MD, Billingsley E, Rubin AI, Haneke E. Onychomatricoma. *J Am Acad Dermatol* 2014;70:395–397.

81. Khelifa E, Tschanz C, Masouyé I, Kerl K, Borradori L. A rare tumour of the nail apparatus: Onychomatricoma. *J Eur Acad Dermatol Venereol* 2008;22:1127–1128.

82. Estrada-Chavez G, Vega-Memije ME, Toussaint-Caire S, Rangel L, Dominguez-Cherit J. Giant onychomatricoma: Report of two cases with rare clinical presentation. *Int J Dermatol* 2007;46:634.

83. Raison-Peyron N, Alirezai M, Meunier L, Barneon G, Meynadier J. Onychomatricoma: An unusual cause of nail bleeding. *Clin Exp Dermatol* 1998;23:138.

84. Fayol J, Baran R, Perrin C, Labrousse F. Onychomatricoma with misleading features. *Acta Derm Venereol* 2000;80:370.

85. Goettman S, Zaraa I, Moulonguet I. Onychomatricoma with pterygium aspect: Unusual clinical presentation. *Acta Derm-Venereol* 2006;86:369–370.

86. Perrin C, Baran R. Onychomatricoma with matricial pterygium. Pathogenetic mechanism in 3 cases. *J Am Acad Dermatol* 2008;59:990–994.

87. Perrin C, Goettmann S, Baran R. Onychomatricoma: Clinical and histopathologic findings in 12 cases. *J Am Acad Dermatol* 1998;39:560–564.

88. Gaertner EM, Gordon M, Reed T. Onychomatricoma: Case report of an unusual subungual tumor with literature review. *J Cutan Pathol* 2009;36(Suppl 1):66–69.

89. Goettmann S, Drape JL, Idy-Peretti I, Bittoun J, Thelen P, Arrive L, Belaich S. Magnetic resonance imaging: A new tool in the diagnosis of tumours of the nail apparatus. *Br J Dermatol* 1994;130:701–710.

90. Tavares G, Di-Chiacchio N, Di-Santis E, Alvarenga L, Stuhr P, de-Farias D, Tosti A, Di-Chiacchio NG. Onychomatricoma: Epidemiological and clinical findings in a large series of 30 cases. *Br J Dermatol.* 2015 May 12. doi: 10.1111/bjd.13900. [Epub ahead of print].

91. Sanchez M, Hu S, Miteva M, Tosti A. Onychomatricoma has channel-like structures on in vivo reflectance confocal microscopy. *J Eur Acad Dermatol Venereol.* 2014;28:1560–1562.

92. Soto R, Wortsman X, Corredoira Y. Onychomatricoma: Clinical and sonographic findings. *Arch Dermatol* 2009;145:1461–1462.

93. Perrin C, Baran R, Balaquer T, Chignon-Sicard B, Cannata GE, Petrella T, Michiels JF. Onychomatricoma: New clinical and histological features. A review of 19 tumors. *Am J Dermatopathol* 2010;32:1–8.

94. Stewart CL, Sobanko JF, Rubin AI. Myxoid onychomatricoma: An unusual variant of a rare nail unit tumor. *Am J Dermatopathol* 2015;37:473–476.

95. Miteva M, Cadore de Farias D, Zaiac M, Romanelli P, Tosti A. Nail clipping diagnosis of onychomatricoma. *Arch Dermatol* 2011;147;1117–1118.

96. Fernández-Sánchez M, Saeb-Lima M, Charli-Joseph Y, Méndez-Flores S, Sánchez-Hernández C, Carbajosa-Martinez J. Onychomatricoma: An infrequent nail tumor. *Indian J Dermatol Venereol Leprol* 2012;78:382–383.

97. Perrin C, Baran R, Pisani A, Ortonne JP, Michiels JF. The onychomatricoma: Additional histologic criteria and immunohistochemical study. *Am J Dermatopathol* 2002;24:199.

98. Lee KJ, Kim WS, Lee JH, Yang J-M, Lee E-S, Lee D-Y, Mun G-H, Jang T-K. CD10, a marker for specialized mesenchymal cells (onychofibroblasts) in the nail unit. *J Dermatol Sci* 2006;42:65–67.

99. Lee DY, Yang JM, Mun GH, Jang KT, Cho KH. Immunohistochemical study of specialized nail mesenchyme containing onychofibroblasts in transverse sections of the nail unit. *Am J Dermatopathol* 2011;33:266–270.

100. Cañueto J, Santos-Briz A, García JL, Robledo C, Unamuno P. Onychomatricoma: Genome-wide analyses of a rare nail matrix tumor. *J Am Acad Dermatol* 2011;64:573–578.

101. Misciali C, Fanti PA, Iorizzo M, Piraccini BM, Tosti A. Onychoblastoma—Hamartoma of the nail unit: A new entity? (Abstr). *J Cut Pathol* 2005;32:104.

102. Misciali C, Iorizzo M, Fanti PA, Piraccini BM, Ceccarelli C, Santini D, Tosti A. Onychoblastoma (hamartoma of the nail unit): A new entity? *Br J Dermatol* 2005;152:1077–1078.

103. Ko CJ, Shi L, Barr RJ, Mölne L, Ternesten-Bratel A, Headington JT. Unguioblastoma and unguioblastic fibroma—An expanded spectrum of onychomatricoma. *J Cutan Pathol* 2004;31:307–311.

104. Petersson F, Tang ALY, Jin ACE, Barr RJ, Lee VK. Atypical cellular unguioblastic fibroma—A rare case with more atypical histological features than previously reported. *Am J Dermatopathol* 2010;32:387–391.

105. Baran R. Is onychoblastoma really a new entity? *Br J Dermatol* 2006;154:384–385.

106. Blatière V, Baran R, Barnéon G, Perrin C. A syringoma of the big toenail. *J Eur Acad Dermatol Venereol* 1999;12(Suppl 2):S128.

107. Barreto CA, Lipton MN, Smith HB, Potter GK. Intraosseous chondroid syringoma of the hallux. *J Am Acad Dermatol* 1994;30:374–378.

108. Yamamoto O, Yasuda H. An immunohistochemical study of the apocrine type of cutaneous mixed tumors with special reference to their follicular and sebaceous differentiation. *J Cutan Pathol* 1999;26:232–241.

109. Theunis A, André J, Forton F, Wanet J, Song M. A case of subungual reactive eccrine syringofibroadenoma. *Dermatology* 2001;203:185–187.

110. Chen S, Palay D, Templeton SF. Familial eccrine syringofibroadenomatosis with associated ophthalmologic abnormalities. *J Am Acad Dermatol* 1998;39:356–358.

111. Arora P, Bansai S, Garg VK, Khurana N, Lai B. Solitary eccrine syringofibroadenoma with nail involvement: A rare entity. *Indian J Dermatol* 2015;60:103.

112. Fouilloux B, Perrin C, Dutoit M, Cambazard F. Clear cell syringofibroadenoma (of Mascaró) of the nail. *Br J Dermatol* 2001;144:625–627.

113. Mascaró JM. Considérations sur les tumeurs fibro-épithéliales: Le syringofibroadénome eccrine. *Ann Dermatol Syphilol* 1963;90:146–153.

114. Odell ID, Lilly E, Reeve K, Bosenberg MW, Milstone LM. Well-differentiated syringofibrocarcinoma in a patient with Clouston syndrome. *JAMA Dermatol* 2016, published online Jan 16, 2016.

115. Arenas R. *Dermatología. Atlas, Diagnostico y Tratamiento.* Mexico: McGraw Hill, 1987;539–540.

116. Goettmann S, Marinho E, Grossin M, Bélaich S. Porome eccrine sous-unguéal. A propos de deux observations. *Ann Dermatol Vénéréol* 1995;122(Suppl 1):S147–S148.

117. Al-Qattan MM, Al-Turaiki TM, Al-Oudah N, Arab K. Benign eccrine poroma of the dorsum of the hand: Predilection for the nail fold and P53 positivity. *J Hand Surg Eur* 2009;34:402–403.

118. Haim H, Chiheb S, Benchikhi H. An unusual case of eccrine poroma. 21st Cong Eur Acad Dermatol Venereol, Prague, Sept 27–30, 2012, P371.

119. Battistella M, Langbein L, Peltre B, Cribier B. From hidroacanthoma simplex to poroid hidradenoma: Clinicopathologic and immunohistochemic study of poroid neoplasms and reappraisal of their histogenesis. *Am J Dermatopathol* 2010;32:459–468.

120. Lin YT, Chen CM, Yang CH, Chuang YH. Eccrine angiomatous hamartoma: A retrospective study of 15 cases. *Chang Gung Med J* 2012;35:167–177.

121. Sanmartin O, Botella R, Alegre V, Martinez A, Aliaga A. Congenital eccrine angiomatous hamartoma. *Am J Dermatopathol* 1992;14:161–164.

122. Sezer E, Koseoglu RD, Filiz N. Eccrine angiomatous hamartoma of the fingers with nail destruction. *Br J Dermatol* 2006;154:1002–1004.

123. Gabrielsen TO, Elgjo K, Sommerschild H. Eccrine angiomatous hamartoma of the finger leading to amputation. *Clin Exp Dermatol* 1991;16:44–45.

124. Man X-Y, Cai S-Q, Zhang A-H, Min Zheng M. Mucinous eccrine naevus presenting with hyperhidrosis: A Case Report. *Acta Derm-Venereol* 2006;86:554–555.

125. Lee H-W, Han S-S, Kang J, Lee M-W, Choi J-H, Moon K-C, Koh J-K. Multiple mucinous and lipomatous variant of eccrine angiomatous hamartoma associated with spindle cell hemangioma: A novel collision tumor? *J Cutan Pathol* 2006;33:323–326.

126. Haneke E. Neuro-arterio-syringeal hamartoma in subungual location. 14th Int Cong Dermatol Surg, Book of Abstracts, Sevilla, Oct 1–4, 1993; 85.

127. Domonkos AN, Suarez IN. Sudoriparous angioma. *Arch Dermatol* 1967;92:552–553.

128. Rositto A, Ranelleta M, Drut R. Congenital hemangioma of eccrine sweat glands. *Pediat Dermatol* 1993;10:341–343.

129. Baran R, Goettmann S. Distal digital keratoacanthoma: A report of 12 cases and review of the literature. *Br J Dermatol* 1998;139:512–515.

130. André J, Richert B. Kératoacanthome sous-unguéal. *Ann Dermatol Venereol* 2012;139:68–72.

131. Haneke E, Mainusch O, Hilker O. Subunguale Tumoren: Keratoakanthom, Neurofibrom, Nagelbett-Melanom. *Z Dermatol* 1998;184:86–102.

132. Gonzales-Ensenat A, Vilalta A, Torras H. Kératoacanthome péri et sous-unguéal. *Ann Dermatol Vénérél* 1988;115:329–331.

133. Hilker O, Winterscheidt M. Familiäre multiple Keratoakanthome. *Z Hautkr* 1987;62:284–289.

134. Haneke E. Multiple subungual keratoacanthomas. XIIth Int Cong Dermatol Surg, Munich 1991. *Zbl Haut- GeschlKr* 1991;159:337–338.

135. Stoebner PE, Fabre C, Delfour C, Joujoux JM, Roger P, Dandurand M, Meunier L. Solitary subungual keratoacanthoma arising in an MSH2 germline mutation carrier: Confirmation of a relationship by immunohistochemical analysis. *Dermatology* 2009;219:174–178.

136. Cecchi R, Troiano M, Buralli L, Innocenti S. Recurrent distal digital keratoacanthoma of the periungual region treated with Mohs micrographic surgery. *Australas J Dermatol* 2012;53:e5–e7.

137. Stoll D, Ackerman AB. Subungual keratoacanthoma. *Am J Dermatopathol* 1980;2:265–271.

138. Connolly M, Narayan S, Oxley J, de Berker DA. Immunohistochemical staining for the differentiation of subungual keratoacanthoma from subungual squamous cell carcinoma. *Clin Exp Dermatol* 2008;33:625–628.

139. Underhill T. Subungual keratoacanthoma: The importance of accurate diagnosis. *J Hand Surg Eur Vol.* 2010;35:599–600.

140. González-Rodríguez AJ, Gutiérrez-Paredes EM, Montesinos-Villaescusa E, Burgués Gasión O, Jordá-Cuevas E. Subungual keratoacanthoma: The importance of distinguishing it from subungual squamous cell carcinoma. *Actas Dermosifiliogr* Jan 23, 2012. [Epub ahead of print].

141. Bowen AR, Burt L, Boucher K, Tristani-Firouzi P, Florell SR. Use of proliferation rate, p53 staining and perforating elastic fibers in distinguishing keratoacanthoma from hypertrophic lichen planus: A pilot study. *J Cutan Pathol* 2012;39:243–250.

142. Miteva L, Broshtilova V, Schwartz RA. Verrucous systemic lupus erythematosus. *Acta Dermatovenereol* 2009;17:301–304.

143. Zedek DC, Smith ET Jr, Hitchcock MG, Feldman SR, Shelton BJ, White WL. Cutaneous lupus erythematosus simulating squamous neoplasia: The clinicopathologic conundrum and histopathologic pitfalls. *J Am Acad Dermatol* 2007;56:1013–1020.

144. Baran R, Tosti A, De Berker D. Periungual keratoacanthoma preceded by a wart and followed by a verrucous carcinoma at the same site. *Acta Derm Venereol* 2003;83:232–233.

145. Kaabipour E, Haupt HM, Stern JB, Kanetsky PA, Podolski VF, Martin AM. p16 expression in keratoacanthomas and squamous cell carcinomas of the skin: An immunohistochemical study. *Arch Pathol Lab Med* 2006;130:69–73.

146. Fujii M, Honma M, Takahashi H, Ishida-Yamamoto A, Iizuka H. The nuclear factor kappa B p50 subunit and cortactin as markers to distinguish between keratoacanthoma and well-differentiated squamous cell carcinoma. *Clin Exp Dermatol* 2011;36: 788–792.

147. Sakiz D, Turkmenoglu TT, Kabukcuoglu F. The expression of p63 and p53 in keratoacanthoma and intraepidermal and invasive neoplasms of the skin. *Pathol Res Pract* 2009;205:589–594.

148. Peternel S, Manestar-Blažić T, Brajac I, Prpić-Massari L, Kaštelan M. Expression of TWEAK in normal human skin, dermatitis and epidermal neoplasms: Association with proliferation and differentiation of keratinocytes. *J Cutan Pathol* 2011;38:780–789.

149. Ribeiro D, Narikawa S, Marques ME. Expression of apoptotic and cell proliferation regulatory proteins in keratoacanthomas and squamous cell carcinomas of the skin. *Pathol Res Pract* 2008;204:97–104.

150. Skyrlas A, Hantschke M, Passa V, Gaitanis G, Malamou-Mitsi V, Bassukas ID. Expression of apoptosis-inducing factor (AIF) in keratoacanthomas and squamous cell carcinomas of the skin. *Exp Dermatol* 2011;20:674–676.

151. Vasiljević N, Andersson K, Bjelkenkrantz K, Kjellström C, Månsson H, Nilsson E, Landberg G, Dillner J, Forslund O. The Bcl-xL inhibitor of apoptosis is preferentially expressed in cutaneous squamous cell carcinoma compared with that in keratoacanthoma. *Int J Cancer.* 2009;124:2361–2366.

152. Tan KB, Lee YS. Immunoexpression of Bcl-x in squamous cell carcinoma and keratoacanthoma: Differences in pattern and correlation with pathobiology. *Histopathology* 2009;55:338–345.

153. Park HR, Min SK, Min K, Jun SY, Seo J, Kim KH, Choi J. Differential expression of ezrin in epithelial skin tumors: Cytoplasmic ezrin immunoreactivity in squamous cell carcinoma. *Int J Dermatol* 2010;49:48–52.

154. Kossard S, Tan KB, Choy C. Keratoacanthoma and infundibulocystic squamous cell carcinoma. *Am J Dermatopathol* 2008;30:127–134.

155. Misago N, Inoue T, Toda S, Narisawa Y. Infundibular (follicular) and infundibulocystic squamous cell carcinoma: A clinicopathological and immuno-histochemical study. *Am J Dermatopathol.* 2011;33:687–694.

156. Potter GK. Neoplasia in the toes and toenail areas. *Clin Podiatr Med Surg* 1995;12:287–297.

157. Feldman SR, Fleischer AB Jr. Progression of actinic keratosis to squamous cell carcinoma revisited: Clinical and treatment implications. *Cutis* 2011;87:201–207.

158. Jung GW, Dover DC, Salopek TG. Risk of second primary malignancies following a diagnosis of cutaneous malignant melanoma or nonmelanoma skin cancer in Alberta, Canada from 1979 to 2009. *Br J Dermatol* 2014;170:136–143.

159. Glogau RG. The risk of progression to invasive disease. *J Am Acad Dermatol* 2000;42:23–24.

160. Quaedvlieg PJ, Tirsi E, Thissen MR, Krekels GA. Actinic keratosis: How to differentiate the good from the bad ones? *Eur J Dermatol* 2006;16:335–339.

161. Parker SG, Diffey BL. The transmission of optical radiation through human nails. *Br J Dermatol* 1983;108:11–16.

162. Stern DK, Creasey AA, Quijije J, Lebwohl MG. UV-A and UV-B penetration of normal human cadaveric fingernail plate. *Arch Dermatol* 2011;147:439–441.

163. Grizzle WE, Srivastava S, Manne U. The biology of incipient, pre-invasive or intraepithelial neoplasia. *Cancer Biomark* 2011;9(1–6):21–39.

164. Ackerman AB. What is the boundary that separates a thick solar keratosis and a thin squamous cell carcinoma? *Am J Dermatopathol* 1984;6:306.

165. Heaphy MR Jr, Ackerman AB. The nature of solar keratosis: A critical review in historical perspective. *J Am Acad Dermatol* 2000;43:138–150.

166. Ackerman AB. Solar keratosis is squamous cell carcinoma. *Arch Dermatol* 2003;139:1216–1217.

167. Proby CM, Churchill L, Purkis PE, Glover MT, Sexton CJ, Leigh IM. Keratin 17 expression as a marker for epithelial transformation in viral warts. *Am J Pathol* 1993;143:1667–1678.

168. Adair BM, Hudgens EE, Schmitt MT, Calderon RL, Thomas DJ. Total arsenic concentrations in toenails quantified by two techniques provide a useful biomarker of chronic arsenic exposure in drinking water. *Environmental Research* 2006;101:213–220.

169. Haneke E. Arsenverbindungen—eine Gefahr für den biologischen Präparator. *Präparator* 1978;24:131–135.

170. Maity JP, Nath B, Kar S, Chen CY, Banerjee S, Jean JS, Liu MY, Centeno JA, Bhattacharya P, Chang CL, Santra SC. Arsenic-induced health crisis in peri-urban Moyna and Ardebok villages, West Bengal, India: An exposure assessment study. *Environ Geochem Health* May 12, 2012. [Epub ahead of print].

171. Khandpur S, Malhotra AK, Bhatia V, Gupta S, Sharma VK, Mishra R, Arora NK. Chronic arsenic toxicity from Ayurvedic medicines. *Int J Dermatol* 2008;47:618–621.

172. Elmariah SB, Anolik R, Walters RF, Rosenman K, Pomeranz MK, Sanchez MR. Invasive squamous-cell carcinoma and arsenical keratoses. *Dermatol Online J* 2008;14(10):24.

173. Ehlers G. Klinische und histologische Untersuchungen zur Frage arzneimittelbedingter Arsen-Tumoren. *Z Hautkr* 1968;43:763–774.

174. Hundeiker M, Petres J. Morphogenese und Formenreichtum der arseninduzierten Präkanzerosen. *Arch Klin Exp Dermatol* 1968;231:355–365.

175. Yeh S. Skin cancer in chronic arsenicism. *Hum Pathol* 1973;4:469–485.

176. Gunjan M, Jacobs AA, Orengo IF, McClunga A, Rosen T. Combination therapy with imiquimod, 5-fluorouracil, and tazarotene in the treatment of extensive radiation-induced Bowen's disease of the hands. *Dermatol Surg* 2009;35:1–7. DOI: 10.1111/j.1524-4725.2009.01325.x.

177. Holgado RD, Ward SC, Suryaprasad SG. Squamous cell carcinoma of the hallux. *J Am Podiatr Assoc* 2000;90:309–312.

178. Riddel C, Rashid R, Thomas V. Ungual and periungual human papillomavirus-associated squamous cell carcinoma: A review. *J Am Acad Dermatol* 2011;64:1147–1153.

179. Haneke E. Morbus Bowen und Plattenepithelkarzinom der Nagelregion - klinisches Spektrum und Therapie. In: Winter H, Bellmann K-P, eds. *Fortschritte der operativen und onkologischen Dermatologie—Operative Dermatologie—Möglichkeiten und Grenzen.* Heidelberg: Springer, 1995;9:187–190.

180. Haneke E. Epidermoid carcinoma (Bowen's disease) of the nail simulating acquired ungual fibrokeratoma. *Skin Cancer* 1991;6:217–221.

181. Haneke E, Bragadini LA, Mainusch O. Enfermedad de Bowen de células claras del aparato ungular. *Act Terap Dermatol* 1997;20:311–313.

182. Baran R, Perrin C. Longitudinal erythronychia with distal subungual keratosis. Onychopapilloma of the nail bed and Bowen's disease. *Br J Dermatol* 2000;143:132–135.

183. Guitart J, Bergfeld WF, Tuthull RJ, Tubbs RR, Zienowicz R, Fleegler EJ. Squamous cell carcinoma of the nail bed: A clinicopathological study of 12 cases. *Br J Dermatol* 1990;123:215–222.

184. Haneke E. Bowen's disease of the nails. 4th Cong Eur Acad Dermatol Venereol, Brussels, Oct 10–15, 1995: Abstracts on CD-ROM EADV 1995;S75.

185. Sachse MM, Schmoll J, Wagner G. Cornu cutaneum-like HPV 45 positive subungual squamous cell carcinoma. *J Dtsch Dermatol Ges* 2011;9:226–228.

186. Baran R, Simon C. Longitudinal melanonychia: A symptom of Bowen's disease. *J Am Acad Dermatol* 1988;18:1359–1360.

187. Lemont H, Haas R. Subungual pigmented Bowen's disease in a nineteen-year-old black female. *J Am Podiatr Med Assoc* 1994;84:39–40.

188. Baran R, Eichmann A. Longitudinal melanonychia associated with Bowen disease. *Dermatology* 1993;18:159–160.

189. Sass U, André J, Stene JJ, Noel JC. Longitudinal melanonychia revealing an intraepidermal carcinoma of the nail apparatus: Detection of integrated HPV-16 DNA. *J Am Acad Dermatol* 1998;39:490–493.

190. Lambiase MC, Gardner TL, Altman CE, Albertini JG. Bowen disease of the nail bed presenting as longitudinal melanonychia: Detection of human papillomavirus type 56 DNA. *Cutis* 2003;72:305–309.

191. Baran R, Gormley D. Polydactylous Bowen's disease of the nail. *J Am Acad Dermatol* 1987;17:201–204.

192. Goodman G, Mason G, O'Brien T. Polydactylous Bowen's disease of the nail bed . *Australas J Dermatol* 1995;36:164–165.

193. Moy RL, Eliezri Y, Nuovo GJ, Zitelli JA, Bennett RG, Silverstein S. Human papillomavirus Type 16 DNA in periungual squamous cell carcinomas. *J Am Med Ass* 1989;261:2669–2673.

194. Ashinoff R, Li JJ, Jacobson M, Friedman-Kien AE, Geronemus RG. Detection of HPV DNA in squamous cell carcinoma of the nail bed and finger determined by polymerase chain reaction. *Arch Dermatol* 1991;127:1813–1818.

195. De Dobbeleer G, André J, Laporte M, Schroeder F, Peny MO, Scarcériaux B, Noël JC. Human papillomavirus type 6/11 and 16 in periungual squamous carcinoma in situ. *Eur J Dermatol* 1993;3:12–14.

196. Grundmeier N, Hamm H, Weissbrich B, Lang SC, Bröcker EB, Kerstan A. High-risk human papillomavirus infection in Bowen's disease of the nail unit: Report of three cases and review of the literature. *Dermatology* 2011;223:293–300.

197. Mii S, Niiyama S, Takasu H, Kosaka S, Hara K, Kitasato H, Sato Y, Katsuoka K. Detection of human papillomavirus type 16 in Bowen's carcinoma of the toe. *Int J Dermatol* 2012;51:804–808.

198. Rüdlinger R, Grob R, Yu YX, Schnyder UW. Human papillomavirus-35 positive bowenoid papulosis of the anogenital area and concurrent with bowenoid dysplasia of the periungual area. *Arch Dermatol* 1989;125:655–659.

199. Uezato H, Hagiwara K, Ramuzi ST, Khaskhely NM, Nagata T, Nagamine Y, Nonaka S, Asato T, Oshiro M. Detection of human papilloma virus type 56 in extragenital Bowen's disease. *Acta Dermatol Venereol* 1999;79:311–313.

200. Ohishi K, Nakamura Y, Ohishi Y, Yokomizo E, Ohara K, Takasaki M, Ueno T, Kawana S, Mitsuishi T. Bowen's disease of the nail apparatus and association with various high-risk human papillomavirus types. *J Dermatol Sci* 2011;63:69–72.

201. Shim WH, Park HJ, Kim HS, Kim SH, Jung DS, Ko HC, Kim BS, Kim MB, Kwon KS. Bowenoid papulosis of the vulva and subsequent periungual Bowen's disease induced by the same mucosal HPVs. *Ann Dermatol* 2011;23:493–496.

202. Turowski CB, Ross AS, Cusack CA. Human papillomavirus-associated squamous cell carcinoma of the nail bed in African-American patients. *Int J Dermatol* 2009;48:117–120.

203. Shimizu A, Tamura A, Abe M, Amano H, Motegi S, Nakatani Y, Hoshino H, Ishikawa O. Human papillomavirus type 56-associated Bowen's disease. *Br J Dermatol* 2012;167:1161–1164.

204. Stetsenko GY, McFarlane RJ, Chien AJ, Fleckman P, Swanson P, George E, Argenyi ZB. Subungual Bowen disease in a patient with epidermodysplasia verruciformis presenting clinically as longitudinal melanonychia. *Am J Dermatopathol* 2008;30:582–585.

205. Ongenae K, Van De Kerckhove M, Naeyart J. Bowen's disease of the nail. *Dermatology* 2002;204: 348–350.

206. Young LC, Tuxen AJ, Goodman G. Mohs' micrographic surgery as treatment for squamous dysplasia of the nail unit. *Australas J Dermatol* 2012;53: 123–127.

207. Coskey RJ, Mehrehan A, Fosnaugh R. Bowen's disease of the nail bed. *Arch Dermatol* 1972;106:79–80.

208. Gordon KB, Garden JM, Robinson JK. Bowen's disease of the distal digit: Outcome of treatment with carbon dioxide laser vaporization. *Dermatol Surg* 1996;22:723–728.

209. Weisenseel P, Prinz J, Korting H. Behandlung eines parungualen HPV73-positiven Morbus Bowen mit Imiquimodcreme. [Treatment of paraungual HPV73-positive Bowen disease with imiquimod cream]. *Hautarzt.* 2006;57:309–312.

210. Yanagishita T, Akita Y, Nakanishi G, Tamada Y, Watanabe D. Pigmented Bowen's disease of the digit successfully treated with imiquimod 5% cream. *Eur J Dermatol* 2011;21:1021–1022.

211. Wong TW, Sheu HM, Lee JY, Fletcher RJ. Photodynamic therapy for Bowen's disease (squamous cell carcinoma in situ) of the digit. *Dermatol Surg* 2001;27:452–456.

212. Usmani N, Stables GI, Telfer NR, Stringer MR. Subungual Bowen's disease treated by topical aminolevulinic acid—Photodynamic therapy. *J Am Acad Dermatol* 2005;53:S273–S276.

213. Baran R, Perrin C. Bowen's disease of the nail bed clinically simulating an onychomatricoma. *J Am Acad Dermatol* 2002;6:947–949.

214. Mikhail GR. Bowen's disease and squamous cell carcinoma of the nail bed. *Arch Dermatol* 1974;110:267–270.

215. Mikhail G. Subungual epidermoid carcinoma. *J Am Acad Dermatol* 1984;11:291–298.

216. Walling HW, Swick BL. Simulation of cutaneous Bowen's disease by freeze artifact in tissue briefly fixed in formalin. *Int J Dermatol* 2011;50:757–758.

217. Santos-Briz A, Cañueto J, del Carmen S, Mir-Bonafe JM, Fernandez E. Pagetoid dyskeratosis in dermatopathology. *Am J Dermatopathol* 2015;37:261–265;quiz 266–268.

218. Nuño-González A, Vicente-Martín FJ, Pinedo-Moraleda F, López-Estebaranz JL. High-risk cutaneous squamous cell carcinoma. *Actas Dermosifiliogr* Jan 17, 2012. [Epub ahead of print].

219. Sung W, Sam H, Deleyiannis FW. Subungual squamous cell carcinoma after organ transplantation. *J Am Podiatr Med Ass* 2010;100:304–308.

220. Bhutoria B, Shome K, Ghosh S, Bose K, Datta C, Bhattacharya S. Lewandowsky and Lutz dysplasia: Report of two cases in a family. *Indian J Dermatol* 2011;56:190–193.

221. Zavos G, Karidis NP, Tsourouflis G, Bokos J, Diles K, Sotirchos G, Theodoropoulou E, Kostakis A. Nonmelanoma skin cancer after renal transplantation: A single-center experience in 1736 transplantations. *Int J Dermatol* 2011;50:1496–1500.

222. Krynitz B, Edgren G, Lindelöf B, Baecklund E, Brattström C, Wilczek H, Smedby KE. Risk of skin cancer and other malignancies in kidney, liver, heart and lung transplant recipients 1970 to 2008—A Swedish population-based study. *Int J Cancer* 2013;132:1429–1438.

223. Lecerf P, Richert B, Theunis A, André J. A retrospective study of squamous cell carcinoma of the nail unit diagnosed in a Belgian general hospital over a 15-year period. *J Am Acad Dermatol* 2013;69:253–261.

224. Perruchoud DL, Varonier C, Haneke E, Hunger RE, Beltraminelli H, Borradori L, Ehnis Pérez A. Bowen disease of the nail unit: A retrospective study of 12 cases and their association with human papillomaviruses. *J Eur Acad Dermatol Venereol* July 13, 2016. doi: 10.1111/jdv.13654. [Epub ahead of print].

225. Patel PP, Hoppe IC, Bell WR, Lambert WC, Fleegler EJ. Perils of diagnosis and detection of subungual squamous cell carcinoma. *Ann Dermatol* 2011;23(Suppl 3):S285–S287.

226. Campbell J, Keokarn T. Squamous-cell carcinoma of the nail bed in epidermal dysplasia. *J Bone Joint Surg* 1966;48A:92–99.

227. Mauro JA, Maslyn R, Stein AA. Squamous-cell carcinoma of nail bed in hereditary ectodermal dysplasia. *N Y State J Med* 1972;72:1065–1066.

228. Fromer JL. Carcinoma of the nail bed: Discussion. *Arch Dermatol* 1970;101:66–67.

229. Morule A, Adamthwaite DN. Squamous carcinoma of the nail bed. *A case report. S Afr Med J* 1984;65:63–64.

230. Lai CS, Lin SD, Tsai CW, Chou CK. Squamous cell carcinoma of the nail bed. *Cutis* 1996;57:341–345.

231. Canovas F, Dereure O, Bonnel F. A propos d'un cas de carcinoma épidermoïde du lit unguéal avec métastase intraneurale du nerf médian. *Ann Chir Main* 1998;17:232–235.

232. Figus A, Kanitkar S, Elliot D. Squamous cell carcinoma of the lateral nail fold. *J Hand Surg [Br]* 2006;31:216–220.

233. Mii S, Amoh Y, Tanabe K, Kitasato H, Sato Y, Katsuoka K. Nestin expression in Bowen's disease and Bowen's carcinoma associated with human papillomavirus. *Eur J Dermatol* 2011;21:515–519.

234. Misago N, Toda S, Narisawa Y. Tricholemmoma and clear cell squamous cell carcinoma (associated with Bowen's disease): Immunohistochemical profile in comparison to normal hair follicles. *Am J Dermatopathol.* 2012;34:394–399.

235. Kim MS, In SG, Park OJ, Won CH, Lee MW, Choi JH, Kim CW, Kim SE, Moon KC, Chang S. Increased expression of activating transcription factor 3 is related to the biologic behavior of cutaneous squamous cell carcinomas. *Hum Pathol* 2011;42:954–959.

236. Corbalán-Vélez R, Oviedo-Ramírez I, Ruiz-Maciá JA, Conesa-Zamora P, Sánchez-Hernández M, Martínez-Barba E, Brufau-Redondo C, López-Lozano JM. Immunohistochemical staining of p16 in squamous cell carcinomas of the genital and extragenital area. *Actas Dermosifiliogr* 2011;102:439–447.

237. Farshchian M, Kivisaari A, Ala-Aho R, Riihilä P, Kallajoki M, Grénman R, Peltonen J, Pihlajaniemi T, Heljasvaara R, Kähäri VM. Serpin peptidase inhibitor clade A member 1 (SerpinA1) is a novel biomarker for progression of cutaneous squamous cell carcinoma. *Am J Pathol* 2011;179:1110–1119.

238. Clausen OPF, Aass HCD, Beigi M, Purdie KJ, Proby CM, Brown VL, Mattingsdal M, Micci F, Kølvraa S, Bolund L, DeAngelis PM. Are keratoacanthomas variants of squamous cell carcinomas? A comparison of chromosomal aberrations by comparative genomic hybridization. *J Invest Dermatol* 2006;126:2308–2315.

239. McKee R, Wilkinson JD, Black MM, Whimster IW. Carcinoma (epithelioma) cuniculatum: A clinico-pathological study of nineteen cases and review of the literature. *Histopathology* 1981;5:425–436.

240. Magnin PH, Label MG, Schroh R, Morales MS. Carcinoma cuniculatum localizado en el ledra subungual. *Rev Argent Dermatol* 1986;67:68–72.

241. Coldiron BM, Brown FC, Freeman RC. Epithelioma cuniculatum of the thumb: A case report and literature review. *J Dermatol Surg Oncol* 1986;12: 1150–1154.

242. Baran R, Haneke E. Epithelioma cuniculatum. XIth Congress of the International Society of Dermatologic Surgery, Florence, Italy, Book of Abstracts 1990.

243. Hitti IF, Sadowski G, Statsinger AL, Frolich SC. Inverted variant of carcinoma cuniculatum of the toe. *Cutis* 1987;39:250–252.

244. Van Geertruyden JP, Olemans C, Laporte M, Noël JC. Verrucous carcinoma of the nail bed. *Foot Ankle Int* 1998;19:327–328.

245. Tosti A, Morelli R, Fanti PA, Morselli PG, Catrani S, Landi G. Carcinoma cuniculatum of the nail apparatus: Report of three cases. *Dermatology* 1993;186:217–221.

246. Chiheb S, Bouziane K, Azzuzi S, Benchikhi H. Carcinome verruqueux de l'orteil. *Ann Dermatol Venereol* 2010;137:169–7.

247. Gallouj S, Harmouch T, Soughi M, Baybay H, Meziane M, Hammas N, Mikou O, Saidi A, Amarti A, Mernissi FZ. [Subungual verrucous carcinoma of the toe]. *Ann Dermatol Venereol* 2010;137:842–843.

248. Chiheb S, Slaoui W, Marnissi F, Zamiaty S, Benchikhi H. Carcinome verruqueux de l'ongle. *Presse Med* 2014;43:1144–1145.

249. Schwartz RA. Verrucous carcinoma of the skin and mucosa. *J Am Acad Dermatol* 1995;32:1–21.

250. Kurashige Y, Kato Y, Hobo A, Tsuboi R. Subungual verrucous carcinoma with bone invasion. *Int J Dermatol* 2013;52:217–219.

251. Haneke E, Baran R. Epithelioma cuniculatum, histopathology, immuno and lectin histochemistry. XIth Congress of the International Society of Dermatologic Surgery, Florence, Italy, Book of Abstracts 1990.

252. Badani H, Abi Ayad Y, Saleh H, Kadi A, Mahammedi M, Zaidi N, Serradj A. Carcinome verruqueux de l'rteil: La difficulté de diagnostic. *Ann Dermatol Vénéréol* 2013;140:S120–S121.

253. Rubin AI, Chen EH, Ratner D. Basal-cell carcinoma. *N Engl J Med* 2005;353:2262–2269.

254. Eisenklam D. Über subunguale Tumoren. *Wien Klin Wochenschr* 1931;44:1192–1193.

255. Forman SB, Ferringer TC, Garrett AB. Basal cell carcinoma of the nail unit. *J Am Acad Dermatol* 2007;56:811–814.

256. Grine RC, Parlette HL, Wilson BB. Nail unit basal cell carcinoma: A case report and literature review. *J Am Acad Dermatol* 1997;37:790–793.

257. Guana AL, Kolbusz R, Goldberg LH. Basal cell carcinoma on the nailfold of the right thumb. *Int J Dermatol* 1994;33:204–205.

258. Kim HJ, Kim YS, Suhr KB, Yoon TY, Lee JH, Park JK. Basal cell carcinoma in the nail bed in a Korean woman. *Int J Dermatol* 2000;39:397–398.

259. Martinelli PT, Cohen PR, Schulze KE, Dorsey KE, Nelson BR. Periungual basal cell carcinoma: Case report and literature review. *Dermatol Surg* 2006;32:320–323.

260. Brasie RA, Patel AR, Nouri K. Basal cell carcinoma of the nail unit treated with Mohs micrographic surgery: Superficial multicentric BCC with jagged borders—A histopathological hallmark for nail unit BCC. *J Drugs Dermatol* 2006;5:660–663.

261. Rudolph RI. Subungual basal cell carcinoma presenting as longitudinal melanonychia. *J Am Acad Dermatol* 1987;16:229–233.

262. Okuyama R, Watanabe H, Aiba S, Tagami H. Subungual basal cell carcinoma in an elderly Japanese woman. *Acta Dermatol Venereol* 2006;86:261.

263. Mikhail GR. Subungual basal cell carcinoma. *J Dermatol Surg Oncol* 1985;11:1222–1223.

264. Waldman MH, Jacobs LA. Malignant tumors of the foot. A report of 2 cases. *J Am Podiatr Med Ass* 1986;76:345.

265. Matsushita K, Kawada A, Aragane Y, Tezuka T. Basal cell carcinoma on the right hallux. *J Dermatol* 2003;30:250–251.

266. Pedro M-B, Pedro V-F, Susana B, Rodrigo C, Alexandre J, Cristina A. Acral basal cell carcinomas in an infant with Gorlin syndrome: Expanding the phenotype? *J Dtsch Ges Dermatol* 2017;15:89–90.

267. Torrelo A, Vicente A, Navarro L, Planaguma M, Bueno E, González-Sarmiento R, Hernández-Martín A et al. Early-onset acral basal cell carcinomas in Gorlin syndrome. *Br J Dermatol* 2004;171:1227–1229.

268. Herzinger T, Flaig M, Diederich R, Röcken M. Basal cell carcinoma of the toenail unit. *J Am Acad Dermatol* 2003;48:277–278.

269. Asada M, Schaart FM, de Almeida HL Jr, Korge B, Kurokawa I, Asada Y, Orfanos CE. Solid basal cell epithelioma (BCE) possibly originates from the outer root sheath of the hair follicle. *Acta Derm Venereol* 1993;73:286–292.

270. Krüger K, Blume-Peytavi U, Orfanos CE. Basal cell carcinoma possibly originates from the outer root sheath and/or the bulge region of the vellus hair follicle. *Arch Dermatol Res* 1999;291:253–259.

271. Sellheyer K, Krahl D. Basal cell (trichoblastic) carcinoma. Common expression pattern for epithelial cell adhesion molecule links basal cell carcinoma to early follicular embryogenesis, secondary hair germ, and outer root sheath of the vellus hair follicle: A clue to the adnexal nature of basal cell carcinoma? *J Am Acad Dermatol* 2008;58:158–167.

272. Tellechea O, Reis JP, Domingues JC, Baptista AP. Monoclonal antibody Ber EP4 distinguishes basal-cell carcinoma from squamous-cell carcinoma of the skin. *Am J Dermatopathol* 1993;15:452–455.

273. Ansai SI, Takayama R, Kimura T, Kawana S. Ber-EP4 is a useful marker for follicular germinative cell differentiation of cutaneous epithelial neoplasms. *J Dermatol* 2012;39:688–692.

274. Krahl D, Sellheyer K. Monoclonal antibody Ber-EP4 reliably discriminates between microcystic adnexal carcinoma and basal cell carcinoma. *J Cutan Pathol* 2007;34:782–787.

275. Perrin C, Langbein L, Ambrossetti D, Erfan N, Schweizer J, Michiels J-F. Onychocytic carcinoma: A new entity. *Am J Dermatopathol* 2013;35:679–684.

276. Perrin C, Cannata GE, Ambrosetti D, Patouraux S, Langbein L, Schweizer J. Acquired localized (monodactylous) longitudinal pachyonychia and onychocytic carcinoma in situ (2 cases): Part II. *Am J Dermatopathol.* May 5, 2016. [Epub ahead of print].

277. Wang L, Gao T, Wang G. Invasive onychocytic carcinoma. *J Cutan Pathol* 2015;42:361–367.

278. Perrin C. Tumors of the Nail Unit. A Review. Part II: Acquired Localized Longitudinal Pachyonychia and Masked Nail Tumors. *Am J Dermatopathol* 2013;35:693–712.

279. Alessi E, Coggi A, Gianotti R, Parafioriti A, Berti E. Onycholemmal carcinoma. *Am J Dermatopathol* 2004;26:397–402.

280. Inaoki M, Makino E, Adachi M, Fujimoto W. Onycholemmal carcinoma. *J Cutan Pathol* 2006; 33:577–580.

281. Rashid RMM, Cutlan JE. Onycholemmal carcinoma. *Dermatol Online J* 2010;16(3):12.

282. Chaser BE, Renszel KM, Crowson N, Osmundson A, Shedrik V, Yob EH, Drew S, Callegaris PR, Campbell S, Pitha JV, Magro CM. Onycholemmal carcinoma: A morphologic comparison of 6 reported cases. *J Am Acad Dermatol* 2013;68:290–295.

283. Perrin C, Kettani S, Ambrosetti D, Apard T, Raimbeau G, Michiels, J-F. "Onycholemmal carcinoma." An unusual case with apocrine and sebaceous differentiation. Are these tumors a microcystic nail bed carcinoma? *Am J Dermatopathol* 2012;34:549–552.

284. Kao GF, Helwig EB, Graham JH. Aggressive digital papillary adenoma and adenocarcinoma. A clinicopathological study of 57 patients with histochemical, immunopathological and ultrastructural observations. *J Cutan Pathol* 1987;14:129–146.

285. Duke WH, Sherod TT, Lupton GP. Aggressive digital papillary carcinoma (aggressive digital papillary adenoma and adenocarcinoma revisited). *Am J Surg Pathol* 2000;24:775–784.

286. Ferrándiz-Pulido C, Fernández-Figueras MT, Marco V, Combalia A, Ferrándiz C. An intertriginous lesion on the foot of a 74-year-old man: Aggressive digital papillary adenocarcinoma. *Clin Exp Dermatol* 2014;39:102–104.

287. Matysik TS, Port M, Black JR. Aggressive digital papillary adenoma: A case report. *Cutis* 1990;46:125–127.

288. Bazil MK, Henshaw RM, Werner A, Lowe EJ. Aggressive digital papillary adenocarcinoma in a 15-year-old female. *J Pediatr Hematol Oncol* 2006;28:529–530.

289. Frey J, Shimek C, Woodmansee C, Myers E, Greer S, Liman A, Adelman C, Rasberry R. Aggressive digital papillary adenocarcinoma: A report of two diseases and review of the literature. *J Am Acad Dermatol* 2009;60:331–339.

290. Inaloz HS, Patel GK, Knight AG. An aggressive treatment for aggressive digital papillary adenocarcinoma. *Cutis* 2002;69:179–182.

291. Gorva AD, Mohil R, Srinivasan MS. Aggressive digital papillary adenocarcinoma presenting as a paronychia of the finger. *J Hand Surg [Br]* 2005; 30:534.

292. Chi CC, Kuo TT, Wang SH. Aggressive digital papillary adenocarcinoma: A silent malignancy masquerading as acquired digital fibrokeratoma. *Am J Clin Dermatol* 2007;8:243–245.

293. Bogner PN, Fullen DR, Lowe L, Paulino A, Biermann JS, Sondak VK, Su LD. Lymphatic mapping and sentinel lymph node biopsy in the detection of early metastasis from sweat gland carcinoma. *Cancer* 2003;97:2285–2289.

294. Singla AK, Shearin JC. Aggressive surgical treatment of digital papillary adenocarcinoma. *Plast Reconstr Surg* 1997;99:2058–2060.

295. Jih DM, Elenitsas R, Vittorio CC, Berkowitz AR, Seykora JT. Aggressive digital papillary adenocarcinoma: A case report and review of the literature. *Am J Dermatopathol* 2001;23:154–157.

296. Cebellos PI, Penneys NS, Acosta H. Aggressive digital papillary adenocarcinoma. *J Am Acad Dermatol* 1990;23:331–334.

297. McCalmont TH. A call for logic in the classification of adnexal neoplasms. *Am J Dermatopathol* 1996;18:103–109.

298. Pinkus H, Mehregan AH. Epidermotropic eccrine carcinoma. *Arch Dermatol* 1963;88:597–606.

299. Mehregan AH, Hashimoto K, Rahbari H. Eccrine adenocarcinoma. A clinicopathologic study of 35 cases. *Arch Dermatol* 1983;119:104–114.

300. Van Gorp J, van der Putte SC. Periungual eccrine porocarcinoma. *Dermatology* 1993;187:67–70.

301. Requena L, Sanchez M, Aguilar P, Ambrojo P, Sánchez Yus E. Periungual porocarcinoma. *Dermatologica* 1990;180:177–180.

302. Moussallem CD, Abi Hatem NE, El-Khouri ZN. Malignant porocarcinoma of the nail fold: A tricky diagnosis. *Dermatol Online* 2008;14:8.

303. Snow SN, Reizner GT. Eccrine porocarcinoma of the face. *J Am Acad Dermatol* 1992;27:306–311.

304. Zina AM, Bundino S, Pippione MG. Pigmented hidroacanthoma simplex with porocarcinoma. Light and electron microscopic study of a case. *J Cutan Pathol* 1982;9:104–112.

305. Landa NG, Winkelmann RK. Epidermotropic eccrine porocarcinoma. *J Am Acad Dermatol* 1991; 24:27–31.

306. Rütten A, Requena L, Requena C. Clear-cell porocarcinoma in situ: A cytologic variant of porocarcinoma in situ. *Am J Dermatopathol* 2002;24: 67–71.

307. Robson A, Green J, Ansari N, Kim B, Seed PT, McKee PH, Calonje E. Eccrine porocarcinoma (malignant eccrine poroma); a clinicopathologic study of 69 cases. *Am J Surg Pathol* 2001;25:710–720.

308. Claudy AL, Garcier F, Kanitakis J. Eccrine porocarcinoma. Ultrastructural and immunological study. *J Dermatol* 1984;11:282–286.

309. Huet P, Dandurand M, Pignodel C, Guillot B. Matastasizing eccrine porocarcinoma: Report of a case and review of the literature. *J Am Acad Dermatol* 1996;35:680–684.

310. Akalin T, Sen S, Yucetürk A, Kandiloglu G. P53 expression in eccrine poroma and porocarcinoma. *Am J Dermatopathol* 2001;23:402–406.

311. Tateyama H, Eimoto T, Toda T, Inagaki H, Nakamura T, Yamauchi R. p53 protein and proliferating cell nuclear antigen in eccrine poroma and porocarcinoma, an immunohistochemal study. *Am J Dermatol* 1995;17:457–464.

312. Gu LH, Ichiki Y, Kitayama Y. Aberrant expression of p16 and RB protein in eccrine porocarcinoma. *J Cutan Pathol* 2002;29:473–479.

313. Gschnait F, Horn F, Lindlbauer R, Sponer D. Eccrine porocarcinoma. *J Cutan Pathol* 1980;7:349–353.

314. Geraci TL, Janis L, Jenkinson S, Stewart R. Mucinous (adenocystic) sweat gland carcinoma of the great toe. *J Foot Surg* 1987;26:520–523.

315. Terada T. Pigmented adenoid cystic carcinoma of the ear skin arising from the epidermis: A case report with immunohistochemical studies. *Int J Clin Exp Pathol* 2012;5:254–259.

316. Fernandez-Acenero MJ, Manzarbeitia F, Mestre de Juan MJ, Requena L. Malignant spiradenoma: Report of two cases and literature review. *J Am Acad Dermatol* 2001;44:395–398.

317. Granter SR, Seeger K, Calonje E, Busam K, McKee PH. Malignant eccrine spiradenoma (spiradenocarcinoma): A clinicopathologic study of 12 cases. *Am J Dermatopathol* 2000;22:97–103.

318. Ishikawa M, Nakanishi Y, Yamazaki N, Yamamoto A. Malignant eccrine spiradenoma: A case report and review of the literature. *Dermatol Surg* 2001;27:67–70.

319. Meyer TK, Rhee JS, Smith MM, Cruz MJ, Osipov VO, Wackym PA. External auditory canal eccrine spiadenocarcinoma: A case report and review of literature. *Head Neck* 2003;25:505–510.

320. Argenyi ZB, Nguyen AV, Balogh K, Sears JK, Whitaker DC. Malignant eccrine spiradernoma. A clinicopathologic study. *Am J Dermatopathol* 1992;14:381–390.

321. Engel CJ, Meads GE, Joeph NG, Stavraky W. Eccrine spiradenoma: A report of malignant transformation. *Can J Surg* 1991;34:477–480.

322. Brenn T. *Distal Phalangeal Spiradenocarcinoma Involving the Nail Apparatus.* XXIII Vars Dermatopathol Sem, Vars, France, January 24–29, 2016.

323. McCluggage WG, Fon LJ, O'Rourke D, Ismail M, Hill CM, Parks TG, Allen DC. Malignant eccrine spiradenoma with carcinomatous and sarcomatous elements. *J Clin Pathol* 1997;50:871–873.

324. Lee HH, Lee KG. Malignant eccrine spiradenoma with florid squamous differentiation. *J Korean Med Sci* 1998;13:191–195.

325. Roetman B, Vakilzadeh F, Krismann M. Ekkrines Spiradenokarzinom mit ungewöhnlicher histiozytoider Riesenzellkomponente. Fallbericht und Literaturübersicht eines seltenen Schweißdrüsentumors. *Pathologe* 202;23:149–155.

326. Wick MR, Swanson PE, Kaye VN, Pittelkow MR. Sweat gland carcinoma ex eccrine spiradenoma. *Am J Dermatopathol* 1987;9:90–98.

327. McKee PH, Fletcher CD, Stavrimos P, Pambakian H. Carcinosarcoma arising in eccrine spiradenoma. A clinicopathologic and immunohistochemical study of two cases. *Am J Dermatopathol* 1990;12:335–343.

328. Fernandez-Acenero MJ, Manzarbeitia F, Mestre MJ, Requena L. p53 expression in two cases of spiradenocarcinomas. *Am J Dermatopathol* 2000;22:104–107.

329. Liu Y. The histogenesis of clear cell papillary carcionoma of the skin. *Am J Pathol* 1949;25:93–103.

330. Mackenzie DH. A clear-cell hidradenocarcinoma with mestastases. *Cancer* 1957;10:1021–1023.

331. Kersting DW. Clear cell hidradenoma and hidradenocarcinoma. *Arch Dermatol* 2003;87:332–333.

332. Keesbey LE, Hadley CG. Clear-cell hidradenoma. Report of three cases with widespread metastases. *Cancer* 1954;7:934–952.

333. Czarnecki DB, Aarons I, Dowling JP, Lauritz B, Wallis P, Taft EH. Malignant clear cell hidradenoma: A case report. *Acta Dermatol Venereol* 1982;62:173–176.

334. Headington JT, Niedrhuber JE, Beals TF. Malignant clear cell acrospiroma. *Cancer* 1978;41:641–647.

335. Ogilvie JW. Malignant eccrine acrospiroma. A case report. *J Bopne Joint Surg Am* 1982;64:780–782.

336. Swanson PE, Cherwitz DL, Neumann MP, Wick MR. Eccrine sweat gland carcinoma: A histologic and immunohistochemical study of 32 cases. *J Cutan Pathol* 1987;14:65–86.

337. Dissanayake RV, Salm R. Sweat-gland carcinomas: Prognosis related to histogical type. *Histopathology* 1980;4:445–466.

338. Berg JW, McDivitt RW. Pathology of sweat gland carcinoma. *Pathol Annu* 1968;3:123–144.

339. Gallager MS, Miller GV, Grampa G. Primary mucoepidermoid carcinoma of the skin. *Report of a case.* *Cancer* 1959;12:286–288.

340. Wenig BL, Sciubba JJ, Goodman RS, Platt N. Primary cutaneous mucoepidermoid carcinoma of the anterior neck. *Laryngoscope* 1983;93:464–467.

341. Nash J, Chaffins M, Krull E. Hidradenocarcinoma. 59th Ann Meet Am Acad Dermatol, Washington, DC, March 2–7, 2001.

342. Wick MR, Goellner JR, Wolfe JT III, Su WP. Adnexal carcinomas of the skin. II. Extraocular sebaceous carcinomas. *Cancer* 1985;56:1163–1172.

343. Pricolo VE, Rodil JV, Vezeridis MP. Extraorbital sebaceous carcinoma. *Arch Surg* 1985;120:853–855.

344. Pickford MA, Hogg FJ, Fallowfield ME, Webster MH. Sebaceous carcinoma of the periorbital and extraorbital regions. *Br J Plast Surg* 1995;48:93–96.

345. Margo CE, Mulla ZD. Malignant tumors of the eyelid: A population-based study of non-basal cell and non-squamous cell malignant neoplasms. *Arch Ophthalmol* 1998;116:195–198.

346. Zurcher M, Hintschich CR, Garner A, Bruce C, Collin JR. Sebaceous carcinoma of the eyelid: A clinicopathological study. *Br J Ophthalmol* 1998;82:1049–1055.

347. Howrey RP, Lipham WJ, Schultz WH, Buckley EG, Dutton JJ, Klintworth GK, Rosoff PM. Sebaceous gland carcinoma: A subtle second malignancy following radiation therapy in patients with bilateral retinoblastoma. *Cancer* 1998;83:767–781.

348. Wolfe JT III, Yeatts RP, Wick MR, Campbell RJ, Waller RR. Sebaceolus carcinoma of the eyelid. Errors in clinical and pathologic diagnosis. *Am J Surg Pathol* 1984;8:597–606.

349. DiLeonardo M. Sebaceous adenoma vs. sebaceoma vs. sebaceous carcinoma. *Dermatopathol Pract Concept* 1997;3:11.

350. Gloor P, Ansari I, Sinard J. Sebaceous carcinoma presenting as a unilateral papillary conjunctivitis. *Am J Ophthalmol* 1999;127:458–459.

351. Kasdan ML, Stutts JT, Kassan MA, Clanton JN. Sebaceous gland carcinoma of the finger. *J Hand Surg* 1991;16A:870–872.

352. Nguyen GK, Mielke BW. Extraocular sebaceous carcinoma with intraepidermal (pagetoid) spread. *Am J Dermatopathol* 1987;9:364–365.

353. Chao AN, Shields CL, Krems H, Shields JA. Outcome of patients with periocular sebaceous gland carcinoma with and without conjunctival intraepithelial invasion. *Ophthalmology* 2001;108:1877–1883.

354. Margo CE, Grossniklaus HE. Intraepithelial sebaceous neoplasia without underlying invasive carcinoma. *Surv Ophthalmol* 1995;39:293–301.

355. Ansai S, Mitsuhashi Y, Kondo S, Manabe M. Immunohistochemical differentiation of extra-ocular sebaceous carcinoma from other skin cancers. *J Dermatol* 2004;31:998–1008.

356. Sinard JH. Immunohistochemical distinction of ocular sebaceous carcinoma from basal cell and squamous cell carcinoma. *Arch Ophthalmol* 1999;117:776–783.

357. Bayer-Garner IB, Givens V, Smoller B. Immuno-histochemical staining for androgen receptors: A sensitive marker of sebaceous differentiation. *J Cutan Pathol* 1999;21:426–431.

358. Wolfe JT, Wick MR, Campbell RJ. Sebaceous carcinoma of the oculo-cutaneous adnexa and extra-ocular skin. In: Wick MR, ed. *Pathology of Unusual Malignant Cutaneous Tumors*. New York: Marcel Dekker, 1985; 77–106.

359. Kazakov DV, Kutzner H, Rütten A, Mukensnabl P, Michal M. Carcinoid-like pattern in sebaceous neoplasms: Another distinctive previously unrecognized pattern in extraocular sebaceous carcinoma and sebaceoma. *Am J Dermatopathol* 2005;27:195–203.

Fibrous tumors

9

There is a vast number of fibrous, sometimes fibrohistiocytic, tumors. Their biological behavior is not always evident from their histopathological appearance as benign tumors may demonstrate considerable cellular atypia and some intermediate and malignant soft tissue neoplasms may display bland cells. For some tumors, particularly spindle cell ones, immunohistochemical examinations are necessary to differentiate them, and sometimes even more sophisticated investigations have to be performed. Whereas (fibrous) histiocytoma is very common on the extremities, it is exceedingly rare in the nail apparatus. True fibrous/fibrohistiocytic tumors are positive for vimentin. Keratinocyte, neural, and melanocyte markers are negative. However, there are exceptions to the rule, particularly in the malignant neoplasms.

9.1 BENIGN FIBROUS TUMORS

9.1.1 Fibrous histiocytoma

Histiocytoma predominantly occurs on the extremities and is very rare in the nail apparatus. Depending on its localization within the nail apparatus the clinical appearance varies.[1] Localization in the nail matrix caused bulging of the nail and thinning of the plate.[2] However, most ungual fibromas described in the literature were in fact acquired fibrokeratomas.

9.1.1.1 Histopathology

Histiocytoma, also called fibrous histiocytoma, dermatofibroma, sclerosing hemangioma, or nodulus cutaneus is usually an ill-defined, firm, mainly dermal lesion of spindle-shaped and round cells some of which may be fibrocytes or macrophages that may extend into the subcutis (Figure 9.1). Early histiocytomas are rich in macrophages

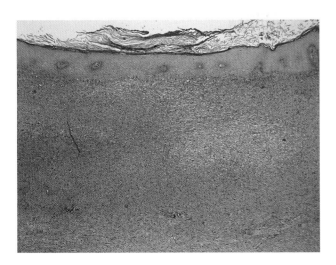

Figure 9.1 Histiocytoma.

that may store lipids or iron. Scattered lymphocytes are seen throughout and particularly at the periphery. Multinucleate cells of the Touton or foreign body type occur. Well-developed lesions exhibit coarse and haphazardly arranged collagen bundles, which may be arranged in a storiform pattern with a sclerotic center. Elastic fibers are markedly reduced or absent. The periphery may be indistinct with so-called collagen trapping. Epidermal hyperplasia is often obvious, but hyperpigmentation is not common in this particular localization although it apparently appeared in one case.[1]

Immunohistochemistry is positive for factor XIIIa, CD68, and stromelysin,[3,4] but negative for CD34. However, with aging of the histiocytoma the positivity of factor XIIIa and CD68 diminishes progressively and may be completely absent in sclerotic histiocytomas. Actin is demonstrated in the myofibroblastic variant.[5]

9.1.1.2 Differential diagnosis

Histiocytoma is one of the most common benign tumors of the skin and usually does not pose problems in making the correct diagnosis. However, valuable distinctive markers for the differentiation of histiocytoma from dermatofibrosarcoma are factor XIIIa, CD68, and stromelysin 3 with the latter displaying a sensitivity of 100% and specificity of 94%, the former of 100% and 71%. In contrast, CD34 has a sensitivity of 94% for dermatofibrosarcoma protuberans and a specificity of 83%.[3,4] Dermatofibrosarcoma protuberans shows positivity for collagen triple helix repeat containing-1 whereas histiocytoma is negative.[6]

9.1.2 Storiform collagenoma

Storiform collagenoma, also termed sclerotic fibroma or plywood fibroma, is a rare form of dermal fibroma arising spontaneously[7] or in association with Cowden's syndrome.[8,9] It mainly occurs in young and middle-aged adults and grows slowly to a size of approximately 1 cm in diameter. It may be a variant of fibrous histiocytoma although collagen I synthesis suggests a fibroblastic origin.[10] Occurrence in the nail has been described.[11]

9.1.2.1 Histopathology

Storiform collagenoma is a well-circumscribed, usually paucicellular dermal lesion mainly composed of collagen bundles with a characteristic interweaving storiform pattern. Clefting between the sclerotic collagen bundles is very characteristic. There are no elastic fibers in the orcein stain, but reticulin fibers are prominent. The cells are often poorly defined with oval to elongated nuclei (Figure 9.2). Giant and pleomorphic cells have not been observed in ungual collagenoma.

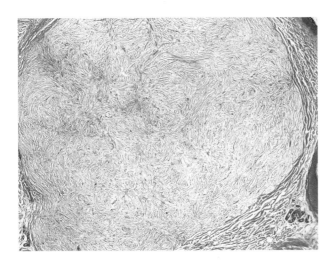

Figure 9.2 Storiform collagenoma.

Immunohistochemistry demonstrates vimentin and focal positivity for CD34; neural and keratinocyte markers are negative; its relation to the medaillion-like CD34+ fibroma has not yet been established. Most of the few scattered dermal dendritic cells are positive for factor XIIIa.

9.1.2.2 Differential diagnosis

The differential diagnosis comprises other well-circumscribed fibrous skin tumors of which an old sclerotic histiocytoma is the most common. Giant cell collagenoma is characterized by two types of cells, one compartment of spindle-shaped mononuclear cells, and the other composed by bizarre multinucleated giant cells; it has not been observed in or around the nail apparatus.[12,13] Sclerotic lipoma has some fat cells interspersed that are positive for S100.[14] Giant cell angiohistiocytoma and fibrotic Spitz nevus may occasionally be encountered.

9.1.3 Keloids

Keloids are elevated scars extending beyond the confines of the original trauma or wound, grow insidiously, and show no tendency to spontaneous involution as compared to hypertrophic scars. They occur mainly in younger individuals and are more frequent in dark-skinned persons. There is a genetic predisposition to develop keloids. They are commonly located on the earlobes, cheeks, and upper thorax, but rare on palms and soles and exceptional in ungual location.[15] They are usually due to trauma, particularly to the heat trauma of electrosurgery for viral warts. However, also so-called spontaneous keloids of the tips of several toes were observed. They may grow to a considerable size and overgrow or even completely destroy the nails. Treatment is challenging as the recurrence rate is between 45% and 95%.[16] Differential diagnostically, they have to be distinguished from chronic sclerotic scar tissue as is often seen in very long-standing ingrown toenails.[17] The etiopathogenesis of keloids is still not fully understood. A plethora of studies has shown an excess of various stimulating cytokines and a decrease of collagen synthesis

downregulating factors including a decreased collagenase activity. However, a synthesis of all these research data to form a reasonable hypothesis leading to a rational treatment is still lacking.

9.1.3.1 Histopathology

Keloids are distinctive for their thick eosinophilic hyalinized collagen type I bundles, which are haphazardly arranged but frequently form nodular or whorled masses. The border is often ill-defined. Thick collagen bundles may extend under normal appearing epidermis.

9.1.3.2 Differential diagnosis

Hypertrophic scars show nodular aggregates of collagen with many fibroblasts, but the collagen bundles are less thick and less homogenous. In hypertrophic scars, there are usually many vessels running perpendicular to the surface epidermis. It has to be stressed, however, that the distinction between keloids and hypertrophic scars, both clinically as well as histologically, is occasionally somewhat arbitrary.

9.1.4 Knuckle pads

Knuckle pads are persistent asymptomatic, slightly hyperpigmented, keratotic plaques mainly occurring on the dorsal surface of the metacarpophalangeal and interphalangeal joints, sometimes extending to the proximal nail fold. Men are predominantly affected. They are most probably a reaction to chronic rubbing and other chronic repeated traumas.[18] Knuckle pad-like keratoses on the finger joints and clubbing of the nails may be associated with epidermolytic palmar and plantar keratoderma of Vörner.[19] Pseudo-knuckle pads, also called chewing pads[20] or pachydermodactyly,[21] may be a sign of obsessive-destructive behavior.[22]

9.1.4.1 Histopathology

The epidermis shows acanthosis, hyperkeratosis, and often some hyperpigmentation. There may be fibroblast proliferation and thickened collagen in the dermis.[23]

9.1.4.2 Differential diagnosis

Knuckle pads are similar to irritation or friction induced acanthomas and lichen simplex chronicus. In pseudo-knuckle pads due to biting, the epidermis shows signs of excessive superficial traumatization. The dermal changes are very similar to those of Dupuytren's contracture and the two disorders may occur in association.[24] In epidermolytic palmoplantar keratoderma due to a keratin 9 mutation, the epidermis shows the characteristic granular clumping of tonofibrils already seen in suprabasal keratinocytes.[25]

9.1.5 Recurrent digital fibrous tumors of childhood

Described in 1965 and also called Reye's tumors or infantile digital fibromatosis, this condition occurs mainly in young children[26,27] but was recently also described in adults.[28] The fibromas are round, smooth, shiny, dome-shaped, usually skin-colored or red, firm to tense nodules on the dorsal and lateral surfaces of the digits 2–5 sparing the thumbs and the big toes. Subungual localization has not been observed, but periungual nodules may interfere with nail growth and joint mobility.[29–32] They may already be present at birth or appear shortly thereafter, but late occurrence is possible. Typically they regress spontaneously;[33] hence, no aggressive surgery is indicated. The digital fibromas seen in terminal osseous dysplasia and pigmentary defects also disappear spontaneously.[34]

Clinical differential diagnoses include hypertrophic lip of the great toe with overgrowth of the lateral nail fold, keloids, superficial fibromatosis,[35] juvenile aponeurotic fibroma, pachydermodactyly, cerebriform connective tissue nevus, proteus syndrome, multiple mucinous periungual tumors in systemic sclerosis, and terminal osseous dysplasia and pigmentary defects.[34,36]

9.1.5.1 Histopathology

Excision specimens usually are covered by a slightly flattened or normal epidermis with mild hyperkeratosis. There is a poorly circumscribed, uniform proliferation of mostly spindle-shaped fibroblasts in a dense stroma of collagen tissue extending from the epidermis to the deep dermis or even subcutis. On close inspection, a variable amount of paranuclear inclusion bodies separated by a narrow clear zone from the nucleus is seen in the cytoplasm of the fibroblasts.[37] However, sometimes they are very few and not easily detected. These inclusion bodies are not membrane-bound, they are eosinophilic, about the size of erythrocytes (3–12 µm) (Figure 9.3). They stand out with phosphotungstic acid—hematoxylin as deep purple, are deep red in Masson's trichrome stain, and red in hematoxylin-eosin stain. PAS, alcian blue, mucin stains, and birefringence are negative.

Immunohistochemistry of the fibroblasts as well as the inclusion bodies is positive for vimentin and actin.[38,39] This has led some authors to believe this condition to be a digital myofibroblastoma.[40] Electron microscopy has

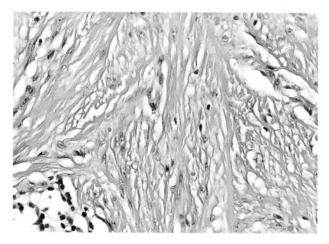

Figure 9.3 Recurring digital fibrous tumor of infancy displaying several nonmembrane bound eosinophilic intracytoplasmic granules.

demonstrated that these inclusion bodies are continuous with microfibrils that are most probably actin fibrils.[41]

9.1.5.2 Differential diagnosis

The digital fibromas of terminal osseous dysplasia and pigmentary defects are virtually identical; however, no paranuclear inclusion bodies are found despite a biological behavior mimicking infantile digital fibromatosis.[42] Myofibroma has to be excluded,[43] but it has not yet been observed at the nail. All other fibrous tumors may have areas similar to infantile digital fibromatosis but lack the characteristic inclusion bodies.

9.1.6 Ungual fibrokeratoma

Ungual fibrokeratomas are common tumors originating from the nail folds, the matrix, nail bed, or hyponychium. Clinically, acquired ungual fibrokeratomas are differentiated from Koenen's tumors. The latter occur in approximately 50% of the patients with tuberous sclerosis from the age of 12 years on, are more common on toes than fingers, and are more frequent in females than in males.[44] They constitute one of the major criteria of the tuberous sclerosis complex (TSC).[45] There is no difference in the clinical and histologic appearance of Koenen's tumors in patients with TSC1 localized on chromosome 9q34 and TSC2 on 16p13.3.[46] Koenen's tumors progressively increase in size and number. They may be the sole sign of tuberous sclerosis. These tumors are usually small round multiple lesions, 1–5 mm long, emerging from under the proximal nail fold, and causing longitudinal depressions in the nail plate; however, when their origin is localized in the matrix, they may cause nail thickening and a honeycomb appearance of the nail on plate avulsion similar to an onychomatricoma.[47] Fibromas of the nail folds may grow to large nodules and plaques. In contrast, acquired ungual fibrokeratomas are usually solitary although they may have a double,[48] triple, or even quadruple tip. They are narrower and more sausage-like than Koenen's tumors. Their tip is either hyperkeratotic or, particularly in long narrow lesions, black as it contains clotted serum, blood, and hyperkeratosis. Fibrokeratomas arising from the depth of the nail pocket cause a longitudinal depression whereas those originating in the mid-matrix run intraungually until the overlying nail lamella breaks off showing the tip of a narrow fibrokeratoma and giving rise to a distal longitudinal depression. Fibrokeratomas arising in the nail bed cause a rim in the nail plate. All fibrokeratomas are easily detachable from the overlying and underlying epithelium or nail plate, respectively, thus allowing the clinical differential diagnosis of onychopapilloma to be made easily. The etiology of acquired ungual fibrokeratomas is not yet elucidated, but trauma may occasionally play a role.[49,50] The clinical differential diagnosis comprises viral warts and a supernumerary digit, particularly when located on one side of the distal phalanx. Bowen's disease and squamous cell carcinoma may mimic fibrokeratoma.[51,52] Other clinical differential diagnoses are keloids, other fibromas, recurring digital fibromas of childhood, exostosis,

(a) (b) (c)

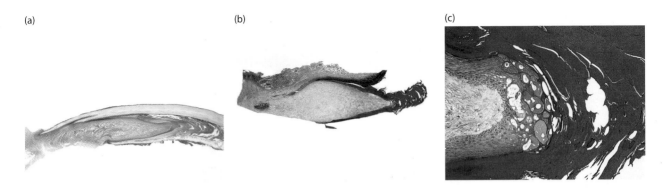

Figure 9.4 (a–c) Ungual fibrokeratoma with parallel arrangement of the collagen fibers.

cutaneous horn, pyogenic granuloma, eccrine poroma, fibrosarcoma, and dermatofibrosarcoma protuberans.[53]

9.1.6.1 Histopathology

There is no clear-cut difference between hereditary and acquired fibrokeratomas.[54] Usually a distal portion, which is loose with edematous connective tissue and abundant, often dilated thin-walled blood vessels, can be distinguished from the proximal part consisting of denser tissue with coarse interwoven eosinophilic collagen bundles.[55] The more distal the section, the more the collagen fibers are oriented in the longitudinal axis of the fibrokeratoma (Figure 9.4). Hair follicles, glial and neural tissue, or arterio-venous anastomoses are not present. The Verhoeff-van Gieson elastin stain reveals a decrease or absence of elastic fibers in the dermis. The covering epidermis is acanthotic at the base, thin on the sides, and may be markedly acanthotic or necrotic and almost lacking on the tip of the lesion. The tip is made up of parakeratotic lamellae and inspissated plasma, which is PAS positive due to its glycoprotein (immunoglobulin M) content.

The morphology is slightly different in epiungual, intraungual (dissecting), and subungual fibrokeratomas. Particularly the intraungual variant may reveal a thin lamella of nail plate dorsally although this depends greatly on the removal technique.

Transverse sections of a fibrokeratoma reveal a round structure with a dense fibrotic core and an epidermal lining in the proximal part, a loose connective tissue with dilated vessels in the distal part.

Three histologic types of acquired fibrokeratomas were described: type I with closely packed, thick dense collagen bundles, type II with an increase in the number of fibroblasts in the dermis, and type III with a loose edematous structure poor in cells.[56] Accessory germinal matrix was also observed at the distal end of some fibrokeratomas.[57] Occasionally, the stroma may contain abundant mucin; however, the tumor architecture allows easy differentiation from superficial acral fibromyxoma.[58] Extraskeletal bone formation has been observed twice at the base of a fibrokeratoma (Figure 9.5).

Koenen's tumors were also classified in three subtypes: a fibrotic, a mixed, and an angiomatous subtype.[59] The fibrotic subtype is the most frequent one, characterized by vertically oriented thick collagen bundles in the dermis and small thick-walled blood vessels. Compared to nonlesional skin, the elastic tissue is significantly decreased. The angiomatous subtype features numerous large dilated vascular spaces lined by plump endothelial cells. Stellate fibroblasts and variable amounts of dense collagen are seen in between the vessels. The mixed subtype displays histologic changes between the fibrotic and the angiomatous

(a) (b)

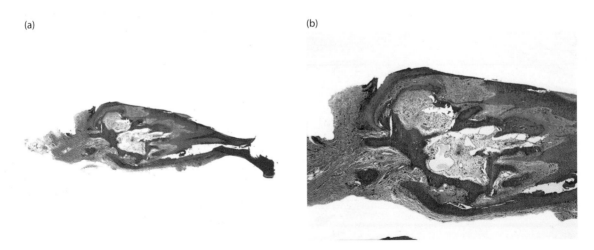

Figure 9.5 (a,b) Ungual fibrokeratoma with marked bone formation at its base.

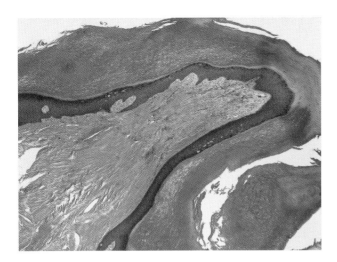

Figure 9.6 Koenen tumor from a 56-year-old woman with tuberous sclerosis. Note the pagetoid dyskeratosis on both the dorsal and ventral surface of the lesion.

subtypes (Figure 9.6). The fibrotic subtype usually has a more hyperkeratotic epidermis at its tip than the angiomatous one. It was suggested that the three subtypes merely reflect a spectrum of the same lesions.

9.1.6.2 Differential diagnosis

Provided the fibrokeratoma is sectioned longitudinally, no difficulties should arise in making the correct diagnosis. However, in transverse sections, this may be delicate. A solitary fibrous tumor of the skin mimicking an accessory nail of the little toe was recently described; it was diffusely positive for vimentin and CD34 and exhibited patchy postivity for bcl-2.[60] A soft fibroma on the proximal nail fold was desribed once.[61] Onychomatricoma has a peculiar cell-rich stroma.[62] When bone formation is seen, the pseudomalignant osseous soft tissue tumor has to be ruled out.[63] Recurring digital fibrous tumors of childhood (Reye's tumors) do not arise directly from the nail unit but in its immediate vicinity and may impair nail growth; their hallmark are small intracytoplasmic nonmembrane bound eosinophilic granules in approximately 2% of the fibroblasts that stain best with phosphotungstic acid–hematoxylin. Giant cell fibroblastoma stands out by its unique fibroblasts with their wreath or floret like nuclei.[64] Dermatofibrosarcoma protuberans and fibrosarcoma are exceedingly rare in the nail region; the former can be ruled out by its immunohistochemical characteristics.

9.1.7 Superficial acral fibromyxoma

Described in 2001,[58] this tumor has now been frequently observed. It occurs in middle-aged adults but with an age range from 4 to 86 years. Men are slightly more often affected. Almost all tumors occur on fingers or toes with a predilection for the big toe, and more than half of them in the periungual or subungual location. The tumor size ranges from 0.5–5 cm. Roughly 40% of the lesions are painful. Clinically, a dome-shaped mass is seen that grows insidiously and finally distorts or even destroys the nail.

About one-third may erode the bone.[65] Complete extirpation is the treatment of choice. Recurrences are observed in approximately one-quarter of the cases, most probably due to insufficient excision. No metastases have been observed thus far.[66–68]

9.1.7.1 Histopathology

Superficial acral fibromyxoma is well circumscribed in four-fifths of the cases, but usually not encapsulated. It is localized in the dermis and subcutis, infiltrating the dermal collagen in 70%, the fat in 27%, and the bone in 3%. There is a proliferation of spindle and stellate cells with pale eosinophilic cytoplasm in a mucinous matrix alternating with dense hyaline collagen (Figure 9.7). They may be arranged in loose fascicles. By far the majority of the digital fibromyxomas show this alternating pattern whereas 11% have a predominantly fibrous and only 3% a mainly myxoid stroma. However, it appears that with long persistence, the myxoid component decreases and the collagenous one prevails.[69] Mast cells are increased. There is some hypervascularity. Cellular atypia is rare and minimal with an occasional "degenerative change." Mitoses are rare. Multinucleate CD34+ cells are exceptional.[70] There is no cellular pleomorphism and no tumor necrosis. Perineural or neural infiltration is absent. Multinucleate cells occur only rarely. Immunohistochemistry shows vimentin positivity in almost all tumor cells, CD34 is seen in more than two-thirds, CD99 is also frequently focally or diffusely positive, but smooth muscle actin and epithelial membrane antigen are rarely positive (5/42 [12%] and 3/40 [7.5%], respectively). CD10 appears to be a specific marker[71,72] although not consistently seen by some authors. Also epithelial membrane antigen was found.[73] Nestin is positive in approximately 30% of the cells, mainly in the myxoid areas.[74] Whereas CD10 is a normal constituent of the onychodermis, nestin is positive in multipotent precursor cells of the dermis able to differentiate into neural and mesodermal progeny.[75,76] Neural, melanocytic, and keratinocyte markers are negative, whereas factor XIIIa may decorate an occasional dendritic cell.

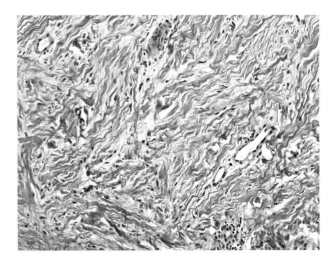

Figure 9.7 Superficial acral fibromyxoma.

Sequencing did not reveal mutations in exon 8 or 9 of GNAS1, which is seen in intramuscular or cellular myxoma. Fluorescence *in situ* hybridization (FISH) for translocation t(17:22) was negative.[77]

9.1.7.2 Differential diagnosis

All fibromyxoid tumors have to be differentiated. Digital fibrokeratoma may occasionally present a myxoid stroma, but expresses factor XIIIa, is CD34 negative and exhibits a specific macroscopic shape. Superficial acral fibromyxoma and myxoid neurofibroma may be similar, but the latter lacks the prominent vasculature and is positive for protein S100, whereas there can also be focal CD34 positivity. Myxoid onychomatricoma is CD34+ and shows the characteristic microarchitecture. Sclerosing perineurioma is more a tumor of the palms than the nails; it expresses epithelial membrane antigen and CD34 is usually negative. Myxoid dermatofibrosarcoma protuberans is very rare, but was also observed on digits. It shows a storiform proliferation of CD34+ tumor cells, which also infiltrate the subcutaneous tissue. FISH reveals the typical t(17:22) translocation. Apolipoprotein D is expressed by dermatofibrosarcoma protuberans, but not by superficial acral fibromyxoma.[78,79] Low-grade fibromyxoid sarcoma has once been observed on the big toe.[80] It shows alternating fibrous and myxoid areas with a swirling growth pattern and the tumor cells have uniform spindle cell morphology with minimal nuclear atypia. It is consistently CD34 negative,[81] but typically shows the fusion transcript FUS/CREB2L3.[82,83] Superficial angiomyxoma is mainly localized in the head and neck region but may exceptionally be observed in a digit. It is commonly ill-defined, multilobular, often hypervascularized, includes an epithelial component in about 20% of the cases, and consists of a proliferation of spindle and stellate cells in a more diffusely myxoid matrix. It is surrounded by a neutrophil-rich infiltrate. CD34 is inconsistently expressed.[84] Monophasic spindle cell variant of synovial sarcoma may also be considered differential diagnostically. However, it can be immunohistochemically characterized by EMA positivity and reactivity for keratins.[85] Myxoinflammatory fibroblastic sarcoma occurs in the soft tissues of the extremities and is usually much larger but has no predilection for the nail apparatus. It can be distinguished thanks to its inflammatory infiltrate and the Sternberg-Reed like cells. When the myxoid component of superficial acral fibromyxoma is lacking, the histological features resemble cellular digital fibroma.[86,87]

9.1.8 Matrix fibroma

Occasionally, fibromas arising from the matrix dermis are seen. The clinical pattern is uncharacteristic; usually a bulging of the nail over the matrix is seen. The lesion is asymptomatic and no nail dystrophy is observed.

9.1.8.1 Histopathology

The tumor consists of a dense stroma of relatively fine collagen fibers and is very cell-rich. Thus, it is virtually identical to the stromal component of onychomatricoma, but

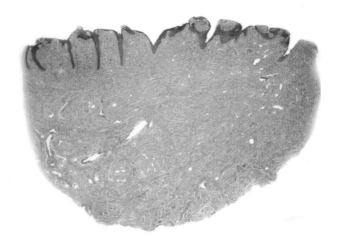

Figure 9.8 Matrix fibroma with slightly proliferated matrix epithelium.

the epithelium covering the lesion shows normal matrix without or with only mild proliferation, deep splits, or digitiform projections (Figure 9.8) and the overlying nail plate is normal.

9.1.8.2 Differential diagnosis

All other fibroblastic proliferations have to be considered. Onychomatricoma can only be ruled out when sufficient material is available.

9.1.9 Pleomorphic fibroma

Pleomorphic fibroma is a rare benign lesion mostly occurring in adults on the trunk, extremities, head, and rarely in the subungual location.[88] The neoplasm is solitary, dome-shaped or polypoid, asymptomatic, slow-growing, and flesh-colored. Its size is between 4 and 16 mm. One subungual pleomorphic fibroma had been present for 40 years.[89] Clinically, acrochordon, dermal nevus, solitary neurofibroma, or angioma may be considered. Incomplete excision may be followed by a recurrence.[90]

9.1.9.1 Histopathology

Pleomorphic fibroma is a well-circumscribed, commonly dome-shaped fibrous tumor with few spindle and irregularly shaped stellate and multinucleate cells. These have scant cytoplasm, the nuclei are large, pleomorphic, and hyperchromatic, the nucleoli are small, and mitoses are rare. Foam cells may occasionally be found. The collagen fibers are hyalinized and haphazardly arranged with some mucin between them. There may be clefting between the collagen.[91] Abundant mucin may occur.

Immunohistochemistry shows positivity for vimentin, rarely also α_1-antichymotrypsin. CD34 and muscle specific actin were positive in one report, negative in the other, and negative for protein S-100, cytokeratin, and factor XIIIa.[92]

9.1.9.2 Differential diagnosis

There are a variety of lesions with large pleomorphic cells that have to be considered in the differential diagnosis:

acrochordon with monster cells, dermatofibroma (histiocytoma) with monster cells, atypical fibroxanthoma, fibrosarcoma, fibrous papule, and desmoplastic Spitz nevus; however, most of them have not yet been observed in the nail apparatus.

9.1.10 Calcifying aponeurotic fibroma

Originally described as juvenile aponeurotic fibroma (calcifying fibroma) in young children and adolescents with a predilection to the palms and soles,[93] this lesion has now also been reported in adults and in nonacral sites.[94] It usually presents as a slow-growing, painless, poorly circumscribed, firm mass. There is no preceding trauma.[95] The subungual location has not been described, but several cases were localized in the distal phalanx, one even with bone invasion[96] and some influence on the nail shape.[97]

9.1.10.1 Histopathology

The lesions are relatively uniform from one to another. There is a fibrous mass extending into the surrounding structure with multiple processes and with calcification and/or cartilage formation in the more central portions. The cellularity is variable. Most fibroblasts are plump with a round to oval nucleus and an ill-defined cytoplasm. They are surrounded by a dense collagenous stroma that may be attached to blood vessels or encircle nerves. Sometimes there is a cartwheel or whorled pattern. Calcifications, which may only be absent in infants, are small to string-like and may be surrounded by radiating cellular columns. These cells may resemble chondrocytes lying in lacunae. An occasional osteoclast-like multinucleate giant cell may be found. Mitoses do not commonly occur.

Electron microscopy shows that the cells are fibroblasts, chondrocytes, and some myofibroblasts. Thus, the lesion somewhat mimics embryonal chondrogenesis with the fibromatous areas representing an overgrowth of the fibrous layer of the perichondrium.[98]

9.1.10.2 Differential diagnosis

With the clinical date and the characteristic calcifications and cartilage formation, the diagnosis is usually obvious. Other fibromas with secondary calcification have to be ruled out. Pseudomalignant ossifying soft tissue tumor is a reactive mesenchymal lesion.

9.1.11 Juvenile hyaline fibromatosis

Juvenile hyaline fibromatosis is a rare autosomal recessive disease of the connective tissue caused by mutations in the gene encoding the anthrax toxin receptor 2 protein, also called capillary morphogenesis gene 2 located on chromosome 4p21.[99,100] The onset is usually between the age of 3 months to 5 years, but may also be later. Hyaline material is deposited in skin, mucous membranes, and other organs causing gingival hypertrophy, flexion contractures of the joints, and skin lesions. The latter are multiple cutaneous papules mainly on the face and neck, nodules, large plaques with a transparent appearance, and gelatinous consistency on ears, around the nose, and on fingers, as well as large firm subcutaneous masses on scalp, trunk, and limbs.[101] Distal onycholysis with nail deformation was described.[102] Periungual lesions have repeatedly been observed,[103] and were clinically similar to recurrent infantile digital fibromatosis.[104] Infantile systemic hyalinosis is an allelic syndrome. It bears some similarity to myofibromatosis; however, the distribution of tumors in the skin, associated clinical features, and histopathology allow it to be differentiated.

9.1.11.1 Histopathology

The lesions are not well delimited. Scattered and cords of spindle-shaped cells are embedded in a hyaline eosinophilic matrix. This stains positive with PAS and alcian blue, but is completely devoid of elastic fibers. Congo red is negative. The older the lesion, the more homogenous matrix is present.

Electron microscopy shows fibroblasts with all signs of very active synthesis of fibrillar and granular material.[105] Immunohistochemically, these cells are actin negative. There may be some CD68 positive macrophages between the tumor cells.

9.1.11.2 Differential diagnosis

Juvenile hyaline fibromatosis and infantile systemic hyalinosis share the same gene defect and many features both clinically as well as histopathologically. It has therefore been proposed to use the common term hyaline fibromatosis syndrome.[106]

9.1.12 Pseudomalignant osseous tumor of soft tissue (digital pseudotumor)

Pseudomalignant osseous tumor of soft tissue is a benign reactive condition. It is characterized by an aggressive periosteal reaction and benign soft-tissue inflammation.[107] It is generally considered rare; however, there are several reports referring to this disease with a variety of different terms such as benign fibro-osseous pseudotumor, digital pseudotumor, florid reactive periostitis, parosteal fasciitis, fasciitis ossificans, myositis ossificans, and bizarre parosteal osteochondromatous proliferation.[108–110] As a consequence of the confusing nomenclature, some authors have placed it into the heterogeneous group of pseudomalignant osseous tumors of soft tissue or proliferative periosteal processes;[111,112] other authors call it metaplastic bone formation in chronic fibroblastic inflammation[113] or classify it into the myositis ossificans group.[114] Most of these lesions occur in the phalanges of the fingers although the subungual location is rare. The term "pseudomalignant" was coined as the speckled appearance on radiographs may resemble that of an extraskeletal osteosarcoma or chondrosarcoma. Clinically, it is a tender or painful, fusiform, often erythematous lesion of the volar aspect of the proximal phalanx of fingers and infrequently the toes. Ulceration is rare. Most patients are young adults with a slight female preponderance. It is thought that repeated minor trauma is the cause. When occurring in the subungual location, its clinical appearance is totally

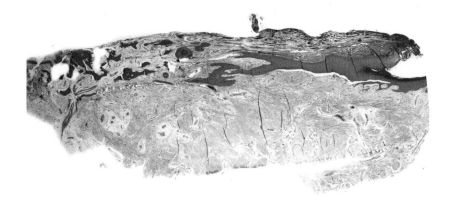

Figure 9.9 Pseudomalignant osseous soft tissue tumor with bone trabeculae and osteoid without accociation with the terminal phalanx bone.

nonspecific with the most common misdiagnosis being pyogenic granuloma.[61] Radiographically, an exostosis may be suspected.[115]

9.1.12.1 Histopathology

Pseudomalignant osseous soft tissue tumor is a fairly well-circumscribed lesion with mature bony trabeculae and osteoid with little portions of woven bone in a fibrous, often edematous, or even myxomatous stroma without direct association with the bone. They are surrounded by active osteoblasts with some osteoclasts. The bone trabeculae are haphazardly distributed with no or an incomplete zoning pattern (Figure 9.9).[116] Cellular atypia, nuclear pleomorphism, and pathologic mitoses are absent. Immunohistochemistry shows that virtually all cells are positive for vimentin and only a few also for actin and calponin[117] thus representing myofibroblasts.[118] Cytokeratin, CD34, protein S-100, and H-caldesmon are negative.

9.1.12.2 Differential diagnosis

Exostosis can usually be ruled out clinically, radiographically, and histopathologically. There is close resemblance with myositis ossificans; however, it does not show the zonal pattern of myositis ossificans; in contrast, the fibroblasts are irregularly distributed in the myxoid stroma of pseudomalignant osseous tumor.[119] Ossifying fibromyxoid tumors of soft tissue are deep, well-defined lesions made up of round and ovoid or sometimes spindle-shaped cells that form cords and nests in a myxoid stroma. An incomplete lamellar bone shell may be seen. Co-expression of protein S-100 and vimentin is unique.[120] Pyogenic granuloma with bone formation, acral angioosteoma cutis, acral myxoinflammatory fibroblastic sarcoma, extraskeletal osteosarcoma, myxochondroma, and myxochondrosarcoma are other differential diagnoses.[121] Extraskeletal osteosarcoma is a rare, highly malignant neoplasm most commonly occurring in the thighs of elderly persons. It is characterized by disorderly growth as well as hyperchromatic and pleomorphic cells that surround lace-like osteoid. Highly cellular areas composed of spindle cells with scant eosinophilic cytoplasm and elongated hyperchromatic nuclei are present

in osteosarcoma. The absence of MDM2 and CDK4 labeling in benign proliferative ossifying lesions permits their differentiation from low-grade osteosarcoma.[122] All these lesions are either extremely rare in ungual location or have not even been observed in a distal phalanx. Instead, the most important clinical differential diagnoses in an oozing onycholysis are subungual squamous cell carcinoma and amelanotic melanoma. The former is rare in toes, but not so uncommon in the thumbs.[123]

9.2 MALIGNANT FIBROUS TUMORS

Sarcomas constitute a heterogeneous group of malignant mesenchymal tumors. Most cases on the tip of the digit and in the nail apparatus are single-case anecdotal reports and occasionally the diagnosis of sarcoma would not be confirmed without using modern diagnostic histopathology methods.

9.2.1 Fibrosarcoma

Fibrosarcomas are the prototype of a malignant fibroblastic tumor. Those of the skin usually arise in the dermis as superficial, hard, often painful neoplasms, but may also be deep-seated and secondarily invade the skin. They often have a long phase of slow growth until they start to increase rapidly and metastasize, mainly to the lung. They are very rare in the nail organ and distal phalanx.[124] Treatment of choice is amputation of the digit.[125]

9.2.1.1 Histopathology

The tumor is mainly composed of spindle cells with varying numbers of mitoses, which often are atypical. Immunohistochemistry is positive for vimentin.

9.2.1.2 Differential diagnosis

All spindle cell tumors have to be included in the differential diagnosis. A case of low-grade myofibroblastic sarcoma of the distal phalanx was seen in a middle-aged woman.[126] This lesion was composed of sheets of spindle cells arranged in short fascicles, bundles, whorls, and in storiform pattern. The spindle cells were plump with vesicular nucleus, inconspicuous nucleoli, and eosinophilic cytoplasm. A mixed inflammatory infiltrate composed of lymphocytes, plasma cells, neutrophils, eosinophils, and few multinucleated foreign body type giant cells were seen. Atypical mitoses and areas of necrosis were also noted. Immunohistochemically, it was positive for vimentin, smooth muscle actin, desmin, Ki-67 index of 20%–30%. CK, ALK, CD117 (c-kit), CD34, and CD23 were negative.

9.2.2 Dermatofibrosarcoma protuberans

Dermatofibrosarcoma protuberans, called Darier-Ferrand tumor in the francophone literature, is a fibroblastic low- to intermediate-grade malignant neoplasm of the dermis and subcutis.[127] Of all sarcomas in dermatology, it is the most frequent one.[128] It typically occurs in young to middle-aged males, but very early onset is not uncommon and slight female preponderance was noted in a Korean cohort.[129] Most neoplasms are located on the trunk, but they also develop on the head, neck, and extremities.[130] Acral localization is more frequent in children.[131] Previous trauma or surgery is occasionally noted. Rapid enlargement during pregnancy was observed.[132] Recurrences after local excision are frequent as the tumor is usually ill-defined. Metastases occur in less than 5%. Clinically, it presents as a firm nodular mass with a slow and insidious growth, in the beginning more plaque-like and later developing into a large lesion or protuberant nodes. Only three cases involving the distal digit were reported, all in women. One tumor appeared as a pink, multilobulated, firm and painful mass involving the palmar aspect of the distal thumb of a 31-year-old black woman.[133] The second case was observed as a dark hyperkeratotic plaque on the proximal nail fold of the big toe in a 55-year-old Japanese female. It was first diagnosed as a wart and treated with cryosurgery, and then a white tumor appeared.[134] The third case presented as a pigmented nail thickening and turned out to be a subungual dermatofibrosarcoma.[135] Clinical diagnoses are keloid, hypertrophic scar, recurrent infantile digital fibromatosis, and chronic fibrotic-sclerotic paronychia.

Dermatofibrosarcoma protuberans is due to a t(17:22)(q22:q13) somatic mutation, which is identical to that of giant cell fibroblastoma; this is therefore often thought to be the juvenile form of dermatofibrosarcoma protuberans.[136,137] It leads even to a ring chromosome in some cases. The t(17:22) translocation fuses the collagen 1A1 gene to the platelet derived growth factor B (PDGFB) chain gene from chromosome 22q13, which results in a chimeric COL1A1-PDGFB gene encoding for a transforming protein, which is biologically very similar to normal PDGFB. Since the tumor cells not only have this mutation but also display receptors for PDGFB on their surface, an autocrine loop is generated whereby the neoplastic cells stimulate their own growth.[138] Treatment of choice is complete extirpation with a safety margin of >3 cm; narrower margins will be followed by a recurrence in roughly 50% of the cases.

9.2.2.1 Histopathology

Dermatofibrosarcoma protuberans is a tumor that diffusely infiltrates the dermis and subcutis of the skin, the latter particularly along the fibrous septa of the cutaneous fat. The epidermis remains intact and often a grenz zone is seen. The tumor center is made up of dense aggregates of uniform, slender, spindle-shaped cells with only mild to moderate cellular atypia. Their arrangement is often whorled, storiform, or in a cartwheel pattern. In specimens from skin, the appendages remain usually intact. There is little nuclear pleomorphism and mitotic activity. The more superficial areas are less cellular with spindle cells being separated by collagen. In the deep part the tumor cells are arranged in very dense sheets, expand the fibrous septa of the fat, and infiltrate the fat lobules mimicking a honeycomb appearance. Giant cells may occur. Occasionally, there may be a myxoid component in the stroma.[139] Peculiar myoid nodules are said to represent a myointimal myofibroblastic proliferation; they are non-neoplastic. Rarely, areas resembling low-grade fibrosarcoma may be seen with more cellular atypia and mitoses, which however, do not exceed 5/10 high-power fields.[140] Immunohistochemically, dermatofibrosarcoma protuberans is positive for vimentin and for CD34; this may be lost in nodular areas. PDGFB expression is seen in more than 90% of the tumors.[141] The low affinity nerve growth factor P75 was also reported to be positive.[137] Some scattered cells may be positive for factor XIIIa. Dermatofibrosarcoma protuberans does not express cytokeratins, smooth muscle actin, desmin, protein S100, and epithelial membrane antigen nor tenascin in the dermoepidermal zone.

9.2.2.2 Differential diagnosis

The most important differential diagnosis is histiocytoma, which is also surprisingly rare in the nail apparatus. In contrast to dermatofibrosarcoma protuberans, histiocytoma exhibits epidermal hyperplasia, often with basal hyperpigmentation, sometimes basal cell hyperplasia mimicking superficial basal cell carcinoma. In histiocytoma, there is a very prominent collagenous stroma with dense eosinophilic bundles. Often, collagen trapping is seen and also involvement of the fibrous fat septa, but not of the fat lobules. It is diffusely CD68 positive whereas dermatofibrosarcoma protuberans is CD68 negative, but CD34 positive, which is only focally positive in histiocytoma, if at all. Stromelysin is negative in dermatofibrosarcoma protuberans and positive in histiocytoma.[3] Tenascin is expressed in the dermoepidermal zone in histiocytoma, but not in dermatofibrosarcoma protuberans.[142] Keloids sometimes miss the typical hyalinized collagen bundles and deep fibrosis may be present.[143]

A subungual soft tissue fibrosarcoma of the big toe was described as an enlarging expansile painless mass that demonstrated no calcifications in X-ray films.[144]

Malignant fibrous histiocytoma shows more cellular atypia, nuclear pleomorphism, and mitoses. Necrotic areas may be present, which is not a feature of dermatofibrosarcoma protuberans.

A giant cell xanthosarcoma secondarily involving the little toe and its nail was described once.[145] Its true nature remains disputable.

Myxoid dermatofibrosarcoma protuberans has to be differentiated from myxoid liposarcoma. The latter shows lipoblasts, is CD34 negative, and usually has a deep invasive component. Acral fibromyxoma stands out by its lack of cellular atypia and mitoses.[146]

Low-grade fibromyxoid sarcoma is a rare deep soft tissue tumor with spindle-shaped cells with no or few mitoses and characteristic, though not specific, areas of myxoid stroma. Local recurrences are frequent and late metastases are observed. It is due to a translocation of the FUS/CREB3L2 gene.[147]

The low-grade myxofibrosarcoma exhibits more cellular atypia and has a uniformly myxoid stroma. It is mainly seen in adult women and seen in the proximal extremities. It grows to several centimeters without causing pain. Its origin is the deep subcutis from where it grows toward the dermis. Histologically, it displays a lobular pattern. Low-grade sarcomas are paucicellular with round to longitudinal pleomorphic cells in their prominently myxoid stroma. The nuclei are irregular and hyperchromatic and mitoses may be frequent. There are plenty of vessels with thin walls with vacuolar cells around them when stained for alcian blue.

A subungual liposarcoma of the right thumb metastasizing to the brain was seen once.[148]

Synovial sarcoma is a relatively frequent malignant soft tissue tumor making up for about 10% of all soft tissue tumors. It is positive for cytokeratins and epithelial membrane antigen and characterized by a chromosomal translocation t(X:18), which results in the expression of SYT-SSX fusion transcripts. This can be demonstrated by PCR and is a valuable marker for synovial sarcoma. Its monomorphic spindle cells may mimic dermatofibrosarcoma protuberans and superficial acral fibromyxoma.

Diffuse neurofibroma has a stroma of fine collagen fibers and its spindle cells have wavy nuclei. The cells are diffusely positive for protein S100. Mast cells are frequent in its stroma.

9.2.3 Epithelioid sarcoma

Epithelioid sarcoma is a slow-growing tumor mainly occurring in the vicinity of joints in young persons.[149] It exhibits no clinical characteristic features and is therefore often diagnosed very late when it is ulcerated[150] and has already metastasized.[151] Bleeding may give it a black appearance. When localized at the distal interphalangeal joint, it appears as a tender swelling or as a hard myxoid pseudocyst. Nail growth may be secondarily affected. Amputation in case of distal digit involvement is indicated, but recurrences may nevertheless occur.[152,153] The 5-year survival rate is about 50%.

9.2.3.1 Histopathology

Epithelioid sarcoma is characterized by granuloma-like proliferations of eosinophilic plump, often epithelioid and spindle-shaped cells. There is frequently necrosis in the center of the nodular proliferations. Immunohistochemistry is positive for vimentin and in some areas for pan-cytokeratins and epithelial membrane antigen as well as in many cases for actin and CD34.[154] It is negative for CD31, HMB45, and protein S-100. The histogenesis is still not clear, but electron microscopy suggests that it originates from primitive mesenchymal cells with a potential for epithelial differentiation.[155]

9.2.3.2 Differential diagnosis

Nodular proliferations with central necrobiosis or necrosis have to be considered: granuloma annulare, necrobiosis lipoidica, necrobiotic xanthogranuloma, and more.

REFERENCES

1. Rupp M, Khalluf E, Toker C. Subungual fibrous histiocytoma mimicking melanoma. *J Am Podiat Med Ass* 1957;3:141–142.
2. Kinoshita Y, Kojima T, Furusato Y. Subungual dermatofibroma of the thumb. *J Hand Surg Br* 1996;21:408–409.
3. Cribier B, Noacco G, Peltre B, Grosshans E. Stromelysin 3 expression: A useful marker for the differential diagnosis dermatofibroma versus dermatofibrosarcoma protuberans. *J Am Acad Dermatol* 2002;46:408–413.
4. Kim HJ, Lee JY, Kim SH, Seo YJ, Lee JH, Park JK, Kim MH, Cinn YW, Cho KH, Yoon TY. Stromelysin-3 expression in the differential diagnosis of dermatofibroma and dermatofibrosarcoma protuberans: Comparison with factor XIIIa and CD34. *Br J Dermatol* 2007;157:319–324.
5. Zelger BW, Zelger BG, Rappersberger K. Prominent myofibroblastic differentiation. A pitfall in the diagnosis of dermatofibroma. *Am J Dermatopathol* 1997;19:138–146.
6. Wang L, Xiang YN, Zhang YH, Tu YT, Chen HX. Collagen triple helix repeat containing-1 in the differential diagnosis of dermatofibrosarcoma protuberans and dermatofibroma. *Br J Dermatol* 2011;164:135–140.
7. Metcalf JS, Maize JC, LeBoit PE. Circumscribed storiform collagenoma (sclerosing fibroma). *Am J Dermatopathol* 1991;13:122–129.
8. Al-Daraji WI, Ramsay HM, Ali RB. Storiform collagenoma as a clue for Cowden disease or PTEN hamartoma tumour syndrome. *J Clin Pathol* 2007;60:840–842.
9. Trufant JW, Greene L, Cook DL, McKinnon W, Greenblatt M, Bosenberg MW. Colonic ganglioneuromatous polyposis and metastatic adenocarcinoma in the setting of Cowden syndrome: A case report and literature review. *Hum Pathol* 2012;43:601–604.
10. Shitabata PK, Crouch EC, Fitzgibbon JF, Swanson PE, Adesokan PN, Wick MR. Cutaneous sclerotic fibroma. Immunohistochemical evidence of a fibroblastic neoplasm with ongoing type I collagen synthesis. *Am J Dermatopathol* 1995;17:339–343.
11. Tosti A, Cameli N, Peluso AM. Storiform collagenoma of the nail. *Cutis* 1999;64:203–204.

12. Rudolph P, Schubert C, Harms D, Parwaresch R. Giant cell collagenoma: A benign dermal tumor with distinctive multinucleate cells. *Am J Surg Pathol* 1998;22:557–563.

13. Brito H, Pereira EM, Reis-Filho JS, Maeda SA. Giant cell collagenoma: Case report and review of the literature. *J Cutan Pathol* 2002;29:48–51.

14. Zelger BG, Zelger B, Steiner H, Rütten A. Sclerotic lipoma: Lipomas simulating sclerotic fibroma. *Histopathology* 1997;31:174–181.

15. Samman PD. *The Nails in Disease*, 3rd edn. London: Heinemann, 1978.

16. Niessen FB, Spauwen PH, Schalkwijk J, Kon M. On the nature of hypertrophic scars and keloids: A review. *Plast Reconstr Surg* 1999;104:1435–1458.

17. Haneke E. Controversies in the treatment of ingrown nails. *Dermatol Res Pract* 2012;2012:1–12 Article ID 783924, doi: 10.1155/2012/783924.

18. Rushing ME, Sheehan DJ, Davis LS. Video game induced knuckle pad. *Pediatr Dermatol* 2006;23:455–457.

19. Küster W, Zehender D, Mensing H, Hennies HC, Reis A. Keratosis palmoplantaris diffusa Vörner. Klinische, formalgenetische und molekularbiologische Untersuchungen bei 22 Familien. *Hautarzt* 1995;46:705–710.

20. Meigel WN, Plewig G. Kauschwielen, eine Variante der Fingerknöchelpolster. *Hautarzt* 1976;27:391–395.

21. Yanguas I, Goday JJ, Soloeta R. Pachydermodactyly: Report of two cases. *Acta Derm Venereol* 1994;74:217–218.

22. Calikoğlu E. Pseudo-knuckle pads: An unusual cutaneous sign of obsessive-compulsive disorder in an adolescent patient. *Turk J Pediatr* 2003;45:348–349.

23. Mackey SL, Cobb MW. Knuckle pads. *Cutis* 1994;54:159–160.

24. Hueston JT. Some observations on knuckle pads. *J Hand Surg Br* 1984;9:75–78.

25. Codispoti A, Colombo E, Zocchi L, Serra V, Pertusi G, Leigheb G, Tiberio R et al. Knuckle pads in an epidermal palmoplantar keratoderma patient with keratin 9 R163W transgrediens expression. *Eur J Dermatol* 2009;19:114–118.

26. Reye RD. Recurring digital fibrous tumors of childhood. *Arch Pathol* 1965;80:228–231.

27. Beckett JH, Jacobs AH. Recurring digital fibrous tumors of childhood: A review. *Pediatrics* 1977;59:401–406.

28. Sarma DP, Hoffmann EO. Infantile digital fibroma-like tumor in an adult. *Arch Dermatol* 1980;116:578–579.

29. Poppen NK, Niebauer JJ. Recurring digital fibrous tumor of childhood. *J Hand Surg Am* 1977;2:253–255.

30. Coskey RJ, Nabai H, Rahbari H. Recurring digital fibrous tumor of childhood. *Cutis* 1979;23:359–362.

31. Mehregan AH. Superficial fibrous tumors in childhood. *J Cutan Pathol* 1981;8:321–334.

32. Burgert S, Jones DH. Recurring digital fibroma of childhood. *J Hand Surg Br* 1996;21:400–402.

33. Niamba P, Léauté-Labrèze C, Boralevi F, Lepreux S, Chamaillard M, Vergnes P, Taieb A. Further documentation of spontaneous regression of infantile digital fibromatosis. *Pediat Dermatol* 2007;24:280–287.

34. Bacino CA, Stockton DW, Sierra RA, Heilstedt HA, Lewandowski R, Van den Veyver IB. Terminal osseous disysplasia and pigmentary defects: Clinical characterization of a novel male lethal X-linked syndrome. *Am J Med Genet* 2000;94:102–112.

35. Jo HJ, Chae SU, Kim GD, Kim YJ, Choi DH, Park JI. Superficial fibromatosis mimicking glomus tumor of the second toe. *Clin Orthop Surg* 2015;7:418–421.

36. Marzano AV, Berti E, Gasparini G, Vespasiani A, Scorza R, Caputo R. Unique digital skin lesions associated with systemic sclerosis. *Br J Dermatol* 1997;136:598–600.

37. Zardawi IM, Earley MJ. Inclusion body fibromatosis. *J Pathol* 1982;137:99–107.

38. Fringes B, Thais H, Böhm N, Altmannsberger M, Osborn M. Identification of actin microfilaments in the intracytoplasmic inclusions present in recurring infantile digital fibromatosis (Reye tumor). *Pediatr Pathol* 1986;6:311–324.

39. Choi KC, Hashimoto K, Setoyama M, Kagetsu N, Tronnier M, Sturman S. Infantile digital fibromatosis: Immunohistochemical and immunoelectron microscopic studies. *J Cutan Pathol* 1990;17:225–232.

40. Bhawan J, Bacchetta C, Joris I, Majno G. A myofibroblastic tumor. Infantile digital fibroma (recurrent digital fibrous tumor of childhood). *Am J Pathol* 1979;94:19.

41. Mukai M, Torikata C, Iri H. Infantile digital fibromatosis. An electron microscopic and immunhistochemical study. *Acta Pathol Jap* 1986;36:1605.

42. Horii E, Sugiura Y, Nakamura R. A syndrome of digital fibromas, facial pigmentary dysplasia, and metacarpal and metatarsal disorganization. *Am J Med Genet* 1998;80:1–5.

43. Navas-Palacios JJ, Conde-Zurita JM. Inclusion body myofibroblasts other than those seen in recurring digital fibroma of childhood. *Ultrastruct Pathol* 1984;7:109–121.

44. Aldrich S, Hong CH, Groves L, Olsen C, Moss J, Darling T. Acral lesions in tuberous sclerosis complex: Insights into pathogenesis. *J Am Acad Dermatol* 2010;63:244–251.

45. Roach ES, Gomez MR, Northrup H. Tuberous sclerosis complex consensus conference: Revised clinical diagnostic criteria. *J Child Neurol* 1998;13:624–628.

46. Sampson JR, Harris PC. The molecular genetics of tuberous sclerosis. *Hum Mol Gen* 1994;3:1477–1480.

47. Haneke E. Intraoperative differential diagnosis of onychomatricoma, Koenen's tumours, and hyperplastic Bowen's disease. *J Eur Acad Dermatol Venereol* 1998;13(Suppl):S119.

48. Göktay F, Altan ZM, Haras ZB, Güneş P, Yaşar Ş, Aytekin S, Haneke E. Multibranched acquired periungual fibrokeratomas with confounding

histopathologic findings resembling papillomavirus infection: A report of two cases. *J Cutan Pathol.* 2015;42:652–656.

49. Baykal C, Büyükbabani N, Yazganoglu KD, Saglik E. Acquired digital fibrokeratoma. *Cutis* 2007; 79:129–132.

50. Sezer E, Bridges AG, Koseoglu D, Yuksek J. Acquired periungual fibrokeratoma developing after acute staphylococcal paronychia. *Eur J Dermatol* 2009;19:636–637.

51. Haneke E. Epidermoid carcinoma (Bowen's disease) of the nail simulating acquired ungual fibrokeratoma. *Skin Cancer* 1991;6:217–221.

52. Dominguez-Cherit J, Garcia C, Vega-Memije ME, Arenas R. Pseudo-fibrokeratoma: An unusual presentation of subungual squamous cell carcinoma in a young girl. *Dermatol Surg* 2003;29:788–789.

53. Cahn RL. Acquired periungual fibrokeratoma. *Arch Dermatol* 1977;113:1564–1568.

54. Zeller J, Friedmann D, Clerici T, Revuz J. The significance of a single periungual fibroma: Report of seven cases. *Arch Dermatol* 1995;131:1465–1466.

55. Kint A, Baran R. Histopathologic study of Koenen tumors. *J Am Acad Dermatol* 1988;18:369–372.

56. Kint A, Baran R, De Keyser H. Acquired (digital) fibrokeratoma. *J Am Acad Dermatol* 1985;12:816–821.

57. Saito S, Ishikawa K. Acquired periungual fibrokeratoma with accessory germinal matrix. *J Hand Surg Br* 2002;27:549–555.

58. Fetsch JF, Laskin WB, Miettinen M. Superficial acral fibromyxoma: A clinicopathologic and immunohistochemical analysis of 37 cases of a distinctive soft tissue tumor with a predilection for the fingers and toes. *Hum Pathol* 2001;32:704–714.

59. Ma D, Darling T, Moss J, Lee C-CR. Histologic variants of periungual fibromas in tuberous sclerosis complex. *J Am Acad Dermatol* 2011;64:442–444.

60. Kemp J, Thomas B. Solitary fibrous tumor of the skin. *J Cut Pathol* 2011;38:134.

61. Guelzim S, Mahfoudi M. Tumeur unguéale rare: le fibrome molluscum ou fibrome mou à propos d'un cas. *Pan Afr J Med* 2015;20:289.

62. Fraga GR, Patterson JW, McHargue CA. Onychomatricoma: Report of a case and its comparison with fibrokeratoma of the nailbed. *Am J Dermatopathol* 2001;23:36–40.

63. Haneke E. Subungual pseudomalignant osseous soft tissue tumor: Treatment for complete cure. *Eur J Clin Med Oncol* 2011;3(2):77–81.

64. Dymock RB, Allen PW, Stirling JW, Gilbert EF, Thornbery JM. Giant cell fibroblastoma. A distinctive, recurrent tumor of childhood. *Am J Surg Pathol* 1987;11:263–271.

65. Oteo-Álvaro A, Meizoso T, Scarpellini A, Ballestín C, Pérez-Espejo G. Superficial acral fibromyxoma of the toe, with erosion of the distal phalanx. A clinical report. *Arch Orthop Trauma Surg* 2008;128:271–274.

66. André J, Theunis A, Richert B, de Saint-Aubain N. Superficial acral fibromyxoma: Clinical and pathological features. *Am J Dermatopathol* 2004;26: 472–474.

67. Kroft EBM, Haneke E, Pruszczinski M, Blokx WAM, Pasch MC. Een zeldzame subunguale tumor. *Ned T Dermatol Venereol* 2007;17:169–172.

68. Hollmann TJ, Bovée JV, Fletcher CD. Digital fibromyxoma (superficial acral fibromyxoma): A detailed characterization of 124 cases. *Am J Surg Pathol* 2012;36:789–798.

69. Goo J, Jung Y-J, Kim J-H, Sung-yul Lee S-Y, Ahn SK. A case of recurrent superficial acral fibromyxoma. *Ann Dermatol* 2010;22:110–113.

70. Luzar B, Calonje E. Superficial acral fibromyxoma: Clinicopathological study of 14 cases with emphasis on a cellular variant. *Histopathology* 2009;54:375–377.

71. Juan C, Tardío JC, Butrón M, Martín-Fragueiro LM. Superficial acral fibromyxoma: Report of 4 cases with CD10 expression and lipomatous component, two previously underrecognized features. *Am J Dermatopathol* 2008;30:431–435.

72. Dohse L, Ferringer T. CD34 negative superficial acral fibromyxoma. *J Cut Pathol* 2010;37:165.

73. Ashby-Richardson H, Rogers GS, Stadecker MJ. Superficial acral fibromyxoma: An overview. *Arch Pathol Lab Med* 2011;135:1064–1066.

74. Misago N, Ohkawa T, Yanai T, Narisawa Y. Superficial acral fibromyxoma on the tip of the big toe: Expression of CD10 and nestin. *J Eur Acad Dermatol Venereol* 2008;22:235–262.

75. Joannides A, Gaughwin P, Schwiening C, Majed H, Sterling J, Compston A, Chandran S. Efficient generation of neural precursors from adult human skin: Astrocytes promote neurogenesis from skin-derived stem cells. *Lancet* 2004;364:172–178.

76. Toma JG, McKenzie IA, Bagli D, Miller FD. Isolation and characterization of multipotent skin-derived precursors from human skin. *Stem Cells* 2005;23:727–737.

77. Cogrel O, Stanislas S, Coindre J-M, Guillot P, Beylot-Barry M, Doutre M-S, Vergier B. Fibromyxome acral superficiel: Trois observations. *Ann Dermatol Vénéréol* 2012;137:789–793.

78. Mentzel T, Schärer L, Kazakov DV, Michal M. Myxoid dermatofibrosarcoma protuberans: Clinicopathologic, immunohistochemical, and molecular analysis of eight cases. *Am J Dermatopathol* 2007;29:443–448.

79. Lisovsky M, Hoang MP, Dresser KA. Apolipoprotein D in CD34-positive and CD34-negative cutaneous neoplasms: A useful marker in differentiating superficial acral fibromyxoma from dermatofibrosarcoma protuberans. *Mod Pathol* 2008;21:31–38.

80. Cabibi D, Mustacchio V, Rodolico V. Rare localization of low-grade fibromyxoid sarcoma of the nail region. *Br J Dermatol* 2005;153:686–688.

81. Billings SD, Giblen G, Fanburg-Smith JC. Superficial low-grade fibromyxoid sarcoma (Evans tumor): A clinicopathologic analysis of 19 cases with a unique observation in the pediatric population. *Am J Surg Pathol* 2005;29:204–210.

82. Kusumi T, Nishikawa S, Tanaka M, Ogawa T, Jin H, Sato F. Low grade fibromyxoid sarcoma arising in the big toe. *Path Int* 2005;55:802–806.

83. Mertens F, Fletcher CDM, Antonescu CR, Coindre JM, Colecchia M, Domanski HA, Downs-Kelly E et al. Clinicopathologic and molecular genetic characterisation of low-grade fibromyxoid sarcoma, and cloning of a novel FUS/CREB3L1 fusion gene. *Lab Invest* 2005;85:408–415.

84. Calonje E, Guerin D, McCormick D, Fletcher CD. Superficial angiomyxoma. Clinicopathologic analysis of a series of distinctive but poorly recognized cutaneous tumors with tendency for recurrence. *Am J Surg Pathol* 1999;23:910–917.

85. Michal M, Fanburg-Smith JC, Lasota J, Fetsch JF, Lichy J, Miettinen M. Minute synovial sarcoma of the hands and feet. A clinicopathological study of 21 tumors less than 1 cm. *Am J Surg Pathol* 2006;30:721–726.

86. McNiff JM, Subtil A, Cowper SE, Lazova R, Glusac EJ. Cellular digital fibromas: Distinctive CD34-positive lesions that may mimic dermatofibrosarcoma protuberans. *J Cutan Pathol* 2005;32:413–418.

87. Guitart J, Ramirez J, Laskin WB. Cellular digital fibromas: What about superficial acral fibromyxoma? *J Cutan Pathol* 2006;33:762–763.

88. Hassenein A, Telang G, Benedetto E, Spielvogel R. Subungual myxoid pleomorphic fibroma. *Am J Dermatopathol* 1998;20:502–505.

89. Hsieh YJ, Lin YC, Wu YH, Su HY, Billings SD, Hood AF. Subungual pleomorphic fibromas. *J Cutan Pathol* 2003;30:569–571.

90. Kamino H, Lee JY, Berke A. Pleomorphic fibroma oft the skin: A benign neoplasm with cytologic atypia. A clinic-pathologic study of eight cases. *Am J Surg Pathol* 1989;13:107–113.

91. Chen TM, Purohit SK, Wang AR. Pleomorphic sclerotic fibroma: A case report and literature review. *Am J Dermatopathol* 2002;24:54–58.

92. Rudolph P, Schubert C, Zelger BG, Zelger B, Parwaresch R. Differential expression of CD34 and KiM1p in pleomorphic fibroma and dermatofibroma with monster cells. *Am J Dermatopathol* 1999;21:414–419.

93. Keasbey LE. Juvenile aponeurotic fibroma (calcifying fibroma): A distinctive tumor arising in the palms and soles of young children. *Cancer* 1953;6:338–346.

94. Fetsch JF, Miettinen M. Calcifying aponeurotic fibroma: A clinicopathologic study of 22 cases arising in uncommon sites. *Hum Pathol* 1998;29:1504–1510.

95. Nishio J, Inamitsu H, Iwasaki H, Hayashi H, Naito M. Calcifying aponeurotic fibroma of the finger in an elderly patient: CT and MRI findings with pathologic correlation. *Exp Ther Med* 2014;8:841–843.

96. Choi S-J, Ahn JH, Kang G, Lee JH, Park MS, Ryu DS, Jung SM. Calcifying aponeurotic fibroma with osseous involvement of the finger: A case report with radiologic and US findings. *Korean J Radiol* 2008;9:91–93.

97. McCurdie I, Jawad SS. Unusual and memorable. Calcifying aponeurotic fibromata. *Ann Rheum Dis* 1998;57:78.

98. Iwasaki H, Kikuchi M, Eimoto T, Enjoji M, Yoh S, Sakurai H. Juvenile aponeurotic fibromas: An ultrastructural study. *Ultrastruct Pathol* 1983;4:75–83.

99. Fong K, Rama Devi AR, Lai-Cheong JE, Chirla D, Panda SK, Liu L, Tosi I, McGrath JA. Infantile systemic hyalinosis associated with a putative splice-site mutation in the ANTXR2 gene. *Clin Exp Dermatol* 2012;37:635–638.

100. Denadai R, Raposo-Amaral CE, Bertola D, Kim C, Alonso N, Hart T, Han S et al. Identification of 2 novel ANTXR2 mutations in patients with hyaline fibromatosis syndrome and proposal of a modified grading system. *Am J Med Genet A* 2012;158A:732–742.

101. Finlay AY, Ferguson SD, Holt PJ. Juvenile hyaline fibromatosis. *Br J Dermatol* 1983;108:609–616.

102. Puretic S, Puretic B, Fišer-Herman M, Adamcic M. A unique form of mesenchymal dysplasia. *Br J Dermatol* 1962;74:8–19.

103. Rimbaud P, Jean R, Meynadier J, Rieu D, Guilhou JJ, Barnéon G. Fibro-hyalinose juvénile. *Bull Soc Fr Dermatol Syphiligr* 1973;80:435–436.

104. Ribeiro SLE, Guedes EL, Botan V, Barbosa A, Guedes de Freitas EJ. Juvenile hyaline fibromatosis: A case report and review of the literature. *Acta Reumatol Port* 2009;34:128–133.

105. Remberger K, Krieg T, Kunze D, Weinmann HM, Hübner G. Fibromatosis hyalinica multiplex (juvenile hyaline fibromatosis). Light microscopic, electron microscopic, immunohistochemical and biochemical findings. *Cancer* 1985;56:614–624.

106. Nofal A, Sanad M, Assaf M, Nofal E, Nassar A, Almokadem S, Attwa E, Elmosalamy K. Juvenile hyaline fibromatosis and infantile systemic hyalinosis: Unifying term and a proposed grading system. *J Am Acad Dermatol* 2009;61:695–700.

107. Moosavi CA, Al-Nahar LA, Murphey MD, Fanburg-Smith JC. Fibroosseous pseudotumor of the digit: A clinicopathologic study of 43 new cases. *Ann Diagn Pathol* 2008;12:21–28.

108. Prevel CD, Hanel DP. Fibro-osseous pseudotumor of the distal phalanx. *Ann Plast Surg* 1996;36:321–324.

109. Abramovici L, Steiner GC. Bizarre parosteal osteochondromatous proliferation (Nora's lesion): A retrospective study of 12 cases, 2 arising in long bones. *Human Pathol* 2002;33:1205–1210.

110. Solana J, Bosch M, Español I. Florid reactive periostitis of the thumb: A case report and review of the literature. *Chir Main* 2003;22:99–103.

111. Patel MR, Desai SS. Pseudomalignant osseous tumor of soft tissue: A case report and review of the literature. *J Hand Surg [Am]* 1986;11:66–70.

112. Dupree WB, Enzinger FM. Fibro-osseous pseudotumor of the digits. *Cancer* 1986;58:2103–2109.

113. Ernstberger H. Metaplastische Knochengewebsbildung bei chronisch-narbenbildender Entzündung der rechten Großzehe. *Hautarzt* 1985;36:248.

114. Schütte HE, van der Heul RO. Reactive mesenchymal proliferation. *J Belge Radiol* 1992;75:297–302.

115. Shin J, Kim EH, Kim YC. A bonelike protrusion on the toe—Fibro-osseous pseudotumor (FOPT) of the digit. *Arch Dermatol* 2011;147 (Aug).

116. Tan KB, Tan SH, Aw DC, Lee YS. Fibro-osseous pseudotumor of the digit: Presentation as an enlarging erythematous cutaneous nodule. *Dermatol Online J* 2010;16(12):7.

117. Chaudhry IH, Kazakov DV, Michal M, Mentzel T, Luzar B, Calonje E. Fibro-osseous pseudotumor of the digit: A clinicopathological study of 17 cases. *J Cut Pathol* 2010;37:323–329.

118. Sleater J, Mullins D, Chun K, Hendricks J. Fibroosseous pseudotumor of the digit: A comparison to myositis ossificans by light microscopy and immunohistochemical methods. *J Cutan Pathol* 1996;23:373–377.

119. De Silva MV, Reid R. Myositis ossificans and fibroosseous pseudotumor of digits: A clinicopathological review of 64 cases with emphasis on diagnostic pitfalls. *Int J Surg Pathol* 2003;11:187–195.

120. Enzinger FM, Weiss SW, Liang CY. Ossifying fibromyxoid tumor of soft parts. A clinicopathological analysis of 59 cases. *Am J Surg Pathol* 1989;13:817–827.

121. Nishio J, Iwasaki H, Soejima O, Naito M, Kikuchi M. Rapidly growing fibro-osseous pseudotumor of the digits mimicking extraskeletal osteosarcoma. *J Orthop Sci* 2002;7:410–413.

122. Yoshida A, Ushiku T, Motoi T, Shibata T, Beppu Y, Fukayama M, Tsuda H. Immunohistochemical analysis of MDM2 and CDK4 distinguishes low-grade osteosarcoma from benign mimics. *Mod Pathol* 2010;23:1279–1288.

123. Dalle S, Depape L, Phan A, Balme B, Ronger-Savle S, Thomas L. Squamous cell carcinoma of the nail apparatus: Clinicopathological study of 35 cases. *Br J Dermatol* 2007;156:871–874.

124. Inoue A, Hasegawa T, Ikata T, Hizawa K. Fibrosarcoma of the toe: A destructive lesion of the distal phalanx. *Clin Orthop Relat Res* 1996;333:239–244.

125. Butler ED, Hamill JP, Seipel RS, de Lorimier AA. Tumors of the hand. *Am J Surg* 1960;100:293–302.

126. San Miguel P, Fernández G, Ortiz-Rey JA, Larrauri P. Low-grade myofibroblastic sarcoma of the distal phalanx. *J Hand Surg Am* 2004;29:1160–1163.

127. Weiss SW, Goldblum JR. Fibrohistiocytic tumors of intermediate malignancy. In: Weiss SW, Goldblum JR, eds. *Enzinger and Weiss's Soft Tissue Tumors*, 4th edn. St Louis: Mosby, 2001: 491–516.

128. Miettinen M. Malignant and potentially malignant fibroblastic and myofibroblastic tumors. In: Miettinen M, ed. *Diagnostic Soft Tissue Pathology*. New York: Churchill Livingston, 2003: 189–204.

129. Kim M, Huh CH, Cho KH, Cho S. A study on the prognostic value of clinical and surgical features of dermatofibrosarcoma protuberans in Korean patients. *J Eur Acad Dermatol Venereol* 2012;26:964–971.

130. Gonzalez Medina EM, Lacy Niebal RM, Ángeles RB, Vega Memije ME. Dermatofibrosarcoma protuberans: una revisión. *Dermatol Cosm Méd Quir* 2015;13:149–158.

131. Tsai YJ, Lin PY, Chew KY, Chiang YC. Dermatofibrosarcoma protuberans in children and adolescents: Clinical presentation, histology, treatment, and review of the literature. *J Plast Reconstr Aesthet Surg* 2014;67:1222–1229.

132. Taylor HB, Helwig EB. Dermatofibrosarcoma protuberans. A study of 115 cases. *Cancer* 1962;15:717–725.

133. Coles M, Smith M, Rankin EA. An unusual case of dermatofibrosarcoma protuberans. *J Hand Surg* 1989;14A:135–138.

134. Hashiro M, Fujio Y, Shoda Y, Okumura M. A case of dermatofibrosarcoma protuberans on the right first toe. *Cutis* 1995;56:281–282.

135. Dumas V, Euvrard S, Ligeron C, Ronger S, Chouvet B, Faure M, Claudy A. Dermatofibrosarcome de Darier–Ferrand sous-unguéal. *Ann Dermatol Vénéréol* 1998;125(Suppl 3):S93.

136. Macarenco RS, Oliveira AM, Nascimento AG, Erickson-Johnson M, Wang X. Ganhos de cópias genômicas de COL1A1-PDFGB ocorrem na progressao de fibroblastoma de células gigantes para dermatofibrossarcoma protuberans. *An Bras Dermatol* 2007;82(Suppl 1):S172–S173.

137. Eminger LA, Shinohara MM, Elenitsas R, Halpern AV, Heymann WR. Giant cell fibroblastoma mimicking a soft fibroma arising within a dermatofibrosarcoma protuberans. *J Am Acad Dermatol* 2012;67:e137–e139.

138. O'Brien KP, Senoussi E, Dal Cin P, Sciot R, Mandahl N, Fletcher JA, Turc-Garet C, Dumanski JP. Various regions within the alpha-helical domain of the COL1A gene are fused to the second exon of the PDGFB gene in dermatofibrosarcoma and giant-cell fibroblastomas. *Genes Chromosomes Cancer* 1998;23:187–193.

139. Calonje E, Fletcher CD. Myxoid differentiation in dermatofibrosarcoma protuberans and its fibrosarcomatous variant: Clinicopathologic analysis of 5 cases. *J Cutan Pathol* 1996;23:30–36.

140. Goldblum JR, Reith JD, Weiss SW. Sarcomas arising in dermatofibrosarcoma protuberans: A reapprasal of biologic behavior in eighteen cases treated by wide local excision with extended clinical follow up. *Am J Surg Pathol* 2000;24:1125–1130.

141. Nakamura I, Kariya Y, Okada E, Yasuda M, Matori S, Ishikawa O, Uezato H, Takahashi K. A novel chromosomal translocation associated with *COL1A2-PDGFB* gene fusion in dermatofibrosarcoma protuberans. PDGF expression as a new diagnostic tool. *JAMA Dermatol* 2015; epub Sept 2.

142. Kahn HJ, Fekete E, From L. Tenascin differentiates dermatofibroma from dermatofibrosarcoma protuberans: Comparison with CD34 and factor XIIIa. *Hum Pathol* 2001;32:50–56.

143. Vanhaecke C Jr, Hickman G, Cavelier-Balloy B, Masson V, Duron J-B, Gorj M, May P et al. Plantar keloids: Diagnostic and therapeutic issues in six patients. *J Eur Acad Dermatol Venereol* 2015;29:1421–1426.

144. Silvers SH, Weinstein S. Soft tissue fibrosarcoma. A case report and review of the literature. *Cutis* 1982;29:195–198.

145. Hartert W. Zur Kenntnis der pigmentierten riesenzellenhaltigen Xanthosarcome an Hand und Fuss. *Beiträge Klin Chirurg* 1913;84:546–562.

146. Carranza C, Molina-Ruiz AM, Pérez de la Fuente T, Kutzner H, Requena L, Santonja C. Subungual acral fibromyxoma involving the bone: A mimicker of malignancy. *Am J Dermatopathol* 2015;37:555–559.

147. Evans HL. Low-grade fibromyxoid sarcoma: A report of two metastasizing neoplasms having a deceptively benign appearance. *Am J Clin Pathol* 1987;88:615–619.

148. Bailey SC, Bailey B, Smith NT, Van Tassel P, Thomas CR Jr. Brain metastasis from a primary liposarcoma of the digit: Case report. *Am J Clin Oncol* 2001;24:81–84.

149. Chase DR, Enzinger FM. Epithelioid sarcoma. *Am J Surg Pathol* 1985;9:241–263.

150. Tsoitis G, Asvesti Z, Papadimitriou C et al. Epithelioid sarcoma. In: *Book of Abstracts*, #86. Rotterdam: EurSoc Pediat Dermatol, 1996: 133.

151. Hwang JS, Fitzhugh VA, Kaushal N, Beebe KS. Epithelioid sarcoma: An unusual presentation in the distal phalanx of the toe. *Am J Orthop (Belle Mead NJ)* 2012;41:223–227.

152. Carloz B, Bioulac P, Gavard J, Baudet J, Doutre MS, Beylot C. Recidives multiples d'un sarcome épithélioïde. *Ann Dermatol Vénéréol* 1991;118:623–628.

153. Khapake DP, Jambhekar NA, Anchan C, Madur BP, Chinoy RF, Agarwal M, Puri A. Epithelioid sarcoma of the foot with subsequent lesion in hand: Metastatic lesion or second primary? *Indian J Pathol Microbiol* 2007;50:563–565.

154. Zanolli MD, Wilmoth G, Shaw JA, Poehling G, White WL. Epithelioid sarcoma, clinical and histologic characteristics. *J Am Acad Dermatol* 1992;26:302–305.

155. Miettinen M, Fanburg-Smith JC, Virolainen M, Shmookler BM, Fetsch JF. Epithelioid sarcoma: An immunohistochemical analysis of 112 classical and variant cases and a discussion of the differential diagnosis. *Hum Pathol* 1999;30:934–942.

Vascular tumors

This chapter deals with tumors and tumor-like proliferations of blood vessels and lymphatics. Not all lesions described here are histogenetically clear; some are reactive lesions, others pseudotumors.[1]

Whereas port-wine stains, other vascular malformations, and hemangiomas are very common in glabrous skin, they are exceptional in the nail region. Glomeruloid hemangioma, reactive angioendotheliomatosis, generalized essential telangiectasia, unilateral nevoid telangiectasia, angioma serpiginosum, nevus araneus, senile angioma, tufted angioma, microvenular hemangioma, targetoid hemosiderotic hemangioma, acquired elastotic hemangioma, cutaneous epithelioid angiomatous nodule, and some other rare angiomatous lesions have not, to our knowledge, been observed in the nail apparatus or its immediate vicinity. Eruptive epithelioid hemangiomas were recently described in a patient with two of them growing under the nail and in the proximal nail fold, respectively.[2]

10.1 BENIGN VASCULAR TUMORS AND PROLIFERATIONS OF THE NAIL UNIT

10.1.1 Intravascular papillary endothelial hyperplasia (pseudoangiosarcoma of Masson)

Intravascular papillary endothelial hyperplasia was originally thought to be an angiosarcoma by Masson. It is a reactive lesion only once described in the nail apparatus. The tip of the index finger was slightly tender, bulbous, and the nail bed was bluish red. The nail appeared enlarged. The lesion was embarrassing with the patient's profession as a hair stylist.[3]

10.1.1.1 Histopathology

Usually, intravascular papillary endothelial hyperplasia is situated within an ectatic thin-walled vein that is often partially thrombotic. Parts of the thrombus may be in organization. The lumen contains villous proliferations of endothelia with an inconspicuous connective tissue core. Mitoses and cellular atypias are absent (Figure 10.1).

10.1.1.2 Differential diagnosis

Low-grade angiosarcoma has to be considered as well as any other thrombosing process.

10.1.2 Acral arteriovenous shunting

This reactive condition may develop posttraumatically or due to autonomic nerve damage as the result of luxury blood supply with relatively high pressure[4] or as a chronic stasis dermatitis associated with venous insufficiency.[5] Clinically, it usually results in a pseudo-Kaposi-like appearance with dark red to almost blackish papules and plaques that may also develop keloid-like areas. Acroangiodermatitis of Mali[6] and Stewart-Bluefarb syndrome[7] are variants. The toes and perionychium may be involved; however, the nails are rarely directly affected, but may show a purple hue or be leukonychotic. One 52-year-old woman with terminal renal insufficiency developed a pincer nail due to a pseudo-Kaposi sarcoma thought to be due to an arteriovenous fistula placed to perform hemodialysis.[8] Doppler ultrasound can diagnose an acral hyperstomy syndrome.[9] The clinical differential diagnoses are Kaposi's sarcoma, stasis dermatitis, lichen purpuricus, purpura pigmentosa, lichen aureus, vasculitis, lichen simplex chronicus, actinic keratosis, basal cell

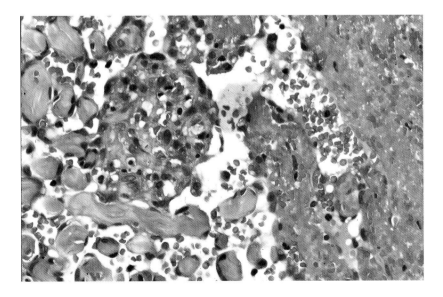

Figure 10.1 Intravascular endothelial papillary hyperplasia under the latral aspect of the index fingernail of a 52-year-old man.

carcinoma, bleeding melanoma, hemangioma, lymphangioma, and lymphangiosarcoma.[10,11]

10.1.2.1 Histopathology

Regularly built capillary vessels with thick walls, edematous stroma, and loosely structured lobuli are found in the papillary and reticular dermis. The epidermis may be acanthotic and hyperkeratotic. Extravasated erythrocytes lead to massive hemosiderin deposits, both within macrophages (siderophages) as well as in the interstitium. With time, the dermis becomes more fibrotic and finally sclerotic. There are no atypical endothelial cells, no strands of spindle cells, and no lymph vessel-like lacunae. Chronic spongiotic dermatitis (stasis eczema) may develop, particularly in acroangiodermatitis.

10.1.2.2 Differential diagnosis

Kaposi's sarcoma does not have regularly developed, thick-walled, capillary vessels in lobular arrangement, it is CD34 negative and HHV8 positive.

10.1.3 Lymphangioma circumscriptum

Lymphangioma circumscriptum is a fairly common developmental anomaly involving the deep muscular lymph collectors.[12] This leads to dilatation of the superficial lymph capillaries clinically simulating frog spawn. Bleeding into the lymphangioma may occur; however, it is one of the functions of lymph vessels to take up extravasated erythrocytes and to reintroduce them into the circulation. Thus, the term "hemangiolymphangioma" is not correct and the term "hematolymphangioma" is probably also unnecessary. Involvement of the tip of the digit is rare, but may lead to nail deformation or even gross enlargement of the digit. Superficial lacerations are common and may lead to recurrent erysipelas finally ending up in elephantiasis nostras. Therapeutically, "circumscribed" lymphangiomas are difficult to extirpate as their limits in the tissue are usually very ill-defined and the

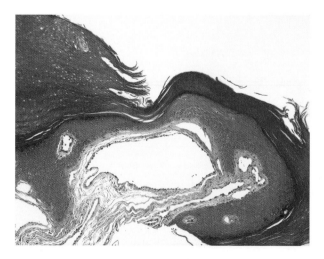

Figure 10.2 Lymphangioma circumscriptum in the free margin of the proximal nail fold of the middle finger.

underlying malformation of the large lymph collectors may be missed or impossible to remove.

10.1.3.1 Histopathology

There are multiple round to oval to irregularly shaped cavities lined with a very thin, sometimes incontinuous appearing endothelium. They are often directly in contact with the epidermis mimicking intraepidermal blisters. Long-standing lesions may develop a variable degree of hyperkeratosis (Figure 10.2). Podoplanin and LYVE-1 (lymphatic vessel endothelial HA receptor 1) are markers of lymphatic endothelium.[13]

10.1.3.2 Differential diagnosis

The lymphatic endothelium may sometimes be difficult to see and the vesicle-like spaces may then be mistaken for artifacts. Lymphatic markers are then very useful.

10.1.4 Naevus flammeus

Port-wine stains very rarely involve the tip of the digit. Extensive involvement may be a sign of Klippel-Trenaunay syndrome. The nail of an involved digital tip may be leukonychotic.

10.1.4.1 Histopathology

In young children, usually no ectatic capillaries are seen until the age of 10 years.[14] Later, they may become obvious and frank telangiectasiae are easily discerned.

10.1.4.2 Differential diagnosis

Telangiectasiae are a frequent nonspecific finding. Without a clinical suspect diagnosis, naevus flammeus is probably not diagnosed histologically in the nail.

10.1.5 Hemangioma

Infantile hemangioma mostly presents as a so-called strawberry angioma. It is the most frequent vascular tumor of infancy and childhood, affecting roughly 1% of all newborns and more than 10% of premature babies. It makes up for approximately one-third of all vascular neoplasms.[15] It has a characteristic course: appearance between the third and sixth week of life, growing for 6–12 months, and slow regression thereafter over a period of several years. Occurrence in the nail organ is extremely rare. It may then present as a reddish to violaceous, soft lesion under the nail and at the tip of the digit. A subungual hemangioma with its ultrasound characteristics was described in the big toe of a 27-year-old woman; however, the exact histopathological classification was not given.[16] An acquired hemangioma caused pseudoclubbing of the nail.[17]

10.1.5.1 Histopathology

Infantile hemangioma has a lobular architecture. During the growth phase, there is endothelial proliferation around small capillary lumina or in solid strands and clusters. The endothelial cells are large and mitoses are frequent. Crystalline intracytoplasmic inclusions may occasionally be seen. Perineural extension may occur.[18] The lumina can be seen more clearly using a reticulin stain. In the maturing phase, the endothelial cells flatten, the lumina become wider, and mitoses decrease in number. In mature hemangiomas, some lumina are grossly dilated mimicking a cavernous hemangioma. Finally, in regressing lesions, there is more and more fibrosis and the blood vessels gradually disappear. At the end, a fibrotic lobular lesion is seen.

Electron microscopic examination has shown a marked cellular heterogeneity. Endothelial cells and pericytes prevail.[19] Many cells are factor XIIIa positive. Infantile hemangioma is typically diffusely positive for the human erythrocyte glucose transporter GLUT-1,[20] which is an antigen of human placenta.[21]

10.1.5.2 Differential diagnosis

Apart from the fact that neither variant of congenital hemangioma—rapidly involuting congenital hemangioma (RICH) and noninvoluting congenital hemangioma (NICH)—has been observed in the nail region, congenital hemangiomas are GLUT-1 negative.[22] However, there may be some overlap between RICH, NICH, and infantile hemangioma and they may occur together in the same subject.

10.1.6 Cirsoid angioma

Cirsoid angiomas are believed to be arteriovenous tumors that are mainly found in the fronto-temporal area as a solitary, dark red nodule, but may be observed in the acral[23] and subungual location.[24] Clinically, a periungual or subungual mass may be observed that is not sufficiently characteristic to make the diagnosis. In the published cases, either a nodular vascular lesion was observed in the lateral nail fold of the little finger or under the nail. In another patient, both thumb nails showed an overcurvature and a central wide split (Haneke, unpublished observation). There is neither clinical nor histological resemblance with pyogenic granuloma.

10.1.6.1 Histopathology

Densely packed thick-walled and some thin-walled vessels are found in the nail bed and matrix connective tissue. They are lined by a single layer of endothelial cells and have a wall of mainly fibrotic tissue with some smooth muscle cells. There may be an internal elastic lamina in some vessels, but most do not contain this and are thus probably of venous origin. Glomus cells are normally not present; however, in the nail bed, there may be a certain component with more glomus cells. The number of mast cells may be increased. Whether this lesion is a purely venous angioma with arterialization of some of the vessels is not clear.[25]

10.1.6.2 Differential diagnosis

In the nail bed and matrix connective tissue, there is often an increase in the number of vessels that have an oval shape with an impression of the lumen on one side due to a thick cushion of smooth muscle-like cells (Figure 1.9). These lesions have apparently no specific clinical

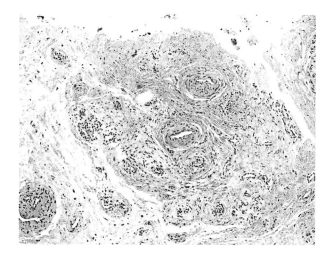

Figure 10.3 Subungual angioma with small arteries and many glomus cells around small vessel lumina.

appearance, but may histologically be seen as related to subungual cirsoid angioma.

Venous malformations show ectatic capillary and venous lumina with normal endothelium.

We have also seen a patient with a subungual angioma, the vessels of which were intermediate between small arteries and beginning glomus bodies (Figure 10.3).

10.1.7 Pyogenic granuloma

Pyogenic granuloma (PG), also called telangiectatic angioma, is in fact an eruptive lobular angioma.[26] It is quite common and often seen in association with a previous trauma. In the nail, a minor penetrating trauma may be remembered by the patient, particularly in the case of transungual growth. Most patients are youngsters and young adults, but PG may occur at any age. Pregnancy appears to be a manifesting factor. Clinically, there is a rapidly growing, bright red papule of 10–20 mm in diameter that often breaks through the horny layer of the skin as a round tumor giving the typical aspect of a collaret around a red and oozing mushroom. The surface then becomes eroded, crusted, and even ulcerated. Some lesions may regress with time, but if this is not the case removal is advocated. Oral and topical propanolol was also found to be efficacious.[27,28] The most common clinical differential diagnosis and misdiagnosis is granulation tissue.[29]

10.1.7.1 Histopathology

Pyogenic granuloma is an eruptive lobular angioma. Most lesions are elevated or polypoid angiomatous tumors either covered by a thinned epidermis or erosive (Figure 10.4). At the base, there is frequently a collaret of acanthotic epidermis sometimes almost completely embracing the base. When the lesion is erosive or ulcerated there may be an inflammatory infiltrate with plenty of neutrophils similar to granulation tissue. The angiomatous component consists of lobular proliferations of capillary vessels with well-developed endothelia and variably dilated lumina, but also solid strands of cells, with prominent connective

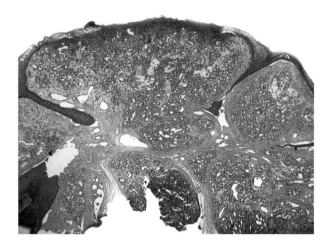

Figure 10.4 Pyogenic granuloma in the lateral nail fold of a middle-aged woman who performed a lot of gardening. The microphotograph shows a characteristic lobular angioma.

tissue septa. The tumor stroma is loose and edematous to myxoid. Here, spindled and stellate fibroblasts can be seen. Mitoses are usually a sign of ongoing progression. Feeder vessels can often be discerned reaching deep into the dermis. In older and regressing lesions, the fibrotic septa become wider and the walls of the capillary vessels thicker.

10.1.7.2 Differential diagnosis

The main differential diagnoses are granulation tissue (Figure 10.5), coccal nail fold angiomatosis, bacillary angiomatosis, but also Kaposi's sarcoma and angiosarcoma. Granulation tissue is quite common around the nails, most frequently as part of an ingrown nail. The surface is eroded, there are commonly vertically oriented vessels, the connective tissue may be very loose at the surface but

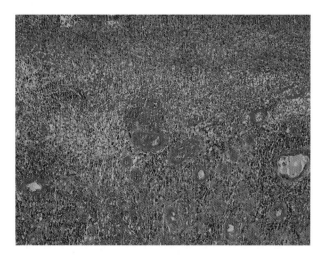

Figure 10.5 Granulation tissue from the lateral nail fold of an ingrown big toe nail patient. There is a very dense inflammatory infiltrate rich in blood vessels but without any lobular or angiomatous structure.

scarry at the base, and there is a mixed inflammatory infiltrate with abundant plasma cells. The so-called periungual pyogenic granulomas[30] under treatment with synthetic retinoids,[31,32] antiretrovirals,[33–36] taxanes,[37] other cytostatic drugs,[38] epidermal growth factor receptor (EGFR) inhibitors,[39,40] and anti-CD20 therapy[41] are, in fact, at least in most cases, granulation tissue. Also, lectitis purulenta et granulomatosa[42] is most probably granulation tissue induced by trauma and nail avulsion. Coccal nail fold angiomatosis[43] is characterized by peculiar, sometimes painful, pyogenic granuloma-like lesions usually occurring on several fingers after a cast was removed, which had been applied for 1 to 3 months to treat a phalanx, metacarpal bone, or wrist fracture. Most patients had mild pain or paresthesia during cast wearing.[44] Between 7 to 30 days after cast removal, oozing small tumors grow out from under the proximal nail fold, which in contrast to classical pyogenic granuloma, are never covered with an epidermis. Later, onychomadesis is seen. Histology shows capillary vessels in a myxoid stroma with lymphoid cells, plasma cells, and some neutrophils; cultures grew β-hemolytic streptococci and *Staphylococcus aureus*. Etiologically, a mild nerve injury and a reaction similar to reflex sympathetic dystrophy (complex regional pain syndrome) were suggested.[45,46] Bacillary angiomatosis is now rarely seen as antibiotic prophylaxis has become the rule in severely immunodepressed patients with HIV infection, leukemia,[47] other malignancies, and in organ transplant recipients.[48] They are angiomatous tumors due to *Bartonella* (*Rochalimaea*) *henselae* or *B. quintana*[49,50] and may be associated with systemic symptoms such as fever, hepatosplenomegaly, lymph node swellings, neuropsychiatric disorders, and lesions in skin, deep soft tissue, and several internal organs.[51,52] The superficial type of bacillary angiomatosis demonstrates eruptive nodules resembling pyogenic granuloma or nodes similar to Kaposi's sarcoma. The lesions are bright red, often eroded and crustous. Histologically, there is a cellular lobular proliferation of very large epithelioid endothelia in an edematous stroma; however, in contrast to pyogenic granuloma there are neither connective tissue septa nor feeder vessels. The endothelial cells may show some nuclear atypia. Abundant neutrophil granulocytes are scattered in the entire lesion with massive karyorrhexis. Amphophilic perivascular granular material around the vessels is pathognomonic. Giemsa as well as Warthin-Starry silver stains show bacterial colonies. In bacteria-poor bacillary angiomatosis, PCR for *Rochalimaea* DNA may help to establish the diagnosis. Cat scratch disease is also caused by *B. henselae*, it is characterized by gradual regional lymph node enlargement, accompanied by a papule that develops in the scratch line after 3–10 days and persists from a few days to 2–3 weeks.[53] Verruga peruana is a late manifestation of Carrion's disease, which is endemic in the Andes and due to *Bartonella bacilliformis*.[54] It is a reactive bacterial lobular capillary hemangioma and resembles bacillary angiomatosis; however, there are extracellular and intracellular bacteria called Rocha-Lima bodies, which stain with Giemsa and Warthin-Starry stains. In late stages, a lympho-plasmocytic infiltrate develops that gradually masks the angiomatous structure. There are only few granulocytes and nuclear dust is not prominent. Whereas its superficial portion resembles pyogenic granuloma, the deeper one displays densely arranged cells with large epithelioid endothelia. Lumina may no longer be visible and vascular stains such as CD31 and/or CD34 may be useful to elucidate its vascular nature.[55]

Acral angioosteoma was described in the subungual location as a dome-shaped ulcerated lesion on the left fourth toe. Another case was seen under the big toenail of a 35-year-old pregnant woman. It is clinically similar to pyogenic granuloma and histologically demonstrates a capillary proliferation with metaplastic bone formation. It lacks the lobular pattern of vascular proliferation typical for pyogenic granuloma allowing it to be distinguished from pyogenic granuloma with bone formation.[56,57]

10.1.8 Histiocytoid hemangioma (pseudopyogenic granuloma)

Histiocytoid hemangioma is now the accepted term[58,59] for a lesion originally described under the term of pseudopyogenic granuloma.[60] Involvement of the distal phalanx and the nail was described several times. In one case, there were angiomatous nodules in the fingertip, nail bed, and lateral nail folds.[61] Another case had involvement of both the skin and bone that caused distal onycholysis, subungual and periungual reddening, longitudinal splitting of the nail, swelling of the nail folds, and purulent secretion.[62] Radiation treatment led to disappearance of the nodules. Yet another case presented with multiple painless lesions of the right middle fingernail, which were mostly small measuring between 1 and 3 mm, and a larger vegetating angiomatous nodule of 5 mm that was bright red, smooth, and eroded destroying the nail plate.[63]

10.1.8.1 Histopathology

Histopathology shows nests and cords of endothelial cells and abnormal vessels that are lined by large endothelial cells. They display vesicular nuclei and prominent nucleoli. Small lumina are usually present within these endothelial cell aggregates, which finally form vessel lumina. The endothelial cells are positive for factor VIII and vimentin. A variable number of inflammatory cells is usually present, which was the reason for the first designation of pseudopyogenic granuloma.

10.1.8.2 Differential diagnosis

Under the collective term of histiocytoid hemangioma, a spectrum of tumorous and reactive lesions are summarized, which are overlapping and which are all characterized by remarkable histiocytoid endothelial cells: atypical pyogenic granuloma, pseudopyogenic granuloma, epithelioid hemangioma, angiolymphoid hyperplasia with eosinophilia, Kimura disease, papular angioplasia, and inflammatory arteriovenous hemangioma.

10.1.9 Angiolymphoid hyperplasia with eosinophilia

Angiolymphoid hyperplasia with eosinophilia is a benign reactive skin lesion characterized by a circumscribed proliferation of blood vessels and a chronic inflammatory infiltrate rich in eosinophils. Synonyms were epithelioid angioma, inflammatory angiomatous nodule, pseudopyogenic granuloma, atypical pyogenic granuloma, and intravenous atypical vascular proliferation.[64–66] Trauma and inflammation are thought to play an etiological role. Clinically, bright red or violaceous nodules are seen, quite often in the head and neck region. Distal digital localization is rare. Nail bed involvement leads to a reddish or bluish-red discoloration or to nail splitting and nail deformity.[67] One case was described in association with pachydermoperiostosis.[68]

10.1.9.1 Histopathology

Histopathologically, a benign vascular proliferation with large endothelial cells and a dense lymphocytic infiltrate with many eosinophils is seen, hence some define it as an epithelioid or histiocytoid hemangioma with prominent eosinophilia.[69,70] Occasionally, a medium-sized vessel is seen in association with the lesion. Arborizing small vessels may be seen around larger ones. Their walls contain smooth muscle cells and/or pericytes and contain mucin. The large eosinophilic cytoplasm often contains small vacuoles and protrudes into the lumina. It was thought that the intracellular small lumina of the endothelial cells might be early vascular lumina. Mitoses may be present. Multinucleate endothelial cells are assumed to be endothelial sprouts.[71] The endothelial cells are positive for CD31, CD34, and factor VIII-related antigen. The proliferation index as determined with Ki67 staining was 5% and cyclin D1 and bcl-2 were negative.[72] No light chain restriction was found.[73]

10.1.9.2 Differential diagnosis

All the lesions discussed above have to be considered. However, often a clear-cut differential diagnosis is not possible and it remains a matter of interpretation and/or preference, which term is given to the lesion in question. Kimura disease presents with similar skin tumors but has a more prominent lymphoid proliferation, less vessels, and the endothelial cells are not epithelioid. Furthermore, it has systemic symptoms such as fever and lymphadenopathy.

10.1.10 Acral pseudolymphomatous angiokeratoma of children

This lesion was originally observed in children and called acral pseudolymphomatous angiokeratoma of children (APACHE), but it has now also been observed in adolescents and adults.[74,75] Characteristically, multiple small hyperkeratotic angiomatoid lesions are seen on the tips of several digits with striking clinical similarity with angiokeratoma of Mibelli.[76] Single digit plus nail involvement is very rare.[77] Its true nature is now debated as some authors believe it to be a form of pseudolymphoma with secondary vessel proliferation.[78]

10.1.10.1 Histopathology

There is usually marked hyperkeratosis and thinning of the epidermis over the lesion itself with elongated rete pegs at the margin of the lesion. A well-circumscribed, dense lymphocytic infiltrate is present around dilated vessels that extends from the papillary dermis down to the subcutaneous tissue. The epidermis is not invaded. Immunohistochemistry shows an equal amount of mature T and B lymphocytes,[79] an argument for pseudolymphoma.[76] CD8+ suppressor cells are more numerous than CD4+ helper cells.[80] One study also found abundant CD20 positive B lymphocytes.[81] Cutaneous lymphocyte antigen was demonstrated in the high venule endothelial cells, which might be the reason for the self-perpetuation of the lymphoid proliferation.[82]

10.1.10.2 Differential diagnosis

The absence of grossly dilated vessels and chilblains as well as the multiple lesions rule out angiokeratoma of Mibelli. The recently described T-cell-rich angiomatoid polypoid pseudolymphoma of the skin[83] is a solitary lesion and presents with a different localization.

10.1.11 Angiokeratoma circumscriptum

Angiokeratoma circumscriptum is a hyperkeratotic lesion with an angiomatous base mainly occurring on the lower extremity in young adults. Involvement of the toes, fingers, and perionychium has been observed.[84] A subungual angiokeratoma gave rise to an irregular dark streak in the nail.[85] Verrucous hemangioma may be indistinguishable clinically. One major clinical differential diagnosis is melanoma.

10.1.11.1 Histopathology

Abundant ectatic, thin-walled capillaries filled with erythrocytes, are found mainly in the papillary dermis bulging the thin epidermis up. There is often acanthosis at the margins and a variable degree of hyperkeratosis. Extension into the deep dermis or even the cutaneous fat is not seen. The subungual angiokertoma demonstrated aggregates of erythrocytes in the middle nail plate layer extending from the matrix to the distal nail margin. The dermis of the middle matrix showed a projection with numerous dilated, thin-walled, blood-filled vessels partly surrounded by matrix epithelium, which upon onychotization takes the blood with it into the newly formed nail plate.[83]

10.1.11.2 Differential diagnosis

By light microscopy, the other three forms of angiokeratoma, namely angiokeratoma corporis diffusum of Fabry, angiokeratoma of Mibelli on the dorsa of the fingers and toes, and angiokeratoma of Fordyce on the scrotum, are identical.[86] In the former, which is an X-linked recessive deficiency of lysosomal A-galactosidase, birefringent lipids are present in cytoplasmic vacuoles of fibroblasts, endothelial cells and pericytes, provided they were not dissolved during the processing in the histopathology lab.

Verrucous angioma is characterized by marked hyperkeratosis, parakeratosis, papillomatosis, and elongation of the rete ridges extending from the dermo-epidermal junction into the deeper dermis, where numerous small to large vascular channels are seen lined by flattened endothelial cells and filled with blood. Intervening dermal fibrosis and chronic inflammatory infiltrate are present.[87]

10.1.12 Aneurysmal bone cyst

Also called arterio-venous fistula, aneurysmal bone cyst is a rare benign, locally aggressive bone lesion that may also occur in the distal phalanx of young individuals. It grows rapidly, is painful, and markedly enlarges the tip of the digit.[88–90] This leads to an enlarged nail. Radiographs show a distension of the bone resembling the secular protrusion of the walls of an aneurysm. The phalanx appears almost completely substituted by an osteolytic process.[91–93] The etiology is not clear; however, one case of an aneurysmal bone cyst of the distal phalanx was described after a crush trauma.[94]

10.1.12.1 Histopathology

The lesion is usually removed by curettage and shows a stroma of proliferating fibroblasts, histiocytes, and multinucleated giant cells. There are dilated, blood-filled vascular spaces without endothelial cells separated by fibrous septa and small osteoid or bone strands. The nuclei of the mononuclear stromal cells and of the multinucleate giant cells are identical. An inflammatory infiltrate may be present.[95] The giant cells express an osteoclast-like phenotype (CD51+, CD14-, HLA DR-, CD163-, cathepsin K+, TRAP+)[96] and are formed from CD14+ macrophage precursors.[97] Genetic and immunohistochemical studies suggest that primary aneurysmal bone cysts are tumors and not reactive tumor-simulating lesions. A neoplastic basis was suggested by the demonstration of clonal chromosome band 17p13 translocations, placing the USP6 oncogene under the regulation of the highly active CDH11 promoter.[98]

10.1.12.2 Differential diagnosis

Giant cell reparative granuloma is a solid aneurysmal bone cyst and thus almost identical except for the lack of blood-filled spaces.[99]

10.1.13 Angioleiomyoma

Cutaneous angioleiomyomas are fairly common tumors mainly observed at the lower leg and the labial mucosa. They are round, elastic to firm nodules that may be tender on vigorous palpation. The first angioleiomyoma of the nail was described in 1889.[100] Since then, more cases were reported,[101] of which several were mistaken for glomus tumor because they were painful.[102,103] Depending on their localization within the nail apparatus, angioleiomyomas of the nail may elevate the nail plate, appear as a small nodule at the tip of the digit just under the hyponychium, or distort the nail.

10.1.13.1 Histopathology

Angioleiomyomas are usually well-circumscribed lesions consisting of a ball of densely packed mature smooth muscle cells with some small blood vessel lumina. Myxoid degeneration of the myoma is possible. However, subungual angioleiomyomas are often much less compact and are more similar to cirsoid angiomas.

10.1.13.2 Differential diagnosis

Cutaneous angiolipoleiomyoma is a solitary, painless, acquired nodule in acral localization. It is a subcutaneous, well circumscribed nodule, and composed of smooth muscle, vascular spaces, connective tissue, and mature fat. In some tumors, the fat is the predominant component, in others smooth muscle predominates. Elastic tissue stain reveals that some blood vessels developed an elastic lamina whereas other blood vessels lacked it. Occasionally, included vascular thrombi, glomus bodies, and focal mucin deposition are observed.[104]

10.1.14 Glomus tumor

Glomus tumor was first described 200 years ago as a painful subcutaneous tubercle.[105] More tumors were later reported as colloid sarcoma or angiosarcoma. Since then it is probably the best-known nail tumor for its highly characteristic symptoms although it is not so frequent. Glomus tumors make up approximately 2% of all hand tumors. They most commonly occur in the fingers, specifically in the nail matrix and proximal nail bed. Most patients consult the dermatologist or surgeon because of the intense pain that is often spontaneous or elicited by minor trauma such as an accidental bump, but also cold may cause pain that can radiate up to the shoulder. A tourniquet at the base of the finger or a blood pressure cuff inflated to 300 mm Hg stops the pain. Most patients are between 30 and 50 years old. Women are more frequently affected than men. The glomus tumor is often seen in the distal matrix as a bluish or violaceous round to oval spot of 3–8 mm in diameter, from which a reddish band extends distally. The nail may be slightly elevated over the lesion or even split distally.[106] Probing provokes intense pain, but can usually localize the tumor very exactly. Dermatoscopy, ultrasound, thermography, dynamic thermography, arteriography, magnetic resonance, and particularly angio-MRI help to visualize the lesion, but are rarely more precise than probing. On X-ray, an impression of the phalangeal bone may be seen in approximately one-fifth to one-third of the cases.[107] Up to 10% of glomus tumors are multiple, which may be the cause for presumed recurrence.[108,109] Surgical removal is not demanding as the glomus tumor is a round, very well delimited, encapsulated lesion standing out by its grayish color from the surrounding connective tissue or fat. The clinical diagnosis is almost always obvious as there are no other lesions with this particular and highly specific symptomatology. The clinical differential diagnosis comprises virtually all painful conditions of the nails

such as subungual warts, keratoacanthoma, subungual exostosis, enchondroma, neuroma, Pacinian neuroma, caliber-persistent artery, leiomyoma, paronychia, osteitis terminalis, subungual felon, herpetic whitlow, causalgia, gout, melanoma,[110] and several more. Glomangioma is often multiple, sometimes in linear distribution involving an extremity including the periungual skin, usually not painful or only tender on deep palpation, and the main clinical differential diagnosis is venous malformation or blue rubber bleb nevus.[110,112] Familial glomangioma has been described.[113] Glomangiomyoma has a more pronounced muscular component. It does not exhibit the typical symptomatology of glomus tumors like pain and cold sensitivity.[114] Minute synovial sarcomas may have some similarity with glomus tumors.[115]

A genetically different subset of glomus tumors occurs in von Recklinghausen's neurofibromatosis I, which is characterized by a bi-allelic mutation in the tumor suppression gene NF1.[116] These patients have a higher risk of developing multiple glomus tumors.[117] In a cohort of glomus tumor patients, 29% had neurofibromatosis I giving an odds ratio of 168:1.[118]

The treatment of choice of subungual glomus tumors is either transungual resection or dissection through the lateral nail fold in case of lateral localization.[119]

10.1.14.1 Histopathology

Histologic examination shows a well-circumscribed lesion with a fibrous capsule. It has an afferent arteriole, efferent veins leading into small veins of the dermis and the glomus tumor in-between. Thus, the glomus tumor is held to be a true hamartoma rather than a tumor. These structures of the glomus tumor are, however, usually not seen in routine sections.

Histological sections show an encapsulated tumor made up of small vessel lumina lined by flat endothelial cells and surrounded by a multilayered sheath of glomus cells (Figure 10.6), which each have their own PAS-positive

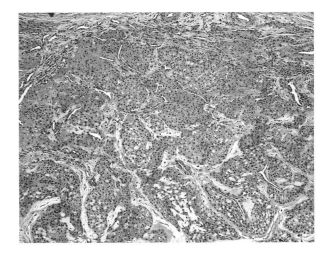

Figure 10.6 Glomus tumor of the matrix dermis. There are densely packed cuboid cells with some vessel lumina lined by a flat endothelium.

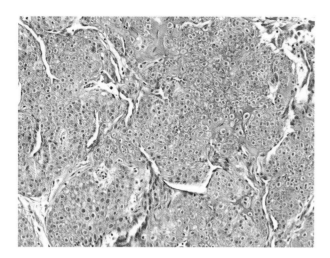

Figure 10.7 Glomus tumor. The PAS stain demonstrates the basal membrane of the glomus cells.

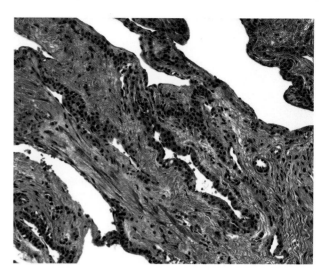

Figure 10.8 Glomangioma. There are large vascular lumina surrounded by a layer of mainly two glomus cells.

basal membrane (Figure 10.7).[120] The stroma is dense and collagenous or shows variable degrees of myxoid changes. Immunohistochemistry demonstrates that the glomus cells are positive for vimentin, smooth muscle actins HHF 35 and CGA7, myosin, and h-caldesmon.[121] Glomus cells stain moderately to substance P and TRPV1.[122] They are negative for desmin, CD117, S-100 protein, creatine kinase, c-KIT, CD99, EMA CD68, collagen type IV, CD34 and p53, factor XIIIa, AE1/AE3, and the lymphatic marker LYVE-1,[123] melanocytic markers, and neural markers including glial fibrillic acid protein, synaptophysin, and chromogranin.[124,125] Apparently, glomus tumors with myxoid areas may coexpress actin and CD34.[126] The markers for neuron-specific enolase, neurofilament, protein S100, and Leu7 stain abundant nerve fibers in the glomus tumors.[127] These myelinated and unmyelinated nerves may be responsible for the pain. The endothelial cells are positive with factor VIII-related antigen, CD34, β-2 microglobulin, claudin-5,[128] and the lectin *Ulex europaeus* agglutinin I (UEA I), whereas only a few endothelial cells bind peanut agglutinin (PNA), which does not stain endothelial cells of normal blood vessels of the matrix and nail bed at all. The expression pattern of the cells of glomus tumors similar to that of epithelioid cells of arteriovenous anastomoses was interpreted as confirmation of the glomus tumor as a benign lesion.[129]

Fine needle aspiration biopsy shows uniform cells with scanty cytoplasm and homogeneous chromatin, which together with the history of a painful subungual tumor was suggestive of a glomus tumor.[130]

One glomus tumor of the distal phalanx was observed in a digital nerve.[131]

10.1.14.2 Differential diagnosis

In general, the histopathologic diagnosis of glomus tumors is obvious. Subungual symplastic glomus tumor exhibits pronounced nuclear pleomorphism, atypia, and multinucleate cells;[132] however, no mitoses; it is important to differentiate it from malignant glomus tumor as it has no

propensity to metastasize.[133] A tumor with a transition of the cuboid glomus cells to more elongated mature smooth muscle cells was termed glomangiomyoma.[134] When there is a marked concentric perivascular proliferation of round-to-spindle cells around the glomus cells, the lesion is called glomangiopericytoma.[135,136] Glomangioma histologically shows wide vascular lumina that are surrounded by one or several layers of glomus cells (Figure 10.8). One malignant glomus tumor was reported in the hand.[137] Epithelioid angioleiomyoma may share some features with glomus tumor and was considered to be an intermediate between angioleiomyoma and glomus tumor.[138] Myopericytoma may rarely exhibit areas of glomoid features. However, it was also claimed that myofibromatosis in adults, glomangiopericytoma, and myopericytoma might be a spectrum of tumors with perivascular myoid differentiation.[139,140]

10.1.15 Caliber-persistent artery

Caliber-persistent artery, also known as Dieulafoy's lesion, cirsoid aneurysm, or submucosal arterial malformation, is not a tumor. It is an acquired or inborn lesion where the terminal artery caliber does not diminish with each branching but remains wide. It is relatively common in the intestinal tract and may be the reason for dramatic or even fatal gastrointestinal bleeding[141–143] with a lethality of 60%,[144] but it is rare in skin. Its main cutaneous localization is the lower lip[145,146] and here its most important differential diagnosis is labial carcinoma.[147,148] A small nodule with chronic superficial ulceration develops. Gentle palpation may reveal pulsation.[148] Ultrasound also helps to make the diagnosis.[150,151] Treatment is ligation of the artery on both ends; however, when the diagnosis was not anticipated brisk arterial bleeding is usually experienced. Two subungual lesions causing a split nail were histologically diagnosed as caliber persistent artery. Magnetic resonance imaging had shown a longitudinal lesion of suspected vascular origin. The diagnosis was completely unexpected; as nail surgery is performed with a tourniquet, bleeding was not an intraoperative feature suggesting the correct diagnosis. A third case was seen in association with a subungual myxoid pseudocyst (unpublished observations).

10.1.15.1 Histopathology

Histopathologic examination of excision specimens from the gastrointestinal tract as well as wedge excisions from the lip show that the walls of the pathologic arteries are of normal structure, in the gastrointestinal tract they are of normal diameter as submucous arteries, in the stomach they are attached to the mucosa by virtue of Wanke's musculoelastic mantle, and at the level of the muscularis mucosae, they are definitely oversized. In the area of the linkage of the artery to the mucosa, a vulnerable mucosal spot develops. The artery is accompanied by a vein of similar caliber. Perforation of the vein takes place before that of the artery.[135] In the specimens from the matrix and nail bed, a disproportionately large and tortuous artery was seen which was otherwise anatomically normal (Figure 10.9). The pathogenesis of the split nail is analogous to the mucosal ulcer formation: pressure from the pulsating artery against the overlying nail plate leads to circumscribed matrix epithelium atrophy, which eventually results in insufficient nail formation and finally in a split nail.

10.1.15.2 Differential diagnosis

The diagnosis of subungual caliber-persistent artery is an unexpected finding. As a split in the nail can have many different causes, caliber-persistent artery should be included in the list of differential diagnoses.

10.2 MALIGNANT VASCULAR TUMORS

There are a great number of angiosarcomas, many of which are also known under different terms. The group of angioendotheliomas is now considered to belong to the low to medium grade angiosarcomas.[152,153] The so-called classical angiosarcoma is mainly seen in the head and neck area of elderly men and not observed in the nail apparatus. Histopathologically, post-mastectomy angiosarcoma and angiosarcoma in congenital or chronic acquired lymphedema as well as after irradiation are not sufficiently different to allow their diagnosis from just a biopsy; they are diagnosed in their clinical setting.[154,155] However, the differentiation of these sarcomas from benign vascular lesions in irradiated skin may be extremely difficult.[156] Most cases published before 1920 as subungual angiosarcoma[157,158] were probably glomus tumors.

10.2.1 Epithelioid hemangioendothelioma

Epithelioid hemangioendothelioma is an uncommon soft tissue tumor having an epithelioid appearance.[159] Originally thought to run a clinical course between that of a hemangioma and that of a conventional angiosarcoma, some authors now consider it to be a true angiosarcoma.[160] It occurs in skin and other sites such as the lung, liver, and bone. It is exceedingly rare in the nail region. One case of epithelioid hemangioendothelioma presented clinically as a paronychia. The left great toe of a 42-year-old female developed a progressive swelling with some tenderness over a period of 6 months. The toe was diffusely swollen, the pulp was bluish-red, and the nail showed an increased curvature. An x-ray film exhibited a large lytic lesion of the distal phalanx without reactive new bone formation and with expansion of the proximal end of the phalanx and an associated large soft tissue mass. A bone isotope scan revealed the typical multicentric neoplasm. Another case that had developed in an arteriovenous fistula and was described as epithelioid angiosarcoma presented with small violaceous nodules of the fingertips as well as under and around the thumbnail.[161] A multifocal epithelioid hemangioendothelioma of the sole of the foot and tip of the toes was seen in a 63-year-old woman. MRI scan and digital subtraction angiography showed multifocal bone involvement. Treatment with interferon-α led to partial regression.[162] One case of a subungual hemangioendothelioma exhibited a scar-like erythematous aspect and nail destruction[163] and yet another one was thought to be due to prolonged professional contact with vinyl chloride.[164]

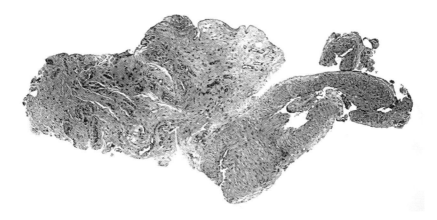

Figure 10.9 Caliber-persistent artery of the nail bed.

10.2.1.1 Histopathology

Epithelioid hemangioendotheliomas are vascular tumors with apparent epithelioid cells. There are both solid as well as vascular components with vessels of varying size that often show papillary proliferations extending into the lumina. Pathologic mitoses and cellular pleomorphism may be marked. Frequently, associated inflammatory infiltrates containing lymphocytes and eosinophils are observed.[165] The diagnosis can be confirmed by endothelial markers such as factor VIII, CD 31, and CD 34. Because of the proliferations of endothelial cells into vascular lumina, a lymphatic differentiation was suggested.

10.2.1.2 Differential diagnosis

Solid areas may be mistaken for carcinoma or metastases. Histopathology of curetted tissue shows abundant vessels of varying size and development, many with large epithelioid endothelial cells.[166]

10.2.2 Kaposi sarcoma

Originally called sarcoma haemorrhagicum multiplex and mainly seen in the lower extremity of elderly men, Kaposi's sarcoma is now subdivided into the classical form, an epidemic form mainly seen in Africa, and a subtype seen in acquired immunodeficiency syndrome and other immunodepressions including drug-induced immunosuppression. Histopathologically, they are virtually identical. The classical form, but also the other types, very often involves the lower legs and feet including the toes. All different forms of Kaposi sarcoma were demonstrated to be associated with human herpes virus (HHV) 8; some authors therefore believe it to be a reactive process.

Kaposi's sarcoma typically grows in phases beginning with a macular lesion clinically often resembling a bruise, which then develops into a plaque with considerable hemorrhage and finally nodules form that may ulcerate and bleed. These phases are, however, usually not seen under or around the nail as the lesions on the feet, lower legs, and elsewhere are much more obvious.

Kaposi's sarcoma often affects the nail folds or even overgrows the nail. Subungual Kaposi's sarcoma was found to cause elevation and deformation of the nail plate.[167] A 61-year-old man with "angiosarcoma multiplex" in the distal phalanges of three toes was described. This patient later developed metastases in the calf.[168] Kaposi sarcoma of the nail region in AIDS patients often appears as a small bruise that may turn brown or violaceous or may cause distal phalanx enlargement due to intraosseous growth.[169] Clinical differential diagnoses comprise pseudo-Kaposi sarcoma in patients with acral hyperstomy syndrome and hyperplastic acroangiodermatitis.

10.2.2.1 Histopathology

In the early phase, the histologic changes are very discrete. There are some slit-like capillary vessels separating the collagen bundles, and extravasated erythrocytes. Cellular atypia is not a predominant feature. These changes are more obvious in the plaque stage with both vascular and some solid tumor portions. In the full-blown lesion, there may be large hemorrhagic solid areas with split-like vessels mainly at their periphery, but some dilated vessels may also be seen. Most cells are spindle-shaped.

Immunohistochemistry is positive for HHV 8; this is thought to be diagnostic in patients with angiomatous lesions. CD34 is usually negative whereas podoplanin as detected with the antibody D2-40 is positive indicating a lymphatic differentiation.[170]

10.2.2.2 Differential diagnosis

Although nonmalignant, a case of acquired pincer nail associated with pseudo-Kaposi sarcoma has been described in a 52-year-old female patient with terminal renal insufficiency and was thought to be due to the presence of an arteriovenous fistula placed to perform hemodialysis.[8]

10.2.3 Glomangiosarcoma

Glomangiosarcoma is a very rare form of a malignant glomus tumor and only one case was observed in the distal phalanx of the thumb.[137] The diagnosis is clinically suspected when the symptomatic lesion is over 20 mm in diameter.

10.2.3.1 Histopathology

There may be a preexisting benign glomus tumor component, but glomangiosarcoma is deeply located and there are cytologic and nuclear atypia and atypical mitoses. The cells are often spindle-shaped or ovoid and arranged in fascicles. The proliferation rate may be as high as 10%.[171]

10.2.3.2 Differential diagnosis

Symplastic glomus tumor is histologically in-between a benign glomus tumor and glomangiosarcoma. Solid glomangioma and glomangiosarcoma have to be differentiated from eccrine spiradenoma, which, however, has the typical two-cell populations, focal ductal differentiation, and is positive for epithelial markers. Intradermal nevi with pseudovascular spaces display nesting and maturation and the cells are positive for protein S-100 and other melanocyte markers.

REFERENCES

1. Mertens F, Unni K, Fletcher DJM. *Pathology and Genetics. Tumours of Soft Tissue and Bone.* Lyon: IACR Press, 2002.
2. Velasco ML. Multifocal Epithelioid Vascular Tumors. XXIII Dermatopathol Sem, Vars, France, January 24–29, 2016.
3. Haneke E. Subungual intravascular papillary endothelial hyperplasia. Diaklinik der Hautklinik Wuppertal. *Z Dermatol* 1997;183:180–195.
4. Landthaler M, Stolz W, Eckert F, Schmoeckel C, Braun-Falco O. Pseudo-Kaposi's sarcoma occurring after placement of arteriovenous shunt. *J Am Acad Dermatol* 1989;21:499–505.

5. Pimentel MIF, Cuzzi T, Azeredo-Coutinho RBG, Vasconcellos ECF, Benzi TSCG, Carvalho LMV. Acroangiodermatitis (Pseudo-Kaposi sarcoma): A rarely recognized condition. A case on the plantar aspect of the foot associated with chronic venous insufficiency. *An Bras Dermatol* 2011;86(S1):S13–S16.

6. Mali JWH, Kuiper JP, Hamers AA. Acroangiodermatitis of the foot. *Arch Dermatol* 1965;92:515–518.

7. Bluefarb SM, Adams LA. Arteriovenous malformation with angiodermatitis. Stasis dermatitis simulating Kaposi sarcoma. *Arch Dermatol* 1967;96:176–181.

8. Hwang SM, Lee SH, Ahn SK. Pincer nail deformity and pseudo Kaposi sarcoma: Complication of an artificial arteriovenous fistula for haemodialysis. *Br J Dermatol* 1999;141:1129–1132.

9. Alioua Z, Lamsyah H, Sbai M, Rimani M, Baba N, Ghfir M, Sedrati O. Pseudo-Kaposi's sarcoma secondary to superficial arteriovenous malformation: Stewart-Bluefarb syndrome. *Ann Dermatol Vénéréol* 2008;135:44–47.

10. Rao B, Unis M, Poulos E. Acroangiodermatitis: A study of ten cases. *Int J Dermatol* 1994;33:179–183.

11. Ozkaya DB, Su O, Onsun N, Ulusal H, Demirkesen C. Non-healing ulcer on the foot: Early onset unilateral Mali-type acroangiodermatitis. *Acta Dermatovenerol Alp Pannonica Adriat* 2013;22(2):49–51.

12. Whimster IW. The pathology of lymphangioma circumscriptum. *Br J Dermatol* 1976;94:473–486.

13. Ji RC, Eshita Y, Xing L, Miura M. Multiple expressions of lymphatic markers and morphological evolution of newly formed lymphatics in lymphangioma and lymph node lymphangiogenesis. *Microvasc Res* 2010;80:195–201.

14. Finley JL, Noe JM, Arndt KA, Rosen S. Port-wine stains: Morphologic variations and developmental lesions. *Arch Dermatol* 1984;120:1453–1455.

15. Coffin CM, Dehner LP. Vascular tumors in children and adolescents: A clinicopathologic study of 228 tumors in 222 patients. *Pathol Annu* 1999;28:97.

16. Baek HJ, Lee SJ, Cho KH, Choo HJ, Lee SM, Lee YH, Suh KJ et al. Subungual tumors: Clinicopathologic correlation with US and MR imaging findings. *Radiographics* 2010;30:1621–1636.

17. De Giorgi V, Sestini S, Massi D, Panelos J, Papi F, Alfaioli B, Lotti T. Acquired pseudoclubbing of a fingernail caused by spontaneous subungual haemangioma. *J Eur Acad Dermatol Venereol* 2008;22:1501–1503.

18. Calonje E, Menzel T, Fletcher CDM. Pseudosarcomatous neural invasion in capillary hemangioma. *Histopathology* 1995;26:159.

19. Gonzales-Crussi F, Reyes-Mugica M. Cellular hemangiomas ("hemangioendotheliomas") in infancy: Light microscopic, immunohistochemical and ultrastructural observations. *Am J Surg Pathol* 1991;15:769.

20. North PE, Waner M, Mizeracki A, Mrak RE, Nicholas R, Kincannon J, Suen JY, Mihm MC Jr. A unique microvascular phenotype shared by juvenile hemangiomas and human placenta. *Arch Dermatol* 2001;137:559–570.

21. North PE, Waner M, Mizeracki A, Mihm MC Jr. GLUT-1: A newly discovered immunohistochemical marker for juvenile hemangioma. *Hum Pathol* 2000;31:11–22.

22. North PE, Waner M, James CA, Mizeracki A, Frieden IJ, Mihm MC Jr. Congenital nonprogressive hemangioma: A distinct clinicopathologic entity unlike infantile hemangioma. *Arch Dermatol* 2001;137:1607–1620.

23. Gurbuz Y, Muezzinoglu B, Apaydin R, Yumbul AZ. Acral arteriovenous tumor (cirsoid aneurysm): Clinical and histopathological analysis of 6 cases. *Adv Clin Path* 2002;6:25–29.

24. Burge SM, Baran R, Dawber RPR, Verret JL. Periungual and subungual arteriovenous tumours. *Br J Dermatol* 1986;115:361–366.

25. Koutlas IG, Jessurun J. Arteriovenous hemangioma: A clinicopathological and immunohistochemical study. *J Cut Pathol* 1994;21:343–349.

26. Mills SE, Cooper PH, Fechner RE. Lobular capillary hemangioma: The underlying lesion of pyogenic granuloma. A study of 73 cases from the oral and nasal mucous membranes. *Am J Surg Pathol* 1980;4:470–479.

27. Wine Lee L, Goff KL, Lam JM, Low DW, Yan AC, Castelo-Soccio L. Treatment of pediatric pyogenic granulomas using β-adrenergic receptor antagonists. *Pediatr Dermatol* 2014;31:203–207.

28. Piraccini BM, Alessandrini A, Dika E, Starace M, Patrizi A, Neri I. Topical propranolol 1% cream for pyogenic granulomas of the nail: Open-label study in 10 patients. *J Eur Acad Dermatol Venereol* 2015 Feb 23, doi: 10.1111/jdv.13071

29. Keles MK, Yosma E, Aydogdu IO, Simsek T, Park TH. Multiple subungual pyogenic granulomas following levothyroxine treatment. *J Craniofac Surg* 2015;26:e476–e477.

30. Piraccini BM, Bellavista S, Misciali C, Tosti A, De Berker D, Richert B. Periungual and subungual pyogenic granuloma. *Br J Dermatol* 2010;163:941–953.

31. Baran R. Action thérapeutique et complications du retinoïde aromatique sur l'appareil unguéal. *Ann Dermatol Vénéréol* 1982;109:367–371.

32. Baran R. Pyogenic granuloma-like lesions associated with topical retinoid therapy. *J Am Acad Dermatol* 2002;47:970.

33. Tosti A, Piraccini BM, D'Antuono A, Marzaduri S, Bettoli V. Periungual inflammation and pyogenic granulomas during treatment with the antiretroviral drugs lamivudine and indinavir. *Br J Dermatol* 1999;140:1165–1168.

34. Williams LH, Fleckman P. Painless periungual pyogenic granulomata associated with reverse transcriptase inhibitor therapy in a patient with human immunodeficiency virus infection. *Br J Dermatol* 2007;156:163–164.

35. Bouscarat F, Bouchard C, Bouhour D. Paronychia and pyogenic granuloma of the great toes in patients treated with indinavir. *N Engl J Med* 1998;338:1776–1777.

36. Calista D, Boschini A. Cutaneous side effects induced by indinavir. *Eur J Dermatol* 2000;10:292–296.

37. Paul LJ, Cohen PR. Paclitaxel-associated subungual pyogenic granuloma: Report in a patient with breast cancer receiving paclitaxel and review of drug-induced pyogenic granulomas adjacent to and beneath the nail. *J Drugs Dermatol* 2012;11:262–268.

38. Curr N, Saunders H, Murugasu A, Cooray P, Schwarz M, Gin D. Multiple periungual pyogenic granulomas following systemic 5-fluorouracil. *Australas J Dermatol* 2006;47:130–133.

39. Segaert S, Van Cutsem E. Clinical signs, pathophysiology and management of skin toxicity during therapy with epidermal growth factor receptor inhibitors. *Ann Oncol* 2005;16:1425–1433.

40. High WA. Gefitinib: A cause of pyogenic granulomalike lesions of the nail. *Arch Dermatol* 2006;142:939.

41. Wollina U. Multiple eruptive periungual pyogenic granulomas during anti-CD20 monoclonal antibody therapy for rheumatoid arthritis. *J Dermatol Case Rep* 2010;4(3):44–46.

42. Eichmann A, Baran R. Lectitis purulenta et granulomatosa (granulomatous purulent nail bed inflammation). *Dermatology* 1998;196:352–353.

43. Davies MG. Coccal nail fold angiomatosis. *Br J Dermatol* 1995;132:162–163.

44. Tosti A, Piraccini BM, Camacho F. Onychomadesis and pyogenic granuloma following cast immobilization. *Arch Dermatol* 2001;137:231–232.

45. Tosti A, Baran R, Peluso AM, Fanti PA, Liguori R. Reflex sympathetic dystrophy with prominent involvement of the nail apparatus. *J Am Acad Dermatol* 1993;29:865–868.

46. Camacho F, Ordoñez E. Reflex sympathetic dystrophy with nail involvement: Its role in atopic dermatitis. *Eur J Dermatol.* 1996;6:172–174.

47. LeBoit PE, Berger TG, Egbert BM, Beckstead JH, Yen TSB, Stoler MH. Bacillary angiomatosis. The histopathology and differential diagnosis of a pseudoneoplastic infection in patients with human immunodeficiency virus disease. *Am J Surg Pathol* 1989;13:909–920.

48. Moulin C, Kanitakis J, Ranchin B, Chauvet C, Gillet Y, Morelon E, Euvrard S. Cutaneous bacillary angiomatosis in renal transplant recipients: Report of three new cases and literature review. *Transpl Infect Dis* 2012 Feb 9, doi: 10.1111/j.1399-3062.2011.00713.x

49. Cockerell CJ. Bacillary angiomatosis and related diseases caused by Rochalimaea. *J Am Acad Dermatol* 1995;32:783–790.

50. Sala M, Font B, Sanfeliu I, Sanfeliu I, Quesada M, Ponts I, Segura F. Bacillary angiomatosis caused by *Bartonella quintana. Ann N Y Acad Sci* 2005;1063:302–307.

51. Webster GF, Cockerell CJ, Friedman-Kien AE. The clinical spectrum of bacillary angiomatosis. *Br J Dermatol* 1992;126:535–541.

52. Psarros G, Riddell J 4th, Gandhi T, Kauffman CA, Cinti SK. *Bartonella henselae* infections in solid organ transplant recipients: Report of 5 cases and review of the literature. *Medicine (Baltimore).* 2012;91:111–121.

53. Sanguinetti-Morelli D, Angelakis E, Richet H, Davoust B, Rolain JM, Raoult D. Seasonality of cat scratch disease, France, 1999–2009. *Emerg Infect Dis* 2011;17:705–707.

54. Seas C, Villaverde H, Maguiña C. A 60-year-old man from the highlands of Peru with fever and hemolysis. *Am J Trop Med Hyg* 2012;86:381.

55. Arias-Stella J, Lieberman PF, Erlandson RA, Arias-Stella J. Histology, immunohistochemistry, and ultrastructure of the verruga in Carrion's disease. *Am J Surg Pathol* 1986;10:595–610.

56. Lee EJ, Lee JH, Shin MK, Lee SW, Haw CR. Acral angioosteoma cutis. *Ann Dermatol* 2011;23(Suppl 1):S105–S107.

57. Wang AL, Vandergriff T, Srivastava D, Nijhawan RI. Recurrent acral angioosteoma cutis in a pregnant patient. *JAAD Case Rep* 2016;2:430–432.

58. Rosai J, Gold J, Landy R. Histiocytoid haemangiomas. *Hum Pathol* 1979;10:707–729.

59. Verret JL, Avenel M, François H, Baudoin M, Alain P. Hémangiomes histiocytoïdes des pulpes digitales. *Ann Dermatol Vénéréol* 1983;110:251–257.

60. Wilson-Jones E, Bleehen SS. Pseudo-pyogenic granuloma. *Br J Dermatol* 1969;81:804–816.

61. Avenel M, Verret JL, Fortier P. Finger localisation of Wilson–Jones pseudo-pyogenic granuloma. XVI Int Congr Dermatol, Tokyo, University of Tokyo Press, Japan, 1982.

62. Dannaker C, Piacquadio D, Willoughby CB, Goltz RW. Histiocytoid hemangioma: A disease spectrum. *J Am Acad Dermatol* 1989;21:404–409.

63. Tosti A, Peluso AM, Fanti PA, Torresan F, Solmi L, Bassi F. Histiocytoid hemangioma with prominent fingernail involvement. *Dermatology* 1994;189:87–89.

64. Wilson Jones E, Bleehen SS. Inflammatory angiomatous nodules with abnormal blood vessels occurring about the ears and scalp (pseudo or atypical pyogenic granuloma). *Br J Dermatol* 1969;81:804–815.

65. Rosai J, Akerman LR. Intravenous atypical vascular proliferation. A cutaneous lesion simulating a malignant blood vessel tumor. *Arch Dermatol* 1974;109:714–717.

66. Bendl BJ, Asano K, Lewis RJ. Nodular angioblastic hyperplasia with eosinophilia and lymphofolliculosis. *Cutis* 1977;19:327–329.

67. Risitano C, Gupta A, Burke F. Angiolymphoid hyperplasia with eosinophilia in the hand. *J Hand Surg* 1990;15B:376–377.

68. Kanekura T, Mizumoto J, Kanzaki T. Pachydermoperiostosis with angiolymphoid hyperplasia with eosinophilia. *J Dermatol* 1994;21:133–134.

69. Imbing FD, Viegas SF, Sánchez RL. Multiple angiolymphoid hyperplasia with eosinophilia of the hand: Report of a case and review of the literature. *Cutis* 1996;58:345–348.

70. Ward KA, Sheehan AL, Kennedy CT. Angiolymphoid hyperplasia with eosinophilia (ALHE) of the digit. *Br J Dermatol* 1996;135(Suppl 47):43.

71. Sakamoto F, Hashimoto T, Takenouchi T, Ito M, Nitto H. Angiolymphoid hyperplasia with eosinophilia presenting multinucleated cells in histology: An ultrastructural study. *J Cutan Pathol* 1998;25:322–326.

72. Arnold M, Geilen CC, Coupland SE, Krengel S, Dippel E, Sproder J, Goerdt S, Orfanos CE. Unilateral angiolymphoid hyperplasia with eosinophilia involving the left arm and hand. *J Cutan Pathol* 1999;26: 436–440.

73. Olsen TG, Helwig EB. Angiolymphoid hyperplasia with eosinophilia. A clinicopathologic study of 116 patients. *J Am Acad Dermatol* 1985;12:781–796.

74. Okada M, Funayama M, Tanita M, Kudoh K, Aiba S, Tagami H. Acral angiokeratoma-like pseudolymphoma: One adolescent and two adults. *J Am Acad Dermatol* 2001;45(Suppl 6):S209–S211.

75. Chedraoui A, Malek J, Tamraz H, Zaynoun S, Kibbi AG, Ghosn S. Acral pseudolymphomatous angiokeratoma of children in an elderly man: Report of a case and review of the literature. *Int J Dermatol* 2010;49:184–188.

76. Ramsay B, Dahl MG, Malcolm AJ, Soyer HP, Wilson-Jones E. Acral pseudolymphomatous angiokeratoma of children (APACHE). *Br J Dermatol* 1983;119(Suppl 33):13.

77. Hara M, Matsunaga J, Tagami H. Acral pseudolymphomatous angiokeratoma of children (APACHE). A case report and immunohistological study. *Br J Dermatol* 1991;124:387–388.

78. Kaddu S, Cerroni L, Pilatti A, Soyer HP, Kerl H. Acral pseudolymphomatous angiokeratoma. A variant of the cutaneous pseudolymphomas. *Am J Dermatopathol* 1994;16:130–133.

79. Hagari Y, Hagari S, Kambe N, Kawaguchi T, Nakamoto S, Mihara M. Acral pseudolymphomatous angiokeratoma of children: Immunohistochemical and clonal analyses of the infiltrating cells. *J Cutan Pathol* 2002;29:313–318.

80. Ramsay B, Dahl MG, Malcolm AJ, Wilson-Jones E. Acral pseudolymphomatous angiokeratoma of children. *Arch Dermatol* 1990;126:1524–1525.

81. Okuyama R, Masu T, Mizuashi M, Watanabe M, Tagami H, Aiba S. Pseudolymphomatous angiokeratoma: Report of three cases and an immunohistological study. *Clin Exp Dermatol* 2009;34:161–165.

82. Fernández-Figueras MT, Puig L, Armengol MP, Juan M, Ribera M, Ariza A. Cutaneous angiolymphoid hyperplasia with high endothelial venules is characterized by endothelial expression of cutaneous lymphocyte antigen. *Hum Pathol* 2001;32:227–229.

83. Dayrit JF, Wang WL, Goh SG, Ramdial PK, Lazar AJ, Calonje E. T-cell-rich angiomatoid polypoid pseudolymphoma of the skin: A clinicopathologic study of 17 cases and a proposed nomenclature. *J Cutan Pathol* 2011;38:475–482.

84. Dolph JL, Demuth RJ, Miller SH. Angiokeratoma circumscriptum of the index finger in a child. *Plast Reconstr Surg* 1981;67:221–223.

85. Hasegawa M, Tamura A. Subungual angiokeratoma presenting as longitudinal pigmented band in the nail. *Acta Derm Venereol* 2015;95:1001–1002.

86. Schiller PI, Itin PH. Angiokeratomas: An update. *Dermatology* 1996;193:275.

87. Pavithra S, Mallya H, Kini H, Pai GS. Verrucous hemangioma or angiokeratoma? A missed diagnosis. *Indian J Dermatol* 2011;56:599–600.

88. Leeson MC, Lowry L, McCue RW. Aneurysmal bone cyst of the distal thumb phalanx. A case report and review of the literature. *Orthopedics* 1988;11: 601–604.

89. Katz MA, Dormans JP, Uri AK. Aneurysmal bone cyst involving the distal phalanx of a child. *Orthopedics* 1997;20:463–466.

90. Sakka SA, Lock M. Aneurysmal bone cyst of the terminal phalanx of the thumb in a child. *Arch Orthop Trauma Surg* 1997;116:119–120.

91. Schajowicz F, Aiello C, Slullitel I. Cystic and pseudocystic lesions of the terminal phalanx with special reference to epidermoid cysts. *Clin Orthop Rel Res* 1970;68:84–92.

92. El-Khoury GY, Seaman RW. Case report 125: Aneurysmal bone cyst terminal phalanx of the first toe. *Skeletal Radiol* 1980;5:201–203.

93. Schmutz JL, Cuny JF, Duprez A. Kyste osseux anévrismal d'un orteil. *Rech Dermatol* 1988;1:679–681.

94. Fuhs SE, Herndon JH. Aneurysmal bone cyst involving the hand: A review and report of two cases. *J Hand Surg Am* 1979;4:152–159.

95. Parashari UC, Khanduri S, Upadhyay D, Bhadury S, Singhal S. Radiologic and pathologic correlation of aneurysmal bone cysts at unusual sites. *J Can Res Ther* 2012;8:103–105.

96. Maggiani F, Forsyth R, Hogendoorn PC, Krenacs T, Athanasou NA. The immunophenotype of osteoclasts and macrophage polykaryons. *J Clin Pathol* 2011;64:701–705.

97. Taylor RM, Kashima TG, Hemingway FK, Dongre A, Knowles HJ, Athanasou NA. CD14- mononuclear stromal cells support (CD14+) monocyte-osteoclast differentiation in aneurysmal bone cyst. *Lab Invest* 2012;92:600–605.

98. Oliveira AM, Chou MM, Perez-Atayde AR, Rosenberg AE. Aneurysmal bone cyst: A neoplasm driven by upregulation of the USP6 oncogene. *J Clin Oncol* 2006;24:e1; author reply e2.

99. Pan Z, Sanger WG, Bridge JA, Hunter WJ, Siegal GP, Wei S. A novel t(6;13)(q15;q34) translocation in a giant cell reparative granuloma (solid aneurysmal bone cyst). *Hum Pathol* 2012;43:952–957.

100. Lebouc L. Etude cliniqude et anatomique sur quelques sur quelques cas de tuneurs sous-ungué-ales. *Med Thesis*, Paris, 1889.

101. Requena L, Baran R. Digital angioleiomyoma: An uncommon neoplasm. *J Am Acad Dermatol* 1993;29:1043–1044.

102. Sawada Y. Angioleiomyoma masquerading as a painful ganglion of the great toe. *Eur J Plast Surg* 1988;11:175–177.

103. Baran R, Requena L, Drapé JL. Angioleiomyoma mimicking glomus tumour in the nail matrix. *Br J Dermatol* 2000;142:1239–1241.

104. Fitzpatrick JE, Mellette JR, Hwang RJ, Golitz LE, Zaim MT, Clemons D. Cutaneous angiolipoleiomyoma. *J Am Acad Dermatol* 1990;23:1093–1098.

105. Wood W. On painful subcutaneous tubercle. *Edinb Med J* 1812;8:28.

106. Vanti AA, Cuce LC, Di Chiacchio N. Subungual glomus tumor: Epidemiological and retrospective study, from 1991 to 2003. *An Bras Dermatol* 2007;82:425–431.

107. Vandenberghe L, De Smet L. Subungual glomus tumours: A technical tip towards diagnosis on plain radiographs. *Acta Orthop Belg* 2010;76:396–397.

108. Parsons ME, Russo G, Fucich L, Millikan LE, Kim R. Multiple glomus tumors. *Int J Dermatol* 1997;36:894–900.

109. Di Chiacchio N, Loureiro WR, Di Chiacchio NG, Bet DL. Synchronous subungueal glomus tumors in the same finger. *An Bras Dermatol* 2012;87(3):475–476.

110. Smalberger GJ, Suszko JW, Khachemoune A. Painful growth on right index finger. Subungual glomus tumor. *Dermatol Online J* 2011;17(9):12.

111. Miyamoto H, Wada H. Localized multiple glomangiomas on the foot. *J Dermatol* 2009;36:604–607.

112. Iliescu OA, Benea V, Georgescu SR, Alice R, Liana Manolache L. Multiple glomus tumors. *Dermatol Case Rep* 2008;2(2):24–27.

113. Namazi MR, Hinckley ML, Jorizzo JL. Multiple collections of soft bluish nodules on the body. *Arch Dermatol* 2008;144:1383–1388.

114. Wollstein A, Wollstein R. Subungual glomangiomyoma: A case report. *Hand Surg* 2012;17:271–273.

115. Michal M, Fanburg-Smith JC, Lasota J, Fetsch JF, Lichy J, Miettinen M. Minute synovial sarcomas of the hands and feet: A clinicopathologic study of 21 tumors less than 1 cm. *Am J Surg Pathol* 2006;30:721–726.

116. Brems H, Park C, Maertens O, Pemov A, Messiaen L, Upadhyaya M, Claes K et al. Glomus tumors in neurofibromatosis type 1: Genetic, functional, and clinical evidence of a novel association. *Cancer Res* 2009;69:7393–7401.

117. Harrison B, Sammer D. Glomus tumors and neuro-fibromatosis: A newly recognized association. *Plast Reconstr Glob Open* 2014;2:e214.

118. Harrison B, Moore AM, Calfee R, Sammer DM. The association between glomus tumors and neurofibro-matosis. *J Hand Surg Am* 2013;38:1571–1574.

119. Jawalkar H, Maryada VR, Brahmajoshyula V, Kotha GKV. Subungual glomus tumors of the hand: Treated by transungual excision. *Indian J Orthop* 2015;49:403–407.

120. Hisa T, Nakagawa K, Wakasa K. Solitary glomus tumour with mucinous degeneration. *Clin Exp Dermatol* 1994;19:227–229.

121. Watanabe K, Kusakabe T, Hoshi N, Saito A, Suzuki T. h-Caldesmon in leiomyosarcoma and tumors with smooth muscle cell-like differentiation: Its specific expression in the smooth muscle cell tumor. *Hum Pathol* 1999;30:392–396.

122. Lee DW, Yang JH, Chang S, Won CH, Lee MW, Choi JH, Moon KC. Clinical and pathological characteristics of extradigital and digital glomus tumours: A retrospective comparative study. *J Eur Acad Dermatol Venereol* 2011;25:1392–1397.

123. Xu H, Edwards JR, Espinosa O, Banerji S, Jackson DG, Athanasou NA. Expression of a lymphatic endothelial cell marker in benign and malignant vascular tumors. *Hum Pathol* 2004;35:857–861.

124. Daugaard S, Jensen ME, Fisher S. Glomus tumours. An immunohistochemical study. *APMIS* 1990;98:983–990.

125. Netscher DT, Aburto J, Koepplinger M. Subungual glomus tumor. *J Hand Surg Am* 2012;37:821–823; quiz 824.

126. Mentzel T, Hügel H, Kutzner H. CD34-positive glomus tumor: Clinicopathologic and immunohistochemical analysis of six cases with myxoid stromal changes. *J Cutan Pathol* 2002;29:421–425.

127. Herbst WM, Nakayama K, Hornstein OP. Glomus tumours of the skin: An immunohistochemical investigation of the expression of marker proteins. *Dermatology* 1991;124:172–176.

128. Miettinen M, Sarlomo-Rikala M, Wang ZF. Claudin-5 as an immunohistochemical marker for angiosarcoma and hemangioendotheliomas. *Am J Surg Pathol* 2011;35:1848–1856.

129. Gölfert F, Kasper M, van Eys GJ, Funk RH. Cytoskeletal characterization of arteriovenous epithelioid cells. *Histochem Cell Biol* 1997;108:513–523.

130. Mukherjee S, Bandyopadhyay G, Saha S, Choudhuri M. Cytodiagnosis of glomus tumor. *J Cytol* 2010;27:104–105.

131. Mitchell A, Spinner RJ, Ribeiro A, Mafra M, Mouzinho MM, Scheithauer BW. Glomus tumor of digital nerve: Case report. *J Hand Surg Am* 2012;37:1180–1183.

132. Kamarashev J, French LE, Dummer R, Kerl K. Symplastic glomus tumor—A rare but distinct benign histological variant with analogy to other "ancient" benign skin neoplasms. *J Cutan Pathol* 2009;36:1099–1102.

133. Chong Y, Eom M, Min HJ, Kim S, Chung YK, Lee KG. Symplastic glomus tumor: A case report. *Am J Dermatopathol* 2009;31:71–73.

134. Quaterman MJ, Lucas JG, Pellegrini AE et al. Subungual glomangioleiomyoma: A case report. *J Cutan Pathol* 1996;23:90.

135. Calonje E. Myopericytoma. Chapter 33. Vascular tumors: Tumors and tumor-like conditions of blood vessels and lymphatics. In: Elder DE, ed. *Lever's Histopathology of the Skin*, 10th edn. Philadelphia: Lippincott Williams & Wilkins, 2009; 1049–1051.

136. Lee YB, Lee KJ, Park HJ, Cho BK. Cutaneous glomangiopericytoma on the tip of the nose. *Acta Derm Venereol* 2011;91:375–376.

137. Wetherington RW, Lyle WG, Sangüeza OP. Malignant glomus tumor to the thumb: A case report. *J Hand Surg* 1997;22A:1098–1102.

138. Liu JY, Liao SL, Zheng J. Cutaneous epithelioid angioleiomyoma with clear-cell change. *Am J Dermatopathol* 2007;29:190–193.

139. Granter SR, Badizadegan K, Fletcher CD. Myofibromatosis in adults, glomangiopericytoma, and myopericytoma: A spectrum of tumors showing perivascular myoid differentiation. *Am J Surg Pathol* 1998;22:513–525.

140. Mentzel T, Dei Tos AP, Sapi Z, Kutzner H. Myopericytoma of skin and soft tissues: Clinicopathologic and immunohistochemical study of 54 cases. *Am J Surg Pathol* 2006;30:104–113.

141. Mikó T, Adler P, Endes P. Simulated cancer of the lower lip attributed to a "caliber persistent" artery. *J Oral Pathol* 1980;9:137–144.

142. Molnár P, Mikó T. Multiple arterial caliber persistence resulting in hematomas and fatal rupture of the gastric wall. *Am J Surg Pathol* 1982;6:83–86.

143. McClave SA, Goldschmid S, Cunningham JT, Boyd WP Jr. Dieulafoy's cirsoid aneurysm of the duodenum. *Dig Dis Sci* 1988;33:801–805.

144. Mikó TL, Thomázy VA. The caliber persistent artery of the stomach: A unifying approach to gastric aneurysm, Dieulafoy's lesion, and submucosal arterial malformation. *Hum Pathol* 1988;19:914–921.

145. Jaspers MT. Oral caliber-persistent artery. Unusual presentations of unusual lesions. *Oral Surg Oral Med Oral Pathol* 1992;74:631–633.

146. Lovas JG, Rodu B, Hammond HL, Allen CM, Wysocki GP. Caliber-persistent labial artery. A common vascular anomaly. *Oral Surg Oral Med Oral Pathol Oral Radiol Endod* 1998;86:308–312.

147. Lovas JG, Goodday RH. Clinical diagnosis of caliber-persistent labial artery of the lower lip. *Oral Surg Oral Med Oral Pathol* 1993;76:480–483.

148. Howell JB, Freeman RG. The potential peril from caliber-persistent arteries of the lips. *J Am Acad Dermatol* 2002;46:256–259.

149. Lewis DM. Caliber-persistent labial artery. *J Okla Dent Assoc* 2003;93(3):37–39.

150. Vazquez L, Lombardi T, Guinand-Mkinsi H, Samson J. Ultrasonography: A noninvasive tool to diagnose a caliber-persistent labial artery, an enlarged artery of the lip. *J Ultrasound Med* 2005;24:1295–1301.

151. Wortsman X, Calderón P, Arellano J, Orellana Y. High-resolution color Doppler ultrasound of a caliber-persistent artery of the lip, a simulator variant of dermatologic disease: Case report and sonographic findings. *Int J Dermatol* 2009;48:830–833.

152. Sangüeza O. Angiosarcoma. Oral comm. XIV World Cong Cancers Skin, São Paulo, Aug 1–4, 2012.

153. Requena L, Sangueza OP. Cutaneous vascular proliferations. Part III. Malignant neoplasms, other cutaneous neoplasms with significant vascular component, and disorders erroneously considered as vascular neoplasms. *J Am Acad Dermatol* 1998;38:143–175; quiz 176–178.

154. Stewart FW, Treves N. Lymphangiosarcoma in postmastectomy lymphedema. *Cancer* 1948;1:64–81.

155. Stokkel MP, Petersen HL. Angiosarcoma of the breast after lumpectomy and radiation therapy for adenocarcinoma. *Cancer* 1992;69:2965–2968.

156. Requena L, Kutzner H, Mentzel T, Duran R, Rodriguez-Peralto JL. Benign vascular proliferations in irradiated skin. *Am J Surg Pathol* 2002;26:328–337.

157. Kolaczeck J. Über das Angio-Sarkom. *Dtsch Zschr Chirurg* 1878;9:1–48.

158. Kraske P. Über subunguale Geschwülste. *Münch Med Wschr* 1887;34:889–891.

159. Weiss SW, Enzinger FM. Epithelioid hemangioendothelioma. A vascular tumor often mistaken for a carcinoma. *Cancer* 1982;50:970–981.

160. Mentzel T, Beham A, Calonje E, Katenkamp D, Fletcher CD. Epithelioid hemangioendothelioma of skin and soft tissues: Clinicopathologic and immunohistochemical study of 30 cases. *Am J Surg Pathol* 1997;21:363–374.

161. Bessis D, Sotto A, Roubert P, Chabrier PE, Mourad G, Guilhou JJ. Endothelin-secreting angiosarcoma occurring at the site of an arteriovenous fistula for haemodialysis in a renal transplant recipient. *Br J Dermatol.* 1998;138:361–363.

162. Laskowski J, Bamberg C, Zimmermann R, Gross G. Multifokales Hämangioendotheliom der unteren Extremität. *Hautarzt* 1999;50(Suppl 1):S74.

163. Kikuchi K, Watanabe M, Terui T, Ohtani N, Ohtani H, Tagami H. Nail-destroying epithelioid hae-mangioendothelioma showing an erythematous scar-like appearance on the finger. *Br J Dermatol* 2003;148:834–836.

164. Davies MFP, Curtis M, Howat JMT. Cutaneous hae-mangioendothelioma, possible link with chronic exposure to vinyl chloride. *Br J Indust Med* 1990; 47:65–67.

165. Kennedy CT, Burton PA, Cook P. Swollen toe due to epithelioid haemangioma of bone. *Br J Dermatol* 1990;123(Suppl 37):85–89.

166. Tsuneyoshi M, Dorfman HD, Bauer TW. Epithelioid hemangioendothelioma of bone. A clinicopathologic, ultrastructural, and immunohistochemical study. *Am J Surg Pathol* 1986;10:754–756.

167. Zaias N. *The Nail in Health and Disease.* Norwalk, CT: Appleton and Lange, 1990.

168. König F. Über multiple Angiosarkome. *Arch Chir* 1899;59:600.

169. Aïm F, Rosier L, Dumontier C. Isolated Kaposi sar-coma of the finger pulp in an AIDS patient. *Orthop Traumatol Surg Res* 2012;98:126–128.

170. Kandemir NO, Barut F, Gun BD, Keser SH, Karadayi N, Gun M, Ozdamar SO. Lymphatic differentia-tion in classic Kaposi's sarcoma: Patterns of D2-40 immunoexpression in the course of tumor progres-sion. *Pathol Oncol Res* 2011;17:843–851.

171. Cecchi R, Pavesi M, Apicella P. Malignant glo-mus tumor of the trunk treated with Mohs micro-graphi surgery. *J Dtsch Dermatol Ges* 2011;9: 391–393.

Tumors with adipocyte, myxoid, muscular, osseous, and cartilaginous features

11

The diagnosis of these lesions in the nail apparatus is difficult and on clinical grounds alone often not possible. Imaging techniques such as radiography, ultrasound, computed tomography, and magnetic resonance imaging may be necessary.[1] In addition, simple examinations like probing, dermatoscopy, and transillumination are often helpful. Palpation is rarely helpful in subungual lesions as the nail covers the tumor and does not allow exact determination of its consistency.

11.1 BENIGN TUMORS

11.1.1 Lipoma

Despite their frequency elsewhere in the skin, lipomas of the nail apparatus are exceptional.[2, 3] The nail is deformed depending on the size of the lipoma, it may lose its shine, and get ridged or develop a split.[4, 5] Also, a tender painful enlargement of the thumb's distal phalanx was described.[6] One lipoma of the lateral nail fold resembled nevus lipomatodes superficialis.[7] Subungual lipoma was also observed in association with a squamous cell carcinoma of the nail bed of the same digit.[8] Magnetic resonance imaging easily allows the diagnosis to be made as there is a very intense signal in T1-weighted images and the fat-suppression technique virtually completely abolishes this feature.[9] Homogeneity usually is a sign of a benign lesion.[10]

11.1.1.1 Histopathology

The lesion is composed of mature adipocytes separated by thin fibrous septa. There may or may not be a thin fibrous capsule. Cellular atypias and mitoses are lacking.

One case of subungual spindle cell lipoma was described.[11] This is a well-circumscribed tumor made up of uniformly spindle-shaped cells in a myxoid matrix and mature fat cells. The spindle cells exhibit vimentin and CD34 positivity.

11.1.1.2 Differential diagnosis

Lipoleiomyoma has to be considered. In case of cellular atypia, liposarcoma should be ruled out.

11.1.2 Myxoma

Myxomas are lesions with mostly stellate fibroblasts embedded in abundant myxoid stroma. Their distinction from focal mucinosis is often arbitrary. Most myxoid lesions of the nail apparatus are, however, so-called myxoid pseudocysts.[12,13] Subungual myxomas either elevate or deform the nail or enlarge the nail and fingertip.[14–20] Whether all lesions described earlier as ungual myxoma[21] were in fact myxomas and not superficial acral fibromyxoma is not clear.

11.1.2.1 Histopathology

Myxomas are characterized by abundant hyaluronic acid rich ground substance, in which stellate or fusiform cells are loosely distributed. Toluidin blue, Giemsa as well as colloidal iron stains are positive for these acid mucopolysaccharides. As the subungual connective stroma may be very rich in mucopolysaccharides, other lesions may contain a variable amount of mucinous tissue, such as subungual angiomyxoma,[22] or they may also contain adipocytes (Figure 11.1).[23]

11.1.2.2 Differential diagnosis

Deposition of mucinous material is a common phenomenon in many tumors, some of which have already been mentioned above. Angiomyxolipoma is a nonencapsulated neoplasm made up of mature fat cells with numerous thin- and thick-walled vessels of various sizes. The stroma is loose and in part myxoid. There are scattered mast cells and myelinated nerves in the periphery. Cellular atypias are absent.[22] Immunohistochemistry may be necessary to rule out a myxoid neurogenic tumor[24–27] or another so-called "ancient" tumor with mucinous stroma degeneration.

11.1.3 Myxoid pseudocyst

Myxoid pseudocysts are known under a variety of synonyms: dorsal finger cyst, digital focal mucinosis, distal

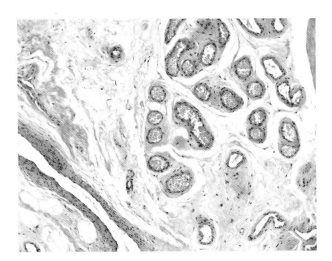

Figure 11.1 Subungual angiolipomyxoma in a middle-aged woman. The lesion was slightly tender prompting the patient to ask for surgical removal.

interphalangeal joint ganglion, mucinous cyst, and so on. The synonyms reflect the different opinions as to their etiology and pathogenesis. Some authors claim that two types of lesions exist: one type is merely a focal mucinosis of the distal phalanx, usually in the proximal nail fold (myxomatous type), the other type has a connection to the distal interphalangeal joint (ganglion type). In about 85% of the lesions, a connection with the joint can be demonstrated by intraarticular injection of 0.05–0.1 mL of sterile methylene blue solution. This connection is, however, most probably secondary to wear-and-tear of the joint capsule in a long-standing lesion. This lesion is one of the most common pseudotumors of the nail apparatus. Women are slightly more often involved than men. Most lesions are solitary although more than one finger can be affected, and very rarely two lesions are found on one finger. When the toes are involved, there is usually a firm protuberant cystic lesion. Almost always, a degenerative distal interphalangeal osteoarthritis with Heberden nodes is present. Three clinical types are distinguished: Type A is localized in the proximal nail fold and is seen as a round dome-shaped skin colored lesion causing a regular longitudinal depression in the nail plate due to pressure on the matrix. Type B is also localized in the proximal nail fold but tends to rupture at the undersurface of the nail fold releasing part of its content into the nail pocket. This leads to an irregular depression in the nail often with narrow transverse ridges in the canaliform depression reflecting the period of diminished pressure on the matrix after rupture. Type C is the submatrical myxoid pseudocyst clinically seen as a hemiovercurvature and a violaceous swelling under the nail. Transillumination is positive. Magnetic resonance imaging usually demonstrates the lesion clearly, sometimes also the connecting stalk to the joint.

11.1.3.1 Histopathology

Systematic histopathologic examination of complete excision specimens shows myxomatous areas in the wall of the pseudocyst in far more than 90% of the cases. In many cases, there is a central lake of mucin surrounded by myxomatous tissue containing scattered stellate and spindle-shaped cells (Figure 11.2). Sometimes the mucin has expanded the surrounding normal connective tissue giving rise to a pseudocapsule. The overlying epidermis is often considerably thinned. The myxoid areas are positive with alcian blue and Hale's colloidal iron stains. In the so-called ganglion type, the myxomatous areas are sparse or not seen in all sections. Although some authors claim that there might be areas of the wall exhibiting a cyst lining, we have never been able to unequivocally demonstrate a synovial lining, not even by electron microscopy.[28] Immunohistochemistry reveals that the cells are positive for vimentin and actin, but negative for desmin.

11.1.3.2 Differential diagnosis

All focal mucinoses as well as myxomas and mucinous tumors have to be considered.

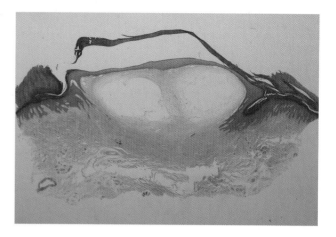

Figure 11.2 Myxoid pseudocyst of the distal portion of the proximal nail fold. The epidermis is thinned and there is a large area of myxoid tissue without any cyst lining.

11.1.4 Chondroma

Three types of subungual chondroma have been observed in the tip of digits: enchondroma, parosteal chondroma, and soft tissue (extraskeletal) chondroma with the former being the most frequent type in ungual location.

11.1.4.1 Enchondroma

Enchondroma is a solitary intraosseous proliferation of cartilage. With up to 90%, it is the most frequent bone tumor of the hand. Multiple enchondromas are observed in enchondromatosis (chondrodysplasia of Ollier, OMIM 166000) and chondrodysplasia with multiple soft tissue and intraosseous hemangiomas (Maffucci–Kast syndrome, OMIM 614569); both syndromes are due to cartilage that fails to undergo normal ossification. Both are also prone to undergo malignant degeneration to chondrosarcoma—almost 25%—and have a higher malignancy rate in general.[29] Solitary enchondromas of the distal phalanx with enlargement of the tip of the digit are, however, rare.[30–32] Roughly one-fifth of the lesions remain asymptomatic, but paronychia, clubbing, and secondary nail changes with longitudinal ridging are seen.[33–35] Pathologic fractures are the result of progressive thinning of the cortical bone. Radiography demonstrates well defined to cloudy radiolucent defects with expansion of the terminal phalanx, in most cases close to the articular surface of the distal interphalangeal joint.[36,37] Curettage of the lesion is the treatment of choice.

11.1.4.2 Parosteal chondroma

Parosteal chondroma of the distal phalanx is very rare. It is a slowly growing lesion that insidiously occupies the subungual or periungual space leading to nail deformation. X-ray may show an impression of the distal phalangeal bone.

11.1.4.3 Extraskeletal chondroma

Extraskeletal or soft tissue chondroma is thought to derive from the connective tissue, not preexisting chondrocytes.[38–43] Its symptomatology is very similar to parosteal chondroma.

The clinical differential diagnoses comprise a number of other chondromatoses, which rarely affect the digits, such as synovial chondromatosis. The common form is mainly seen in large joints of men between the ages of 20 and 50 years, but when it occurs in the small digital joints it predominantly occurs in young women.[44,45] Its malignant potential is debated, but one group estimates it at around 5%.[46]

11.1.4.4 Histopathology

All chondromas are characterized by a proliferation of hyaline cartilage. The cells are irregularly arranged, but there are no mitoses and no cellular atypias (Figure 11.3). There may be a fine connective tissue capsule in soft tissue chondroma. Small areas of calcification and ossification are rarely present; however, they have to prompt a search for malignancy. Staining for the proliferation marker Ki67 (MiB 1) shows a very low proliferation rate. P53 is negative.[41]

11.1.4.5 Differential diagnosis

Chondroid differentiation, active mitoses, multinucleate giant cells, calcification, and necrosis were seen in a case of subungual chondroblastoma of the little toe.[47] Increased cellularity, nuclear pleomorphism, the presence of chondroblasts and epithelioid cells, as well as the proliferation of multinucleated giant cells may be a hint at a malignant tumor. Mild atypical histopathologic findings may also be seen in benign chondromas. Using proliferation markers like Ki-67 and p53 may help to delineate chondroma from chondrosarcoma.[41] Synovial chondromatosis shows well-circumscribed nodules of cartilage and bone with some fragments being surfaced by a thin layer of synovium. The cartilage is of low-to-moderate cellularity and has unremarkable chondrocytes lying individually within the lacunae, indicative of primary synovial chondromatosis. Areas of ossification may be present.[48]

11.1.5 Osteoma cutis

True osteomas of the skin are usually small round to oval nodules with all characteristics of normal bone. They are very rare in the distal digit.[49-51] They may present merely as a splinter hemorrhage extending from the site of the osteoma to the hyponychium.[52] When they occur under the nail, they can only be suspected radiographically.

11.1.5.1 Histopathology

Osteoma cutis is seen as a round to oval, usually well-demarcated lesion of mature bone with a few osteocytes in the bone trabeculae. There may be a few osteoblasts at the margin and rarely an osteoclast is seen.

11.1.5.2 Differential diagnosis

The main differential diagnoses are subungual calcifications, which according to some authors are very common both under the toe as well as the fingernails. They usually present as irregular basophilic von Kossa-positive deposits of clumpy material. Some calcifications may have been erroneously termed osteoma or may be difficult to diagnose.[53, 54]

11.1.6 Subungual exostosis

Subungual exostosis is one of the most frequent reactive bony lesions of the toes,[55] but is relatively rare in fingers.[56-58] The differentiation from osteochondroma[59] depends on its localization[60] though there are some differential diagnostic features including the magnetic resonance image: hyaline cartilage exhibits a high signal as compared to the low signal of the fibrocartilage cap of the typical exostosis.[61-63] Trauma may be an etiologic factor.[64,65] The most common localization is the distal dorsal medial aspect of the distal phalanx of the hallux, but all other digits may occasionally be involved. Usually, the nail plate is lifted and slightly deformed. A small onycholytic area is often present. The overlying epidermis is smooth, shiny, stretched out and often shows a collaret-like delimitation to the ridged skin of the tip of the toe. Superficial ulceration may occur spontaneously or be trauma-induced. The clinical diagnosis is obvious in most cases as there is hardly any other lesion as hard on palpation as an exostosis; however, the list of misdiagnoses reaches from viral wart to pyogenic granuloma to even onychomycosis.[66] Therefore, a radiograph usually showing a bony projection is recommended not only to confirm the diagnosis but also to allow its extension to be made visible to plan the removal, which consists of generous extirpation at the base of the lesion. Malignant degeneration of solitary subungual exostoses has not been observed in contrast to the hereditary multiple exostoses syndrome (diaphyseal aclasis), which rarely affects the distal phalanx.[67] Radiographically, bone fragments after fracture of the distal subungual tuft, subungual calcifications as seen quite frequently in elderly women,[68] posttraumatic subungual calcifications, primary osteoma cutis, and calcified subungual epidermoid inclusions have to be ruled out. Clinical differential diagnoses are melanoma, squamous cell carcinoma, pyogenic granuloma, warts, Nora's lesion,[69] and other tumorous lesions.

The recent finding of chromosomal translocation t(X;6) (q13-14;q22) in subungual exostoses has shed another light

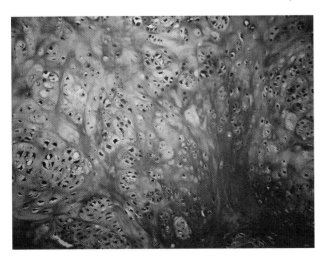

Figure 11.3 Subungual soft tissue chondroma.

on this lesion. Some consider it therefore to be a true benign tumor.[70–73] However, it has also been found in osteochondroma, bizarre parosteal proliferation,[74] and chondromyxoid fibroma.[75] This anomaly leads to increased production of insulin receptor substrate 4, which has a profound effect on cell growth and survival.[71]

11.1.6.1 Histopathology

In the beginning, mucopolysaccharide deposition and osteoid formation are seen close to the periosteum. Then there is a gradual continuum of highly cellular chondroid and osteoid. Eventually the cartilage becomes hyaline and is eroded at its deep part by osteoclast-like giant cells. Enchondral bone apposition follows around all cartilage remnants. Finally cancellous bone develops. This process continues as long as the fibroblasts keep on modulating into matrix-producing cells.[76] The mature subungual exostosis reveals a three-zonal pattern: a fibrocartilaginous cap on its surface, a rim of hyaline cartilage, and below trabeculae of bone with a rim of osteoblasts and some osteoclasts (Figure 11.4). In between the bone lamellae there is some lipomatous medulla, but blood formation is not seen. The proliferation rate is low as seen with Ki67.

11.1.6.2 Differential diagnosis

Subungual osteochondroma is a common tumor that arises from the epiphyseal cartilage and is therefore generally seen in adolescents.[77] However, the terms of subungual exostosis and subungual osteochondroma are often used interchangeably.[78–80]

11.1.7 Osteochondroma

Osteochondroma is a benign bone tumor arising from the epiphyseal cartilage. When located subungually, the signs and symptoms are virtually indistinguishable from subungual exostosis although it originates from the juxtaepiphyseal bone in contrast to subungual exostosis, which arises

from the distal portion of the terminal phalanx.[81] Magnetic resonance shows a cap of hyaline cartilage in contrast to subungual exostosis with its fibrocartilaginous cap.

11.1.7.1 Histopathology

Except for the cap of hyaline cartilage (Figure 11.5), the histologic features are virtually identical to those of subungual exostosis.

11.1.7.2 Differential diagnosis

The histologic differential diagnoses of subungual osteochondroma and subungual exostoses are the same.

11.1.8 Subungual calcifications

Subungual calcifications are a common phenomenon and usually remain unnoticed by the patient and his physician. Women are affected considerably more frequently and earlier than men. Even a congenital tumorous calcification of the distal lateral nail fold was observed.[82] Of the three different types of calcifications, primary calcinosis, metastatic calcinosis, and dystrophic calcinosis, probably the latter is the most frequent type in and around the nail.[83–85]

11.1.8.1 Histopathology

Calcifications are not neoplastic, but in most cases dystrophic lesions, and rarely metastatic in case of disturbances of calcium metabolism. There are deposits of calcium of various size and shape. Most often, they are scattered in the dermis without an inflammatory reaction, but some may be partly surrounded by macrophages and an occasional giant cell.

Calcifications may also arise from onycholemmal cysts (Figure 11.5).

11.1.8.2 Differential diagnosis

The deposition of structureless calcium deposits is typical. Whether cutaneous calculi can be differentiated from

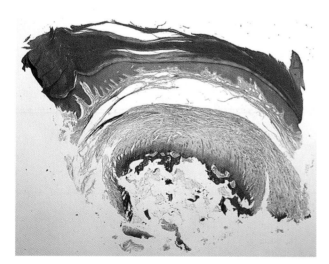

Figure 11.4 Subungual exostosis with the typical fibrous cap. This lesion was taken from the tip of the distal phalanx of the big toe of a 12-year-old girl.

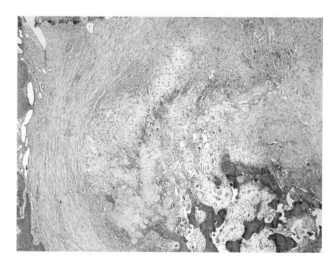

Figure 11.5 Subungual osteochondroma with a cap of hyaline bone; the lesion was located under the nail in the middle of the distal phalanx.

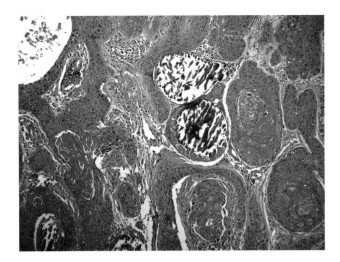

Figure 11.6 Calcifications in subungual onycholemmal cysts.

cutaneous calcifications and calcinosis cutis circumscripta has not been examined in detail.[86,87] Onycholemmal cysts may undergo calcification similar to scrotal epidermal cysts (Figure 11.6).

11.1.9 Osteoid osteoma

Osteoid osteoma is a peculiar bone lesion with a characteristic pattern of pain independent of physical activity.[88] Nagging to pulsating pain at night, reacting promptly to nonsteroidal anti-inflammatory agents or acetylsalicylic acid (Aspirin®) is characteristic.[89,90] The pain has been attributed to the effect on nerves and vessels by the prostaglandin E2 produced by the osteoblasts.[91] They occur in virtually all bones. Approximately 1%–2% of all hand tumors are osteoid osteomas, 8% of them occur in the phalanges, but localization in the distal phalanx is rare.[92,93] Most of these tumors develop in young adults, but there was also one probable congenital case.[94] Osteoid osteomas of the nail region lead to enlargement of the tip of the digit, clubbing, nail thickening, and enlargement of the nail.[95–97] Osteoid osteomas of the distal phalanx often present diagnostic difficulties due to the atypical radiological appearance, the presence of soft tissue enlargement and nail deformity, the small size of the distal phalanx, and consequent close approximation of lesions to the nail plate and distal interphalangeal joint.[98,99] Subperiosteal localization may mimic an exostosis.[100,101] Probing may elicit pain and help to localize the tumor. Radiography exhibits a small area of contrast rarefaction surrounded by a narrow sclerotic ring.[102–104] Arteriography,[105] thermography,[106] scintigraphy,[107] color-coded duplex ultrasonography,[108] fine layer computed tomography, and magnetic resonance imaging[109] help to make the diagnosis and to find the lesion. Preoperative administration of a tetracycline and examination of the lesion under UV light during surgery allows the nidus to be visualized intraoperatively.[110] Treatment is complete extirpation, either by surgery or radiofrequency ablation.[111]

11.1.9.1 Histopathology

Histologic sections show a sharply delimited central growth area, the nidus, consisting of a meshwork of trabeculae of osteoid with a variable degree of calcification. They are surrounded by plump osteoblasts and dispersed in a very vascular connective tissue usually without any sign of inflammation.[112] Most of the osteoid osteomas are positive for CD138 (syndecan-1), which is a surface proteoglycan and specific for plasmocytic differentiation in hematologic disorders, but also in the majority of epithelial tumors.[113] Most osteoid osteomas express nuclear Runx2 (runt-related transcription factor 2) and Osterix (Sp7 transcription factor), two master transcription factors for bone formation, whereas they are negative for Sox9, which is positive in chondromyxoid fibromas and chondroblastoma.[114]

11.1.9.2 Differential diagnosis

Osteoblastoma is histologically almost identical to osteoid osteoma, but it usually lacks the characteristic pain. The nidus is larger, and there is no or only an inconspicuous rim of reactive sclerotic bone formation. On the other hand, the differential diagnosis of osteoblastoma and well-differentiated osteosarcoma can pose extreme difficulties.[115,116] Aggressive or epithelioid osteoblastoma has not been described in the distal phalanx.

11.1.10 Giant cell tumor of the bone

Giant cell tumor of the bone (GCTB), also called osteoclastoma, is an uncommon benign bone tumor accounting for roughly 4% of all primary bone tumors. Usually, the long bones of young adults over 20 years of age are involved. It appears to be more frequent in Asian persons and there are more women than men with GCTB. Distal phalanx affection is exceedingly rare.[117–122] The distal phalanx is massively enlarged and radiographically lytic with a very thin bone lamella but without sclerosis or periosteal reaction. Pain is a leading symptom and probing virtually always reveals a very tender lesion. Spontaneous fracture is not uncommon. The surgical specimen is solid, tan or light brown, often with small hemorrhagic areas. The clinical differential diagnosis is intraosseous epidermal cyst, other intraosseous cysts, enchondroma, and intraosseous glomus tumor.

11.1.10.1 Histopathology

Despite its synonym osteoclastoma, GCTB is a predominantly stromal tumor.[123] There are two main tumor cell components, the stromal cells, which are now thought to constitute the "real neoplastic and proliferative component," and the obvious osteoclast-like giant cells. The giant cells have often 20–30 oval nuclei with light chromatin and a small nucleolus, most being arranged in the center of the cells. Microscopically, enzymatically, ultrastructurally, and immunohistochemically they resemble osteoclasts and derive from fusioned macrophages. The neoplastic stromal cells are probably of mesenchymal origin resembling fibroblasts and osteoblasts and they are able to make osteoid. They secrete monocyte chemoattractant protein (MCP-1) and SDF-1 both attracting blood monocytes and stimulate their migration into the tumor. In the common GCTB, there are abundant osteoclast-like giant cells in between small stromal cells (Figure 11.6) and often some hemorrhage. Immunohistochemistry of the giant cells is positive for microphthalmia associated transcription factor (Mitf), lysozyme, α-antichymotrypsin as well as a number of other histiocytic cell markers. The stromal cells do not express histiocytic surface markers, but cytoplasmic lysozyme and α₁-antitrypsin as well as TP63.[109]

11.1.10.2 Differential diagnosis

Giant cell tumor of soft tissue is virtually identical to GCTB (Figure 11.7). There are several other giant cell lesions of bones and adjacent tissues such as chondromyxoid fibromas, chondroblastoma, nonossifying fibromas, metaphyseal fibrous defect, Langerhans cell histiocytosis, solitary bone cyst, osteitis fibrosa cystica in hyperparathyroidism, giant cell reparative granuloma, aneurysmal bone cyst, osteoid osteoma, and osteoblastoma. Their giant cells may be osteoclast-like. In GCTB, the giant cells are evenly distributed among the stromal cells whereas they tend to be clumped in the simulators of GCTB.[124]

11.1.11 Solitary bone cysts

Solitary bone cysts are reactive pseudotumorous lesions of the long bones mainly seen in young males. A single case of solitary bone cyst was described in the distal phalanx of the second left toe. The phalanx was tender and enlarged and the nail clubbed. X-ray showed a cystic loss of bone with only an extremely thin bone lamella left.[125]

11.1.11.1 Histopathology

The cyst contains a clear yellowish fluid. It is usually lined by a smooth membrane-like material. There are well-vascularized connective tissue, often hemosiderin in

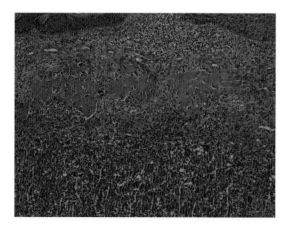

Figure 11.7 Giant cell tumor of soft tissue with the characteristic shell of osteoid and bone.

macrophages and cholesterol clefts. The surrounding bone may be dense with irregular cement lines.[126–128]

11.1.11.2 Differential diagnosis

Some authors claim that the solitary bone cyst is a variant of aneurysmal bone cyst. Secondary cyst formation after bleeding or inflammation has to be ruled out.

11.1.12 Giant cell tumor of the tendon sheath (synovialoma)

This lesion is also called benign xanthomatous giant cell tumor or villonodular pigmented synovitis. It derives from the tendon sheath or synovial membrane of the joints. It is frequent in the hand and occurs more frequently in women. When located on the dorsal aspect of the distal digit, it appears as a solitary or lobulated, firm to hard, skin-colored tumor, to which the skin is firmly attached. In contrast, when the tumor is located volarly in the digital pulp it is easily movable and when being extirpated it appears as a corymbiform yellow to brownish lesion. It is not tender except when pressed too hard and usually does not interfere with nail growth. When localized in the lateral nail fold, it may look similar to a paronychia-like inflammation.[129,130] Subungual localization may cause nail deformity.[131,132] Radiographs of benign synovialoma do not show calcifications in contrast to its very rare malignant counterpart. Clinical differential diagnoses comprise a variety of pseudotumorous, neoplastic and inflammatory lesions such as myxoid pseudocyst, epidermal cyst, neuroma, rheumatoid nodules and Heberden nodes, fibrokeratoma, epidermal cyst, tendon sheath fibroma, multicentric reticulohistiocytosis, reticulohistiocytoma with a virtually identical histopathological picture, tendinous xanthoma, epithelioid sarcoma and other sarcomas as well as metastases, but in rare cases also granuloma annulare and erythema elevatum diutinum.[133]

11.1.12.1 Histopathology

The earliest lesion is a projection of a villous structure into the tendon sheath; this is not seen in nail pathology. When a giant cell tumor of the tendon sheath around the nail is biopsied or removed, it is a lobulated mass extending into the subcutaneous tissue around the tendon in volar location and more into the lower dermis in dorsal location. In the former site, there is usually a dense fibrous capsule that often also divides the tumor into lobules. The microscopic aspect of the lesion varies according to the amount of mononuclear cells, giant cells, hemosiderin deposition, xanthomatous cells, and collagen. There are sheets of mononuclear cells, which when in a collagenized stroma are more spindle-shaped. Intermingled giant cells thought to arise by fusion of the mononuclear cells[134] are large with many nuclei, some of which are more or less evenly distributed in the cytoplasm, but they may also be concentrated in the center of the cells or at the periphery. Clefts are seen predominantly in juxtaarticular location. Xanthoma cell-rich areas are irregularly distributed

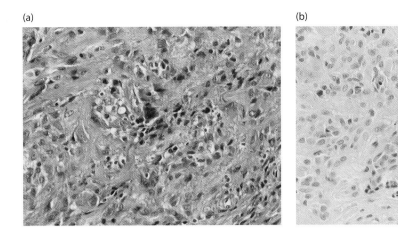

Figure 11.8 (a) Synovialoma of the proximal nail fold clinically diagnosed as a myxoid pseudocyst. (b) Embedded in a fibrotic stroma there are many macrophages, some giant cells with an irregular outline, occasional extravasated erythrocytes, and small hemosiderin deposits.

and may even contain cholesterol clefts. The xanthoma cells also often contain fine hemosiderin granules (Figures 11.8). Normally, mitoses do not occur although they have been observed even in benign lesions.[135] Immunohistochemistry of synovialoma shows a histiocytic pattern of the mononuclear cells: CD68+, HAM56+, MAC387+, PG-M1+, whereas the giant cells are positive for CD68 and LCA (CD45), the latter only being occasionally positive in the mononuclear cells.[136,137] The giant cells also express a variety of osteoclast characteristic markers such as tartrate-resistant acid phosphatase, calcitonin and vitronectin receptor, parathyroid hormone related peptide, and its receptor.[138,139] The tumor is negative for keratins, weakly positive for actin, and some tumors also stain weakly for desmin. Electron microscopy confirms the similarity with synovial cells.[140]

11.1.12.2 Differential diagnosis

A variety of nodular lesions adjacent to tendons or the distal interphalangeal joint may have to be differentiated from giant cell tumor of tendon sheath. Granulomatous lesions with or without necrobiotic or xanthomatous changes are less well circumscribed. Foreign body granulomas have a different type of giant cell. Tendinous xanthomas were not seen in the distal phalanx. Fibromas of the tendon sheath may be similar to a collagenized giant cell tumor of tendon sheath;[141] however, the cells are more fibroblastic and are distributed in a more hyaline stroma.[142] Epithelioid sarcoma with many giant cells shows a monomorphic population with dense eosinophilic cytoplasm and diffuse strong keratin positivity.

11.2 MALIGNANT TUMORS

11.2.1 Leiomyosarcoma

Cutaneous leiomyosarcoma is a malignant tumor of the smooth muscles of the dermis, mainly of the arrector pilorum and vascular muscles. Males are more often affected. It mostly occurs in elderly persons on the extensor surfaces of the extremities as a usually painless tumor of 5 mm to

3 cm in diameter.[143] Subungual location is exceedingly rare. One case of subungual epithelioid leiomyosarcoma was described in a 63-year-old man who had lost his right great toenail after a 3-week history of pain.

11.2.1.1 Histopathology

Dermal leiomyosarcoma is mainly located in the skin. Its delimitation is irregular with the tumor cells blending in with the fibroblasts and collagen fibers of the surrounding tissue. The neoplasm itself shows interlacing bundles of spindle cells. Their cytoplasm is homogeneously eosinophilic and their nuclei are fusiform with blunt ends. Nuclear palisading is a rare event. Mitoses are usually seen, commonly 1 per 10 high-power fields, but areas with higher mitotic activity do occur and are designated as mitotic hot spots.[144] In PAS stains, most tumor cells exhibit their own PAS-positive basal membrane. There are rare variants such as epithelioid, granular cell, desmoplastic and inflammatory leiomyosarcomas.[145]

The subungual epithelioid leiomyosarcoma was mainly composed of interlacing bundles of large spindle cells with indistinct cell borders, eosinophilic cytoplasm, and pleomorphic nuclei.[145]

Immunohistochemical stains are mostly positive for smooth muscle actin, desmin, and focally for pan-muscle actin (HHF-35); they are negative for protein S100, HMB 45, cytokeratin, carcinoembryonic antigen, epithelial membrane antigen, and factor VIII-related antigen.[146]

A specific gene alteration for leiomyosarcoma has not yet been identified.[147]

11.2.1.2 Differential diagnosis

Histopathologically, mainly fibrosarcoma and malignant fibrous histiocytoma as well as other spindle cell tumors have to be ruled out.

11.2.2 Chondrosarcoma

Chondrosarcoma is the most common primary malignant bone neoplasm of the hand with about 4% of all malignant hand tumors; it is thus much less frequent than its benign counterpart enchondroma.[148] Whereas roughly half of the chondrosarcomas of the hand are localized in the proximal and middle phalanges, the distal phalanx is extremely rarely affected.[149–152] It is exceptional in the distal phalanx of toes;[153–155] one developed from a chondroma.[156] The prognosis of distal phalanx chondrosarcoma appears to be better than that of other hand chondrosarcomas.[157] In contrast to benign chondromas, chondrosarcomas usually present with swelling and pain.[158,159] A chronic paronychia may be mimicked.[160] X-ray films show large and relatively well-circumscribed lesions with endosteal scalloping and expanded bone contours. Extraosseous extension, small calcifications, and destruction of the cortical bone are thought to be signs of active growth.[161] Magnetic resonance imaging may be more diagnostic in early lesions. The malignant potential of distal phalanx chondrosarcoma is estimated as being low.[162] Chondrosarcomas are seen in hereditary multiple exostosis syndrome,[67] in up to 50% of multiple enchondroma syndrome of Ollier,[163] and in 18% of Maffucci–Kast syndrome.[29] Chronic radiation was supposedly the cause of one chondrosarcoma.[164]

11.2.2.1 Histopathology

Chondrosarcomas are subdivided into grade 1–3 according to the severity of cellular atypias. In grade 1 chondrosarcoma, there is only slight atypia of the chondrocytes, which are seen in an almost even hyaline ground substance. Grade 2 has more cellular atypia and the ground substance is less homogeneous.[152] Grade 3 shows frankly atypical chondrocytes irregularly scattered in an inhomogeneous ground substance. There may be mitoses and foci of calcification. Clear-cell chondrosarcoma in the distal phalanx is very rare and stands out by large tumor cells with a clear cytoplasm and distinct cell membranes.[165]

11.2.2.2 Differential diagnosis

Low-grade chondrosarcoma is extremely difficult to distinguish from chondroma.[166] Chondrosarcoma may metastasize to the nails.[167] A combination of chondrosarcoma with basaloid squamous cell carcinoma of the distal nail bed of the right middle finger was observed.[168] Cartilaginous differentiation was also observed in a subungual melanoma.[169] A "pseudoanaplastic" chondromyxoid fibroma was first thought to be high-grade chondrosarcoma or osteosarcoma.[170]

REFERENCES

1. Ragsdale BD. Tumors with fatty, muscular, osseous, and/or cartilaginous differention. In: Elder DE, ed. *Lever's Histopathology of the Skin*, 10th edn. Philadelphia: Wolters Kluwer Lippincott Williams & Wilkins, 2009; 1057–1106.
2. Richert B, André J, Choffray A, Rahier S, de la Brassinne M. Periungual lipoma: About three cases. *J Am Acad Dermatol* 2004;51(Suppl 2):S91–S93.
3. Bardazzi F, Savoia F, Fanti PA. Subungual lipoma. *Br J Dermatol* 2003;149:418.
4. Higashi N. Subungual lipoma. *Hifu* 1988;30:447–448.
5. Vélez NF, Telang GH, Robinson-Bostom L, Jellinek NJ. Subungual lipoma: Presenting as longitudinal nail splitting. *Dermatol Surg* 2014;40:1435–1437.
6. Stein AH. Benign neoplastic and nonneoplastic destructive lesions in the long bones of the hand. *Surg Gynec Obstet* 1959;109:189–197.
7. Baran R. Periungual lipoma, an unusual site. *J Dermatol Surg Oncol* 1984;10:32–33.
8. Failla JM. Subungual lipoma, squamous carcinoma of the nail bed, and secondary chronic infection. *J Hand Surg A* 1996;21:512–514.
9. Bancroft LW, Kransdorf MJ, Peterson JJ, O'Connor MI. Benign fatty tumors: Classification, clinical course, imaging appearance, and treatment. *Skeletal Radiol* 2006;35:719–733.
10. Toirkens J, De Schepper AM, Vanhoenacker F, Van Dyck P, Gielen J, Creytens D, Wouters K, Eiber M, Wörtler K, Parizel PM. A comparison between histopathology and findings on magnetic resonance imaging of subcutaneous lipomatous soft-tissue tumors. *Insights Imaging* 2011;2:599–607.
11. Kwon NH, Kim HS, Kang H, Lee JY, Kim HO, Kang SJ, Park YM. Subungual spindle cell lipoma. *Int J Dermatol* 2013;52:636–638.
12. Armijo M. Mucoid cysts of the fingers. *J Dermatol Surg Oncol* 1981;7:317–322.
13. Haneke E. Operative Therapie der myxoiden Pseudozyste. In: Haneke E, ed. *Gegenwärtiger Stand der operativen Dermatologie. Fortschritte der operativen Dermatologie 4*, Heidelberg: Springer, 1988; 221–227.
14. Eisenklam D. Über subunguale Tumoren. *Wien Klin Wschr* 1931;44:1192–1193.
15. Kaehr D, Klug MS. Subungual myxoma. *J Hand Surg Am* 1986;11:73–76.
16. Sanusi D. Subungual myxoma. *Arch Dermatol* 1982;118:612–614.
17. Winke BM, Blair WF, Benda JA. Myxomas in the fingertips. *Clin Orthop Relat Res* 1988;237:271–274.
18. Donzel JP, Martel J. Myxome digital du pouce droit. *Nouv Dermatol* 1991;10:706–707.
19. Gourdin IW, Lang PG. Cylindrical deformity of the nail plate secondary to subungual myxoma. *J Am Acad Dermatol* 1996;35:846–848.
20. Rozmaryn LM, Schwartz MA. Treatment of subungual myxoma preserving the nail matrix: A case report. *J Hand Surg* 1998;23A:178–180.
21. Carvajal L, Uraga E, Garcia I. Tumours of the hallux; myxoma, osteochondroma and enchondroma. *Skin Cancer* 1987;2:197–201.
22. Falidas E, Rallis E, Vlachos C, Konstantoudakis S, Villias C. Superficial subungual angiomyxoma: Case report and review of the literature. *J Cutan Med Surg* 2011;15:180–182.
23. Sánchez Sambucety P, Alonso TA, Agapito PG, Moran AG, Rodríguez Prieto MA. Subungual angiomyxolipoma. *Dermatol Surg* 2007;33:508–509.

24. Baran R, Haneke E. Subungual myxoid neurofibroma on the thumb. *Acta Derm Venereol* 2001;81:210–211.

25. Baran R, Perrin C. Subungual perineurioma: A peculiar location. *Br J Dermatol* 2002;146:125–128.

26. Connolly M, Hickey JR, Intzedy L, Pawade J, de Berker DA. Subungual neurothekeoma. *J Am Acad Dermatol* 2005;52:159–162.

27. Wiemeyer S, Hafer G. Neurothekeoma of the toe. *Foot Ankle Spec* 2013;6:479–481.

28. Haneke E. Dorsal finger cyst. 13th Ann Meet Soc Cutan Ultrastruct Res & Eur Soc Comp Skin Biol, Paris, May 28–31, 1986, Abstract.

29. Cremer H, Gullotta F, Wolf L. The Maffucci–Kast syndrome. Dychondroplasia with hemangiomas and frontal lobe astrocytoma. *J Cancer Res Oncol* 1981;101:231–237.

30. Takigawa K. Chondroma of the bones of the hand. *J Bone Jt Surg* 1971;53A:1591–1600.

31. Wawrosch W, Rassner G. Monströses Enchondrom des Zeigefingerendgliedes mit Nageldeformierung. *Hautarzt* 1985;36:168–169.

32. Koff AB, Goldberg LH, Ambergel D. Nail dystrophy in a 35-year-old man. Subungual enchondroma. *Arch Dermatol* 1996;132:223–226.

33. Shelley WB, Ralston EL. Paronychia due to enchondroma. *Arch Dermatol* 1964;90:412–413.

34. Pastinszky I, Dévai J. Paronychia et onchodystrophia enchondromatosa. *Börgyógy Venereol Szemle* 1968;44:176–178.

35. Dumontier CA, Abimelec P. Nail unit enchondromas and osteochondromas: A surgical approach. *Dermatol Surg* 2001;27:274–279.

36. Monsees B, Murphy AW. Distal phalangeal erosive lesions. *Arthr Rheum* 1984;27:449–455.

37. Baek HJ, Lee SJ, Cho KH, Choo HJ, Lee SM, Lee YH, Suh KJ et al. Subungual tumors: Clinicopathologic correlation with US and MR imaging findings. *Radiographics* 2010;30:1621–1636.

38. Ayala F, Lembo G, Montesano M. A rare tumor: Subungual chondroma. Report of a case. *Dermatologica* 1983;167:339–340.

39. Bauer HI, Kaatz M, Kluge WH, Elsner P. Subunguales Chondrom, ein Fallbericht. *Z Rheumatol* 2002;61:58–61.

40. Cho SB, Kim S-C. Subungual extra skeletal chondroma mimicking glomus tumour. *J Dermatol* 2003;30:492–494.

41. Connolly M, Intzedy L, Collins C, de Berker DA. Lateral views and subungual soft-tissue chondromas. *J Am Acad Dermatol* 2008;58(Suppl 2):S58–S59.

42. Ishii T, Ikeda M, Oka Y. Subungual extraskeletal chondroma with finger nail deformity: Case report. *J Hand Surg* 2010;35A:296–299.

43. Eun YS, Kim MR, Cho BK, Yoo G, Park HJ. Subungual soft tissue chondroma with nail deformity in a child. *Pediatr Dermatol* 2015;32:132–134.

44. Malhotra R, Gaur S, Dave PK, Dinda AK. Synovial chondromatosis of interphalangeal joint of the thumb: A case report. *J Hand Surg* 1994;19A:460–461.

45. Kumar A, Thomas AP. Recurrent synovial chondromatosis of the index finger—Case report and literature review. *Hand Surg* 2000;5:181–183.

46. Davis RI, Hamilton A, Biggart JD. Primary synovial chondromatosis. A clinico-pathologic review and assessment of malignant potential. *Human Pathol* 1998;29:683–688.

47. Castanedo-Cazares JP, Lepe V, Moncada B. Subungual chondroblastoma in a 9-year-old girl. *Pediatr Dermatol* 2004;21:452–453.

48. Gottschalk HP, Newbury R, Wallace CD. Synovial chondromatosis in a child's thumb: A case report and review of the literature. *Hand* 2012;7:98–102.

49. Moeller FA. Ulcerative subungual osteoma. A case report. *J Am Podiatry Assoc* 1964;54:33–34.

50. Duggar GE. Subungual osteoma. A case report. *J Am Podiatry Assoc* 1970;60:324–325.

51. Burgdorf W, Nasemann T. Cutaneous osteomas: A clinical and histopathologic review. *Arch Dermatol Res* 1977;260:121–135.

52. Blatière V, Baran R, Barneon G. An osteoma cutis of the nail matrix. *J Eur Acad Dermatol Venereol* 1999;12(Suppl 2):126.

53. Cambiaghi S, Imondi D, Gangi S, Vegni C. Fingertip calcinosis cutis. *Cutis* 2000;66:465–467.

54. Saavedra MJ, Ambrosio C, Malcata A, Matucci-Cerinic M, da Silva JA. Exuberant calcinosis and acroosteolysis. A diagnostic challenge. *Clin Exp Rheumatol* 2009;27:55–58.

55. Di Giovanni C, Laudati A. L'esostosi subungueale dell'alluce. *Arch Putti Chir Organi Mov* 1986;36:137–142.

56. Hodgkinson DJ. Subungual osteochondroma. *Plast Reconstr Surg* 1984;74:833–834.

57. Stieler W, Reinel D, Jänner M, Haneke E. Ungewöhnliche Lokalisation einer subungualen Exostose. *Akt Dermatol* 1989;15:32–34.

58. Hoehn JG, Coletta C. Subungual exostosis of the fingers. *J Hand Surg Am* 1992;17:468–471.

59. Apfelberg DB, Druker D, Maser M, Lash H. Subungual osteochondroma. *Arch Dermatol* 1979;115:472–473.

60. De Palma L, Gigante A, Specchia N. Subungual exostosis of the foot. *Foot Ankle Int* 1996;17:758–763.

61. Richert B, Baghaie M. Medical imaging and MRI in nail disorders: Report of 119 cases and review of the literature. *Dermatol Ther* 2002;15:159–164.

62. Higuchi K, Oiso N, Yoshida M, Kawada A. Preoperative assessment using magnetic resonance imaging for subungual exostosis beneath the proximal region of the nail plate. *Case Rep Dermatol* 2011;3:155–157.

63. Murphey MD, Choi JJ, Kransdorf MJ, Flemming DJ, Gannon FH. Imaging of osteochondroma: Variants and complications with radiologic-pathologic correlation. *Radiographics* 2000;20:1407–1434.

64. Sebastian G. Subunguale Exostosen der Großzehe, Berufsstigma bei Tänzern. *Dermatol Mschr* 1977;163:998–1000.

65. Davis DA, Cohen PR. Subungual exostosis: Case report and review of the literature. *Pediatr Dermatol* 1996;13:212–218.

66. Ippolito E, Falez F, Tudisco C, Balus L, Fazio M, Morrone A. Subungual exostosis. Histological and clinical considerations on 30 cases. *Ital J Orthop Traumatol* 1987;13:81–87.

67. Solomon L. Chondrosarcoma in hereditary multiple exostosis. *S Afr Med J* 1974;48:671–676.

68. Fischer E. Subunguale Verkalkungen. *Fortschr Röntgenol* 1982;137:580–584.

69. Unlu S, Demirkale I, Kalkan T, Tunc B, Bozkurt M. Large subungual exostosis of the great toe: A case report. *J Am Podiatr Med Ass* 2010;100:296–298.

70. Dal Cin P, Pauwels P, Poldermans LJ, Sciot R, Van den Berghe H. Clonal chromosome abnormalities in a so-called Dupuytren's subungual exostosis. *Genes Chromosomes Cancer* 1999;24:162–164.

71. Mertens F, Möller E, Mandahl N, Picci P, Perez-Atayde AR, Samson I, Sciot R, Debiec-Rychter M. The t(X;6) in subungual exostosis results in transcriptional deregulation of the gene for insulin receptor substrate 4. *Int J Cancer* 2011;128:487–491.

72. Zambrano E, Nosé V, Perez-Atayde AR, Gebhardt M, Hresko MT, Kleinman P, Richkind KE, Kozakewich HP. Distinct chromosomal rearrangements in subungual (Dupuytren) exostosis and bizarre parosteal osteochondromatous proliferation (Nora lesion). *Am J Surg Pathol* 2004;28:1033–1039.

73. Storlazzi CT, Wozniak A, Panagopoulos I, Sciot R, Mandahl N, Mertens F, Debiec-Rychter M. Rearrangement of the COL12A1 and COL4A5 genes in subungual exostosis: Molecular cytogenetic delineation of the tumor-specific translocation t(X;6)(q13-14;q22). *Int J Cancer* 2006;118:1972–1976.

74. Endo M, Hasegawa T, Tashiro T, Yamaguchi U, Morimoto Y, Nakatani F, Shimoda T. Bizarre parosteal osteochondromatous proliferation with a t(1;17) translocation. *Virchows Arch* 2005;447:99–102.

75. Yasuda T, Nishio J, Sumegi J, Kapels KM, Althof PA, Sawyer JR, Reith JD, Bridge JA. Aberrations of 6q13 mapped to the COL12A1 locus in chondromyxoid fibroma. *Mod Pathol* 2009;22:1499–1506.

76. Ragsdale BD. Morpholgic analysis of skeletal lesions: Correlation of imaging studies and pathologic findings. In: Reynaldo A, Weinstein RS, eds. *Advances in Pathology and Laboratory Medicine*, St Louis: Mosby-Year Book, 1993; 445–490.

77. Kim SW, Moon SE, Kim JA. A case of subungual osteochondroma. *J Dermatol* 1998;25:60–62.

78. Sherman BD, Sherman RE. Subungual osteochondroma: A case report. *J Am Podiatry Ass* 1971;61: 434–436.

79. Cavolo DJ, D'Amelio JP, Hirsch AL, Patel T. Juvenile subungual osteochondroma: Case presentation. *J Am Podiatry Ass* 1981;71:81–83.

80. Woo TY, Rasmussen JE. Subungual osteocartilaginous exostosis. *J Dermatol Surg Oncol* 1985;11: 534–536.

81. Schulze KE, Hebert AA. Diagnostic features, differential diagnosis, and treatment of subungual osteochondroma. *Pediatr Dermatol* 1994;11:39–41.

82. Winer LH. Solitary congenital nodular calcification of the skin. *Arch Dermatol Syphil* 1952;66:204–211.

83. Fischer E. Subunguale Verkalkungen im normalen Nagelbett der Finger. *Hautarzt* 1983;34:625–627.

84. Fischer E. Weichteilverkalkungen am Rand der Tuberositas phalangis distalis der Finger. *Fortschr Röntgenther* 1983;139:150–157.

85. Fischer E. Subunguale Verkalkungen im normalen Nagelbett der Zehen. *Radiologie* 1984;24:31–34.

86. Woods B, Kellaway TB. Cutaneous calculi. *Br J Dermatol* 1963;75:1–11.

87. Mendoza LE, Lavery LA, Adam RC. Calcinosis cutis circumscripta. A literature review and case report. *J Am Podiatr Med Assoc* 1990;80:97–99.

88. Jaffé HL. Osteoid osteoma. A benign osteoblastic tumor composed of osteoid and atypical bone. *Arch Surg* 1935;31:709–728.

89. Saville PD. A medical option for the treatment of osteoid osteoma. *Arthritis Rheum* 1980;23:1409–1411.

90. Rosborough D. Osteoid osteoma, report of a lesion in the terminal phalanx of a finger. *J Bone Joint Surg* 1966;48B:485–487.

91. Wold LE, Pritchard DI, Bergert I, Wilson DM. Prostaglandin synthesis by osteoid osteoma and osteoblastoma. *Mod Pathol* 1988;1:129–131.

92. Aulicino PL, DuPuy TE, Moriarity RP. Osteoid osteoma of the terminal phalanx of finger. *Orthoped Rev* 1981;10:59–63.

93. Nakatsuchi Y, Sugimoto Y, Nakano M. Osteoid osteoma of the terminal phalanx. *J Hand Surg Br* 1984;9:201–203.

94. Szabó RM, Smith B. Possible congenital osteoid osteoma of a phalanx; case report . *J Bone Joint Surg* 1985;67A:815–816.

95. Becce F, Jovanovic B, Guillou L, Theumann N. Painful finger tip swelling of the middle finger. Osteoid osteoma of the distal phalanx of the middle finger. *Skeletal Radiol* 2011;40:1479–1480.

96. Turkmen I, Alpan B, Soylemez S, Ozkan FU, Unay K, Ozkan K. Osteoid osteoma of the great toe mimicking osteomyelitis: A case report and review of the literature. *Case Rep Orthop* 2013;2013:234048.

97. Sonntag J, Engelund D. Osteoid osteoma in the distal phalanx of the thumb. *Ugeskr Laeger* 2014;176(42):ii, V12130711.

98. Bowen CVA, Dzus AK, Hardy DA. Osteoid osteomata of the distal phalanx . *J Hand Surg* 1987;12B:387–390.

99. Burger IM, McCarthy EF. Phalangeal osteoid osteomas in the hand: A diagnostic problem. *Clin Orthop Relat Res* 2004;427:198–203.

100. Crosby LA, Murphy RP. Subperiosteal osteoid osteoma of the distal phalanx of the thumb. *J Hand Surg* 1988;13A:923.

101. Shankman S, Desai P, Beltran J. Subperiosteal osteoid osteoma: Radiographic and pathologic manifestations. *Skeletal Radiol* 1997;26:457–462.

102. Foucher G, Lemarechal P, Citron N, Merle M. Osteoid osteoma of the distal phalanx. A report of four cases and review of the literature. *J Hand Surg* 1987;12B:382–386.

103. Meng Q, Watt I. Phalangeal osteoid osteoma. *Br J Radiol* 1989;62:321–325.

104. Sullivan M. Osteoid osteoma of the fingers. *Hand* 1971;3:175–178.

105. Lindbom A, Lindvall N, Sodenberg G, Spujt H. Angiography in osteoid osteoma . *Acta Radiol Stockh* 1960;54:327–333.

106. O'Hara JP, Tegmeyer C, Sweet DE, MacCue FC. Angiography in the diagnosis of osteoid osteoma of the hand. *J Bone Joint Surg* 1975;57A:163–166.

107. Braun S, Chevrot A, Tomeno B, Delbarre F, Pallardy G, Moutounet J, Kulas-Durand R. Les ostéomes ostéoides phalangiens. *Méd Hyg (Genève)* 1980;38: 1222–1229.

108. Gil S, Marco SF, Arenas J, Irurzun J, Agullo T, Alonso S, Fernandez F. Doppler duplex color localization of osteoid osteomas. *Skelet Radiol* 1999;28:107–110.

109. Thomas L, Zook EG, Haneke E, Drapé J-L, Baran R (with participation of Kreusch JF). Tumors of the nail apparatus and adjacent tissues. In Baran R, de Berker DAR, Holzberg M, Thomas L, eds. Baran & Dawber's Diseases of the Nails and Their Management. 4th ed. Wiley-Blackwell, Oxford 2012:637–743.

110. Ayala AG, Murray JA, Erling MA, Raymond AK. Osteoid osteoma: Intraoperative tetracycline fluorescence demonstration of the nidus. *J Bone Jt Surg* 1986;68A:747–751.

111. Mohsen M, Ilaslan H, Davis A, Murali Sundaram M. Subungual osteoid osteoma of the distal phalanx of the great toe. *Orthopedics* 2015;38;344:398–399.

112. Di Gennaro GL, Lampasi M, Bosco A, Donzelli O. Osteoid osteoma of the distal thumb phalanx: A case report. *Chir Organi Mov* 2008;92:179–182.

113. Nunez AL, Siegal GP, Reddy VV. CD138 (syndecan-1) expßression in bone-forming tumors. *Am J Clin Pathol* 2012;137:423–428.

114. Dancer JY, Henry SP, Bondaruk J, Lee S, Ayala AG, de Crombrugghe B, Czerniak B. Expression of master regulatory genes controlling skeletal development in benign cartilage and bone forming tumors. *Human Pathol* 2010;41:1788–1793.

115. Bertoni F, Unni KK, McLeod RA, Dahlin DC. Osteosarcoma resembling osteoblastoma. *Cancer* 1985;55:416–426.

116. Cheung FMF, Wu WC, Lam CK, Fu YK. Diagnostic criteria for pseudomalignant osteoblastoma. *Histopathology* 1997;31:196–200.

117. Averill RM, Smith RJ, Campbell CJ. Giant-cell tumors of the bones of the hand. *J Hand Surg* 1980;5:39–50.

118. Goettmann S, Baran R, Fraitag S, Salon A, Drapé JL, Belaich S. Tumeurs à cellules géantes osseuses avec atteinte unguéale. *Ann Dermatol Vénéréol* 1995;122(Suppl 1):S148–S149.

119. Fujisawa Y, Takahashi T, Kawachi Y, Otsuka F. Giant cell tumor of the distal phalanx of the foot. *Eur J Dermatol* 2006;16:204–205.

120. Yin Y, Gilula LA, Kyriakos M, Manske P. Giant-cell tumor of the distal phalanx of the hand in a child. *Clin Orthop Relat Res* 1995;310:200–207.

121. Kiatisevi P, Thanakit V, Boonthathip M, Sukanthananak B, Witoonchart K. Giant cell tumor of the distal phalanx of the biphalangeal fifth toe: A case report and review of the literature. *Foot Ankle Surg* 2011;50:598–602.

122. Bachhal V, Rangdal S, Saini U, Sament R. Giant cell tumor of distal phalanx of great toe. A case report. *Foot (Edinb)* 2011;21:198–200.

123. Kim Y, Nizami S, Goto H, Lee FY. Modern interpretation of giant cell tumor of bone: Predominantly osteoclastogenic stromal tumor. *Clin Orthop Surg* 2012;4:107–116.

124. Rosai J. Bone and joints. In: Rosai J, ed. *Rosai and Ackerman's Surgical Pathology*, 10th ed. Ch 24. Edinburgh: Elsevier Mosby, 2011;2:2043–2046.

125. Goldsmith E. Solitary bone cyst of the distal phalanx. A case report. *J Am Podiatr Ass* 1966;5:69–70.

126. Amling M, Werner M, Posl M, Maas R, Korn U, Delling G. Calcifying solitary bone cyst. Morphologic aspects and differential diagnosis of sclerotic bone tumours. *Virchows Arch* 1995;426:235–242.

127. Milbrandt T, Hopkins J. Unicameral bone cyst: Etiology and treatment. *Curr Opin Orthop* 2007;18: 555–560.

128. Afshar A. Simple bone cyst as a sequel of forearm plate osteosynthesis. *J Hand Microsurg* 2011;3:38–41.

129. Wright CJE. Benign giant-cell synovioma. An investigation of 85 cases. *Br J Surg* 1951;38:257–271.

130. Richert B, André J. Laterosubungual giant cell tumor of the tendon sheath: An unusual location. *J Am Acad Dermatol* 1999;41:347–348.

131. Abimelec P, Cambiaghi S, Thioly D, Moulonguet I, Dumontier C. Subungual giant cell tumor of the tendon sheath. *Cutis* 1996;58:273–275.

132. Batta K, Tan CY, Colloby P. Giant cell tumour of the tendon sheath producing a groove deformity of the nail plate and mimicking a myxoid cyst. *Br J Dermatol* 1999;140:720–728.

133. Pulitzer DR, Martin PC, Reed RJ. Fibroma of tendon sheath. A clinicopathologic study of 32 cases. *Am J Surg Pathol* 1989;13:472–479.

134. Hosaka M, Hatori M, Smith R, Kokubun S. Giant cell formation through fusion of cells derived from a human giant cell tumor of tendon sheath. *J Orthop Sci* 2004;9:581–584.

135. Rao AS, Vigorita VJ. Pigmented villonodular synovitis (giant cell tumor of the tendon sheath and synovial membrane). A review of eighty-one cases. *J Bone Jt Surg* 1984;66:76–94.

136. O'Connell JY, Fanburg JC, Rosenberg AE. Giant cell tumor of tendon sheath and pigmented villonodular synovitis: Immunophenotype suggests a synovial cell origin. *Hum Pathol* 1995;26:771–775.

137. Maluf HM, DeYoung BR, Swanson PE, Wick MR. Fibroma and giant cell tumor of tendon sheath: A comparative histological and immunohistological study. *Mod Pathol* 1995;8:155–159.

138. Wood GS, Beckstead JH, Medeiros LJ, Kempson RL, Warnke RA. The cells of giant cell tumor of tendon sheath resemble osteoclasts. *Am J Surg Pathol* 1988;12:444–452.

139. Neale SD, Kristelly R, Gundle R, Quinn JM, Athanasou NA. Giant cells in pigmented villonodular synovitis express an osteoclast phenotype. *J Clin Pathol* 1997;50:605–608.

140. Alguacil-Garcia A, Unni K, Goellner JR. Giant cell tumor of tendon sheath and pigmented villonodular synovitis: An ultrastructural study. *Am J Clin Pathol* 1978;69:6–17.

141. Satti MB. Tendon sheath tumors, a pathological study of the relationship between giant cell tumour and fibromas of tendon sheath. *Histopathology* 1992;20:213–220.

142. Park SY, Jin SP, Yeom B, Kim SW, Cho SY, Lee JH. Multiple fibromas of tendon sheath: Unusual presentation. *Ann Dermatol* 2011;23(Suppl 1):S45–S47.

143. Davidson LL, Frost ML, Hanke CW, Epinette WW. Primary leiomyosarcoma of the skin. Case report and review of the literature. *J Am Acad Dermatol* 1989;21:1156–1160.

144. Kaddu S, Beham A, Cerroni L, Humer-Fuchs U, Salmhofer W, Kerl H, Soyer HP. Cutaneous leiomyosarcoma. *Am J Surg Pathol* 1997;21:979–987.

145. Weedon D. *Skin Pathology*, 2nd edn. London: Churchill Livingstone, 2002.

146. Bryant J. Subungual epithelioid leiomyosarcoma. *South Med J* 1992;85:560–561.

147. Shmulevich I, Hunt K, El Naggar A, Taylor E, Randas L, Laborde P, Hess KR, Pollock R, Zhang W. Tumor specific gene expression profiles in human leiomyosarcoma: An evaluation of intratumor heterogeneity. *Cancer* 2002;94:2069–2075.

148. Palmieri TJ. Chondrosarcoma of the hand. *J Hand Surg Am* 1984;9A:332–338.

149. Patil S, De Silva MVC, Crossan J, Reid R. Chondrosarcama of small bones of the hand. *J Hand Surg Br* 2003;28-B:602–608.

150. Sivridis E, Verettas D. Chondrosarcoma in the distal phalanx of the ring finger. A case report. *Acta Orthop Scand* 1990;61:183–184.

151. Debruyne PR, Dumez H, Demey W, Gillis L, Sciot R, Schöffski P. Recurrent low- to intermediate-grade chondrosarcoma of the thumb with lung metastases: An objective response to trofosfamide. *Onkologie* 2007;30:201–204.

152. Tos P, Artiaco S, Linari A, Battiston B. Chondrosarcoma in the distal phalanx of index finger: Clinical report and literature review. *Chir Main* 2009;28:265–269.

153. Masuda T, Otuka T, Yonezawa M, Kamiyama F, Shibata Y, Tada T, Matsui N. Chondrosarcoma of the distal phalanx of the second toe: A case report. *J Foot Ankle Surg* 2004;43:110–112.

154. Hatori M, Watanabe M, Kokubun S. Chondrosarcoma of the distal phalanx of the great toe. *J Am Podiatr Med Assoc* 2007;97:156–159.

155. Mondal SK. Chondrosarcoma of the distal phalanx of the right great toe: Report of a rare malignancy and review of literature. *J Cancer Res Ther* 2012;8:123–125.

156. Koak YP, Patil PS, Mackenny RP. Chondrosarcoma of the distal phalanx of a toe. A case report. *Acta Orthop Belg* 2000;66:286–288.

157. Mittermayer F, Dominkus M, Krepler P, Schwameis E, Sluga M, Toma C, Lang S, Grampp S, Kotz R. Chondrosarcoma of the hand. Is a wide surgical resection necessary? *Clin Orthop Relat Res* 2004;424:211–215.

158. Gargan TJ, Kanter W, Wolfort FG. Multiple chondrosarcomas of the hand. *Ann Plast Surg* 1984;12:542–546.

159. Dahlin DC, Salvador AH. Chondrosarcomas of the bones of the hands and feet. A study of 30 cases. *Cancer* 1974;34:755–760.

160. Marcove RC, Charosky CB. Phalangeal sarcomas simulating infections of the digits. *Clin Orthop Relat Res* 1972;83:224–231.

161. Bellinghausen HW, Weeks PM, Young LV, Gilula LA. Roentgen Rounds 64. Chondrosarcoma. *Orthoped Rev* 1983;XII:97–100.

162. Bovée JV, van der Heul RO, Taminiau AH, Hogendoorn PC. Chondrosarcoma of the phalanx: A locally aggressive lesion with minimal metastatic potential: A report of 35 cases and a review of the literature. *Cancer* 1999;86:1724–1732.

163. Nakajima H, Ushigome S, Fukuda J. Case report 482: Chondrosarcoma (grade 1) arising from the right second toe in patient with multiple enchondroma. *Skelet Radiol* 1988;17:289–292.

164. Carroll RE, Godwin JT. Osteogenic sarcoma of phalanx after chronic Roentgen-ray irradiation. *Cancer* 1956;9:753–755.

165. Engels C, Werner M, Delling G. Clear-cell chondrosarcoma. *Pathologe* 2000;21:449–455.

166. Gottschalk RG, Smith RT. Chondrosarcoma of the hand. *J Bone Joint Surg* 1963;45A:141–150.

167. Ramseier LE, Dumont CE, Exner GU. Multiple subungual soft tissue metastases from a chondrosarcoma. *Scand J Plast Reconstr Surg Hand Surg* 2007;41:332–333.

168. Lee EK, Yoon DH, Tim TY, Kim CW, Lee HK, Kang SJ. Carcinosarcoma of the skin. A new combination of squamous cell carcinoma and chondrosarcoma. *Ann Dermatol* 1998;10:81–85.

169. Cachia AR, Kedziora AM. Subungual malignant melanoma with cartilaginous differentiation . *Am J Dermatopathol* 1999;21:165–169.

170. Bahk WJ, Mirra JM, Sohn KR, Shin DS. Pseudoanaplastic chondromyxoid fibroma. *Ann Diagn Pathol* 1998;2:241–246.

Neurogenic tumors

12

There are many different tumors of the peripheral nerves that can be found in and around the nail organ. The diagnosis is sometimes difficult and based on morphologic similarity with structures of the peripheral nerves, on the development of their neurocristic precursors, and reactions of nerves to injury and regeneration.[1] Various cells like neurosustentacular, some mesenchymal cells, and melanocytes are of neuroectodermal origin and share a common progenitor. Thus, they have a number of cell markers in common but they can also, in part, be differentiated with other immunohistochemical markers. Protein S100 is expressed by Schwann cells, glial cells, melanocytes, secretory cells of eccrine sweat glands, fat cells, and chondrocytes. Neurofilaments can only be demonstrated in axons, which are also demonstrable by silver impregnation. Neuron-specific enolase is produced by Schwann cells, neurons, and axons. Myelin is demonstrated with antibodies to myelin basic protein, CD57 (Leu 7), and Luxol fast blue stain. Glial fibrillary acidic protein is a constituent of glial cells, but it is also positive in some Schwann cells of large soft tissue schwannomas and in some salivary gland tumor cells.[1] Perineurial cells as well as sebaceous cells are positive for epithelial membrane antigen.

Whereas some tumors of neural tissue may be tender or painful, others are completely asymptomatic.

This is not the place for a systematic review of neurogenic tumors; in contrast, the relatively few of them occurring in the nail are listed more according to their morphology.

12.1 BENIGN NEUROGENIC TUMORS

12.1.1 Neuroma

Neuromas of the distal phalanx of the digits usually occur posttraumatically or postoperatively.[2] They occur at any age. Being under the nail they may elevate the nail plate and cause nail dystrophy and tenderness. Neuromas after surgery of the distal phalanx are palpated as tender areas or firm papules in or next to the scar. Lancinating pain may indicate an amputation neuroma.[3,4]

An encapsulated palisaded neuroma of the proximal nail fold resembled a myxoid pseudocyst.[5]

In the multiple mucosal neuroma syndrome,[6] probably multiple endocrine neoplasia syndrome (MEN) type 2B, thickening of the proximal nail fold was observed. Clinical differential diagnosis is glomus tumor and a variety of other painful nail lesions.

12.1.1.1 Histopathology

Traumatic neuromas are not true tumors, but usually a reparative process. They consist of an increased and disorganized number of myelinated nerve fascicles of different sizes and shapes running in various directions. Mucin may be found in the nerves (Figure 12.1). They are embedded in a fibrotic stroma, which may sometimes even be myxoid,[7] but this is not a consistent feature. A true capsule does not exist. The distal end of the regenerating nerve may infiltrate the fibrous tissue. The cells are slender spindle cells and constitute of Schwann cells, perineurial cells, and endoneural fibroblasts. Silver impregnation exhibits the axons showing a 1:1 ratio of axons and Schwann cells. Neural markers such as protein S100 and neurofilament are strongly positive: neurofilament stain highlights the axons, the myelin is positive for myelin basic protein and CD57 (Leu-7), whereas S100 as well as collagen IV stain the Schwann cells. Neurofilament stain may appear as a fine dot when the axon is cut perpendicularly or as a slender long thread-like structure when cut longitudinally. Epithelial membrane antigen is positive in the perineurial cells around the nerve bundles.

Neuromas in the multiple mucosal neuroma syndrome exhibit multiple small nodules of numerous tortuous nerve fibers without an evident capsule.

Encapsulated palisaded neuroma is a well circumscribed, round or oval nodule in the dermis surrounded by a thin fibrous capsule, which is less pronounced or absent at the portion facing the epidermis. It shows large and well-delimited nerve fascicles that are separated by cleft-like spaces. The cells have oval nuclei with an evenly distributed chromatin and their cytoplasm is eosinophilic. Rarely, the nuclei may be arranged in a palisading pattern reminiscent of Verocay bodies (Figure 12.2). Mitoses are absent. Silver impregnation reveals abundant axons. Immunohistochemistry confirms that the tumor is composed of nerves.[8]

12.1.1.2 Differential diagnosis

The neurofilament positivity allows distinguishing neuromas from neurofibromas and schwannomas. Supernumerary

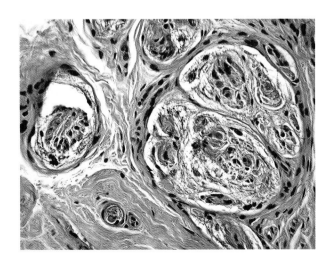

Figure 12.1 Traumatic neuroma.

(a)

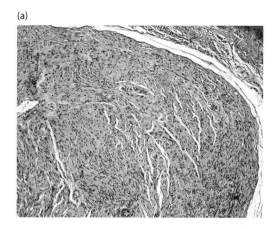

(b)

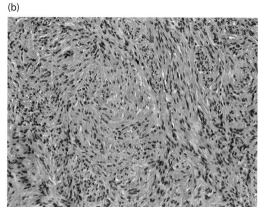

Figure 12.2 (a,b) Palisaded neuroma.

rudimentary digit also shows an increased number of nerves per square unit. Multiple systematized fibrillar neurofibromas were only described once under the nail and in the fingertip;[9] they are not unequivocally distinguishable. Solitary circumscribed neuroma and palisaded encapsulated neuroma are extremely rare in the nail region. In the multiple mucosal neuroma syndrome, there are more scattered individual nerve fibers in the dermis. When they form small nodules, there are no intersecting fascicles and no clefts, but they can have a mucin-rich stroma.[10] Schwannoma has a thick collagenous capsule[11] whereas the neuromas are surrounded by a somewhat thinner perineurium.[12,13]

12.1.2 Rudimentary supernumerary finger

The rudimentary supernumerary finger is usually localized at the lateral aspect of the fifth metacarpo-phalangeal joint and is seen as a small, slightly hyperkeratotic or verrucous nodule. It is usually symmetrical. Rarely, it may cause pain.[14] It is often treated by suture ligation and left for auto-amputation; hence, it may develop an amputation neuroma. Early excision and removal of the accessory digital nerve can prevent the development of this peculiar type of amputation neuroma.[15]

12.1.2.1 Histopathology

The supernumerary digit presents as a polypoid lesion with hyperkeratotic epidermis and a proliferation of myelinated nerves at its base around a fibrous core. Bone is not present. In addition, a large number of Meissner corpuscles are seen in the dermal papillae. They are thought to play a role in the development of cutaneous nerve plexus.[16]

12.1.2.2 Differential diagnosis

The main differential diagnosis is neuroma, particularly when the location of the excision specimen was not indicated.

12.1.3 Pacinian neuroma

Pacinian neuroma or hyperplasia is a rare observation and mostly occurs where Pacini bodies are found normally.[17] It may grow as an asymptomatic lesion[18] or cause tenderness and pain spontaneously or on probing.[19,20] On extirpation,

many tiny sand grain-like ivory colored structures can be seen with the naked eye that seem to fall apart when removed from their "host site." About half of the cases were seen to develop after a trauma.[21]

12.1.3.1 Histopathology

Histologically, four types of Pacinian neuroma were described: (1) a single enlarged corpuscle, (2) a grape-like structure of normal-sized Pacinian corpuscles, (3) slightly enlarged corpuscles arranged in tandem, and (4) hyperplastic Pacinian corpuscles arranged along the entire length of a digital nerve.[22] Types 3 and 4 were considered later as the same category.[23] In the nail region, mainly type 3 is observed. Pacinian neuroma or Pacinian hyperplasia is rare. Vater-Pacini bodies are mainly found in the subdermal tissue of the pulp of the finger and are virtually never seen in the nail bed or nail folds. When they are seen there they probably represent an abnormal event. Pacinian neuromas are made up of myelinated nerve fibers and many Pacini bodies that appear structurally normal. There is no capsule formation (Figure 12.3).

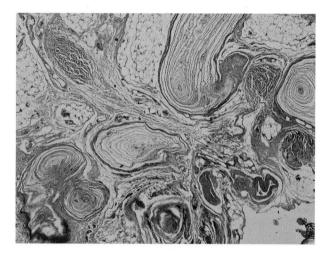

Figure 12.3 Pacinian neuroma in proximal-lateral nail fold junction of the thumb of a 58-year-old man. The lesion was tender and painful on probing.

12.1.3.2 Differential diagnosis

Plexiform perineurioma was misdiagnosed as a Pacinian neuroma.[24]

12.1.4 Neurofibroma

Neurofibromas are common tumors of the Schwann cells of cutaneous nerves. They occur as solitary lesions or there may be hundreds or thousands of neurofibromas in neurofibromatosis. In the nail, however, virtually all the few neurofibromas observed were isolated, so-called extraneural sporadic cutaneous neurofibromas, and not in association with any type of neurofibromatosis.[25] Clinically, they may appear as a Koenen tumor-like lesion, grow subungually elevating the nail, or causing nail dystrophy.[26–28] Those of the proximal nail fold cause a longitudinal depression in the nail.[29,30] Location in the lateral nail fold may imitate paronychia.[31] Ulcerated neurofibromas look like periungual pyogenic granuloma. Enlargement of the distal phalanx is a rare aspect.[32] Pain is uncommon.[33]

12.1.4.1 Histopathology

Neurofibromas of the nail are identical with neurofibromas of the skin elsewhere. They are faintly eosinophilic, circumscribed, but not encapsulated lesions. They consist of loosely and often haphazardly arranged thin spindle cells with elongated wavy nuclei that are regularly spaced in a meshwork of fine wavy collagen fibers. There may be a heterogeneous appearance due to multiple cell populations including Schwann cells, fibroblasts, and mast cells (Figure 12.4). PAS stain shows that all cells have a fine basal membrane. Mast cells can easily be discerned and are moderately increased in number. This is also seen in the myxoid variant.[32] Immunohistochemistry is positive for protein S100 and a variety of other neural and Schwann cell markers, but some axons may also be seen with silver impregnation as well as neurofilament and neuron-specific enolase stains; the latter also lightly decorates the enveloping Schwann cells.

12.1.4.2 Differential diagnosis

Neuromas and schwannomas are the main differential diagnosis in neurofibromas of the nail apparatus. Schwannoma is an intraneural encapsulated lesion not containing axons; they are characterized by Antoni A and Antoni B patterns, the former being part of the Verocay body. Neurotized melanocytic nevi present with Meissner body-like structures in the deep part, but they have not been observed in the nail apparatus.

12.1.5 Schwannoma

Schwannoma is also called neurilemmoma. It is an expansile benign tumor that extends along peripheral nerves. Localization in digits[34,35] and the nail is rare.[36–41] Occasionally, neurilemmomatosis is seen characterized by multiple disseminated benign schwannomas.

12.1.5.1 Histopathology

Schwannoma is a well-circumscribed Schwann cell tumor that often displaces its nerve to the periphery. Two patterns are differentiated: In the Antoni A type, uniform spindle cells are arranged back to back and each cell is surrounded by a delicate basement membrane identified by PAS staining. These cells cluster in stacks with their nuclei often forming columns. Two neighboring palisades with the intervening Schwann cell cytoplasm form a Verocay body; this pattern was also seen in a subungual schwannoma. The Antoni B tissue is made up of end to end arranged Schwann cells and single cells that are loosely spaced in a clear or myxoid matrix (Figure 12.5). Vascular changes were not seen under the nail. Immunohistochemically, the Schwann cells are positive for neural markers such as S100, but also for collagen type IV and laminin. The cells in the capsule are positive for EMA. Axons are usually not seen.

12.1.5.2 Differential diagnosis

Neurofibroma and palisaded encapsulated neuroma contain axons not seen in schwannoma.

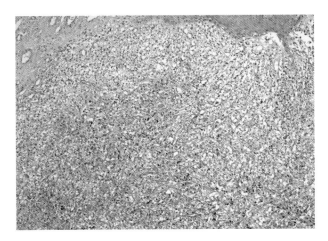

Figure 12.4 Subungual neurofibroma of the second toe.

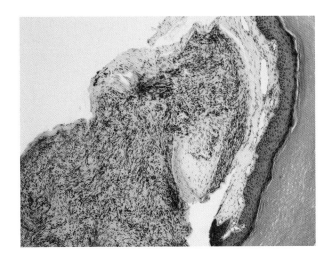

Figure 12.5 Subungual schwannoma, B type. (Courtesy of Dr. N. G. Di Chiacchio, Sao Paulo, Brazil.)

12.1.6 Cellular neurothekeoma

Neurothekeomas are tumors of the nerve sheath. They occur mainly in the upper body of children and young adults. In skin, they are firm, pink to red-brown papules or nodules of 5–30 mm in diameter. One case was described under the nail of the little toe.[42] This lesion was incompletely resected but did not recur.

12.1.6.1 Histopathology

The classification of neurothekeomas is somewhat confusing.[43,44] Cellular neurothekeoma consists of fascicles of closely packed, mostly spindle-shaped cells with a clear cytoplasm and plump rounded nuclei. Occasional mitoses and multinucleate cells may occur; the latter phenomenon is reminiscent of plexiform fibrous histiocytoma. The so-called B pattern shows admixed myxoid components.

Immunohistochemically, the phenotype is inconsistent. Vimentin and CD10 are positive, but S100 and EMA are generally nonreactive. Smooth muscle actin, collagen type IV, NK1/C3, and CD57 are weak or negative.[45] Its exact histogenesis is still not known, but most probably not neurogenic.

12.1.6.2 Differential diagnosis

Cellular neurothekeoma has to be differentiated from nerve sheath myxoma. Granular cell tumor is more epithelioid and positive for S100. Nerve sheath myxoma is positive for S100 and glial fibrillary acidic protein.

12.1.7 Nerve sheath myxoma

This benign neural tumor is clinically nonspecific. Most cases occur in middle-aged persons in the extremities, particularly on digits, as painless firm nodules. Nail involvement is rare and has been erroneously diagnosed as cellular neurothekeoma in one case.[46]

12.1.7.1 Histopathology

Generally, it is well delimited and consists of several round to oval lobules that are separated from each other and occupy the whole dermis. The overlying epidermis may be thinned. Low magnification reveals a light but basophilic tumor. This is due to an Alcian blue positive mucinous substance in which fusiform cells with elongated nuclei abound. They are often arranged in parallel and frequently show small clear vacuoles. The cells have a very light cytoplasm that stains strongly for protein S100 and neuron-specific enolase but is negative for EMA and CD34 allowing the tumor to be distinguished from cellular neurothekeoma.[47] It is estimated to be of Schwann cell origin.

12.1.7.2 Differential diagnosis

Of the other neurogenic tumors occurring on digits, schwannoma has a different morphology and architecture. Neurofibroma is less myxoid even though myxoid neurofibroma has been observed under the nail. Traumatic neuroma contains nerve bundles often in a myxoid stroma. Perineuriomas are much denser and cellular and are positive for EMA.[47]

12.1.8 Granular cell tumor

Granular cell tumor is predominantly a tumor of middle-aged adults. It is about three times more frequent in women. Almost three-quarters are localized in the head and neck region. Most commonly, the skin and subcutis are involved; particularly typical is its localization in the tongue. Granular cell tumor of the nail was observed as a verrucous periungual growth in the deep medial portion of the proximal nail fold of a big toe causing a longitudinal depression in the nail[48] or as an enlargement of the middle toe overgrowing the nail.[49] There may be tenderness of the lesion.

12.1.8.1 Histopathology

Granular cell tumor, originally called granular cell myoblastoma or Abrikosoff's tumor, is an indistinctly circumscribed lesion often observed in the tongue where its cells seemingly mix with, or were thought to derive from, the striated muscle cells. It is now clear that the tumor cells are large granular Schwann cells. They are arranged in poorly cohesive nests, strands, and sheets of large cells. They may infiltrate the dermis and perineural spread is not uncommon. The cell clusters may or may not be surrounded by collagen fiber strands. The tumor cells are large with an indistinct cell membrane, centrally positioned nuclei, pale cytoplasm filled with light eosinophilic round granules. These granules are weakly PAS positive and PAS stain renders the cell boundaries well discernible as it stains their individual basal membrane. Bright, intensely eosinophilic ovoid bodies in a clear halo are occasionally present and thought to be residual giant lysosomes. Spindle cells with a fibroblast-like appearance are scattered between the granular cells. Histiocyte-like cells with triangular granular eosinophilic lysosomes are called angulate bodies. The overlying epidermis often exhibits a pseudo-epitheliomatous hyperplasia. The tumor stains positive with Schwann cell markers such as protein S100 (Figure 12.6), PGP9.5, neuron-specific enolase, nerve-growth factor receptor, P2-P0, calretinin, myelin basic protein, and

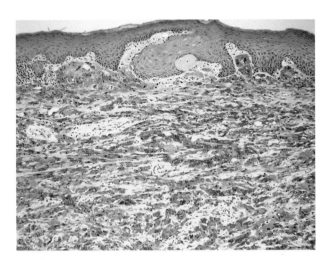

Figure 12.6 Granular cell tumor (Protein S100 demonstration).

CD57, but also some histiocytic markers such as CD68 and α1-antitrypsin. In addition, vimentin is consistently positive. However, neurofilaments and glial fibrillary acidic protein cannot be demonstrated.[50–54]

12.1.8.2 Differential diagnosis

Rhabdomyoma may have a strikingly similar cytology.

12.1.9 Perineurioma

Perineurioma is an uncommon tumor thought to derive from perineurial cells. It is a solitary, well-circumscribed tumor with symmetrical growth, most frequently in the subcutaneous tissue. It is in fact a fibroma that expresses the immunocytochemical markers of perineurial cells, that is, epithelial membrane antigen. Subungual location is very rare.[55,56] One case caused clubbing of the involved digit.[57]

12.1.9.1 Histopathology

Perineurioma is a well-circumscribed lesion separated from its surrounding tissue by a thin fibrous capsule, which may not be seen when the tumor is shelled out meticulously. Within this capsule, a delicate fibrous matrix is formed by fine collagen fibers. This matrix harbors slender fusiform cells with bipolar cytoplasmic processes and plump angulated basophilic nuclei. Small nerves may be seen in concentrically arranged cell formations. Storiform areas may be present.[58] The myxoid component can be important. Immunohistochemistry shows a strong positivity for vimentin, epithelial membrane antigen, and in some cases also CD34. S100 protein, α-smooth muscle actin, desmin, and keratins are negative.

12.1.9.2 Differential diagnosis

Sclerosing perineurioma has a predilection for the fingers and palms. It is very small and heavily collagenized. Its perineurial cells are epithelioid and grow in strands or trabeculae.[59]

12.2 MALIGNANT NEUROGENIC AND NEUROENDOCRINE TUMORS

12.2.1 Merkel cell carcinoma

Merkel cell carcinoma is a rare cutaneous malignant neoplasm first described as trabecular carcinoma.[60] Other synonyms are cutaneous neuroendocrine carcinoma, cutaneous APUDoma, and primary small cell carcinoma of the skin. Most patients are Caucasians;[61] it is exceptional in black individuals. It is about double as frequent in men as in women. Sun-exposed skin is the main location. Etiologically, chronic sun damage and immunosuppression were thought to be responsible, but recently a specific virus, the Merkel cell polyomavirus (MCPyV), was identified in about 80% of the cases.[62–65] Head and neck as well as extremities are mainly involved whereas digital localization is very rare. The tumors are solitary, dome-shaped, painless, red to violaceous, and have a fast growth rate. Most nodules are around 2 cm in diameter,

but larger tumors may occur.[66] Merkel cell carcinomas have a high local recurrence rate and tend to metastasize to the regional lymph nodes until they finally spread hematogenously and/or via the lymphatics.[67] Early and radical surgery is indicated, and many authors recommend postoperative radiotherapy.

Merkel cell carcinoma was seen on the left big toe of a teenage girl.[68] The tumor mimicked granulation tissue associated with an ingrown nail on the medial aspect of the toe. At the junction of the lateral nail fold and the nail bed, a deep red, focally ulcerated, granular nodule was observed. The section of the surgical specimen showed a poorly delineated tumor consisting of brown hemorrhagic tissue measuring 0.7 cm in diameter. We have seen a case of an ulcerated violaceous tumor clinically diagnosed as a giant pyogenic granuloma on the distal dorsal aspect of the middle phalanx of the left middle finger in a 73-year-old woman.

12.2.1.1 Histopathology

The histopathology of Merkel cell carcinoma is sufficiently characteristic in most cases to make the diagnosis on hematoxylin and eosin stained sections alone. It is a blue tumor that may extend into the subcutaneous fat. Although first described as trabecular carcinoma of the skin, this tumor pattern (Figure 12.7) is not so common in contrast to diffuse sheets and solid tumor cell nests. It is composed of uniform small cells with a round to oval nucleus. The cytoplasm is scant and a cell membrane is often not seen. The nuclear membrane, however, is distinct. The chromatin is finely dispersed. The nucleoli are small and inconspicuous. There are numerous mitoses, often nuclear fragments and apoptotic cells. Focally, spindle cells may be seen. Rarely a pagetoid pattern of epidermal involvement is seen.[69] Epidermal necrosis is not common. Lymphatic invasion is occasionally seen. Sometimes regression occurs.[70] An association with a superficial or even invasive squamous cell carcinoma has repeatedly been described,[71] though this is not a feature of Merkel cell carcinoma of the nail apparatus.

Immunohistochemistry exhibits both epithelial as well as neuroendocrine differentiation (Figure 12.7). Low molecular weight cytokeratins as demonstrated by the Merkel cell-characteristic CK 20[72,73] and pan-cytokeratin antibodies such as AE1/AE3 and CAM5.2, as well as epithelial membrane antigen and BER-EP4, are positive. The keratin staining is typically a paranuclear dot, but other patterns may rarely be observed. Neuroendocrine markers are neuron-specific enolase, chromogranin, synaptophysin, bombesin, calcitonin, gastrin, and somatostatin. The KIT receptor tyrosine kinase CD117 and in about 30% also CD99 are expressed.[74] These markers are particularly useful to trace single carcinoma cells that may be seen outside the tumor masses. As mentioned above, MCPyV can be demonstrated in the majority of tumors with the antibody CM2B4.[62,65]

Electron microscopy shows the paranuclear clumps of cytokeratin filaments even in formalin-fixed tissue.[75] Flow

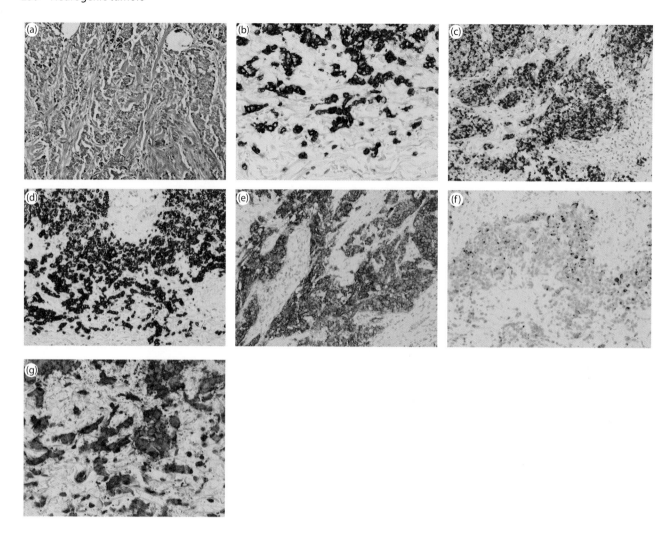

Figure 12.7 Merkel cell carcinoma: (a) H&E stain shows densely packed cells mostly without discernible cell membrane. The nuclei are oval, often with light chromatin. (b) Immunostain for pan-cytokeratin (AE1/AE3) exhibits a diffuse positivity of virtually all tumor cells. (c) Cytokeratin 20 demonstration marks most tumor cells often as a paranuclear dot. (d) CAM5.2 is an antibody marking a portion of low molecular weight cytokeratins and intensely stains MCC cells. (e) CD56 demonstration shows a diffuse positivity of most of the Merkel cell carcinoma. (f) Neurofilament staining is restricted to paranuclear dots. (g) Most tumor cells are intensely positive for neuron-specific enolase.

cytometry revealed a polyclonal pattern.[76] Comparative genomic hybridization showed a number of chromosomal losses and gains, deletions of 5q12-21 and 13q14-21 as well as focal amplification at 1p34.[77]

12.2.1.2 Differential diagnosis

There are many small cell tumors that may be similar to Merkel cell carcinoma. Basal cell carcinoma has a characteristic palisading of its peripheral cells, shows peripheral clefting between the tumor cells and the connective tissue, is usually well delimited, does not have so many mitoses, apoptotic cells are not commonly identified, and cytokeratins of trichilemmal sheath are positive, but no neuroendocrine markers. Small cell undifferentiated squamous cell carcinoma is positive for pan-cytokeratin, but negative for neuroendocrine markers. Amelanotic small cell melanoma usually has a distinctive cell membrane and is positive for the melanocyte markers like protein S100,

Melan-A, Mart 1, and HMB45, which are negative in Merkel cell carcinoma. Lymphomas usually express leukocyte common antigen. Metastatic neuroblastoma is protein S100 positive. Metastatic neuroendocrine carcinoma is mostly cytokeratin 20 negative and thyroid transcription factor-1 positive whereas Merkel cell carcinoma is positive for CK20 and negative for TTF-1.[78] Small cell lung carcinoma is negative for Merkel cell polyoma virus.[79,80] Ewing sarcoma/primary malignant peripheral primitive neuroectodermal tumor is positive for CD99, β-microglobulin, FLI-1, some more neuroendocrine markers, and Leu-7, but negative for chromogranin.

12.2.2 Ewing sarcoma

Two forms of Ewing sarcoma are distinguished: skeletal and extraskeletal. The latter is cytogenetically and molecular genetically identical to primary malignant peripheral primitive neuroectodermal tumor (PNET) with Ewing sarcoma being less differentiated than PNET. Ewing sarcomas and PNET have been observed on the head, trunk, and extremities. They present as commonly painless, sometimes tender nodules with a diameter of 5–10 cm that are not ulcerated. Polypoid form is possible.[81,82] Multiple tumors are very rare.[83] One case of probably skeletal Ewing sarcoma was described in the tip of a toe. X-ray film showed a lytic lesion in the distal phalanx. Clinically, a swelling with ulceration of the digital pulp was seen.[84,85] Another case was seen in a patient with nail patella syndrome.[86] A subungual Ewing sarcoma was observed by F. Facchetti (personal communication 2012). Distal phalanx Ewing sarcoma of the bone was successfully treated by amputation.[87]

12.2.2.1 Histopathology

Extraskeletal Ewing sarcoma occupies the dermis but may extend into the subcutis. The margins are infiltrative or pushing. The epidermis may be necrotic. The tumor cells are arranged in lobules, nests, trabeculae, or sheets. They are uniformly small, round to oval with vesicular or hyperchromatic nuclei. The cytoplasm is scant, pale eosinophilic, or vacuolated with no clearly visible cell membrane. Nucleoli are often not seen or small. There are varying numbers of mitoses and many dark apoptotic cells. Fibrovascular septa may demonstrate a pseudopapillary or epitheliomatous cell arrangement with occasional glomeruloid tufts of the stromal blood vessels. Intracytoplasmic glycogen can be seen in PAS stains. Some tumors contain larger and pleomorphic cells with prominent nucleoli as well as groups of rhabdoid or plasmocytoid cells. Reticulin stain demonstrates fibers around cell groups.

Immunohistochemistry reveals positivity for vimentin, strong diffuse and membrane CD99, a MIC2 gene product, β2-microglobulin, nuclear FLI-1 gene product, and some more neural/neuroendocrine markers such as neuron-specific enolase, neurofilament proteins, Leu-7, PGP9.5, and synaptophysin whereas chromogranin is usually negative. Some scattered cells may show aberrant positivity for cytokeratins, glial fibrillary acidic protein, desmin, protein S100, and NKIC3. The tumor does not exhibit leukocyte common antigen, B and T lymphocyte markers, myeloperoxidase, muscle-specific actin, myogenin, MYO-D1, HMB45, or epithelial membrane antigen.[79]

Electron microscopy of Ewing sarcoma exhibits cells with round to slightly oval nuclei and few organelles.[79]

Approximately 85% of both skeletal and extraskeletal Ewing sarcomas as well as PNETs show the characteristic chromosomal translocation t(11;22)(q24;q12) leading to fusion of the Ewing sarcoma gene on chromosome 22q12 with the FLI-1 gene on 11q24.[88]

12.2.2.2 Differential diagnosis

The tumor cells may mimic lymphoma, leukemia, diffuse Merkel cell carcinoma, amelanotic melanoma, metastatic neuroblastoma, metastases of small cell neuroendocrine carcinoma, rhabdosarcoma, eccrine spiradenocarcinoma, and other types of small cell carcinoma. Most of these tumors can be ruled out on careful evaluation of cellular details and characteristic immunohistochemical findings. The markers CD79a, CD43, TdT, CD10, and CD34 are useful if lymphoma is suspected, as none of them are seen in Ewing sarcoma. Gene rearrangement by PCR can be of great value in controversial cases. Positive IgH-R or TCR-R, never positive in Ewing's sarcoma, will support the diagnosis of lymphoma or lymphoblastic leukemia. Similarly demonstration of EWS/FL-1 fusion transcript by RT-PCR will support the diagnosis of ES/PNET.[89]

12.2.3 Malignant schwannoma

Malignant schwannoma is rare. It is usually not diagnosed clinically. The main sign is an uncharacteristic swelling. When occurring in the distal digit, nail dystrophy is the leading sign.[90]

12.2.3.1 Histopathology

Most cases are low-grade malignant schwannomas with occasional Verocay bodies and fusiform cells and a mitotic count of 2–3 per 10 high-power fields.

12.2.3.2 Differential diagnosis

Benign schwannoma (neurilemmoma) and neurofibroma have to be distinguished.

12.2.4 Malignant granular cell tumor

Granular cell tumors are defined as proliferations of large cells with a characteristic granular cytoplasm. Most derive from modified Schwann cells but other granular cell origins are also known. Malignant granular cell tumor is exceedingly rare. Most cases occur on the extremities. They grow rapidly with local invasion and may ulcerate. Extensive metastases are the rule. One subungual case was seen in the right index finger of a 51-year-old woman. It recurred two years after surgery and was then eroded and 2.5 cm in diameter. Despite finger amputation, the patient developed metastases and died shortly thereafter.[91]

12.2.4.1 Histopathology

Malignant granular cell tumor may be almost identical to its benign counterpart with only minimal cellular atypia and few mitoses. It is then the clinical size, its rapid growth, and ulceration that should raise suspicion. More than 2 mitoses per 10 high-power fields may be a hint at malignancy. Another type even less frequent than the first one is frankly malignant with cytologic atypia of the granular tumor cells and many mitoses. The subungual malignant granular cell tumor exhibited polygonal eosinophilic granular cells with mitoses and some multinucleated giant cells. In the metastasis, anaplastic cells were seen in addition. Immunohistochemistry (protein S100, Leu 7, vimentin) and electron microscopy confirmed the diagnosis of malignant granular cell tumor.

Immunohistochemistry is similar to the benign granular cell tumor, which is positive for the neural markers protein S100, neuron specific enolase, nerve growth factor receptor,[51] PGP9.5,[92] calretinin,[93] myelin basic protein and peripheral myelin proteins, CD57, and P2-P0, but also for the histiocytic markers CD68 and α-antitrypsin.[94,95] The proliferation marker Ki67 is increased and p53 expression is more prominent.[96]

REFERENCES

1. Reed RJ, Pulitzer DR. Tumors of neural tissue. In: Elder DE, ed. *Lever's Histopathology of the Skin*, 10th edn. Philadelphia: Wolters Kluwer Lippincott Williams & Wilkins, 2009;1107–1149.

2. Zook EG. Complications of the perionychium. *Hand Clin* 1988;2:407–427.

3. Conolly WB, Goulston E. Problems of digital amputations: A clinical review of 260 patients and 301 amputations. *Aust N Z J Surg* 1973;43:118–123.

4. Sreedharan S, Teoh LC, Chew WY. Neuroma of the radial digital nerve of the middle finger following trigger release. *Hand Surg* 2011;16:95–97.

5. Jokinen CH, Ragsdale BD, Argenyi ZB. Expanding the clinicopathologic spectrum of palisaded encapsulated neuroma. *J Cutan Pathol* 2010;37:43–48.

6. Runne U. Syndrom der multiplen Neurome mit metastasierendem medullärem Schilddrüsenkarzinom ("Multiple mucosal neuroma-syndrome"). *Z Hautkr* 1977;52:299–301.

7. Argenyi ZsB, Santa Cruz D, Bromley C. Comparative light microscopic and immunohistochemical study of traumatic and palisaded encapsulated neuromas of the skin. *Am J Dermatopathol* 1992;14:504–510.

8. Argenyi ZsB. Immunohistochemical characterization of palisaded, incapsulated neuroma. *J Cutan Pathol* 1990;17:329–335.

9. Altmeyer P, Merkel KH. Multiple systematisierte Neurome der Haut und der Schleimhaut. *Hautarzt* 1981;32:240–244.

10. Schaffer JV, Kamino H, Witkiewicz A, McNiff JM, Orlow SJ. Mucocutaneous neuromas: An underrecognized manifestation of PTEN hamartoma-tumor syndrome. *Arch Dermatol* 2006;142:625.

11. Scheithauer BW, Woodruff JM, Erlandson RA. Tumors of the peripheral nervous system. In: Rosai J, Sobin LH, eds. *Atlas of Tumor Pathology, Series 3*, Washington, DC: Armed Forces Institute of Pathology, 1999.

12. Reed RJ, Fine RM, Meltzer HD. Palisaded, encapsulated neuromas of the skin. *Arch Dermatol* 1972;106:865.

13. Dover JS, From L, Lewis A. Palisaded encapsulated neuromas. A clinicopathologic study. *Arch Dermatol* 1989;125:386.

14. Hartzell TL, Taylor H. Traumatic amputation of a supernumerary digit: A 16-year-old boy's perspective of suture ligation. *Pediatr Dermatol* 2009;26:100–102.

15. Leber GE, Gosain AK. Surgical excision of pedunculated supernumerary digits prevents traumatic amputation neuromas. *Pediatr Dermatol* 2003;20:108–112.

16. Ban M, Kitajima Y. The number and distribution of Merkel cells in rudimentary polydactyly. *Dermatology* 2001;202:31–34.

17. Fletcher CDM, Theaker JM. Digital Pacinian neuroma: A distinctive hyperplastic lesion. *Histopathology* 1989;15:249–256.

18. Altmeyer H. Histologie eines Rankenneuroms mit Vater-Pacini-Lamellenkörper-ähnlichen Strukturen. *Hautarzt* 1979;30:248–252.

19. Kumar A, Darby AJ, Kelly CP. Pacinian corpuscles hyperplasia—An uncommon cause of digital pain. *Acta Orthop Belg* 2003;69:74–76.

20. Haneke E. Pacinian neuroma of the nail apparatus. 19th Sem Dermatopathol, Vars, France, 2012.

21. Zanardi F, Cooke RM, Maiorana A, Curti S, Farioli A, Bonfiglioli R, Violante FS, Mattioli S. Is this case of a very rare disease work-related? A review of reported cases of Pacinian neuroma. *Scand J Work Environ Health* 2011;37:253–258.

22. Rhode CM, Jennings WD Jr. Pacinian corpuscle neuroma of digital nerves. *South Med J* 1975;68:86–89.

23. Cho HH, Hong JS, Park SY, Park HS, Cho S, Lee JH. Tender papule rising on the digit: Pacinian neuroma should be considered in differential diagnosis. *Int J Med Sci* 2012;9:83–85.

24. Zelger B, Weinlich G, Zelger B. Perineuroma. A frequently unrecognized entity with emphasis on a plexiform variant. *Adv Clin Path* 2000;4:25–33.

25. Stolarczuk Dde A, Silva AL, Filgueiras Fda M, Alves Mde F, Silva SC. Solitary subungual neurofibroma: A previously unreported finding in a male patient. *An Bras Dermatol* 2011;86:569–572.

26. Runne U, Orfanos CE. The human nail. *Curr Prob Dermatol* 1981;9:102–149.

27. Bhushan M, Telfer NR, Chalmers RJG. Subungual neurofibroma, an unusual cause of nail dystrophy. *Br J Dermatol* 1999;140:777–778.

28. Huajun J, Wei Q, Ming L, Chongyang F, Weiguo Z, Decheng L. Solitary subungual neurofibroma in the right first finger. *Int J Dermatol.* 2012;51:335–338.

29. Fröhlich W. Fibromatosis subungualis. *Dermatol Wochenschr* 1939;109:1211–1212.

30. Niizuma K, Iijima KN. Solitary neurofibroma: A case of subungual neurofibroma on the right third finger. *Arch Dermatol Res* 1991;283:13–15.

31. Fleegler J, Zeinowicz RJ. Tumors of the perionychium. *Hand Clin* 1990;6:113–133.

32. Baran R, Haneke E. Subungual myxoid neurofibroma on the thumb. *Acta Derm Venereol* 2001;81:210–211.

33. Shelley ED, Shelley WB. Exploratory nail plate removal as a diagnostic aid in painful subungual tumours: Glomus tumour, neurofibroma, and squamous cell carcinomas. *Cutis* 1986;38:310–312.

34. Tisa VN, Pauli CD. Neurilemmoma of a digit: A case report. *J Am Podiatr Assoc* 1980;70:524–526.

35. Wolpa ME, Johnson JD. Schwannoma of the fifth digit. *J Foot Surg* 1989;28:421–424.

36. Moon SE, Cho YJ, Kwon OS. Subungual schwannoma: A rare location. *Dermatol Surg* 2005;31:592–594.

37. Ishida N, Watanabe D, Yokoo K, Tamada Y, Matsumoto Y. Schwannoma of a digit. *Eur J Dermatol* 2006;16:453–454.

38. Huntley JS, Davie RM, Hooper G. A subungual schwannoma. *Plast Reconstr Surg* 2006;117:712–713.

39. Oudhriri L, Chiheb S, Benchikhi H. Subungual schwannoma: An exceptional tumor. 1st Int Nail Summit, Athens, 2010, Poster 0877.

40. Kulkarni J, Moholkar A, Patil A. Subungual schwannoma: An uncommon location. *J Hand Surg Am.* 2013;38:1258–1259.

41. Soto R, Aldunce MJ, Wortsman X, Sazunic I. Subungual schwannoma with clinical, sonographic, and histologic correlation. *J Am Podiatr Med Assoc* 2014;104:302–304.

42. Wiemeyer S, Hafer G. Neurothekeoma of the toe. *Foot Ankle Spec* 2013;6:479–481.

43. Audring H, Sterry W. Bindegewebstumoren der Haut. In: Kerl H, Garbe C, Cerroni L, Wolff HH, eds. *Histopathologie der Haut*, Berlin: Springer, 2003;739.

44. Hügel H, Rudolph P. Mesenchymale Tumoren der Haut. Zellreiches Neurothekeom. In: Klöppel G, Kreipe HH, Remmele W, eds. *Pathologie*, 3rd edn. Cardesa A, Mentzel T, Rudolph P, Slootweg PJ, Vol-eds. Kopf-Hals-Region, Weichteiltumoren, Haut. Springer, Berlin Heidelberg, 2009; 966–967.

45. Laskin WB, Fetsch JF, Miettinen M. The "neurothekeoma": Immunohistochemical analysis distinguishes the true nerve sheath myxoma from its mimics. *Hum Pathol* 2000;31:1230.

46. Connolly M, Hickey JR, Intzedy L, Pawade J, de Berker DA. Subungual neurothekeoma. *J Am Acad Dermatol* 2005;52:159–162.

47. Cribier B, Baran R, Varini J-P. Myxome des gaines nerveuses de l'hyponychium. *Ann Dermatol Vénéréol* 2013;140:535–539.

48. Hasson A, Arias MC, Gutierrez A, Requena L. Periungual granular cell tumour. A light microscopic, immunohistochemical and ultrastructural study. *Skin Cancer* 1991;6:41–46.

49. Peters JS, Crowe MA. Granular cell tumor of the toe. *Cutis* 1998;62:147–148.

50. Nikkels AF, Arrese Estrada J, Piérard-Franchimont C, Piérard GE. CD68 and factor XIIIa expressions in granular cell tumor of the skin. *Dermatology* 1993;186:106–108.

51. Hoshi N, Tsu-ura Y, Watanabe K, Suzuki T, Kasukawa R, Suzuki T. Expression of immunoreactivities to 75 kDa nerve growth factor receptor, trk gene product and phosphotyrosine in granular cell tumors. *Pathol Int* 1995;45:748–756.

52. Billeret-Lebranchu V, Martin de la Salle E, Vandenhaute B, Lecomte-Houcke M. Tumeur à cellules granuleuses et épulis congénitale. Etude histochimique et immunohistochimique de 58 cas. *Arch Anat Cytol Pathol* 1999;47:31–37.

53. Mahalingam M, LoPiccolo D, Byers HR. Expression of PGP 9.5 in granular cell nerve sheath tumors: An immunohistochemical study of six cases. *J Cutan Pathol* 2001;28:282–286.

54. Fine SW, Li M. Expression of calretinin and the alpha-subunit of inhibin in granular cell tumors. *Am J Clin Pathol* 2003;119:259–264.

55. Baran R, Perrin C. Perineurioma: A tendon sheath fibroma-like variant in a distal subungual location. *Acta Derm Venereol* 2003;83:60–61.

56. Wortsman X, Merino D, Catalan V, Morales C, Baran R. Perineurioma of the nail on sonography. *J Ultrasound Med* 2010;29:1379–1382.

57. Baran R, Perrin C. Subungual perineurioma: A peculiar location. *Br J Dermatol* 2002;146:125–128.

58. Mentzel T, Dei Tos AP, Fletcher CDM. Perineurioma (storiform perineurial fibroma). Clinico-pathological analysis of four cases. *Histopathology* 1994;25:261.

59. Fetsch JF, Miettinen M. Sclerosing perineurioma: A clinicopathologic study of 19 cases of a distinctive soft tissue lesion with a predilection for the fingers and palms of young adults. *Am J Surg Pathol* 1997;21:1433–1442.

60. Toker C. Trabecular carcinoma of the skin. *Arch Dermatol* 1972;105:107–110.

61. Miller RW, Rabkin CS. Merkel cell carcinoma and melanoma: Etiological similarities and differences. *Cancer Epidemiol Biomarkers Prev* 1999;8:153–158.

62. Feng H, Shuda M, Chang Y, Moore PS. Clonal integration of a polyomavirus in human Merkel cell carcinoma. *Science* 2008 22;319(5866):1096–1100.

63. Hausen H. Novel human polyomaviruses—Re-emergence of a well known virus family as possible human carcinogens. *Int J Cancer* 2008;123:247–250.

64. Kassem A, Schöpflin A, Diaz C, Weyers W, Stickeler E, Werner M, Zur Hausen A. Frequent detection of Merkel cell polyomavirus in human Merkel cell carcinomas and identification of a unique deletion in the VP1 gene. *Cancer Res* 2008;68:5009–5013.

65. Helmbold P, Lahtz C, Enk A, Herrmann-Trost P, Marsch WCh, Kutzner H, Dammann RH. Frequent occurrence of RASSF1A promoter hypermethylation and Merkel cell polyomavirus in Merkel cell carcinoma. *Mol Carcinog* 2009;48:903–909.

66. Engelmann L, Kunze J, Haneke E. Giant neuroendocrine carcinoma of the skin (Merkel cell tumour). *Skin Cancer* 1991;6:211–216.

67. Coit DG. Merkel cell carcinoma. *Ann Surg Oncol* 2001;8:99S–102S.

68. Goldenhersh MA, Prus D, Ron N, Rosenmann E. Merkel cell tumor masquerading as granulation tissue on a teenager's toe. *Am J Dermatopathol* 1992;14:560–563.

69. LeBoit PE, Crutcher WA, Shapiro PE. Pagetoid intraepidermal spread in Merkel cell (primary neuroendocrine) carcinoma of the skin. *Am J Surg Pathol* 1992;16:584–592.

70. Connelly TJ, Cribier B, Brown TJ, Yangas I. Complete spontaneous regression of Merkel cell carcinoma: A review of the 10 reported cases. *Dermatol Surg* 2000;26:853–856.

71. Walsh NM. Primary neuroendocrine (Merkel cell) carcinoma of the skin: Morphologic diversity and implications thereof. *Hum Pathol* 2001;32:680–689.

72. Miettinen M. Keratin 20: Immunohistochemical marker for gastrointestinal, urothelial and Merkel cell carcinomas. *Mod Pathol* 1995;8:384–388.

73. Jensen K, Kohler S, Rouse RV. Cytokeratin staining in Merkel cell carcinoma: An immunohistochemical study of cytokeratins 5/6, 7, 17, and 20. *Appl Immunohistochem Mol Morphol* 2000;8:310–315.

74. Haneke E, Schulze H-J, Mahrle G. Immuno-histochemical and immunoelectron microscopic demonstration of chromogranin A in formalin-fixed tissue of Merkel cell carcinoma. *J Am Acad Dermatol* 1993;28:222–226.

75. Haneke E. Electron microscopy of Merkel cell carcinoma from formalin-fixed tissue. *J Am Acad Dermatol* 1985;12:487–492.

76. Deinlein E, Gassenmaier A, Haneke E, Grässel-Pietrusky R. Clonal heterogeneity in a case of Merkel cell carcinoma demonstrated by flow cytometry. *Dermatologica* 1985;170:1–5.

77. Paulson KG, Lemos BD, Feng B, Jaimes N, Peñas PF, Bi X, Maher E et al. Array-CGH reveals recurrent genomic changes in Merkel cell carcinoma including amplification of L-Myc. *J Invest Dermatol* 2009;129:1547–1555.

78. Cheuk W, Kwan MY, Suster S, Chan JK. Immunostaining for thyroid transcription factor 1 and cytokeratin 20 aids in the distinction of small cell carcinoma from Merkel cell carcinoma, but not pulmonary from extrapulmonary small cell carcinoma. *Arch Pathol Lab Med* 2001;125:228–231.

79. Wetzels CT, Hoefnagel JG, Bakkers JM, Dijkman HB, Blokx WA, Melchers WJ. Ultrastructural proof of polyomavirus in Merkel cell carcinoma tumour cells and its absence in small cell carcinoma of the lung. *PLoS One* 2009;4(3):e4958.

80. Touzé A, Gaitan J, Maruani A, Le Bidre E, Doussinaud A, Clavel C, Durlach A et al. Merkel cell polyomavirus strains in patients with Merkel cell carcinoma. *Emerg Infect Dis* 2009;15:960–962.

81. Banerjee SS, Agbamu DA, Eyden BP, Harris M. Clinicopathological characteristics of peripheral primitive neuroectodermal tumour of skin and subcutaneous tissue. *Histopathology* 1997;31:355–366.

82. Hasegawa SL, Davison JM, Rütten A, Fletcher JA, Fletcher JC. Primary cutaneous Ewing's sarcoma: Immunophenotypic and molecular cytogenetic evaluation of five cases. *Am J Surg Pathol* 1998;22:310–318.

83. Sangüeza OP, Sangüeza P, Valda KLR, Meshul CK, Requena L. Multiple primitive neuroectodermal tumors. *J Am Acad Dermatol* 1994;31:356–361.

84. Dick HM, Francis KC, Johnston AD. Ewing's sarcoma of the hand. *J Bone Joint Surg* 1971;53A:345–348.

85. Steens SC, Kroon HM, Taminiau AH, de Schepper AM, Watt I. Nail-patella syndrome associated with Ewing sarcoma. *J Belge Radiol—Belg T Radiol* 2007;90:214–215.

86. Lee CS, Southey MC, Slater H, Auldist AW, Chow CW, Venter DJ. Primary cutaneous Ewing's sarcoma/peripheral primitive neuroectodermal tumors in childhood. A molecular, cytogenetic, and immunohistochemical study. *Diagn Mol Pathol* 1995;4:174–181.

87. San-Juan M, Dölz R, Garcia-Barrecheguren E, Noain E, Sierrasesumaga L, Canadell J. Limb salvage in bone sarcomas in patients younger than 10 years. A 20-year experience. *J Pediatr Orthop* 2003;23:753–762.

88. Piganeau M, Ghezraoui H, De Cian A, Guittat L, Tomishima M, Perrouault L, René O et al. Cancer translocations in human cells induced by zinc finger and TALE nucleases. *Genome Res* 2013;23:1182–1193.

89. Ozdemirli M, Fanburg-Smith JC, Hartmann DP, Azumi N, Miettinen M. Differentiating lymphoblastic lymphoma and Ewing's sarcoma: Lymphocyte markers and gene rearrangement. *Mod Pathol* 2001;14:1175–1182.

90. Wood MK, Erdmann MW, Davies DM. Malignant schwannoma mistakenly diagnosed as carpal tunnel syndrome. *J Hand Surg Br* 1993;18:187–188.

91. Urabe A, Imayama S, Yasumoto S, Nakayama J, Hori Y. Malignant granular cell tumor. *J Dermatol* 1991;18:161–166.

92. Mahalingam M, LoPiccolo D, Byers HR. Expression of PGP9.5 in granular cell nerve sheath tumors: An immunohistochemical study of six cases. *J Cutan Pathol* 2001;28:282–286.

93. Fine SW, Li M. Expression of calretinin and the alpha-subunit of inhibin in granular cell tumors. *Am J Clin Pathol* 2003;119:259–264.

94. Mazur MT, Shultz JJ, Myers JL. Granular cell tumor. Immunohistochemical analysis of 21 benign and one malignant tumor. *Arch Pathol Lab Med* 1990;114:692–694.

95. Billeret-Lebranchu V, Martin de la Salle E, Vandenhaute B, Lecomte-Houcke M. Granular cell tumor and congenital epulis. Histochemical and immunohistochemal analysis of 58 cases. *Arch Anat Cytol Pathol* 1999;47:31–37.

96. Scheithauer BW, Woodruff JM, Erlandson RA. *Atlas of Tumor Pathology.* Tumors of the Peripheral Nervous System, 3rd edn. Washington DC: AFIP, 1999.

Histiocytic lesions

13

Under this heading, a few lesions will be summarized that are mainly composed of histiocytes with variable specialization. However, the differentiation of histiocytic and nonhistiocytic lesions is somewhat arbitrary as many cells, particularly those of bone and synovial tumors, often display histiocytic markers. Histiocytoma although CD68-positive is traditionally dealt with in Chapter 9 on fibrous lesions.

There are some useful markers for histiocytes: CD14 is a marker for monocytes from which all other histiocytes are derived. Macrophages stain with CD14, CD68, and CD163. Dermal and interstitial dendritic cells are positive for CD14, CD163, factor XIIIa, and fascin. Langerhans cells stain with antibodies to CD1a, langerin (CD207), and protein S100 and are also demonstrable with peanut agglutinin (PNA).[1,2]

13.1 BENIGN LESIONS

13.1.1 Juvenile xanthogranuloma

This benign proliferative disorder is most frequently seen in children as a yellow to reddish-tan, painless, dome-shaped nodule in the face and on the trunk. Other localizations are rare, especially subungual xanthogranuloma.[3,4] This leads to elevation and deformation of the nail plate. Another juvenile xanthogranuloma was observed on the proximal nail fold covering the proximal third of the nail plate.[5] The clinical diagnosis, among others, concerns Spitz's nevus.

13.1.1.1 Histopathology

Histopathology of juvenile xanthogranuloma is characteristic. There is a granuloma-like infiltrate composed of lymphocytes, some eosinophils, foam cells, and giant cells both of foreign and Touton type. The latter typically exhibit a central homogeneously eosinophilic cytoplasm, a wreath of nuclei, and an outer ring of foamy cytoplasm. Cell atypias are not seen. An occasional mitosis may be present.

13.1.1.2 Differential diagnosis

The typical giant cells with the wreath of nuclei are considered pathognomonic. When foamy cells are lacking or sparse, generalized eruptive histiocytosis has to be ruled out. A case of melanoma clinically and dermatoscopically similar to a xanthomatous lesion was described; the yellow color was thought to be due to lipofuscin that stained positive with Sudan black.[6]

13.1.2 Xanthoma

A case of hyperlipidemic xanthomas of the nail folds of two toes was described that clinically mimicked Koenen tumors of tuberous sclerosis.[7] Xanthomas may be arranged in a coral bead-like fashion at the free margin of the proximal nail fold similar to multicentric reticulohistiocytosis.[8]

13.1.2.1 Histopathology

Histopathology is identical with hyperlipidemic xanthomatosis elsewhere. The nodules contain masses of foamy cells and Touton giant cells. They were negative for protein S100 and CD68 in one case.[8]

13.1.2.2 Differential diagnosis

The histopathology of the various types of xanthomatoses is virtually identical.

13.1.3 Verruciform xanthoma

Verruciform xanthoma is a reactive lesion seen mainly in conditions with chronic inflammation such as lupus erythematosus, pemphigus vulgaris, skin trauma, in hyperplastic epidermis such as inflammatory linear verrucous nevus, congenital hemidysplasia with ichthyosiform erythroderma and limb defects (CHILD syndrome), and in patients with graft-versus-host disease and after organ transplantation. Most cases were observed in the oral mucosa, but anogenital involvement is also common. Skin lesions are rare. One case involving the toenails was observed in a female patient with lymphedema.[9] Another patient had multiple lesions and an almost complete nail dystrophy in the involved digit;[10] this is also a pathognomonic feature of the CHILD nevus, in which nail involvement is usually accompanied by a bulbous swelling of the tip of the digit (see Chapter 6).[11,12] We have observed a truly subungual verruciform xanthoma clinically mimicking subungual fibrokeratoma.[13]

13.1.3.1 Histopathology

Scanning magnification of skin and mucosal lesions gives the impression of a wart. The epidermal rete ridges are slender and elongated. Most commonly, xanthoma cells are seen in elongated dermal papillae. The suprapapillary epidermis is thinned and may be parakeratotic. Hypercholesterolemia and hyperlipidemia are not observed. In the subungual case, which was severely superinfected, an exophytic papilloma was seen with a scale crust of parakeratosis and necrotic keratinocytes on top and marked neutrophilic exocytosis leading to large areas of spongiform pustulation. The dermal papillae contained dilated capillaries and were filled with foamy macrophages (Figure 13.1). The overlying nail plate showed a bacterial biofilm at its undersurface.

13.1.3.2 Differential diagnosis

Common warts are the most important differential diagnosis when the xanthoma cells are not so prominent or overlooked.

(a) (b)

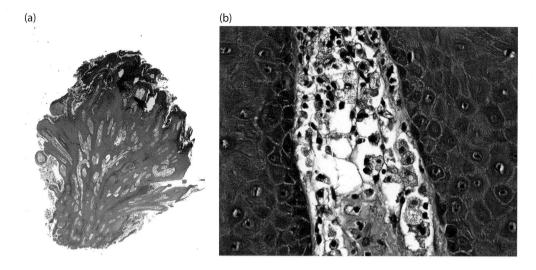

Figure 13.1 Subungual verruciform xanthoma in a 34-year-old woman. (a) The fan-like structure of the lesion is seen and (b) the connective tissue papillae are stuffed with xanthoma cells and dilated vessels.

13.1.4 Multicentric reticulohistiocytosis (see Chapter 5)

The first detailed description from 1936 used the term nodular nondiabetic cutaneous xanthomatosis.[14] Multicentric reticulohistiocytosis is characterized by nodules of skin and synovial membranes, an erosive polyarthritis, various local and systemic symptoms, and a typical histopathology.[15] Approximately at the same time, pain appears in different joints and bones and nodules develop on various skin areas. Women are preferentially affected. The course of the disease is protracted, and it may even be fatal.[16] Typical lesions of the nail organ are small firm nodules at the margin of the proximal nail fold causing the so-called coral bead sign. The nail bed is rarely affected.[17]

13.1.4.1 Histopathology

Histology shows granulomas consisting of a proliferation of oncocytic histiocytes with granular eosinophilic cytoplasm and many large giant cells. The latter containing 3–10 or sometimes more nuclei in irregular distribution, are about 50–100 μ in diameter and their cytoplasm is ground-glass like, weakly eosinophilic, and often contains PAS positive substances, but is negative for fat stains.[18] There are only a few lymphocytes at the margin. The overlying epidermis is moderately atrophic. The tumors are positive for vimentin and CD45. Factor XIIIa is usually negative.

13.1.4.2 Differential diagnosis

Solitary giant cell reticulohistiocytoma is said to be histologically identical, although some differential features were also postulated, particularly that the giant cells are larger.[17] Histological differential diagnoses may be dermatomyositis, rheumatoid arthritis, gout, sarcoidosis, and lepromatous leprosy.[19]

13.1.5 Other tumor-like depositions

Whether their classification into histiocytic lesions is justified remains questionable. Some represent typical metabolic diseases.

13.1.5.1 Mucin

Mucin deposition is a characteristic feature in pretibial myxedema, which rarely can be so extensive as to involve the toes and overgrow the nails. Histopathology of a biopsy is identical with focal mucinosis and myxoma (see Section 11.1.2); an early myxoid pseudocyst presents also as a focal mucinosis.

13.1.5.2 Urate

Urate crystal deposition is a typical feature of gout and described in Chapter 5 on nail changes in general diseases.

13.1.5.3 Oxalate

Oxalate deposition may occur in chronic renal failure. A case of so-called oxalate granuloma was described in a 46-year-old man who had been hemodialysed for 20 years and developed tender, grouped, yellow to tan nodules at the fingertips. Histopathology revealed crystalloid calcium oxalate needles in corymbiform arrangement and surrounded by foreign body granulomas. Foreign body giant cells may be scattered among the oxalate depositions. Polarization microscopy shows intense birefringence.[20]

13.2 MALIGNANT HISTIOCYTOSIS

13.2.1 Langerhans cell histiocytosis

Once called histiocytosis X, this disease is now defined as a proliferation of Langerhans cells. Three main forms with many overlaps are seen: Acute disseminated Langerhans cell histiocytosis (LCH) of Abt-Letterer-Siwe usually occurring in infants but occasionally also in children and adults; chronic multifocal LCH of Hand-Schüller-Christian with

(a)   (b)

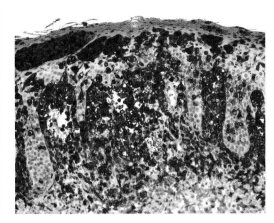

Figure 13.2 (a) Diffuse systemic type of Langerhans cell histiocytosis. This biopsy from the proximal nail fold shows huge amounts of Langerhans cells filling the papillary dermis and invading the epidermis and forming large cell collections. (b) CD1a demonstrations shows that only a certain percentage is positive.

the classical triad of multiple bone defects, diabetes insipidus, and exophthalmus; and eosinophilic granuloma or chronic focal LCH.[21] Nail changes are rare,[22,23] but may be seen as a marker of multisystem disease[24–27] although they were also observed in disseminated cutaneous Langerhans cell histiocytosis.[28,29] Even less frequently, they precede systemic lesions.[30,31] They may be seen as periungual small nodules in acute disseminated LHC,[32] onycholysis, nail thickening, subungual hyperkeratosis, onychorrhexis, pitting, longitudinal grooving, subungual hyperkeratosis, purpuric striae, hemorrhages, subungual pustules, deformity, loss of nail plate, paronychia, and nail fold destruction in fingernails and toenails.[33–35]

13.2.1.1 Histopathology

A dense infiltrate of relatively large cells with a reniform nucleus and a slightly eosinophilic cytoplasm is characteristic. They may invade the epidermis and form intraepidermal aggregates (Figure 13.2). Sometimes, hemorrhage is observed. The cells are positive for S100, CD1a, langerin (CD207), and the lectin peanut agglutinin.[36,37] Electron microscopically, the tumor cells contain Birbeck granules. Lesions in the matrix cause nail dystrophy whereas those in the nail bed are seen as hemorrhages or subungual pustules.

13.2.1.2 Differential diagnosis

In the beginning, a superficial perivascular dermatitis may be mimicked.

REFERENCES

1. Burgdorf WHC, Zelger B. The histiocytoses. In: Elder DE, ed. *Lever's Histopathology of the Skin*, 10th ed. Philadelphia: Lippincott Williams & Wilkins, 2009;667–688.
2. Peters K-P, Vigneswaran N, Hornstein OP, Haneke E. Peanut agglutinin in the diagnosis of skin tumours. *17th World Congr Dermatol, Vol Abstr* 1987;II:368.
3. Frumkin A, Roytan M, Johnson S. Juvenile xanthogranuloma underneath a toenail. *Cutis* 1987;40: 244–245.
4. Chang P, Baran R, Villanueva C, Samayoa M, Perrin C. Juvenile xanthogranuloma beneath a finger nail. *Cutis* 1996;58:173–174.
5. Piraccini BM, Fanti PA, Iorizzo M, Tosti A. Juvenile xanthogranuloma of the proximal nail fold. *Pediatr Dermatol* 2003;20:307–308.
6. Penouil MHJ, Gourhant JY, Segretin C, Weedon D, Rosendahl C. Non-choroidal yellow melanoma showing positive staining with Sudan Black consistent with the presence of lipofuscin: A case report. *Dermatol Pract Concept* 2014;4:45–49, doi: 10.5826/dpc.0402a09. eCollection 2014.
7. Keller PH. Hypercholesterinämische Xanthomatose. *Dermatol Wochenschr* 1960;14:336–337.
8. Yaşar S, Aslan C, Güneş P. Nail fold xanthomas: The coral bead sign revised. *J Dtsch Dermatol Ges* 2011;9:387–388.
9. Chyu J, Medenica M, Whitney DH. Verruciform xanthoma of the lower extremity: Report of a case and review of literature. *J Am Acad Dermatol* 1987;17:695–697.
10. Mountcastle EA, Lupton GP. Verruciform xanthomas of the digits. *J Am Acad Dermatol* 1989;20: 313–317.
11. Happle R, Mittag H, Küster W. The CHILD nevus: A distinct skin disorder. *Dermatology* 1995;191: 210–216.
12. Bittar M, Happle R. CHILD syndrome avant la lettre. *J Am Acad Dermatol* 2004;50(Suppl 2):S34–S37.
13. Haneke E. Subungual verruciform xanthoma. In preparation.
14. Weber FP, Freudenthal W. Nodular nondiabetic cutaneous xanthomatosis with hypercholesterolaemia and atypical histologic features. *Proc Roy Soc Med* 1936;30:522.

15. Orkin M, Goltz RW, Good RA, Michael A, Fisher I. A study of multicentric reticulophistiocytosis. *Arch Dermatol Syph* 1964;89:640–654.

16. Korthaus A. Bericht über einen Fall von multizentrischer Reticulohistiocytose mit letalem Ausgang. *Z Haut-GeschlKr* 1972;47:875–880.

17. Simpson EM, Goeckeritz BE, Teague DJ, Oliver AM. Multicentric reticulohistiocytosis: Diagnosis at the nailbeds. *J Rheumatol.* 2008;35:2272–2273.

18. Zelger B, Cerio R, Soyer HP, Misch K, Orchard G, Wilson-Jones E. Reticulohistiocytoma and multicentric reticulohistiocytosis. Histopathologic and immunophenotypic distinct entities. *Am J Dermatopathol* 1994;16:577–584.

19. Muñoz-Santos C, Sàbat M, Sáez A, Gratacós J, Luelmo J. Multicentric reticulohistiocytosis-mimicking dermatomyositis. Case report and review of the literature. *Dermatology* 2007;214:268–271.

20. Sina B, Lutz LL. Cutaneous oxalate granuloma. *J Am Acad Dermatol* 1990;22:316–317.

21. Arico M, Egeler RM. Clinical aspects of Langerhans cell histiocytosis. *Hematol Oncol Clin N Am* 1998;12:247.

22. Kahn G. Nail involvement in histiocytosis-X. *Arch Dermatol* 1969;100:699–701.

23. Alsina MM, Zamora E, Ferrando J, Mascaro J, Conget JI. Nail changes in histiocytosis X. *Arch Dermatol.* 1991;127:1741.

24. Querings K, Starz H, Balda BR. Clinical spectrum of cutaneous Langerhans' cell histiocytosis mimicking various diseases. *Acta Derm Venereol* 2006;86:39–43.

25. Chander R, Jaykar K, Varghese B, Garg T, Seth A, Nagia A. Pulmonary disease with striking nail involvement in a child. *Pediatr Dermatol* 2008;25:633–634.

26. Sabui TK, Purkait R. Nail changes in Langerhans cell histiocytosis. *Indian Pediatr* 2009;46:728–729.

27. Uppal P, Bothra M, Seth R, Iyer V, Kabra SK. Clinical profile of Langerhans cell histiocytosis at a tertiary centre: A prospective study. *Indian J Pediatr* 2012;79:1463–1467.

28. Munro CS, Morton R. Nail and scalp lesions in a man with diabetes insipidus. Langerhans cell histiocytosis (LCH). *Arch Dermatol* 1998;134:1477–1478, 1480–1481.

29. Moravvej H, Yousefi M, Barikbin B. An unusual case of adult disseminated cutaneous Langerhans cell histiocytosis. *Dermatol Online J.* Oct. 31, 2006;12(6):13.

30. Yazc N, Yalçn B, Ciftci AO, Orhan D, Haliloglu M, Büyükpamukçu M. Langerhans cell histiocytosis with involvement of nails and lungs in an adolescent. *J Pediatr Hematol Oncol* 2008;30:77–80.

31. Ashena Z, Alavi S, Arzanian MT, Eshghi P. Nail involvement in Langerhans cell histiocytosis. *Pediatr Hematol Oncol* 2007;24:45–51.

32. Tallon B, Rademaker M. Asymptomatic papules over the proximal nail fold in a child. *Arch Dermatol* 2008;144:105–110.

33. Berker DL, Lever LR, Windebank K. Nail features in Langerhans cell histiocytosis. *Br J Dermatol* 1994;130:523–527.

34. Jain S, Sehgal VN, Bajaj P. Nail changes in Langerhans cell histiocytosis. *J Eur Acad Dermatol Venereol* 2000;14:212–215.

35. Mataix J, Betlloch I, Lucas-Costa A, Pérez-Crespo M, Moscardó-Guilleme C. Nail changes in Langerhans cell histiocytosis: A possible marker of multisystem disease. *Pediatr Dermatol* 2008;25:247–251.

36. Ree HJ, Kadin ME. Peanut agglutinin. A useful marker for histiocytosis X and interdigitating reticulum cells. *Cancer* 1986;57:282–287.

37. Hajdu I, Zhang W, Gordon GB. Peanut agglutinin binding as a histochemical tool for diagnosis of eosinophilic granuloma. *Arch Pathol Lab Med* 1986;110:719–721.

Hematogenous tumors

14

Under this heading, cutaneous lymphomas and leukemias involving the nails and periungual skin are described. Lesions of the nails secondary to their treatment are not discussed here (see Chapter 5).

14.1 BENIGN HEMATOGENOUS LESIONS

These lesions are generally called pseudolymphomas. They are rare in the nail organ. Acral pseudolymphomatous angiokeratoma has already been discussed in Chapter 10.

14.2 MALIGNANT LYMPHOMAS AND LEUKEMIA

In recent years, malignant lymphomas have gained much interest in pathology, internal medicine, and dermatology. This is not the place to describe all lymphomas as many excellent monographs have appeared describing the manifold aspects of malignant lymphomas of the skin. Whereas the number of publications concerning hair follicle involvement, often called pilotropic or folliculotropic lymphomas, is vast, those affecting the nail, ungueotropic lymphomas, are rare.[1] B cell lymphomas involving the nail are even less frequent. Lymphoma patients often have mutations in the perforin gene that can be found both in the peripheral blood as well as in DNA of nails.[2]

14.2.1 T cell lymphomas

T cell lymphomas, particularly mycosis fungoides and Sézary syndrome, are the most common cutaneous lymphomas. Nail changes in cutaneous T cell lymphomas are unpredictable, often occur later in disease, affect several digits, and are mostly nonspecific, particularly in erythrodermic forms.[3] One- to almost two-thirds of the patients suffering from Sézary's syndrome exhibit atrophic nail alterations.[4,5] They may be indistinguishable from onychodystrophy due to erythrodermic psoriasis or pityriasis rubra pilaris.[6,7] It is often not possible to decide on clinical grounds whether the changes observed are nonspecific or due to specific nail infiltration, particularly in cutaneous T cell lymphomas.[8,9] The nails are brittle, ridged, often thickened, intransparent, yellow[10] with subungual hyperkeratosis[11,12] and occasionally flat or even koilonychotic. Pterygium formation and anonychia have been observed.[13] Isolated involvement of one or two nails is possible.[14] Massive lymphomatous involvement is rare.[15] Long-term onychomadesis[16] and gross nail destruction may occur. Tumor-stage mycosis fungoides of a single fingertip with nail involvement is exceptional.[17] Nail alterations were also seen in childhood mycosis fungoides.[18] Periungual blisters were seen in a case of bullous mycosis fungoides.[19]

14.2.1.1 Histopathology

The specific histopathologic nail alterations in the different cutaneous T cell lymphomas are identical and do not allow further subclassification. However, there are tremendous differences in the severity of the infiltrate explaining at least in part the degree of clinical nail changes. Commonly there is a subepithelial infiltrate of lymphocytes that may exhibit slightly larger and convoluted nuclei. Epitheliotropism is pronounced and Pautrier microabscesses may be numerous (Figure 14.1). When this occurs in the matrix region, the T lymphocytes and whole microabscesses may be included in the nail plate. Serious matrix involvement also interferes with correct nail substance production yielding a rough, ridged, lusterless, brittle nail. However, there may be severe clinical nail damage and only a very mild lymphomatous infiltrate (Figure 14.2). One case of ungual mucinosis was described.

Bullous mycosis fungoides around the nail showed large Pautrier microabscesses and detachment of the epidermis from the dermis.[19]

Immunohistochemistry is usually positive for CD1, CD2, CD3, and various amounts of CD4 and CD8.[20] In Sézary syndrome, the same clone of T cells is found by T cell receptor rearrangement in the blood and the nail infiltrate.[20]

14.2.1.2 Differential diagnosis

Nail involvement in cutaneous T cell lymphomas may look very bland and be mistaken for mild inflammation, psoriasis, pityriasis rubra, eczema, or actinic reticuloid.[5,7] A patient with HTLV-1 infection developed an ungual lymphoma, which was indistinguishable from classical mycosis fungoides.[21] There was a dense subepithelial band of T lymphocytes with unusually pronounced epidermotropism and large Pautrier's microabscesses that were eliminated transepidermally and transungually. The nail was imbibed with hemorrhage. There was an increased number of CD3+ cells and an increased ratio of CD4+/CD8+ cells. Small cell anaplastic carcinomas and melanomas

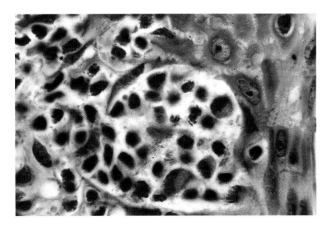

Figure 14.1 Pautrier's microabscess in a case of dyshidrosiform mycosis fungoides. Biopsy from the lateral nail fold shows a dense agglomeration of lymphcytes with dark, often cerebriform nuclei in the epidermis.

(a)

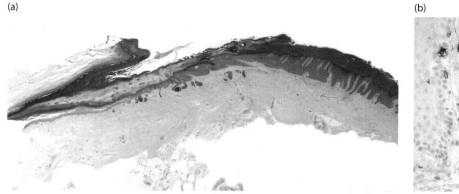

(b)

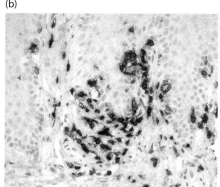

Figure 14.2 Nail involvement in Sézary syndrome: (a) Lateral longitudinal nail biopsy showing a scattered infiltrate in the mid- and distal nail bed despite considerable nail plate alterations. (b) CD8 demonstration exhibits cell clusters in the papillary dermis and epidermis.

may sometimes mimic a lymphoma. Common lymphocyte antigen positivity will rule them out whereas keratinocyte and melanocyte markers allow carcinomas and melanomas to be diagnosed.

14.2.2 B cell lymphoma

Chronic lymphocytic leukemia typically occurs in elderly people and usually runs a protracted, relatively benign appearing course. Specific skin infiltrates on acral sites such as the hands, ears, or nose are common. They form large, soft, and red nodules that occasionally may ulcerate spontaneously or on trauma. When affecting the nail apparatus, it often looks like chronic paronychia.[22-24] Subungual infiltrates cause an overcurvature[25] and elevation of the nail plate.[26] Clubbing and periosteal bone destruction of the distal phalanx were also seen.[27] Nonspecific nail dystrophy occurs in up to one-quarter of the patients.[28] The specific infiltrates respond well to irradiation.

14.2.2.1 Histopathology

Specific infiltrates of chronic lymphatic leukemia show very dense infiltrates of mature lymphocytes with round hyperchromatic nuclei and inconspicuous nucleoli in the dermis often reaching into the subcutis. The epidermis and a narrow grenz zone are spared. Germinal centers are not seen (Figure 14.3).[29]

Immunohistochemistry is positive for common lymphocyte antigen, BCL2, CD5, CD19, CD23, CD43, and CD79a whereas CD20 is only weakly positive.[30] The majority shows chromosomal abnormalities.

14.2.2.2 Differential diagnosis

The main differential diagnoses are benign pseudolymphomas of the B cell type[31] and lupus erythematosus profundus. Irregularity of the nuclear contour may resemble mantle cell lymphoma.

14.2.3 Plasmocytoma

Plasmocytomas are proliferations of malignant cells differentiated toward plasma cells. Most originate in the bones, but soft tissue plasmocytomas also occur. The

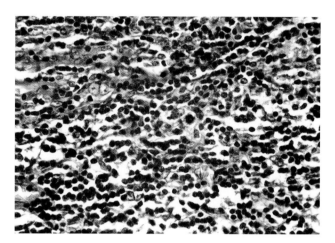

Figure 14.3 Dense infiltrate of the proximal nail fold in chronic lymphocytic leukemia.

former may evolve into multiple myeloma and produce paraproteins. Skin infiltrates commonly appear as asymptomatic reddish plaques or nodules. Involvement of the nail apparatus is rare and may cause nail elevation.[32] One patient developed the clinical features of hyalinosis cutis et mucosae with severe onychoschizia and onycholysis.[33] Clubbing was observed in a patient with POEMS (Crow-Fukase) syndrome (polyneuropathy with organomegaly, endocrinopathy, M proteins, and skin changes) associated with a plasmocytoma.[34] Systemic amyloidosis with lichen planus-like nail changes was seen in a patient with multiple myeloma.[35]

14.2.3.1 Histopathology

A dense infiltrate of immature and mature plasma cells occupies both the dermis as well as the adjacent subcutaneous tissue. The epidermis and papillary dermis remain free. Occasionally, the cells are multinucleated. Immunohistochemistry reveals a monoclonal proliferation of plasma cells producing one type of immunoglobulin. B lymphocyte markers are usually positive. Solitary lesions respond to radiotherapy or may be excised.

14.2.3.2 Differential diagnosis

This depends on the maturity of the plasma cells and includes chronic lymphocytic leukemia as well as plasmocytoid immunocytoma, but also reactive plasma cell-rich immune reactions.

14.2.4 Hodgkin's disease

Hodgkin's disease of the skin is rare but nail involvement appears to be exceptional. It is not clear whether the observed cases of nail changes were due to specific infiltration by the disease or nonspecific.[36,37]

14.2.5 Leukemia

Many nonspecific nail signs of leukemia including pallor, splitting as well as a tendency to bleed with splinter, and periungual hemorrhages were described in the nail.[38] In the preleukemic phase of myelomonocytic leukemia, pernio-like lesions were observed in the acral parts including the fingers and toes.[39–41] Acute myeolomonocytic leukemia was observed to infiltrate the distal thumb phalanx with bone involvement[42] and also causing pachydermoperiostosis.[43] We have seen a brownish spot on the proximal nail fold of the left middle finger in a patient with chronic myeloic leukemia (unpublished observation).

14.2.5.1 Histopathology

In the beginning, acute myelogenic leukemia usually starts with an angiocentric plus interstitial infiltrate of relatively monotonous myeloperoxidase positive cells. Their nuclei are round to oval with inconspicuous nucleoli. Epidermotropism is not seen.

The infiltrating cells of both acute and chronic myelogenous leukemia are bone marrow derived and positive for myeloperoxidase, chloroacetate esterase, Leder stain, and Sudan black B as well as for the myeloid markers CD13, CD15, CD33, and CD117.

14.2.5.2 Differential diagnosis

All monotonous round cell infiltrates may be considered. Myeloperoxidase is a very reliable stain to exclude T and B cell lymphomas. Sweet syndrome, particularly its variant neutrophilic dermatosis of the dorsal hands,[44] may mimic skin lesions of acute myelogenous leukemia and vice versa.[45]

REFERENCES

1. Harland E, Dalle S, Balme B, Dumontet C, Thomas L. Ungueotropic T-cell lymphoma. *Arch Dermatol* 2006;142:1071–1073.
2. Ding Q, Yang LY. Perforin gene mutations in 77 Chinese patients with lymphomas. *World J Emerg Med* 2013;4:128–132.
3. Bishop BBE, Wulkan A, Kerdel F, El-Sharawi-Caelen L, Tosti A. Nail alterations in cutaneous T-cell lymphoma: A case series and review of nail manifestations. *Skin Appendage Disord* 2015;1:82–86.
4. Wieselthier JS, Koh HK. Sézary syndrome: Diagnosis, prognosis, and critical review of treatment options. *J Am Acad Dermatol* 1990;22:381–401.
5. Booken N, Nicolay JP, Weiss C, Klemke CD. Cutaneous tumor cell load correlates with survival in patients with Sézary syndrome. *J Dtsch Dermatol Ges* 2013;11:67–79.
6. Toonstra J, van Weelden H, Gmelin Meylin FH, van der Putte SC, Schiere SI, Baart de la Faille H. Actinic reticuloid mimicking Sézary's syndrome. Report of two cases. *Arch Dermatol Res* 1985;277:159–166.
7. Sonnex TS, Dawber RP, Zachary CB, Millard PR, Griffiths AD. The nails in adult type 1 pityriasis rubra pilaris. A comparison with Sézary syndrome and psoriasis. *J Am Acad Dermatol* 1986;15:956–960. Comment in *J Am Acad Dermatol* 1989;21:811–812.
8. Dalziel KL, Telfer NR, Dawber RP. Nail dystrophy in cutaneous T-cell lymphoma. *Br J Dermatol* 1989;120:571–574.
9. Ogilvie C, Jackson R, Leach M, McKay P. Sezary syndrome: Diagnosis and management. *J R Coll Physicians Edinb* 2012;42:317–321.
10. Toritsugi M, Satoh T, Higuchi T, Yokozeki H, Nishioka K. A vesiculopustular variant of mycosis fungoides palmaris et plantaris masquerading as palmoplantar pustulosis with nail involvement. *J Am Acad Dermatol* 2004;51:139–141.
11. Tomsick RS. Hyperkeratosis in mycosis fungoides. *Cutis* 1982;29:621–623.
12. Trathner A, Ingber A, Sandbank M. Nail pigmentation resulting from PUVA treatment. *Int J Dermatol* 1990;29:310.
13. Bakar O, Seçkin D, Demirkesen C, Baykal C, Büyükbabani N. Two clinically unusual cases of folliculotropic mycosis fungoides: One with and the other without syringotropism. *Ann Dermatol* 2014;26:385–391.
14. Mazzurco JD, Schapiro BL, Fivenson DP. Localized mycosis fungoides of the bilateral thumbs and nail units treated with orthovoltage radiation. *Int J Dermatol* 2010;49:1334–1335.
15. Tosti A, Fanti PA, Varotti C. Massive lymphomatous nail involvement in Sézary syndrome. *Dermatologica* 1990;181:162–164.
16. Fleming CJ, Hunt MJ, Barnetson RSC. Mycosis fungoides with onychomadesis. *Br J Dermatol* 1996;135:1012.
17. Grande-Sarpa H, Callis Duffin KP, Florell SR. Onychodystrophy and tumor-stage mycosis fungoides confined to a single digit: Report of a case and review of nail findings in cutaneous T-cell lymphoma. *J Am Acad Dermatol* 2008;59:154–157.
18. Wilson KG, Cotter FE, Lowe DG, Stansfeld AG, Kirby JD. Mycosis fungoides in childhood: An unusual presentation. *J Am Acad Dermatol* 1992;25:370–372.
19. Fränken J, Haneke E. Mycosis fungoides bullosa. *Hautarzt* 1995;46:186–189.
20. Parmentier L, Dürr C, Vassella E, Beltraminelli H, Borradori L, Haneke E. Specific nail alterations in cutaneous T-cell lymphoma: Successful treatment with topical mechlorethamine. *Arch Dermatol.* 2010;146:1287–1291.

21. Wolter M, Schleussner-Samuel P, Marsch WC. HTLV-I-Infektion: Unguales T-Zell-Lymphom als Primärmanifestation. *Hautarzt* 1991;42:50–52.

22. High DA, Luscombe HA, Kauh YC. Leukemia cutis masquerading as chronic paronychia. *Int J Dermatol* 1985;24:595–597.

23. Yagci M, Sucak GT, Haznedar R. Red swollen nail folds and nail deformity as presenting findings in chronic lymphocytic leukaemia. *Br J Haematol* 2001; 112:1.

24. Saburi Y, Gotoh K, Ohtsuka E, Yamaguchi K. Swollen nail folds due to leukemic cell infiltration in a case of chronic lymphocytic leukemia. *Intern Med* 2004;43:1008.

25. Stanway A, Rademaker M, Kennedy I, Newman P. Cutaneous B-cell lymphoma of nails, pinna and nose treated with chlorambucil. *Australas J Dermatol* 2004;45:110–113.

26. Simon CA, Su WP, Li CY. Subungual leukemia cutis. *Int J Dermatol* 1990;29:636–639.

27. Calvert RJ, Smith E. Metastatic acropachy in lymphatic leukaemia. *Blood* 1955;10:545–549.

28. Beck CH. Skin manifestations associated with lymphatic leukemia. *Dermatologica* 1948;96:350–356.

29. Pedersen LM, Nordin H, Nielsen H, Lisse I. Non-Hodgkin malignant lymphoma in the nails in the course of a chronic lymphocytic leukaemia. *Acta Derm Venereol* 1992;72:277–278.

30. Jackson M, Lee R, Lortscher D, Broome E, Wang H. Chronic lymphocytic leukemia simulating chronic paronychia. *J Cut Pathol* 2011;38:83.

31. Creusy C, Saout J, Audouin J, Diebold J, Duflos M, Callens J, Giaux G, Sion G. Dermo-hypodermic lymphoid pseudotumors with follicular hyperplasia. Apropos of a case. *Arch Anat Cytol Pathol* 1989;37:213–218.

32. Borrego L, Rodríguez J, Bosch JM, Castro V, Hernández B. Subungual nodule as manifestation of multiple myeloma. *Int J Dermatol* 1996;35:661–662.

33. Von der Helm D, Ring J, Schmoeckel C, Braun-Falco O. Erworbene Hyalinosis cutis et mucosae bei Plasmozytom mit monoklonaler IgG-lambda-Gammopathie. *Hautarzt* 1989;40:153–157.

34. Dispenzieri A, Kyle RA, Lacey MQ, Rajkumar SV, Therneau TM, Larson DR, Greipp PR et al. POEMS syndrome: Definitions and long-term outcome. *Blood* 2003;101:2496–2506.

35. Mancuso G, Fanti PA, Berdondini RM. Nail changes as the only skin abnormality in myeloma-associated amyloidosis. *J Am Acad Dermatol* 1997;137:471–472.

36. Shahani RT, Blackburn EK. Nail anomalies in Hodgkin's disease. *Br J Dermatol* 1973;89:457–458.

37. Raffle EJ. Letter: Nail anomalies in Hodgkin's disease. *Br J Dermatol* 1974;90:585–586.

38. Hirschfeld H. Leukämie und verwandte Zustände. In: Schittenhelm A, ed. *Handbuch der blutbildenden Organe*, Berlin: Springer, 1925; vol 1.

39. Marks R, Lim CC, Borrie PF. A perniotic syndrome with monocytosis and neutropenia: A possible association with a preleukaemic state. *Br J Dematol* 1969;81:327–332.

40. Kelly JW, Dowling JP. Pernio: A possible association with chronic myelomonocytic leukemia. *Arch Dermatol* 1985;121:1048–1052.

41. Cliff S, James SL, Mercieca JE, Holden CA. Perniosis: A possible association with a preleukemic state. *Br J Dermatol* 1996;135:330–345.

42. Chang DY, Whitaker LA, La Rossa D. Acute monomyelocytic leukemia presenting as a felon. *Plast Reconstr Surg* 1975;56:623–624.

43. Mackenzie CR. Pachydermoperiostosis: A paraneoplastic syndrome. *N Y State J Med* 1986;86:153–154.

44. Walling HW, Snipes CJ, Gerami P, Piette W. The relationship between neutrophilic dermatosis of the dorsal hands and Sweet syndrome. *Arch Dermatol* 2006;142:57–63.

45. Hirai I, Sakiyama T, Konohana A, Takae Y, Matsuura S. A case of neutrophilic dermatosis of the back of the hand in acute leukemia—A distributional variant of Sweet's syndrome. *J Dtsch Ges Dermatol* 2015;13:1033–1035.

Melanocytic lesions

Much attraction has been focused on melanocytic lesions as melanoma is certainly the most important tumor of the nail unit and often poses considerable diagnostic challenges. The list of differential diagnoses is long and diagnostic delay is unfortunately still very common. Traditionally, melanocytic lesions of the nail are divided into functional melanonychia (melanocyte activation), lentigo, nevus, and melanoma. Particular problems arise in children. Morphologically, melanin pigmentation of the nail is classified as diffuse, longitudinal, and transverse.

15.1 BENIGN MELANOCYTIC LESIONS OF THE NAIL UNIT

Pigmentations due to melanocyte hyperfunction, lentigines, nevi, and melanomas are relatively frequent. Age, race, localization, profession, hobbies, and sun exposure may play a role though to very different degrees. What may be entirely normal in dark-brown and black people can be an alarming sign in light-skinned Caucasians.

15.1.1 Functional hyperpigmentation

This is a frequent phenomenon that may be caused by a variety of events: Racial (ethnic) pigmentation is the most frequent cause of melanin pigmentation of the nails with almost all black people having some degree of nail pigmentation at the age of 50–60 years and functional melanonychia being seen in up to 20% of Asians. Pregnancy may be another physiologic cause.[1] Chronic rubbing leads to hyperpigmentation of the proximal nail fold and frictional melanonychia.[2] A similar mechanism can be assumed in melanonychia due to chronic nail biting,[3] onychotillomania,[4] and some occupational traumas. Photochemotherapy with psoralens and other ultraviolet sensitizers plus UV-A may lead to multidigital brown streaks.[5–7] Many drugs, including cytostatics, cause melanocyte activation with subsequent multiple melanonychias.[8] Nail, skin, and mucous membrane pigmentation are common in Addison's and Nelson's syndromes.[9,10]

Vitamin B_{12} deficiency was associated with multiple brown streaks of the nails.[11,12] Several diseases cause melanocyte proliferation.[13–15] Some authors list more than 100 causes for melanonychias.[16]

Functional melanonychia is seen as a brown band made up of fine brown lines on a gray background under the dermatoscope. Occasionally, a periungual pigmentation may be seen, particularly in black persons on the proximal and lateral nail fold; this is, however, not sharply delimited in contrast to Hutchinson's sign in melanoma.

15.1.1.1 Histopathology

By definition, this is only a functional hyperactivity without a numerical increase of melanocytes. A faint pigmentation by barely visible melanin granules is often the only sign seen in nail clippings. A biopsy of the matrix is also frequently disappointing as it may be impossible to see the hyperpigmentation of the matrix epithelium. However, Fontana's argentaffin reaction shows a strong pigmentation both in the nail plate as well as in the matrix. Here, dendritic melanocytes are usually seen. Immunohistochemical staining for matrix melanocytes with antibodies to protein S100, Melan-A, and HMB45 shows a normal number with a surprising variability of positivity with the different antibodies. Both MITF and Sox10 demonstration do show a normal number of melanocytes (Table 15.1). Cytologically, the melanocytes are normal and no mitoses are seen (Figure 15.1).

The histopathological diagnosis of a melanocyte activation can neither elicit its etiology nor distinguish between diffuse, longitudinal, or transverse melanonychia.

15.1.1.2 Differential diagnosis

Because of the obvious discrepancy between the clinically evident melanonychia and the difficulty to see the melanin and melanocytes in routine histological sections, special stains are necessary to make the diagnosis. Most nonmelanin brown streaks of the nail do not

Table 15.1 Differential diagnosis of melanonychias

	Functional melanonychia	Lentigo	Nevus	Melanoma
H&E stain	Often very inconspicuous	Hyperpigmentation usually visible	Hyperpigmentation usually visible	Pigmentation very variable, cellular atypia
Argentaffin reaction	Increase in pigmentation, normal number of melanocytes	Obvious increase in pigmentation, increased number of dendritic melanocytes	Obvious increase in pigmentation, increased number of dendritic melanocytes, some nests	Melanocytes with plump dendrites
Immunohistochemistry with melanocyte markers	Normal melanocyte number	Increased number of melanocytes	Increased number of melanocytes	Increased number of melanocytes

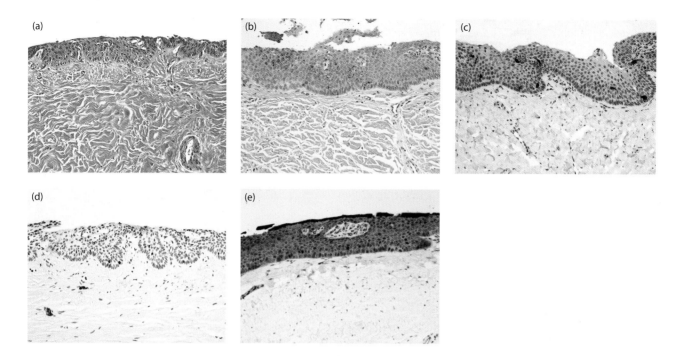

Figure 15.1 Tangential matrix biopsy of a functional melanonychia. (a) H&E stain shows some barely recognizable melanocytes and very little pigment (b) whereas Fontana stain reveals abundant melanin granules. (c) Immunohistochemistry with Melan-A demonstrates a normal number of dendritic melanocytes in the matrix epithelium. (d) Protein S100 shows a slightly lower number of melanocytes than Melan-A. (e) Sox10 is a nuclear stain for melanocytes (e).

show a granular pigment. Fungal melanonychia is characterized by a diffuse yellowish to light brown staining of the nail plate and PAS usually reveals the fungi (see Chapter 4). Exogenous staining is seen on the nail plate surface. Silver nitrate gives a jet-black stain clinically and is seen as black round globules in the upper third of the nail plate (see Chapter 7). Bacterial nail stain is also commonly restricted to either the upper or undersurface of the nail plate and most commonly a bacterial biofilm can be demonstrated.

15.1.2 Lentigo of the nail

Lentigines of the nail matrix are probably the most frequent cause of longitudinal melanonychia in fair-skinned young individuals. They present as brown streaks in the nail that dermatoscopically show regularly spaced narrow bands on a gray to brown background. The intensity of the brown color varies from very light to almost black; it tends to be darker in dark-skinned individuals. After nail avulsion, an oval brown spot is seen in the matrix that may rarely extend to the nail bed.

15.1.2.1 Histopathology

A matrix lentigo is characterized by a numerical increase of melanocytes. These are usually markedly pigmented, which can be seen in H&E sections. Specimens containing both the matrix and the overlying nail plate show pigment in all layers of the matrix epithelium and in the plate; it is present as fine granules staining positive with Fontana's argentaffin reaction. The melanocytes have slender dendrites and they often populate the basal and suprabasal

epithelial layers. However, a pagetoid spread is not a feature of matrix lentigines. Epithelial hyperplasia is not pronounced (Figure 15.2). Melanophages may be present, sometimes in large amounts. Melanocyte markers such as S100, Melan-A, and HMB45 are usually positive, but S100 is often less marked. Sox10 and MITF stain the melanocyte nuclei.

A lentiginous proliferation of melanocytes is also seen in some cases of the Laugier-Hunziker-Baran syndrome.[17,18]

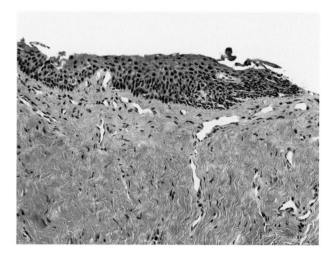

Figure 15.2 Tangential excision of a lentigo of the matrix exhibiting heavily pigmented melanocytes in the matrix epithelium and very intense pigmentary incontinence.

15.1.2.2 Differential diagnosis

The most important and often extremely difficult challenge is to rule out early *in situ* melanoma or the margin of a melanoma of the matrix. It was therefore recommended to use melanocyte markers for the identification of dendrites that are said to be plump in malignant melanocytes.[19]

15.1.3 Nevi

Virtually all types of melanocytic nevi occur under and around the nail apparatus. Periungual melanocytic nevi are surprisingly rare. Most of them are moderately pigmented, slightly elevated, or papular. A pigmented melanocytic nevus of the matrix gives rise to a brown streak in the nail. However, the clinical differentiation of a matrix nevus from a lentigo is often impossible[20-22] except when brown clumps are seen within the melanonychia that represent intraungual nests of nevus cells. Congenital nevi are rare and do not pose a diagnostic challenge.[23-26] They often show periungual pigmentation or extension of the nevus.[27-29] Ungual blue nevi are also rare and mostly of the common type.[30] Congenital blue nevi stand out by their deep pigmentation.[31] Combined nevi of the nail are surprisingly rare. A subungual Spitz nevus was seen in a Hispanic infant.[32]

15.1.3.1 Histopathology

Nevi of the nail matrix are usually markedly pigmented and exhibit both a lentiginous as well as a proliferation in nests. These may range from very few to abundant. Particularly in small children, the nevus nests may migrate upward in the epithelium and become included in the nail plate. The intraungual nevus cell nests may be pyknotic and resemble large clumps of condensed melanin. In addition, pigment may be seen to ascend obliquely upward in a distal direction showing the natural growth direction of matrix cells (Figure 15.3). Most matrix nevi are junctional; compound nevi appear to be very rare.

Periungual nevi may be junctional, compound, and dermal. Transcorneal elimination of small melanocyte groups is relatively common, particularly in junctional nevi.

Congenital nevi are mostly characterized by a heavy pigmentation. Nevus cells often penetrate deep into the dermis, distinguishing them from acquired nail nevi.

Blue nevi represent a proliferation of melanocytes in the dermis of the matrix, nail bed, and periungual skin. In the common type, the cells are spindled and distributed in a loose and haphazard fashion (Figure 15.4). Pigment is easily identified. There is a free zone between the ill-defined lesion and the epithelium. In the cellular type, the cells may be larger, often slightly epithelioid with heavy pigmentation. They frequently penetrate deeply into the nail dermis. Mixed phenotype of blue nevus cells was described.[33] As they have no epithelial nests, the pigment remains in the dermis and is not transferred to the nail, hence no longitudinal nail pigmentation develops. However, when this is seen it is a sign of a combined nevus consisting of a junctional and

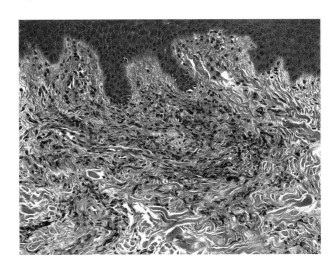

Figure 15.4 Blue nevus, simplex type, of the nail bed with dendritic, intensely pigmented melanocytes in the nail bed dermis.

(a)

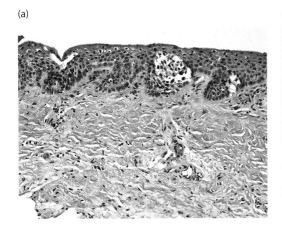

(b)

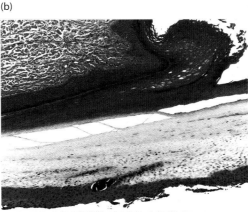

Figure 15.3 Junctional nevus of the matrix. (a) Melanocyte nests in the matrix epithelium. (b) Transungual elimination of a heavily pigmented nest of melanocytes. The direction of melanin incorporation into the nail plate is clearly seen. There are many intraungual melanocytes, which are not a sign of malignancy in children.

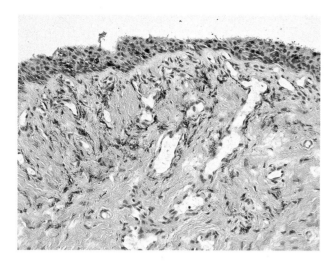

Figure 15.5 Subungual combined nevus showing a junctional component and a simplex type of blue nevus.

a blue nevus component (Figure 15.5). So-called benign lymph node metastasis of a congenital blue nevus of the nail unit was observed.

15.1.3.2 Differential diagnosis

The most important differential diagnosis is nail unit melanoma. Cellular blue nevus has to be separated from a melanoma metastasis. The presence of nests allows nevi to be differentiated from lentigines.

15.2 MALIGNANT MELANOCYTIC TUMORS
15.2.1 Melanoma of the nail unit

Ungual melanomas have attracted considerable attention in the last three decades although the first report dates back to 1834.[34] Melanomas still have the air of a somehow mystic tumor in dermatology and dermatopathology and quite a number of misconceptions have been carried from publication to publication, also and particularly for this special site.[35]

Ungual melanomas are localized either under or around the nail unit and belong to the subgroup of acral lentiginous melanomas. It is generally held that nail melanomas are rare; however, about 1.5%–2.5% of all melanomas in light-skinned Caucasians are ungual melanomas[36,37] and the entire surface of all nails taken together is far below 1%—thus the nail is overrepresented as a localization for melanoma.[38] In darkly pigmented individuals that develop much less cutaneous melanomas, the absolute number of ungual melanomas is comparable to that of Caucasians, but this accounts for about 20% of their melanomas.[39,40] Acral melanomas make up for 50%–77% of all melanomas in Japanese,[41,42] Koreans,[43] and Chinese[44] in contrast to only 4%—7% of the German population.[45,46]

The incidence of cutaneous melanoma is increasing steadily, but has been stable for most populations concerning acral lentiginous and nail melanomas.[47]

The peak age of nail melanoma patients is between 50 and 70 years with a very wide age range, and several cases of subungual melanoma in children have been published.[48,49]

In light-skinned individuals, no clear-cut gender dominance can be found; some publications reported more women, other more men affected.[50]

The thumb and the great toenail are the most common localizations with roughly 70% of all nail melanomas. This gave rise to the assumption that trauma plays a major role in the initiation of nail melanoma.[51–53] However, most reports are not convincing as the time between the perceived trauma and the nail melanoma was too short.[54] On the other hand, trauma is certainly an important factor negatively influencing the prognosis[55] and nail melanomas detected after a trauma were thicker.[50] Artificial nails may hide a subungual melanoma or even promote its growth.[56] In contrast to cutaneous melanomas, those of the nail are not associated with ultraviolet exposure. The nail only permits a fraction of UV to penetrate through the nail plate.[57–59] The big toenail is usually protected from UV irradiation by shoes.

The clinical diagnosis of ungual melanoma may be difficult for the physician not trained in diagnosing nail conditions. Although between two-thirds and three-quarters of them are pigmented, many of these tumors are overlooked and not diagnosed in time. Apparently, it is the lack of suspicion that is the most important factor for not making the correct diagnosis. It is important to know that any melanin pigmentation in the nail must evoke the suspicion of nail melanoma, independent of the patient's age and the digit involved. A rule of thumb is that an acquired melanotic longitudinal streak in the nail of a light-skinned adult is rather malignant than benign.[60] This is particularly true if the streak is

- Wider than 5 mm
- Located on the thumb, index, middle finger, or big toe
- Involves a single digit
- Widening proximally indicating growth of the lesion in the matrix
- Is associated with nail dystrophy even if this is minute
- Is accompanied by periungual pigmentation, the Hutchinson sign
- Develops a tumefaction

However, ungual melanomas were also observed in children[61–63] and even concurrently in two thumbs.[64]

Analogous to the ABC rule of cutaneous melanomas, an ABCDEF rule was proposed for nail melanomas:[65]

A. **A**ge and race—most nail melanomas occur between the ages of 40 and 70 and most patients are **A**sians, **A**fricans, **A**frican-Americans, and native **A**mericans
B. **B**rown to **b**lack band, **b**roader than 3–5 mm, **b**order irregular or blurred
C. **C**hange: rapid increase in width and growth rate, nail dystrophy does not improve despite "adequate treatment"
D. **D**igit: Thumb > big toe > index finger; usually single digit involvement, more fingers rarely affected

E. Extension of pigmentation: periungual pigmentation = Hutchinson sign

F. Family or personal history of melanoma or so-called dysplastic nevi

These criteria are valid for most lesions originating in the nail matrix. However, no melanocytic lesion deriving from the nail bed can give a longitudinal streak as this is due to incorporation of the melanin into the growing nail plate and the nail bed does not add to it. Furthermore, most nail bed melanomas are amelanotic. Thus, the diagnosis of nonpigmented nail melanomas is a real challenge and requires a very high degree of clinical suspicion. It is self-evident and good clinical practice to always submit every piece of a surgical specimen from the nail region for histopathologic examination, even when the clinical diagnosis was just granulation tissue or an ingrown nail. As the absolute number of nail melanomas is not different between light-skinned Caucasians and Africans and Asians, the statement that most patients are from dark-skinned races is not true. Strict adherence to the ABCDEF rule might even delay the diagnosis, as many patients are younger than 30 years.[66] This rule is also not adequate to diagnose childhood nail melanoma.

The list of clinical differential diagnoses is enormous with warts, hematoma, pyogenic granuloma, ingrown toenail, onychomycosis,[67] keratoacanthoma, squamous cell carcinoma, foreign body granuloma, or mole, to mention just a few.[68–71] There are even more disorders to be considered in amelanotic nail melanoma.[72,73] However, onychomycosis may coexist with melanoma.[74]

It is often claimed that ungual melanomas have a particularly poor prognosis; large series of 100 or more cases showed a mean Breslow thickness of 4 mm and more[75, 76] hinting at an enormous neglect both from the patient as well as his physician. The five-year survival for invasive subungual melanoma was only 51%.[36] Several publications of ungual melanomas misdiagnosed and mistreated as onychomycosis give evidence that even pigmented nail melanomas are not correctly diagnosed. Sixty percent of the initially unrecognized acral lentiginous melanomas were nail melanomas, and 30% of them were amelanotic.[50] Thus, the assumption that amelanotic nail melanomas have a poorer prognosis only reflects the fact that they are diagnosed and treated even later than non-nail acral lentiginous melanomas.[77,78] However, long-term survival of stage IV subungual melanoma with spontaneous regression of metastases[79] and even complete regression of an advanced subungual melanoma with a tumor thickness of 4 mm were observed.[80]

It is also not true that subungual melanomas grow faster than those in other locations as there are many reports of decade-long histories of ungual melanomas[81] and many of our cases were still *in situ* even after 10 years or more that a brown streak had been noticed.

The diagnosis of nail melanomas should be straightforward if there is a recently acquired pigmented streak in the nail or a Hutchinson sign in an individual over 30–35

years. This is unfortunately often not the case as briefly mentioned above. The most important is to think of the possibility of melanoma. Two-thirds to three-quarters of nail melanomas are pigmented. Human pigment reaches the free edge of the nail, is granular, and can be identified histologically in Fontana-stained sections as is explained later in detail. Fungal melanin is diffuse and usually forms a narrow wedge with its broad base distally. Blood virtually never reaches the free margin of the nail plate, is deposited in large clumps of erythrocytes, and can easily be demonstrated using the benzidine test: A tiny piece of the nail with the pigment in question is cut or the pigment is scraped into a small test tube, a few drops of water are added, and after a few minutes a Hemostix® such as used for the demonstration of blood in urine is dipped into the test tube: Even a very few erythrocytes give a positive test.[82] Another possibility is to wipe the pigmented nail with 3% hydrogen peroxide, which removes the blood while producing white foam due to the release of atomic oxygen. It must be stressed that the demonstration of blood does not rule out a bleeding melanoma or another bleeding tumor.

Dermatoscopy is a very valuable adjunct to clinical diagnosis. It should be started "dry," that is, without an immersion medium, then "wet." Dry dermatoscopy allows surface irregularities to be seen whereas wet dermatoscopy permits a better look into the nail plate. As the nail surface is curved, a transparent gel staying on the curvature is recommended. The fine melanin granules are not visible whereas blood agglomerates are seen both with a magnifier lens as well as the dermatoscope. However, there may be transungual elimination of nevus cells and nests that look like brown dots. In melanomas, the brown band is built by stripes of pigment, which are irregular in width, spacing, and color. Further, tiny pigmentations of the skin surrounding the nail are seen; this micro-Hutchinson sign is very rare in benign nevi. Dermatoscopy, like clinical inspection, of a melanonychia cannot render the responsible melanocyte focus to be seen. This means that the two-dimensional dermatoscopy of a cutaneous melanocytic lesion is reduced to one-dimension only and that it is not the lesion itself, but its product melanin incorporated in the nail plate, which has to be evaluated. The pigmented lesion is covered by the nail plate and in most instances also by the proximal nail fold. The melanonychia is due to overproduction of melanin that cannot completely be degraded by the matrix keratinocytes and remains included in the upper matrix keratinocytes and finally the nail plate cells. Whereas an increase in the width of the melanocyte lesion will lead to a wider band, a longitudinal increase may lead to a more intense pigmentation of the streak. Growth in the transverse diameter of the melanocyte lesion within a certain time period is visible as a streak wider proximally than distally. This is usually seen as a sign of malignancy. Very even pigmentation of a melanonychia is the rule for benign lesions, but in general, dermatoscopy only gives a hint at the dignity of the lesion. Nail bed melanomas are usually amelanotic, but even if they produce melanin this remains under the nail plate and is not included in it making the diagnosis even more difficult. Independent of the safety of a dermatoscopic diagnosis, histopathology is always a must.[83]

Intraoperative matrix dermatoscopy is an invasive method but it permits direct bidimensional observation of the pigmented lesion in the matrix and nail bed with a multicomponent pattern of brown-black pigmentation, globules, dots, structureless areas, and thick streaks being suspicious for melanoma.[84–86] One study was able to reliably distinguish 7 of 8 matrix melanomas from a benign lentigo by immediate postoperative confocal laser scanning microscopy (CLSM) thus speeding up the diagnostic delay between extirpation and histopathology, and the one lesion not safely diagnosable by CLSM also required immunohistochemistry to make the diagnosis.[87]

X-ray fiber diffraction was claimed to be able to differentiate eight different malignancies from a single nail clipping.[88] This technique still awaits confirmation by an independent group.

The gold standard of diagnosis is histopathology,[89] which requires a biopsy. This is often insufficient, not allowing a diagnosis to be made. Again, the responsible lesion for a longitudinal streak in the nail is the matrix. Thus, an optimal biopsy of the matrix must be obtained. This can be a longitudinal biopsy including the proximal nail fold, the matrix, nail bed, hyponychium, and nail plate. It is the method of choice for laterally located melanonychias. A streak in the center of the nail may be biopsied with a punch with a maximal diameter of 3 mm in order not to leave a nail dystrophy in case the lesion is benign, or with a fusiform or crescentic biopsy of the matrix which is oriented transversely in order to prevent a post-biopsy split nail. Nail bed biopsies are fusiform and performed longitudinally because of the unique longitudinal arrangement of the nail bed rete ridges. We have developed a tangential matrix and nail bed biopsy that prevents post-biopsy nail dystrophy and allows large superficial excisions.[90–92] Briefly, the proximal nail fold is detached from the nail, incised at its both sides and reflected, the proximal third of the nail is detached from the matrix and lifted up to permit the melanocytic lesion to be seen, and a shallow incision is carried around it with an adequate safety margin. Using a #15 scalpel blade, the lesion is then tangentially removed with sawing motions. The nail plate is laid back and the proximal nail fold reclined and stitched. The surgical specimen is about 0.7–1 mm thick[93] and has to be transferred on a piece of filter paper to stretch it out and both are immersed in formalin.

The treatment of ungual melanomas is still somewhat controversial. Whereas amputation was and still is the rule for most surgeons,[94] this is only necessary for frankly invasive nail melanomas. Since 1978, we have adopted a strategy of functional surgery: in situ and early invasive melanomas are widely excised locally and the defect repaired with a free full-thickness graft or other methods;[95, 96] this has proven to be very safe[97–99] and is now more and more accepted also by other dermatosurgeons[100–102] and plastic surgeons.[103] However, a Korean study measuring the distance from the matrix to the underlying bone doubted the safety of this treatment approach whereas another one found that dermal invasion of the matrix is a late event in matrix melanoma.[104, 105] Amputation is held to be the treatment of choice for invasive melanomas. The role of sentinel lymph node biopsy in nail melanomas is still disputed.

15.2.1.1 Histopathology

The histopathologic diagnosis of clinically typical nail melanomas does usually not pose any difficulties. Doubtful cases often require serial and step sections, best from a total excision. This is well achieved using the tangential biopsy technique as it is always the in situ melanoma and intraepithelial component that challenge the diagnostic capabilities of the dermatopathologist. It is important to know that normal matrix melanocytes are often in the suprabasal layer of the lower matrix epithelium, that they are normally dormant, that is, do not produce melanin, are positive for HMB45, and their number is about 6.5 per mm stretch of basal layer.[106,107] Higher melanocyte counts were yielded when counting matrix segments.[108] Melanocyte density was counted 59/mm (39–136) for melanoma as compared to 15 (5–31) in benign melanocytic hyperplasia.[106] Another method found approximately 200 melanocytes/mm² in the matrix that are usually dormant, particularly in the proximal matrix whereas about half of the melanocytes in the distal matrix are active. In the nail bed, there are only up to 50/mm² and they are quiescent. In contrast, about 1150 melanocytes are present per mm² in the epidermis.[109]

Ungual melanomas vary in histologic appearance depending on their exact location within the nail unit, even when a melanoma involves different areas of the same nail unit. Those of periungual skin are similar to acral lentiginous melanoma of the palm and sole, but in the periphery of lesions extending from the proximal nail fold to the dorsum of the digit, it may mimic lentigo maligna melanoma except for the epidermis usually remaining of normal thickness or being slightly acanthotic.

In the beginning, most nail melanomas are lentiginous with their cells being arranged singly at the dermo-epithelial junction and just above it (Figure 15.6). This is particularly obvious at the advancing margin of the lesion. Some melanoma cells may be found in clear-cut suprabasal position and sometimes migrate upward and be included into the nail plate;[110] intraungual melanoma cells (Figure 15.7) always come from the matrix and not from the nail bed as was wrongly stated.[111] Although this underlines the potential importance of attached nail plate for the diagnosis of subungual melanoma,[112] we recline the detached plate and fix it as this facilitates wound healing. Usually the diagnosis is more obvious in the center of the lesion and over invasive portions. Here, cellular atypia is seen, rarely a mitosis. In contrast to many publications, most subungual melanomas we have seen did not have an inflammatory infiltrate although this may be present focally or at the entire lesion and occasionally be so dense as to mask the

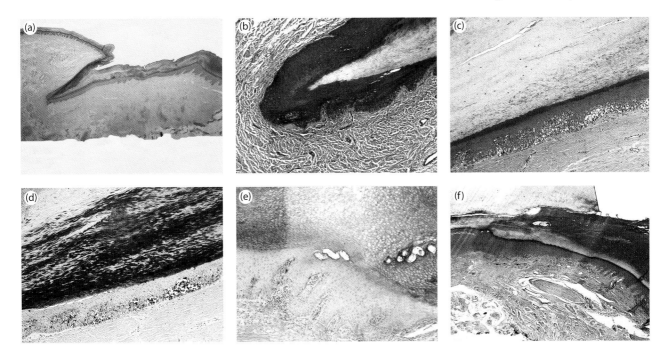

Figure 15.6 Subungual melanoma. (a) Scanning magnification of the surgical specimen of complete nail unit extirpation. There is virtually no inflammatory infiltrate. (b) Apical matrix showing an elevated number of melanocytes. (c) Mid-matrix with huge increase in the number of melanocytes many of which are slightly atypical. H&E. (d) Fontana-Masson stain demonstrates the pigmented melanoma cells. (e) Distal nail bed of the same patient exhibiting very few melanoma cells. Fontana-Masson stain. (f) *In situ* component of the hyponychium, slight sublesional inflammatory infiltrate.

true nature of the lesion. It may display a lichenoid pattern. The melanoma cells are both rounded and spindle-shaped, they often demonstrate long dendrites that may in addition be very plump. Most SUMs deriving from the matrix are pigmented and melanophages may be abundant. The degree of pigmentation is well seen in Fontana stained sections. The localization of the melanin in the nail plate allows its origin to be suggested: Pigment in the uppermost layer derives from melanocytes of the apical matrix, that in the middle of the nail plate from the middle of the

matrix, melanin in the lowermost layers from the distal matrix, and pigment in all layers reflects melanocytes in the entire length of the matrix. In contrast, melanomas originating from the nail bed often, but not always, remain amelanotic (Figure 15.8) and they cannot give pigment into the growing nail.

Nail dystrophy is common in long-standing lesions. This is due to the gradual substitution of nail producing matrix epithelium by melanoma cells.[113,114] As outlined above, any longitudinal melanonychia be it very light or

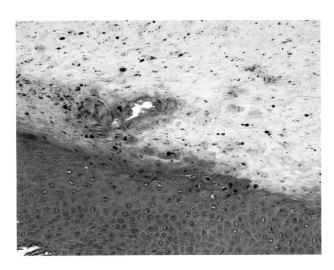

Figure 15.7 Intraungual melanoma cells in a long-standing though still *in situ* melanoma.

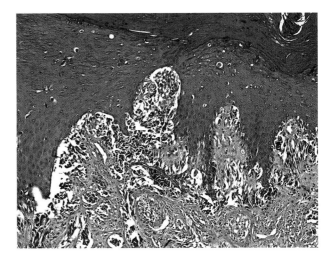

Figure 15.8 Invasive amelanotic nail bed melanoma in a 43-year-old woman with a 5-year history of a swelling of her left thumb nail.

dark, narrow or wide, exhibiting a slight nail dystrophy is suspicious for melanoma.[73,115,116]

The basal and suprabasal layers of the nail bed epithelium are invaded by an excessive number of melanocytes often displaying cellular atypia. Areas of invasion show subepithelial atypical melanocytes, sometimes with mitoses. Even a pigmented nail bed melanoma cannot produce a longitudinal streak as the nail bed keratinocytes do not produce the nail plate despite one contradictory assumption.[117] Three cases of *in situ* amelanotic melanoma clinically mimicking lichen planus were observed. They all had a marked increase of melanocyte density in the matrix and nail bed, which was located in the basal layer and arranged in a lentiginous fashion with only a few nests. In one case, some nuclei were hyperchromatic whereas in another case there was a dense and haphazard intraepithelial spread of atypical melanocytes. The third case exhibited densely packed melanocytes without pagetoid spread. No inflammatory infiltrate was present.[118]

Melanomas originating from the hyponychium are similar to palmar and plantar acral lentiginous melanomas. The basal and suprabasal epidermal layers are populated with more or less atypical melanocytes that are often densely pigmented. Pagetoid spread and transepidermal elimination of single and sometimes small groups of melanoma cells is frequent (Figure 15.9). Mitoses are usually rare. In invasive areas, spindle-shaped cells usually predominate.

Desmoplastic areas and completely desmoplastic acral lentiginous melanomas (ALMs) do occur. They are more often amelanotic and the cells are more often spindle-shaped.[39] The entire dermis may show an alteration of its architecture.[119] Together with focal infiltrates of lymphocytes and occasional plasma cells in or at the periphery, this may be a clue to the diagnosis at scanning magnification. Higher magnification exhibits spindle cells in a markedly fibrotic stroma. In subungual localization, they are often negative for S-100 and only the superficial cells are positive for Melan-A; HMB-45 is often negative. Sox10 was found to be a reliable marker for desmoplastic melanoma. Neurotropism may be seen and neurotropic melanoma may be a variant of desmoplastic melanoma.[120] Spindle cell melanoma fascicles invade the perineurial and intraneurial structures; this may be very difficult to be observed, often only giving the aspect of hypercellularity of the nerves. These melanomas tend to be positive for p75 and other neurotrophins.[121] The neurotropism is often associated with a higher risk of metastasis.

Hutchinson's sign is the periungual extension of an *in situ* component of subungual melanoma. It is often characterized by a seemingly bland proliferation of melanocytes in a lentiginous pattern (Figure 15.10). Equidistant melanocyte distribution is rather the rule than an exception making the diagnosis of clear-cut melanoma *in situ* very difficult although rarely it may be histologically more obvious than the matrix or nail bed melanoma.[122] Immunohistochemistry may be helpful to outline the long and plump dendrites.[19] For cases where the diagnosis is not unequivocal, crowding and nesting are lacking and melanocytic atypia is not convincing like in most cases of the advancing edge of an *in situ* subungual melanoma or Hutchinson sign, the term atypical melanocytic hyperplasia was coined.[123]

In our experience, even long-standing subungual melanomas with a decade long history are often still *in situ*. However, there is frequently an extension on the entire matrix, all along the adjacent ventral surface of the proximal nail fold, the nail bed, and the hyponychium. In these instances, the nail bed often appears to be relatively devoid of melanoma cells as compared to the matrix and the hyponychium (Figure 15.11). As is known from melanomas of the palms and soles, the intraepidermal component may be more extensive than clinically anticipated and in the marginal area, it may be very difficult to see single melanocytes between the keratinocytes. This is where immunohistochemical demonstration of melanocytes is indicated.[19,66]

Immunohistochemistry is a diagnostic adjunct for nail melanomas.[124–128] The most commonly used antibodies are MART-1, Melan-A, HMB45, and S-100p. MART-1 and

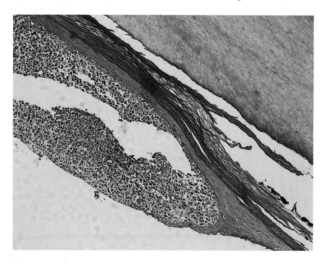

Figure 15.9 Invasive melanoma of the distal nail bed.

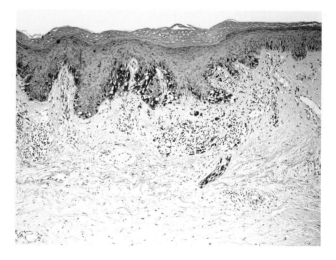

Figure 15.10 Hutchinson sign of the proximal nail fold shows a lentiginous proliferation of melanoma cells in the periungual skin including invasion of the sweat duct (HMB45).

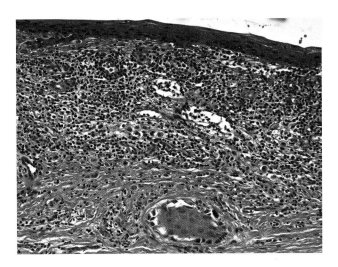

Figure 15.11 Invasive subungual melanoma showing surprisingly few melanoma cells in the nail bed epithelium although a small subungual onycholemmal cyst exhibits melanoma cells in its basal layer.

Melan-A are two slightly different clones of melanosomal proteins recognized by T cells and are cytoplasmic markers for melanocytes with very similar staining profiles; however, they may also stain melanosomes in keratinocytes and melanophages. S-100 has a sensitivity of 90% and specificity of 70%. Melan-A (Figure 15.12a) is more sensitive. HMB45 (Figure 15.12b) has a specificity of 97% and sensitivity of 75% in cutaneous melanoma. Junctional cells are more intensely marked than dermal cells.[129] HMB45 or Melan-A do not stain 83% of spindle cell and desmoplastic melanoma. S-100p is less specific as it stains many other cells derived from the neural crest, but in nail melanomas, this antigen appears to be lost not infrequently.[130] Furthermore, they are not really specific also staining other neural crest derived tumors, adenocarcinomas, and even lymphomas.[131] Microphthalmia transcription factor 1 (MITF-1) is less frequently used[132, 133] although the staining with MITF-1 is more specific as it does not stain melanin or melanosomes, but the nuclei. Sox10 (Figure 15.12c) is a transcription factor necessary for the development of the neurocrest and of melanocytes. It is expressed in the nuclei of melanocytes, melanoma cells, peripheral nerve sheath cells, and secretory sweat gland portions, but also

some other tissues, particularly breast.[134] It is useful for the diagnosis of desmoplastic melanoma since fibroblasts and histiocytes remain unstained.[135,136] Using Melan-A together with Sox10 staining, benign reactive dermal melanocytes were identified in approximately 10% of melanoma *in situ* cases and nearly one-third of squamous and basal cell carcinomas.[137] Sox10 is upregulated with melanoma progression.[138] Both Sox10 and MITF-1 allow easy distinction of pigmented keratinocytes from melanocytes and melanoma cells, but none distinguishes benign from malignant melanocytic lesions.[139]

Recently, new monoclonal antibodies against melanocytic differentiation antigens (MAGE, NKI/C3, NKI/beteb, KBA 62, BNL2) and melanocyte antibody cocktails were developed that virtually stain all melanoma cells; however, they are not melanoma-specific.[140,141] It appears that Ki67 (MiB1) is the most useful adjunct in differentiating benign from malignant melanocytic tumors.[126]

Whereas most of our patients presented with *in situ* and early invasive melanomas, large numbers of patients from other centers showed appallingly thick and advanced tumors.[75,106,142] These cases do not present the diagnostic difficulties outlined above.

Two cases of subungual melanoma with chondroid differentiation were observed.[143] This phenomenon is exceptional, but can be explained by the fact that both melanocytes and chrondrocytes derive from the neural crest.[144]

Melanomas are heterogeneous tumors. At least in part, they are characterized by DNA mutations leading to the activation of oncogenes and inactivation of tumor suppressor genes and by gains, losses, and amplifications of whole or partial chromosomes. These genomic aberrations lead to mutational and karyotypic profiles that differ among different subtypes of melanoma.[145–148]

Approximately one-third of acral and mucosal melanomas as well as melanomas of chronically sun-damaged skin have c-KIT, 10% of acral melanomas have NRAS, and 10%–15% BRAF^{V600} mutations.[149,150] Fluorescence *in situ* hybridization (FISH) and comparative genomic hybridization (CGH) studies have shown that molecular genetically altered cells can be found in the epidermis up to 9 mm from the visible margin of pigmented acral lentiginous melanoma, but this phenomenon was restricted to the *in situ* melanocytes; they were called field cells.[151] This is probably

(a)   (b)   (c)

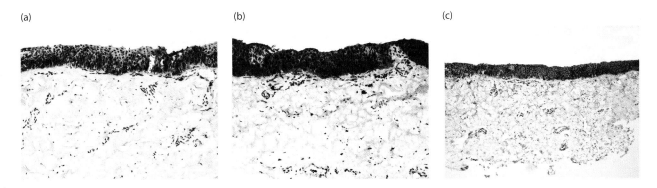

Figure 15.12 Comparative staining of subungual melanoma with antibodies to (a) Melan-A, (b) HMB45, and (c) Sox10.

the reason that acral melanomas seemingly excised *in toto* were observed to recur. Immunohistochemical demonstration of cKIT/CD117 may be useful to identify patients that could benefit from imatinib therapy.[152]

There is now much research on potential melanoma stem cells;[153,154] however, this has not yet arrived at nail unit melanomas.

The histogenetic type of melanoma—acral lentiginous melanoma (ALM), superficial spreading melanoma (SSM), or nodular melanoma (NM)—is difficult to define in the nail. It is, however, not really important as the molecular genetic investigations have not shown differences among them, but among melanomas of different localizations. Clark level and Breslow thickness are also very difficult to ascertain. This is not only due to the fact that most biopsies are only partial, but that the nail anatomy itself is different from skin. The papillary and reticular dermis are not clearly separated, and there is no cutaneous fat between the distal matrix-nail bed and the periosteum.[37] Clark level I is therefore intraepidermal, II is very superficial, III is invasion into the mid- to deep dermis, IV almost reaches the periosteum, and V is invasion to or into the bone. Measuring the vertical tumor thickness according to Breslow is challenging as there is normally no granular layer in the matrix and nail bed and the epithelium may be acanthotic and grossly thickened giving large numbers that do not really reflect the prognosis. Therefore, a division into melanomas thinner or thicker than 2.5 mm has been proposed; this gave statistically significant differences in survival after 5 years: 88% versus 40%.[36] Old age, ulceration, higher mitotic index, amelanotic tumor, and higher stage of disease are further negative prognostic factors.[142]

Melanomas often show characteristic gene alterations seen in fluorescent *in situ* hybridization (FISH) and comparative genomic hybridization. KIT mutations are more frequent in acral lentiginous melanomas than in those of light-exposed skin. Gene amplifications were seen in all ALMs investigated, most commonly on chromosome 11q13 where cyclin D1 is a potential candidate gene. In contrast, mutations of the BRAF oncogene are less frequent.[145,155–159] These changes were typical for melanomas of the palms, soles, and nail independent of their histological growth pattern.[160]

Erosive oozing tumors of the nail may be adequate for cytological diagnosis of smears. This is easily performed with a glass slide that is gently scraped over the tumor and then over another slide to spread the cells. After drying and short alcohol-acetone fixation, the cytosmear can be stained for H&E and a melanocyte marker (Figure 15.13).

15.2.1.2 Nail melanoma in children

Longitudinal melanonychia is not an uncommon finding in children,[20,22] particularly in Asians, Africans, native Americans, and Afro-Americans. Most cases are due to melanocyte activation, lentigo, or junctional nevi in the matrix. In attempts to use dermatoscopy of longitudinal melanonychia, great uncertainty was found.[161] In small children, the nevus may show broad pigmentation with some

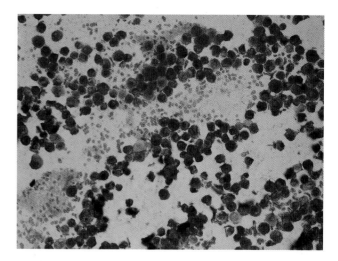

Figure 15.13 Cytosmear of an erosive nail bed melanoma stained for HMB45.

variegation of the brown color similar to that seen in adult nails with melanoma. The parents usually are not only concerned because of the faint risk of being an infant nail melanoma, but also the embarrassing esthetic effect. In children, the pigmentation first exhibits a rapid increase in color intensity and width and then characteristically stabilizes. At adolescence, there is often a regression or even complete disappearance.[162,163] Thus, in general, a brown streak in the nail of a child should be taken as a benign lesion. However, when the streak suddenly widens after having been present and stable for years, becomes markedly darker and wider proximally than distally, a diagnostic excision is recommended.

There are some reports in the literature on nail melanomas in children. This is generally a rare event and most dermatopathologists hesitate to make this diagnosis in children as there may be considerable nuclear atypia in infantile matrix nevi (Figure 15.14). One of our cases sent to a panel of melanoma and nail pathology specialists was not diagnosed as melanoma but as atypical melanocytic hyperplasia.[49,62] Not all lesions described in children were unanimously accepted as nail melanoma, for example, the first case described in a child that was probably fair-skinned[164] and in some of the cases reported from Japan.[165] In fact, most cases were described from Japan,[166] but also from other countries with more intensely pigmented people such as the Philippines,[167] Argentina, Brazil,[49] Colombia,[61] and the United States.[168] Two cases had positive lymph nodes.[164,169]

15.2.1.3 Rare melanocytic tumors

A case of a collision tumor of subungual squamomelanocytic tumor was observed with a positive sentinel lymph node. Whereas the biopsy had only shown a melanoma *in situ*, total nail unit resection revealed a squamous cell carcinoma in a melanoma occupying the entire matrix and nail bed with ulceration and many mitoses.[170]

15.2.1.4 The melanonychia problem

As outlined above, the diagnosis of ungual melanoma in children is often not made. It is well known that lentigines

(a)   (b)

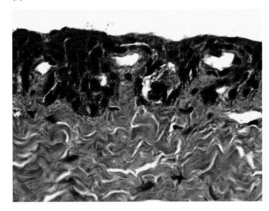
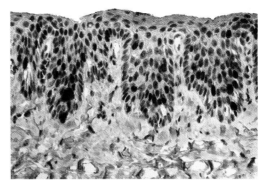

Figure 15.14 *In situ* subungual melanoma in a fair-skinned 11-year-old girl displaying nests and lentiginous proliferation of (a) severely atypical melanocytes (b) that are positive for Ki67 (MiB1).

and junctional nevi of the matrix in children may exhibit very worrying features that when present in an adult nail would be diagnosed as melanoma without hesitation.

Another problem is the acquired, histopathologically often barely noticeable melanonychia in adults. As is known from the advancing edge of subungual *in situ* melanomas, the correct diagnosis can be extremely difficult; indeed, it is often challenging to recognize melanocytes at all.[19] In our experience, an acquired melanonychia in an adult fair-skinned Caucasian should always be considered of potential biologic malignancy despite appearing morphologically bland with the exception of functional melanonychia (Table 15.2).

15.2.1.5 Differential diagnoses

Generally accepted criteria for the diagnosis of early nail melanoma do not (yet) exist. A clinicopathologic correlation is necessary. However, in general, the clinical appearance of a pigmented streak is of little help in establishing the correct diagnosis.[171] The most important differential diagnosis of ungual melanoma is a benign melanocytic proliferation.[172] In longitudinal melanonychia, the responsible melanocytic lesion may be an activation of normal matrix melanocytes without a higher number of melanocytes, called functional melanonychia, or a numerical increase in the number of normal melanocytes, that is, a lentigo or a nevus. The histopathologic changes seen in functional melanonychia may be very subtle and require immunohistochemistry to visualize the melanocytes and

special pigment stains such as Fontana-Masson to see the melanin. A lentigo is usually visible in H&E stained sections as it contains more melanin and some single melanophages may be seen in the superficial matrix dermis. A melanocytic nevus of the matrix is defined by the presence of nests of melanocytes without cellular atypia and with slender dendrites. Whereas some authors claim that a melanonychia in a child as well as a very light-brown band in adults does not require histopathologic examination, it is our policy to excision-biopsy all cases as the tangential matrix biopsy avoids postoperative nail dystrophy.

Particularly in subjects with dark skin, an ungual Bowen's disease may cause a longitudinal pigmentation.[173–177] This is histopathologically seen as a population of the lesion by normal melanocytes. Also squamous cell carcinoma may be pigmented.[178]

Fungal melanonychia presents a diffuse light yellow-brown staining of the nail. Many different species have been isolated; *Trichophyton rubrum* is the most common cause in Central Europe, but a number of nondermatophytic molds were also found to produce brown to black nails.[179] One case of longitudinal melanonychia in three toenails with fumagoid cells (Medlar bodies), a peculiar pattern of chromoblastomycosis, was described.[180]

REFERENCES

1. Fryer JM, Werth VP. Pregnancy-associated hyperpigmentation: Longitudinal melanonychia. *J Am Acad Dermatol* 1992;26:493–494.
2. Baran R. Frictional longitudinal melanonychia: A new entity. *Dermatologica* 1987;174:280–284.
3. Anolik RB, Shah K, Rubin AI. Onychophagia-induced longitudinal melanonychia. *Pediatr Dermatol* 2012;29:488–489.
4. Baran R. Nail biting and picking as a possible cause of longitudinal melanonychia. A study of 6 cases. *Dermatologica* 1990;181:126–128.
5. MacDonald KJ, Hargreaves GK, Ead RD. Longitudinal melanonychia during photochemotherapy. *Br J Dermatol* 1986;114:395–396.

Table 15.2 Melanonychia and age of onset in light-skinned individuals

Babies and children	Benign
Adolescents	Usually benign
Adults < 30 years	Probably benign
Adults > 30 years	Suspicious
Adults > 40 years	Probably malignant
Adults > 50 years	Usually malignant

6. Hann SK, Hwang SY, Park YK. Melanonychia induced by systemic photochemotherapy. *Photodermatol* 1989;6:98–99.

7. Kaptanoglu AF, Oskay T. Symmetrical melanonychia of the thumbnails associated with PUVA in psoriasis. *J Dermatol* 2004;31:148–150.

8. Utaş S, Kulluk P. A case of hydroxyurea-induced longitudinal melanonychia. *Int J Dermatol* 2010; 49:469–470.

9. Prat C, Viñas M, Marcoval J, Jucglà A. Longitudinal melanonychia as the first sign of Addison's disease. *J Am Acad Dermatol* 2008;58:522–524.

10. Chang P, Román V, Monterroso MA, Castro Benincasa ML, Cordón C, Rivera S. Síndrome de Nelson. Reporte de un caso. *Dermatol Cosm Med Quir* 2013;11:199–202.

11. Ridley CM. Pigmentation of fingertips and nails in vitamin B12 deficiency. *Br J Dermatol* 1977; 97:105–106.

12. Noppakun N, Swasdikul D. Reversible hyperpigmentation of skin and nails with white hair due to vitamin B12 deficiency. *Arch Dermatol* 1986;122:896–899.

13. Halaban R, Moellmann G. Proliferation and malignant transformation of melanocytes. *Crit Rev Oncog* 1991;2:247–258.

14. Shoji T, Cockerell CJ, Koff AB, Bhawan J. Eruptive melanocytic nevi after Stevens–Johnson syndrome. *J Am Acad Dermatol* 1997;37:337–339.

15. Alaibac M, Piaserico S, Rossi CR, Foletto M, Zacchello G, Carli P, Belloni-Fortina A. Eruptive melanocytic nevi in patients with renal allografts: Report of 10 cases with dermoscopic findings. *J Am Acad Dermatol* 2003;49:1020–1022.

16. Daniel RC III. Nail pigmentation abnormalities. *Dermatol Clin* 1985;3:431–443.

17. Haneke E. Laugier-Hunziker-Baran syndrome. *Hautarzt* 1991;42:512–515.

18. Moore RT, Chae KA, Rhodes AR. Laugier and Hunziker pigmentation: A lentiginous proliferation of melanocytes. *J Am Acad Dermatol* 2004; 50(Suppl 5):S70–S74.

19. Weedon D, Van Deurse M, Rosendahl C. "Occult" melanocytes in nail matrix melanoma. *Am J Dermatopathol* 2012;34:855.

20. Tosti A, Baran R, Piraccini BM, Cameli N, Fanti PA. Nail matrix nevi: A clinical and histopathologic study of twenty-two patients. *J Am Acad Dermatol* 1996;34:765–771.

21. Léauté-Labrèze C, Bioulac-Sage P, Taïeb A. Longitudinal melanonychia in children. A study of eight cases. *Arch Dermatol* 1996;132:167–169.

22. Goettmann-Bonvallot S, André J, Belaich S. Longitudinal melanonychia in children: A clinical and histopathologic study of 40 cases. *J Am Acad Dermatol* 1999;41:17–22.

23. Ohtsuka H, Hori Y, Ando M. Nevus of the little finger with a remarkable nail deformity: Case report. *Plast Reconstr Surg* 1978;61:108–111.

24. Coskey RJ, Magnell TD, Bernacki EG Jr. Congenital subungual nevus. *J Am Acad Dermatol* 1983;9:747–751.

25. Libow LF, Casey TJ, Varela CD. Congenital subungual nevus in a black infant. *Cutis* 1995;56:154–156.

26. Lazaridou E, Giannopoulou C, Fotiadou C, Demiri E, Ioannides D. Congenital nevus of the nail apparatus—Diagnostic approach of a case through dermoscopy. *Pediatr Dermatol* 2013;30(6):e293–e294.

27. Agusti-Mejias A, Messeguer F, Febrer I, Alegre V. Congenital subungual and periungual melanocytic nevus. *Actas Dermosifiliogr* 2013;104:446–448.

28. Goldminz AM, Wolpowitz D, Gottlieb AB, Krathen MS. Congenital subungual melanocytic nevus with a pseudo-Hutchinson sign. *Dermatol Online J* 2013; 19(4):8.

29. Sawada M, Ishizaki S, Kobayashi K, Dekio I, Tanaka M. Longterm digital monitoring in the diagnosis and management of congenital nevi of the nail apparatus showing pseudo-Hutchinson's sign. *Dermatol Pract Concept* 2014 30;4:37–40.

30. Lee E-J, Shin M-K, Lee M-H. A subungual blue naevus showing expansile growth. *Acta Derm Venereol* 2012;92:162–163.

31. Gershtenson PC, Krunic A, Chen H, Konanahalli M, Worobec S. Subungual and periungual congenital blue naevus. *Australas J Dermatol* 2009;50:144–147.

32. Dominguez-Cherit J, Toussaint-Caire S, Kamino H, Iorizzo M, Tosti A. Subungual Spitz nevus in a Hispanic infant. *Dermatol Surg* 2008;34:1571–1573.

33. Naylor EMT, Ruben BS, Robinson-Bostom L, Telang GH, Jellinek NJ. Subungual blue nevus with combined phenotypic features. *J Am Acad Dermatol* 2008;58:1021–1024.

34. Boyer M. Fongus hématodes du petit doigt. *Gaz Méd Paris* 1834;212.

35. Haneke E. Ungual melanoma—Controversies in diagnosis and treatment. *Dermatol Ther* 2012;25:510–524.

36. Banfield CC, Redburn JC, Dawber RP. The incidence and prognosis of nail apparatus melanoma. A retrospective study of 105 patients in four English regions. *Br J Dermatol* 1998;139:276–279.

37. O'Leary JA, Berend KR, Johnson JL, Levin LS, Seigler HF. Subungual melanoma. A review of 93 cases with identification of prognostic variables. *Clin Orthop Relat Res* 2000;378:206–212.

38. Ragnarsson-Olding BK. Spatial density of primary malignant melanoma in sun-shielded body sites: A potential guide to melanoma genesis. *Acta Oncol* 2011;50:323–328.

39. Kato T, Suetake T, Sugiyama Y, Tabata N, Tagami H. Epidemiology and prognosis of subungual melanoma in 34 Japanese patients. *Br J Dermatol* 1996;134:383–387.

40. Thai KE, Young R, Sinclair RD. Nail apparatus melanoma. *Australas J Dermatol* 2001;42:71–81.

41. Seui M, Takematsu H, Hosokawa M, Obata M, Tomita Y, Kato T, Takahashi M, Mihm MC Jr.

Acral melanoma in Japan. *J Invest Dermatol* 1983; 80(Suppl 1):56s–60s.

42. Ishihara K, Saida T, Otsuka F, Yamazaki N. Prognosis and statistical investigation committee of the Japanese Skin Cancer Society. Statistical profiles of malignant melanoma and other skin cancers in Japan: 2007 update. *Int J Clin Oncol* 2008;13:33–41.

43. Roh MR, Kim J, Chung KY. Treatment and outcomes of melanoma in acral location in Korean patients. *Yonsei Med J* 2010;51:562–568.

44. Chang JW-C. Cutaneous melanoma: Taiwan experience and literature review. *Chang Gung Med J* 2010;33:602–612.

45. Lichte V, Breuninger H, Metzler G, Haefner HM, Moehrle M. Acral lentiginous melanoma: Conventional histology vs. three-dimensional histology. *Br J Dermatol* 2009;160:591–599.

46. Haenssle HA, Hofmann S, Buhl T, Emmert S, Schön MP, Bertsch HP, Rosenberger A. Assessment of melanoma histotypes and associated patient related factors: Basis for a predictive statistical model. *J Dtsch Dermatol Ges* 2015;13:37–45.

47. Bradford PT, Goldstein AM, McMaster ML, Tucker MA. Acral lentiginous melanoma: Incidence and survival patterns in the United States, 1986–2005. *Arch Dermatol* 2009;145:427–434.

48. Kiryu H. Malignant melanoma *in situ* arising in the nail unit of a child. *J Dermatol* 1998;25:41–44.

49. Tosti A, Piraccini BM, Cagalli A, Haneke E. In situ melanoma of the nail unit in children: Report of 2 cases in Caucasian fair skinned children. *Pediatr Dermatol* 2012;29:79–83.

50. Phan A, Touzet S, Dalle S, Ronger-Savlé S, Balme B, Thomas L. Acral lentiginous melanoma: A clinicoprognostic study of 126 cases. *Br J Dermatol* 2006;155:561–569.

51. Möhrle M, Häfner HM. Is subungual melanoma related to trauma? *Dermatologica* 2002;204:259–261.

52. Rangwala S, Hunt C, Modi G, Krishnan B, Orengo I. Amelanotic subungual melanoma after trauma: An unusual clinical presentation. *Dermatol Online J* 2011;17(6):8.

53. Lesage C, Journet-Tollhupp J, Bernard P, Grange F. Mélanome acral post-traumatique: une réalite sousestimée? *Ann Dermatol Venereol* 2012;139:727–731.

54. Fanti PA, Dika E, Misciali C, Vaccari S, Barisani A, Piraccini BM, Cavrin G, Maibach HI, Patrizi A. Nail apparatus melanoma: Is trauma a coincidence? Is this peculiar tumor a real acral melanoma? *Cutan Ocul Toxicol* 2013;32:150–153.

55. Bormann G, Marsch WC, Haerting J, Helmbold P. Concomitant traumas influence prognosis in melanomas of the nail apparatus. *Br J Dermatol* 2006;155:76–80.

56. Keitea M, Keita AM, Traoré B, Thiam I, Soumah MM, Diané BF, Tounkara TM et al. Mélanome du pouce et faux ongles chez une fille de 29 ans infectée par le VIH. *Ann Dermatol Vénéréol* 2013;140:S112–S113.

57. Stern DK, Creasey AA, Quijije J, Lebwohl MG. UV-A and UV-B penetration of normal human cadaveric fingernail plate. *Arch Dermatol* 2011;147:439–441.

58. Micu E, Baturaite Z, Juzeniene A, Bruland ØS, Moan JE. Superficial-spreading and nodular melanomas in Norway: A comparison by body site distribution and latitude gradients. *Melanoma Res* 2012;22:460–465.

59. Moan J, Baturaite Z, Porojnicu AC, Dahlback A, Juzeniene A. UVA, UVB and incidence of cutaneous malignant melanoma in Norway and Sweden. *Photochem Photobiol Sci* 2012;11:191–198.

60. Kopf AW, Waldo E. Melanonychia striata. *Australas J Dermatol* 1980;21:59–70.

61. Motta A, López C, Acosta A, Peñaranda C. Subungual melanoma *in situ* in a Hispanic girl treated with functional resection and reconstruction with onychocutaneous toe free flap. *Arch Dermatol* 2007;143:1600–1602.

62. Iorizzo M, Tosti A, Di Chiacchio N, Hirata SH, Misciali C, Michalany N, Dominguez J, Toussaint S. Nail melanoma in children: Differential diagnosis and management. *Dermatol Surg* 2008;34:974–978.

63. Bonamonte D, Arpaia N, Cimmino A, Vestita M. In situ melanoma of the nail unit presenting as a rapid growing longitudinal melanonychia in a 9-year-old white boy. *Dermatol Surg* 2014;40:1154–1157.

64. Rotunda AM, Graham-Hicks S, Bennett RG. Simultaneous subungual melanoma *in situ* of both thumbs. *J Am Acad Dermatol* 2008;58:S42–S44.

65. Levit EK, Kagen MH, Scher RK, Grossman M, Altman E. The ABC rule for clinical detection of subungual melanoma. *J Am Acad Dermatol* 2000;42:269–274.

66. Rosendahl C, Cameron A, Wilkinson D, Belt P, Williamson R, Weedon D. Nail matrix melanoma: Consecutive cases in a general practice. *Dermatol Pract Concept* 2012;2(2):13:63–70.

67. Elloumi-Jellouli A, Triki S, Driss M, Derbel F, Zghal M, Mrad K, Rhomdhnane KhB. A misdiagnosed nail bed melanoma. *Dermatol Online J* 2010;16(7):13.

68. Wallberg B, Hansson J. Delayed diagnosis of subungual melanoma. Two cases were misjudged as onychomycosis [In Swedish]. *Läkartidningen* 1997;94:2543–2544.

69. Braham C, Fraiture AL, Quatresooz P, Piérard-Franchimont C, Piérard GE. Des "dermatomycoses banales" qui ne pardonnent pas. "Banal onychomycosis" that cannot be overlooked [In French]. *Rev Med Liège* 2002;57:317–319.

70. Soon SL, Solomon AR Jr, Papadopoulos D, Murray DR, McAlpine B, Washington CV. Acral lentiginous melanoma mimicking benign disease: The Emory experience. *J Am Acad Dermatol* 2003;48:183–188.

71. De Giorgi V, Sestini S, Massi D, Panelos J, Papi F, Dini M, Lotti T. Subungual melanoma: A particularly invasive "onychomycosis." *J Am Geriatr Soc* 2007;55:2094–2096.

72. Shukla VK, Hughes LE. Differential diagnosis of subungual melanoma from a surgical point of view. *Br J Surg* 1989;76:1156–1160.

73. Gosselink CP, Sindone JL, Meadows BJ, Mohammadi A, Rosa M. Amelanotic subungual melanoma: A case report. *J Foot Ankle Surg* 2009;48:220–222.

74. Blum A. Onychomykose mit Onychodystrophie oder akrolentiginöses Melanom mit Onychomykose und Onychodystrophie? *Hautarzt* 2012;63:341–343.

75. Blessing K, Kernohan NM, Park KG. Subungual malignant melanoma: Clinicopathological features of 100 cases. *Histopathology* 1991;19:425–429.

76. Cohen T, Busam KJ, Patel A, Brady MS. Subungual melanoma: Management considerations. *Am J Surg* 2008;195:244–248.

77. Chow WT, Bhat W, Magdub S, Orlando A. In situ subungual melanoma: Digit salvaging clearance. *J Plast Reconstr Aesthet Surg* July 16, 2012. [Epub ahead of print].

78. Graf RM, Tolazzi AR, Colpo PG, de Oliveira e Cruz GA. Sentinel lymph node detection in a patient with subungual melanoma after transaxillary breast augmentation. *Plast Reconstr Surg* 2011;127:65e–66e.

79. Wantz M, Antonicelli F, Derancourt C, Bernard P, Avril MF, Grange F. Long-term survival and spontaneous tumor regression in stage IV melanoma: Possible role of adrenalectomy and massive tumor antigen release. *Ann Dermatol Venereol* 2010;137:464–467.

80. Dominguez-Cherit J. Spontaneous regression of subungual melanoma. XXVI Cong Soc Mex Dermatol, Leon Gto, Aug 5–9 2014.

81. Sundell J. Mystery of the swollen leg [Finnish]. *Duodecim* 2010;126:1827–1830.

82. Haneke E, Baran R. Subunguale Tumoren. *Z Hautkr* 1982;57:355–362.

83. Braun RP, Gutkowicz-Krusin D, Rabinovitz H, Cognetta A, Hofmann-Wellenhof R, Ahlgrimm-Siess V, Polsky D et al. Agreement of dermatopathologists in the evaluation of clinically difficult melanocytic lesions: How golden is the "gold standard?" *Dermatology* 2012;224:51–58.

84. Hirata SH, Yamada S, Almeida FA, Almeida FA, Tomomori-Yamashita J, Enokihara MY, Paschoal FM, Enokihara MM, Outi CM, Michalany NS. Dermoscopy of the nail bed and matrix to assess melanonychia striata. *J Am Acad Dermatol* 2005;53:884–886.

85. Hirata SH, Yamada S, Almeida FA, Enokihara MY, Rosa IP, Enokihara MM, Michalany NS. Dermoscopic examination of the nail bed and matrix. *Int J Dermatol* 2006;45:28–30.

86. Di Chiacchio N, Hirata SH, Enokihara MY, Michalany MS, Fabbrocini G, Tosti A. Dermatologists' accuracy in early diagnosis of melanoma of the nail matrix. *Arch Dermatol* 2010;146:382–387.

87. Debarbieux S, Hospod V, Depaepe L, Balme B, Poulalhon N, Thomas L. Perioperative confocal microscopy of the nail matrix in the management of *in situ* or minimally invasive subungual melanomas. *Br J Dermatol* 2012;167:828–836.

88. James VJ. Fiber diffraction of skin and nails provides an accurate diagnostic test for 8 malignancies. *Int J Cancer* 2009;125:133–138.

89. Ruben BS. Pigmented lesions of the nail unit: Clinical and histopathology features. *Semin Cutan Med Surg* 2010;29:148–158.

90. Haneke E. Operative Therapie akraler und subungualer Melanome. In: Rompel R, Petres J, eds. *Operative und onkologische Dermatologie. Fortschritte der operativen und onkologischen Dermatologie*, Berlin: Springer, 1999;15:210–214.

91. Haneke E, Lawry M. Nail surgery. In: Robinson JK, Hanke WC, Sengelmann RD, Siegel DM, eds. *Surgery of the Skin*, Philadelphia, PA: Elsevier, 2005;719–742.

92. Haneke E. Cirugía ungueal. In: Torres Lozada V, Camacho Martínez FM, Mihm MC, Sober AJ, Sánchez Carpintero I, eds. *Dermatología práctica Ibero-Latinoamericana. Atlas, enfermedades sistémicas asociadas y terapéutica*. Chapter 142. México, DF: Nieto Editores, 2005;1643–1652.

93. Di Chiacchio N, Refkalefsky Loureiro W, Schwery Michalany N, Kezam Gabriel FV. Tangential biopsy thickness versus lesion depth in longitudinal melanonychia: A pilot study. *Dermatol Res Pract* 2012;2012, Article ID 353864.

94. Glat PM, Spector JA, Roses DF, Shapiro RA, Harris MN, Beasley RW, Grossman JA. The management of pigmented lesions of the nail bed. *Ann Plast Surg* 1996;37:125–134.

95. Haneke E, Binder D. Subunguales Melanom mit streifiger Nagelpigmentierung. *Hautarzt* 1978;29:389–391.

96. Duarte AF, Correia O, Barros AM, Azevedo R, Haneke E. Nail matrix melanoma *in situ*: Conservative surgical management. *Dermatology* 2010;220:173–175.

97. Möhrle M, Metzger S, Schippert W, Garbe C, Rassner G, Breuninger H. "Functional" surgery in subungual melanoma. *Dermatol Surg* 2003;29:366–374.

98. Möhrle M, Lichte V, Breuninger H. Operative therapy of acral melanomas. *Hautarzt* 2011;62:362–367.

99. Duarte AF, Correia O, Ventura F, Barros M, Haneke E. Nail melanoma *in situ*: Clinical, dermoscopic, pathologic clues, and steps for minimally invasive treatment. *Dermatol Surg* 2015; Epub ahead of print.

100. Lacey LB, Niebla RM, Guevara Sanginés E. Subungual melanoma: Functional treatment with Mohs Surgery. *Dermatol Cosm Med Quir* 2007;5:136–143.

101. Sohl S, Simon JC, Wetzig T. Finger stall technique skin graft for reconstruction of fingers after extensive excisions of acral lentiginous melanomas. *J Dtsch Dermatol Ges* 2007;5:525–526.

102. Sureda N, Phan A, Poulalhon N, Balme B, Dalle S, Thomas L. Conservative surgical management of subungual (matrix derived) melanoma: Report of seven cases and literature review. *Br J Dermatol* 2011;165:852–858.

103. Smock ED, Barabas AG, Geh JL. Reconstruction of a thumb defect with Integra following wide local

excision of a subungual melanoma. *J Plast Reconstr Aesthet Surg* 2010;63:e36–e37.

104. Kim JY, Jung HJ, Lee WJ, Kim DW, Yoon GS, Kim DS, Park MJ, Lee SJ. Is the distance enough to eradicate *in situ* or early invasive subungual melanoma by wide local excision? From the point of view of matrix-to-bone distance for safe inferior surgical margin in Koreans. *Dermatology* 2011;223:122–123.

105. Shin HT, Jang KT, Mun GH, Lee DY, Lee JB. Histopathological analysis of the progression pattern of subungual melanoma: Late tendency of dermal invasion in the nail matrix area. *Mod Pathol* 2014;27:1461–1467.

106. Amin B, Nehal KS, Jungbluth AA, Zaidi B, Brady MS, Coit DC, Zhou Q, Busam KJ. Histologic distinction between subungual lentigo and melanoma. *Am J Surg Pathol* 2008;32:835–843.

107. Tosti A, Piraccini BM, Cadore de Farias D. Dealing with melanonychia. *Semin Cutan Med Surg* 2009;28:49–54.

108. Perrin C. Tumors of the nail unit. A review. Part I. Acquired localized longitudinal melanonychia and erythronchia. *Am J Dermatopathol* 2013;35:621–636.

109. Perrin C, Michiels JF, Pisani A, Ortonne JP. Anatomic distribution of melanocytes in normal nail unit: An immunohistochemical investigation. *Am J Dermatopathol* 1997;19:462–467.

110. Lee D-Y. Variable sized cellular remnants in the nail plate of longitudinal melanonychia: Evidence of subungual melanoma. *Ann Dermatol* 2015;27:328–329.

111. Kerl H, Trau H, Ackerman AB. Differentiation of melanocytic nevi from malignant melanomas in palms, soles, and nail beds solely by signs in the cornified layer of the epidermis. *Am J Dermatopathol* 1984;6(Suppl):159–160.

112. Ruben BS, McCalmont TH. The importance of attached nail plate epithelium in the diagnosis of nail apparatus melanoma. *J Cut Pathol* 2010;37:1028–1029.

113. Haneke E. Pathogenese der Nageldystrophie beim subungualen Melanom. *Verhandlungen der Deutschen Gesellschaft für Pathologie* 1986;70:484.

114. Ohata C, Nakai C, Kasugai T, Katayama I. Consumption of the epidermis in acral lentiginous melanoma. *J Cutan Pathol* 2012;39:577–581.

115. Baran R, Haneke E. Diagnostik und Therapie der streifenförmigen Nagelpigmentierung. *Hautarzt* 1984;35:359–365.

116. Haneke E, Baran R. Longitudinal melanonychia. *Dermatol Surg* 2001;27:580–584.

117. Johnson M, Shuster S. Continuous formation of nail along the bed. *Br J Dermatol* 1993;128:277–280.

118. André J, Moulonguet I, Goettmann-Bonvallot S. In situ amelanotic melanoma of the nail unit mimicking lichen planus: Report of 3 cases. *Arch Dermatol* 2010;146:418–421.

119. Ha JM, Yoon JH, Cho EB, Park GH, Park EJ, Kim KH, Kim KJ. Subungual desmoplastic malignant melanoma. *J Eur Acad Dermatol Venereol* 2016;30:360–362.

120. Quinn MJ, Crotty KA, Thompson JF, Coates AS, O'Brien CJ, McCarthy WH. Desmoplastic and desmoplastic neurotropic melanoma: Experience with 280 patients. *Cancer* 1998;83:1128–1135.

121. Innominato PF, Libbrecht I, van den Oord JJ. Expression of neurotrophins and their receptors in pigment cell lesions of the skin. *J Pathol* 2001;194:95–100.

122. Miranda BH, Haughton DN, Fahmy FS. Subungual melanoma: An important tip. *J Plast Reconstr Aesthet Surg* 2012;65:1422–1424.

123. Cho KH, Kim BS, Chang SH, Lee YS, Kim KJ. Pigmented nail with atypical melanocytic hyperplasia. *Clin Exp Dermatol* 1991;16:451–454.

124. Sheffield MV, Yee H, Dorvault CC, Weilbaecher KN, Eltoum IA, Siegal GP, Fisher DE, Chhieng DC. Comparison of five antibodies as markers in the diagnosis of melanoma in cytologic preparations. *Am J Clin Pathol* 2002;118:930–936.

125. Mahmood MN, Lee MW, Linden MD, Nathanson SD, Hornyak TJ, Zarbo RJ. Diagnostic value of HMB-45 and anti-Melan A staining of sentinel lymph nodes with isolated positive cells. *Mod Pathol* 2002;15:1288–1293.

126. Ohsie SJ, Sarantopoulos GP, Cochran AJ, Binder SW. Immunohistochemical characteristics of melanoma. *J Cutan Pathol* 2008;35:433–444.

127. Jing X, Michael CW, Theoharis CG. The use of immunocytochemical study in the cytologic diagnosis of melanoma: Evaluation of three antibodies. *Diagn Cytopathol* 2013;41:126–130.

128. Orchard GE. Comparison of immunohistochemical labelling of melanocyte differentiation antibodies melan-A, tyrosinase and HMB 45 with NKIC3 and S100 protein in the evaluation of benign naevi and malignant melanoma. *Histochem J* 2000;32:475–481.

129. Pluot M, Joundi A, Grosshans E. Contribution of monoclonal antibody HMB45 in the histopathologic diagnosis of melanoma. *Ann Dermatol Venereol* 1990;117:691–699.

130. Kiuru M, McDermott G, Berger M, Halpern AC, Busam KJ. Desmoplastic melanoma with sarcomatoid dedifferentiation. *Am J Surg Pathol* 2014; 38:864–870.

131. Friedman HD, Tatum AH. HMB-45-positive malignant lymphoma. A case report with literature review of aberrant HMB-45 reactivity. *Arch Pathol Lab Med* 1991;115:826–830.

132. Stalkup JR, Orengo IF, Katta R. Controversies in acral lentiginous melanoma. *Dermatol Surg* 2002;28:1051–1059.

133. Theunis A, Richert B, Sass U, Lateur N, Sales F, André J. Immunohistochemical study of 40 cases of longitudinal melanonychia. *Am J Dermatopathol* 2011;33:27–34.

134. Mohamed A, Gonzalez RS, Lawson D, Wang J, MD, Cohen C. SOX10 expression in malignant melanoma, carcinoma, and normal tissues. *Appl Immunohistochem Mol Morphol* 2013;21:506–510.

135. Palla B, Su A, Binder S, Dry S. SOX10 expression distinguishes desmoplastic melanoma from its histologic mimics. *Am J Dermatopathol* 2013;35:576–581.

136. Shin S, Vincent JG, Cuda JD, Xu H, Kang S, Kim J, Taube JM. Sox10 is expressed in primary melanocytic neoplasms of various histologies but not in fibrohistiocytic proliferations and histiocytoses. *J Am Acad Dermatol* 2012;67:717.

137. Danga ME, Yaar R, Bhawan J. Melan-A positive dermal cells in malignant melanoma *in situ*. *J Cutan Pathol* 2015, doi: 10.1111/cup.12473

138. Rönnstrand, Phung B. Enhanced SOX10 and KIT expression in cutaneous melanoma. *Med Oncol* 2013;30:648–649.

139. Buonaccorsi JN, Prieto VG, Torres-Cabala C, Suster S, Plaza JA. Diagnostic utility and comparative immunohistochemical analysis of MITF-1 and SOX10 to distinguish melanoma *in situ* and actinic keratosis: A clinicopathological and immunohistochemical study of 70 cases. *Am J Dermatopathol* 2014;36:124–130.

140. Kaufmann O, Koch S, Burghardt J, Audring H, Dietel M. Tyrosinase, melan-A, and KBA62 as markers for the immunohistochemical identification of metastatic amelanotic melanomas on paraffin sections. *Mod Pathol* 1998;11:740–746.

141. Kazakov DV, Kutzner H, Rütten A, Michal M, Requena L, Burg G, Dummer R, Kempf W. The anti-MAGE antibody B57 as a diagnostic marker in melanocytic lesions. *Am J Dermatopathol* 2004;26:102–107.

142. Tan KB, Moncrieff M, Thompson JF, McCarthy SW, Shaw HM, Quinn MJ, Li L-XL, Crotty KA, Stretch JR, Scolyer RA. Subungual melanoma: A study of 124 cases highlighting features of early lesions, potential pitfalls in diagnosis, and guidelines for histologic reporting. *Am J Surg Pathol* 2007;31:1902–1912.

143. Cachia AR, Kedziora AM. Subungual malignant melanoma with cartilaginous differentiation. *Am J Dermatopathol* 1999;21:165–169.

144. Shakhova O. Neural crest stem cells in melanoma development. *Curr Opin Oncol* 2014;26:215–221.

145. Curtin JA, Fridlyand J, Kageshita T, Patel HN, Busam KJ, Kutzner H, Cho KH et al. Distinct sets of genetic alterations in melanoma. *N Engl J Med* 2005;353:2135–2147.

146. Blokx WA, van Dijk MC, Ruiter DJ. Molecular cytogenetics of cutaneous melanocytic lesions—Diagnostic, prognostic and therapeutic aspects. *Histopathology* 2010;56:121–132.

147. Pleasance ED, Cheetham RK, Stephens PJ, McBride DJ, Humphray SJ, Greenman CD, Varela I et al. A comprehensive catalogue of somatic mutations from a human cancer genome. *Nature* 2010;463:191–196.

148. Glitza IC, Davies MA. Genotyping of cutaneous melanoma. *Chin Clin Oncol* 2014;3(3):27.

149. Curtin JA, Busam K, Pinkel D, Bastian BC. Somatic activation of KIT in distinct subtypes of melanoma. *J Clin Oncol* 2006;24:4340–4346.

150. Yeh I, Bastian BC. Genome-wide associations studies for melanoma and nevi. *Pigment Cell Melanoma Res* 2009;22:527–528.

151. North JP, Kageshita T, Pinkel D, Leboit PE, Bastian BC. Distribution and significance of occult intraepidermal tumor cells surrounding primary melanoma. *J Invest Dermatol* 2008;128:2024–2030.

152. Junkins-Hopkins JM. Malignant melanoma: Molecular cytogenetics and their implications in clinical medicine. *J Am Acad Dermatol* 2010;63:329–332.

153. Lang D, Mascarenhas JB, Shea CR. Melanocytes, melanocyte stem cells, and melanoma stem cells. *Clin Dermatol* 2013;31:166–178.

154. Redmer T, Welte Y, Behrens D, Fichtner I, Przybilla D, Wruck W, Yaspo M-L, Lehrach H, Schäfer R, Regenbrecht CRA. The nerve growth factor receptor CD271 is crucial to maintain tumorigenicity and stem-like properties of melanoma cells. *PLoS ONE* 2014;9(5):e92596.

155. Bastian BC, Kashani-Sabet M, Hamm H, Godfrey T, Moore DH 2nd, Bröcker EB, LeBoit PE, Pinkel D. Gene amplifications characterize acral melanoma and permit the detection of occult tumor cells in the surrounding skin. *Cancer Res* 2000;60:1968–1973.

156. Bauer J, Bastian B. Genomic analysis of melanocytic neoplasia. *Adv Dermatol* 2005;21:81–99.

157. Bauer J, Bastian BC. Distinguishing melanocytic nevi from melanoma by DNA copy number changes: Comparative genomic hybridization as a research and diagnostic tool. *Dermatol Ther* 2006;19:40–49.

158. Fargnoli MC, Pike K, Pfeiffer RM, Tsang S, Rozenblum E, Munroe DJ, Golubeva Y et al. MC1R variants increase risk of melanomas harboring BRAF mutations. *J Invest Dermatol* 2008;128:2485–2490.

159. Gerami P, Jewell SS, Morrison LE, Blondin B, Schulz J, Ruffalo T, Matushek P 4th et al. Fluorescence *in situ* hybridization (FISH) as an ancillary diagnostic tool in the diagnosis of melanoma. *Am J Surg Pathol* 2009;33:1146–1156.

160. Viros A, Fridlyand J, Bauer J, Lasithiotakis K, Garbe C, Pinkel D, Bastian BC. Improving melanoma classification by integrating genetic and morphologic features. *PLoS Med* 2008;5(6):e120.

161. Di Chiacchio N, Farias DC de, Piraccini DM, Hirata SH, Richert B, Zaiac M, Daniel R et al. Consensus on melanonychia nail plate dermoscopy. *An Bras Dermatol* 2013;88:309–313.

162. Kikuchi I, Inoue S, Sakaguchi E, Ono T. Regressing nevoid nail melanosis in childhood. *Dermatology* 1993;186:88–93.

163. Koga H, Saida T, Uhara H. Key point in dermoscopic differentiation between early nail apparatus melanoma and benign longitudinal melanonychia. *J Dermatol* 2011;38:45–52.

164. Lyall D. Malignant melanoma in infancy. *J Am Med Assoc* 1967;202:93.

165. Kato T, Usuba Y, Takematsu H, Kumasaka N, Tanita Y, Hashimoto K, Tomita Y, Tagami H. A rapidly

growing pigmented nail streak resulting in diffuse melanosis of the nail. A possible sign of subungual melanoma *in situ*. *Cancer* 1989;64:2191–2198.

166. Hori Y, Yamada A, Tanizaki T. Pigmented small tumors. *Jpn J Pediatr Dermatol* 1988;7:117–120.

167. Antonovich DD, Grin C, Grant-Kels JM. Childhood subungual melanoma *in situ* in diffuse nail melanosis beginning as expanding longitudinal melanonychia. *Ped Dermatol* 2005;22:210–212.

168. Jean-Gilles J Jr, Bercovitch L, Jellinek N, Robinson-Bostom L, Telang G. Subungual melanoma in-situ arising in a 9-year-old child. *J Cut Pathol* 2011;38:185.

169. Uchiyama M, Minemura K. Two cases of malignant melanoma in young persons. *Nippon Hifuka Gakkai Zasshi* 1979;89:668.

170. Haenssle HA, Buhl T, Holzkamp R, Schön MP, Kretschmer L, Bertsch HP. Squamomelanocytic tumor of the nail unit metastasizing to a sentinel lymph node: A dermoscopic and histologic investigation. *Dermatology* 2012;225:127–130.

171. Husain S, Scher RK, Silvers DN, Ackerman AB. Melanotic macule of nail unit and its clinicopathologic spectrum. *J Am Acad Dermatol* 2006;54: 664–667.

172. Tomizawa K. Early malignant melanoma manifested as longitudinal melanonychia: Subungual melanoma may arise from suprabasal melanocytes. *Br J Dermatol* 2000;143:431–434.

173. Baran R, Simon C. Longitudinal melanonychia: A symptom of Bowen's disease. *J Am Acad Dermatol* 1988;18:1359–1360.

174. Lemont H, Haas R. Subungual pigmented Bowen's disease in a nineteen-year-old black female. *J Am Podiatr Med Assoc* 1994;84:39–40.

175. Baran R, Eichmann A. Longitudinal melanonychia associated with Bowen disease. *Dermatology* 1993;18:159–160.

176. Sass U, André J, Stene JJ, Noel JC. Longitudinal melanonychia revealing an intraepidermal carcinoma of the nail apparatus: Detection of integrated HPV-16 DNA. *J Am Acad Dermatol* 1998;39:490–493.

177. Lambiase MC, Gardner TL, Altman CE, Albertini JG. Bowen disease of the nail bed presenting as longitudinal melanonychia: Detection of human papillomavirus type 56 DNA. *Cutis* 2003;72:305–309.

178. Ruben BS. Pigmented lesions of the nail unit: Clinical and histopathologic features. *Semin Cutan Med Surg* 2010;29:148–158.

179. Kim DM, Suh MK, Ha GY, Sohng SH. Fingernail onychomycosis due to *Aspergillus niger*. *Ann Dermatol* 2012;24:459–463.

180. Ko CJ, Sarantopoulos GP, Pai G, Binder SW. Longitudinal melanonychia of the toenails with presence of Medlar bodies on biopsy. *J Cutan Pathol* 2005;32:63–65.

Metastases of the digital tip

16

Acrometastases are an uncommon event. Men are almost twice as often affected as women. The mean age is 58 years. The mean survival time is 6 months. Metastases to the tip of the digit or to the nail region are even less frequent with approximately 150 cases reported.[1] In the beginning, they are often wrongly diagnosed as acute or chronic paronychial infection[2] and treated by antibiotics and incisions. Sometimes, metastases to the nail region may be the first manifestation of an internal malignancy.[3–5] Most metastatic neoplasms involve the bone first and grow into the soft tissues later,[6] but the reverse may also be seen. The clinical appearance of these metastases varies considerably. The tip of the digit may be swollen, violaceous red, painful, slightly tender, or painless. Pseudoclubbing is another common sign, sometimes with expansile pulsation. Nail dystrophy follows direct matrix damage or overstretching of the matrix and nail bed due to the sheer volume of the metastasis. Simulation of acute or chronic infection,[7] such as a whitlow or osteomyelitis,[8] is common. When pain is very intense, a glomus tumor[9] or rheumatoid arthritis[10] may be mimicked. A metastatic hypopharynx carcinoma imitated necrotizing vasculitis and ulcerating subungual metastases of lung squamous cell carcinoma looked like vasculitic nodules.[11,12] It is characteristic that the signs of metastatic growth increase much more than the relatively mild pain would suggest. The absence of injury or infection hints at the possibility of a metastasis, even when ulceration occurs. Acrometastases were also observed after the use of frozen gloves during adjuvant chemotherapy of breast carcinoma.[13] X-rays usually show an osteolytic focus, which may resemble spina ventosa or osteitis. Distal phalangeal metastases usually do not cross the articular surface. In fact, they characteristically preserve a thin margin of subchondral cortical bone and sometimes a blown-out cortical shell.[14]

16.1 HISTOPATHOLOGY

Lung,[15,16] kidney, and breast carcinoma are the most frequent causes of acrometastases. Colon, stomach, liver, prostate, and rectum carcinoma[17] follow. Approximately 20% of these acrometastases are found in the distal phalanx. The middle finger, followed by the thumb and ring finger, are most frequently affected.

Fine needle aspiration cytology or, better, incisional biopsy is necessary to classify the tumor and exclude a primary bone tumor but even this may fail to reveal the true nature of the primary neoplasm. Bronchial carcinoma makes up for almost 50% of phalangeal metastases,[18] followed by carcinomas of the breast (15% in females),[1] kidney,[19] colon, rectum and parotid gland,[20] seminoma,[21] melanoma,[22–24] neuroblastoma, plasmocytoma, chondrosarcoma, nonmelanoma skin, bladder, thyroid,[4] endometrial,[25] and adrenal gland cancers. In general, very few

subungual metastases allow their origin to be determined with certainty (Figure 16.1) except for clear-cell renal carcinoma and melanoma that can usually be diagnosed. Most other carcinomas are just diagnosed as an adenocarcinoma (Figures 16.2 through 16.4) or keratinizing squamous cell carcinoma. Occasionally, immunohistochemistry may help to determine the primary tumor.

16.2 DIFFERENTIAL DIAGNOSIS

Most metastases of the digit tip derive from adenocarcinomas. Some group antigens may be able to limit the number of malignancy potentially responsible for the metastasis, such as keratins, vimentin, neural antigens, lymphocyte markers, carcinoembryonic antigen, specific enzymes, hormones,

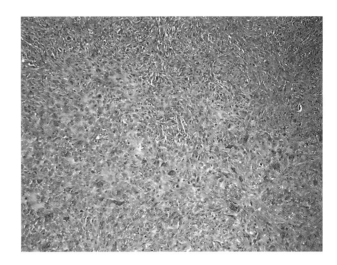

Figure 16.1 Subungual metastasis of an undifferentiated squamous cell carcinoma.

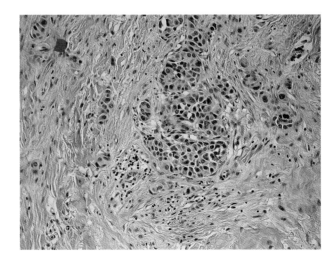

Figure 16.2 Nail bed metastasis of an adenocarcinoma. H&E.

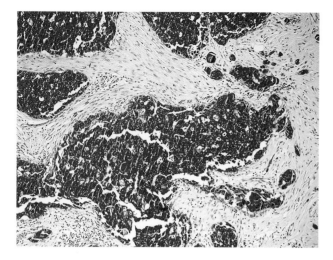

Figure 16.3 Adenocarcinoma metastasis. Keratin demonstration.

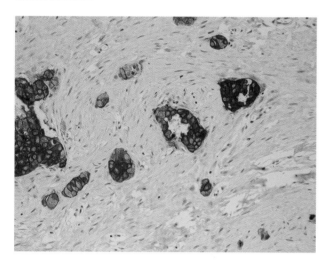

Figure 16.4 CEA demonstration in the metastasis of an adenocarcinoma.

and so on. Some primary carcinomas have tumor-specific antigens that may be demonstrated by immunohistochemical methods and allow a specific diagnosis to be made.

REFERENCES

1. Baran R, Tosti A. Metastatic bronchogenic carcinoma to the terminal phalanx of the toe. Report of 2 cases and review of the literature. *J Am Acad Dermatol* 1994;31:259–263.
2. Basora J, Fery A. Metastatic malignancy of the hand. *Clin Orthop Relat Res* 1975;108:182–186.
3. Camiel MR, Aron BS, Alexander LL, Benninghoff DL, Minkowitz S. Metastases to palm, sole, nailbed, nose, face, and scalp from unsuspected carcinoma of the lung. *Cancer* 1969;23:214–220.
4. Seth R, Athanassopoulos A, Mir S. First presentation of lung adenocarcinoma as a subungual metastasis. *Hand (NY)* 2008;3:69–71.
5. Kattepur AK, Gopinath KS. Metastasis from thyroid carcinoma. *N Engl J Med* 2014;370:2131.
6. Cohen PR. Metastatic tumors to the nail unit: Subungual metastases. *Dermatol Surg* 2001;27:280–293.
7. Hsu CS, Hentz VR, Yao J. Tumours of the hand. *Lancet Oncol* 2007;8:157–166.
8. Marmor C, Horner R. Metastasis to a phalanx simulating infection in a finger. *Am J Surg* 1959;97:236–237.
9. Wu KK, Guise ER. Metastatic tumours of the hand, a report of six cases. *J Hand Surg* 1978;3:271.
10. Karten I, Bartfeld H. Bronchogenic carcinoma simulating early rheumatoid arthritis. *J Am Med Ass* 1962;179:162–164.
11. Nigro MA, Chieregato G, Castellani L. Metastatic hypopharyngeal carcinoma mimicking necrotizing vasculitis of the skin. *Cutis* 1992;49:187–188.
12. Babacan NA, Kiliçkap S, Sene S, Kacan T, Yucel B, Eren MF, Cihan S. A case of multifocal skin metastases from lung cancer presenting with vasculitic-type cutaneous nodule. *Indian J Dermatol* 2015;60:213.
13. Brygger L, Cold S. Acrometastasis from breast cancer after the use of frozen gloves by adjuvant chemotherapy. *Ugeskr Laeger* 2015;177(2A)26–27.
14. Monsees B, Murphy WA. Distal phalangeal erosive lesions. *Arthritis Rheum* 1984;27:449–455.
15. Vanhooteghem O, Dumont M, André J, Leempoel M, de la Brassinne M. Bilateral subungual metastasis from squamous cell carcinoma of the lung: A diagnostic trap! *Rev Méd Liège* 1999;54:653–654.
16. Ryu JS, Cho JW, Moon TH, Lee HL, Han HS, Choi GS. Squamous cell lung cancer with solitary subungual metastasis. *Yonsei Med J* 2000;41:666–668.
17. Gallagher B, Yousef G, Bishop L. Subungual metastasis from a rectal primary: Case report and review of the literature. *Dermatol Surg* 2006;32:592–595.
18. Hödl S. Fingermetastasen bei Bronchuskarzinom. *Akt Dermatol* 1980;6:249–254.
19. Vine JE, Cohen PR. Renal cell carcinoma metastatic to the thumb: A case report and review of subungual metastases from all primary sites. *Clin Exp Dermatol* 1996;21:377–380.
20. Falkinburg LW, Fagan JH. Malignant mixed tumor of the parotid gland with a rare metastasis. *Am J Surg* 1956;91:279–282.
21. Gartmann H. Seminommetastasen der Haut. *Dermatol Wochenschr* 1958;138:828–829.
22. Kolmsee I, Schultka O. Keratoma palmare et plantare dissipatum hereditarium, Pachyonychia congenita und Hypotrichosis lanuginosa, malignes Melanom, Möller-Huntersche Glossitis, Vasculitis allergica superficialis (Bildberichte). *Hautarzt* 1972;23:459–460.
23. Retsas S, Samman PD. Pigment streaks in the nail plate due to secondary malignant melanoma. *Br J Dermatol* 1983;108:367–370.
24. Zaun H, Dill-Müller D. *Krankhafte Veränderungen des Nagels*, 7th edn. Balingen: Spitta Verlag, 1997; 74.
25. Amiot RA, Wilson SE, Reznicek MJ, Webb BS. Endometrial carcinoma metastasis to the distal phalanx of the hallux: A case report. *J Foot Ankle Surg* 2005;44:462–465.

Index